SMALL ANIMAL
Clinical Diagnosis by
Laboratory Methods

SMALL ANIMAL Clinical Diagnosis by Laboratory Methods

2ND EDITION

MICHAEL D. WILLARD, DVM, Dipl ACVIM
Professor of Small Animal Medicine
Department of Small Animal Medicine and Surgery
College of Veterinary Medicine
Texas A&M University
College Station, Texas

HAROLD TVEDTEN, DVM, PhD, Dipl ACVP
Professor of Pathology
Department of Pathology
College of Veterinary Medicine
Michigan State University
East Lansing, Michigan

GRANT H. TURNWALD, BVSc, MS, Dipl ACVIM
Professor of Small Animal Medicine and Head
Department of Veterinary Medicine and Surgery
College of Veterinary Medicine
Oklahoma State University
Stillwater, Oklahoma

W.B. SAUNDERS COMPANY
A Division of Harcourt Brace & Company
Philadelphia □ London □ Toronto □ Montreal □ Sydney □ Tokyo

W.B. SAUNDERS COMPANY
A Division of
Harcourt Brace & Company

The Curtis Center
Independence Square West
Philadelphia, Pennsylvania 19106

Library of Congress Cataloging-in-Publication Data

Small animal clinical diagnosis by laboratory methods /
[edited by] Michael D. Willard, Harold Tvedten,
Grant H. Turnwald.—2nd ed.

p. cm.

Includes bibliographical references and index.

ISBN 0–7216–5202–6

1. Dogs—Diseases—Diagnosis.   2. Cats—Diseases—Diagnosis.
   3. Veterinary clinical pathology.   I. Willard, Michael D.
   II. Tvedten, Harold.   III. Turnwald, Grant H.

SF991.S59 1994   636.7'08960756—dc20   93–31784

Small Animal Clinical Diagnosis by Laboratory Methods, 2nd edition   ISBN 0–7216–5202–6

Printed in the United States of America

Last digit is the print number: 9   8   7   6   5   4   3   2   1

Contributors

Ota Barta, MVDr, PhD
Professor of Immunology, Department of Pathobiology, Virginia–Maryland Regional College of Veterinary Medicine, Virginia Polytechnical Institute and State University, Blacksburg, Virginia

Helio S. Autran de Morais, MV, MS, Dipl ACVIM
Clinical Instructor, Department of Veterinary Clinical Sciences, Ohio State University; Clinical Instructor, Veterinary Teaching Hospital, Ohio State University, Columbus, Ohio

Stephen P. DiBartola, DVM, Dipl ACVIM
Professor, Department of Veterinary Clinical Science, College of Veterinary Medicine, and Small Animal Medicine Clinician, Veterinary Teaching Hospital, Ohio State University, Columbus, Ohio

Robert A. Green, DVM, Dipl ACVP
Professor, Department of Veterinary Pathobiology, and Director, Clinical Pathology Laboratory, Veterinary Teaching Hospital, Texas A&M University, College Station, Texas

Cheri A. Johnson, DVM, MS, Dipl ACVIM
Professor, Department of Small Animal Clinical Sciences, College of Veterinary Medicine, and Chief of Staff, Small Animal Hospital, Veterinary Teaching Hospital, Michigan State University, East Lansing, Michigan

Michael R. Lappin, DVM, PhD, Dipl ACVIM
Associate Professor, Department of Clinical Sciences, College of Veterinary Medicine and Biomedical Sciences, Colorado State University, Fort Collins, Colorado

George E. Lees, DVM, MS, Dipl ACVIM (Internal Medicine)
Professor of Medicine, Small Animal Medicine and Surgery, College of Veterinary Medicine; and Small Animal Clinic, Veterinary Teaching Hospital, Texas Veterinary Medical Center, Texas A&M University, College Station, Texas

Richard W. Nelson, DVM, Dipl ACVIM
Associate Professor, School of Veterinary Medicine, Department of Medicine, University of California at Davis, Davis, California

N. Bari Olivier, DVM, PhD, Dipl ACVIM
Associate Professor of Medicine, Department of Small Animal Clinical Sciences and Department of Physiology, College of Veterinary Medicine, Michigan State University, East Lansing, Michigan

Joane Parent, BSc, DMV, MVSc, Dipl ACVIM
Professor of Neurology, Department of Veterinary Clinical Studies, Archibald Small Animal Clinic, Ontario Veterinary College, University of Guelph, Guelph, Ontario, Canada

Grant H. Turnwald, BVSc, MS, Dipl ACVIM
Professor of Small Animal Medicine and Head, Department of Veterinary Medicine and Surgery, College of Veterinary Medicine, Oklahoma State University, Stillwater, Oklahoma

Harold Tvedten, DVM, PhD, Dipl ACVP
Professor of Pathology, Department of Pathology, College of Veterinary Medicine, Michigan State University, East Lansing, Michigan

David C. Twedt, DVM, Dipl ACVIM
Professor, Veterinary Teaching Hospital, College of Veterinary Medicine and Biomedical Sciences, Small Animal Medicine Section Chief, Colorado State University, Fort Collins, Colorado

Linda L. Werner, DVM, PhD
Lecturer, Department of Pathology, Microbiology and Immunology, School of Veterinary Medicine, University of California at Davis, Davis, California

Michael D. Willard, DVM, Dipl ACVIM
Professor of Small Animal Medicine, Department of Small Animal Medicine and Surgery, College of Veterinary Medicine, Texas A&M University, College Station, Texas

Alice M. Wolf, DVM, Dipl ACVIM
Associate Professor of Small Animal Medicine, Department of Small Animal Medicine and Surgery, Texas A&M University, College Station, Texas

Preface

The first edition of this book was intended to address questions often asked by students and primary care veterinary practitioners that reflect common problems veterinarians encounter with laboratory tests. The second edition has the same goal, but we have attempted to enhance the text by incorporating several new authors. In most cases the previous chapter was not rewritten completely, but rather was extensively updated as the new author sought to keep what was still current, add what was new, and also add his or her personal feelings about the most appropriate and cost-effective manner in which to follow up a given problem or laboratory abnormality. Suggestions are sometimes provided regarding where the clinician should look in diagnostically confusing cases. The goal has been to present a system of how to select and use laboratory tests in as simple and rapid a way as possible. This book emphasizes diagnostic approach, why something is done, and conclusions instead of a detailed description of pathophysiology. Too often, clinicians expect an answer that a particular test cannot provide; consequently, they and the client are disappointed. Techniques and instruments are discussed as appropriate to explain the limitations of the test or instrument. Most of the techniques discussed are commonly performed in small animal clinics. We have sought to be sure that new tests and techniques have been included so that the text is as current as possible. By the same token, tests that are now rarely used and those of dubious value have been given minimal space. Despite their value, references have been kept to a minimum because of the difficulty of using them in practice situations.

Acknowledgments

The help, support, and tolerance of our families, friends, colleagues, and students, as well as of the W. B. Saunders Company, are gratefully acknowledged. Matthew 6:25–33.

Contents

SMALL ANIMAL
Clinical Diagnosis by
Laboratory Methods

Harold Tvedten

1 Referral and In-Office Laboratories

Medicine relies heavily on laboratory testing to diagnose, monitor, and make prognostic statements about disease, but what testing procedures belong in one's clinic, and what testing procedures should be done elsewhere? No standard correct answer fits all situations. The approach to laboratory testing by a veterinarian practicing in a large city near a full-service veterinary diagnostic laboratory differs greatly from that of a rural veterinarian who must tolerate the delays of mailing samples to referral laboratories. Veterinarians appropriately should rely on referral laboratories, when conveniently available, for most of their testing because of better accuracy, lower cost, and greater variety and to avoid the problems of performing laboratory procedures themselves.

Although comments are made about the purchase or use of certain products and referral laboratories, readers should not favor one particular company's products discussed in this chapter or a particular referral laboratory listed in Appendix I over ones unintentionally excluded. The products and laboratories discussed are those the author has had experience with and are not necessarily better than those not mentioned. Costs are subject to change and so should be considered as guidelines only.

THE BASIC VETERINARY LABORATORY

Veterinary clinics routinely have the laboratory capacity to analyze urine, to examine parasitology specimens (e.g., feces and heartworms), and to do some microscopic work on hematology and cytology specimens. Testing procedures included in in-office laboratories must be simple, inexpensive, accurate, and necessary. Testing procedures that require relatively expensive equipment or complex procedures that require significant amounts of time in preparation of materials or training of personnel are usually inappropriate. Veterinarians are not medical technologists, and if something can go wrong with a laboratory procedure, it will.

The unstable nature of many substances in urine requires that urine samples be analyzed quickly in-office instead of sent to a referral laboratory. Since the urine chemistry test strips (i.e., dipsticks) are cheap, easy, accurate, and

1

useful, they are routinely used in clinical laboratories. For example, 6 to 10 chemistry tests for substances in urine are on a test strip (Ames* Multistix), which costs only about $0.45 per strip (Fischer Scientific Co.†). A test strip with two tests like the Keto-Diastix for urinary ketones and glucose is only about $0.12 per strip.

Parasitology testing (e.g., heartworms, ecto- and endoparasites) similarly is inexpensive and simple. Immediate test results allow treatment for the parasitism to begin with the office call, avoiding the owner's inconvenience of returning the pet. A good quality microscope is necessary for in-office laboratories. Poor quality instruments barely able to distinguish *Toxocara canis* ova are ineffective for evaluation of blood smears and cytologic preparations. The microscope section in Chapter 16 discusses purchase, care, and use of microscopes.

New "quick" stains provide easy and consistent staining characteristics of blood smears, bacteria and fungi, and cytologic smears. New methylene blue is even easier to use for urine sediments, cytology smears, and reticulocytes in blood (see stain section in Chapter 16).

Cell counts in blood and other fluids have been made easy by the simplicity and consistency of diluting samples with Unopette containers (Becton-Dickinson‡). Erythrocyte and leukocyte counting techniques are discussed in Chapter 2, and platelet counting in Chapter 5.

A refractometer is needed for determination of urine specific gravity and total protein in plasma or various body fluids. Many small animals with possible renal failure have urine sample volumes too small to determine the specific gravity by the cheaper urinometer. A refractometer requires only a drop of urine to determine the specific gravity, which is essential for evaluating renal function. Similarly, only the volume of plasma in a microhematocrit tube is needed for an accurate estimate of plasma protein. The veterinary TS Meter is a refractometer calibrated for cats and dogs (Reichert§).

Two good quality centrifuges are needed in most laboratories. A single-purpose centrifuge for microhematocrit tubes is needed to ensure consistent packed cell volume determinations; cost is about $1145. A basic centrifuge capable of centrifuging blood to obtain serum or plasma

costs about $720. Serum or plasma may need to be stored in a refrigerator ($-4°C$) or freezer ($-20°C$) before mailing to a referral laboratory. Freezers included in refrigerators and many home freezers may not maintain a temperature below $-20°C$. Frost-free freezers may have fluctuating temperatures.

QUALITY CONTROL

Quality control (QC) becomes the veterinarian's responsibility if chemistry testing is done in the clinic. QC test results must be performed and recorded as proof of the validity of the answers sold to the client. Practices with low test volume should analyze control serum with each patient's sample and for each type of test performed. This is an additional expense, so the frequency and extent of QC testing in many practices have often been less than recommended. The frequency of QC testing may be reduced if, based on a written log, a testing procedure has proved to remain consistent between QC checks.

A routine in-house QC program is required since instruments, reagents, or people develop problems after some time. These problems must be detected and corrected as soon as possible. Intralaboratory QC is performed by repeated analysis of control reagents containing known amounts of various substances (i.e., analyte) like glucose or blood urea nitrogen (BUN). Results of analysis of the control serum should match the expected QC results that are included with the control sera. Control sera with high, low, and normal levels of each substance to be tested should be used. In laboratories with a large volume, all three control sera (i.e., high, normal, and low) are analyzed with each batch of patient samples. The results for the patient samples are not reported if the control sera's results are out of range. The control serum's (QC) values are recorded daily in a log or a computer to seek sudden shifts or gradual trends of results that suggest instrument, personnel, or reagent problems. Gradual changes may be due to slow deterioration of a reagent or slowly decreasing light intensity in an instrument. Rapid changes are caused by introducing a new reagent, sudden change in a component in the instrument, or human error. Control serum can be divided into portions and preserved for later use to reduce the cost per test.

Laboratories performing tests on human patients are required to have outside testing programs to prove the validity and quality of their test results at frequent intervals. Veterinary lab-

---

*Ames Division, Miles Laboratories, P.O. Box 70, Elkhart, IN 46515.

†Fisher Scientific Co., 1991–1992, P.O. Box 2249, 32231 Schoolcraft, Livonia, MI 48151.

‡Unopette, Becton-Dickinson and Co., Rutherford, NJ 07070.

§Reichert, Division of Warner-Lambert Technologies, Inc., P.O. Box 123, Buffalo, NY 14240.

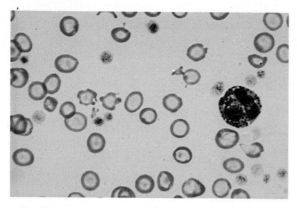

Color Plate 1A Canine iron deficiency anemia. The erythrocytes have marked central pallor (hypochromasia) with only thin rims of hemoglobin. Erythrocyte fragmentation is also seen.

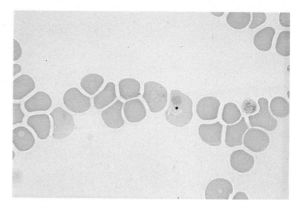

Color Plate 1D Canine distemper. There is a round, distemper inclusion body in five erythrocytes. Two are reddish and three are gray inclusion bodies. The most obvious inclusion is near a small, dark Howell-Jolly body.

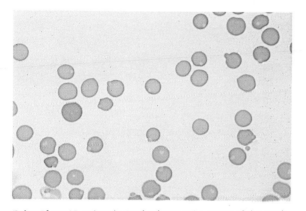

Color Plate 1B Feline Heinz body anemia. Many of the erythrocytes have a round, usually lighter staining Heinz body at the margin, with about half of the Heinz body extending above the surface. One free, round Heinz body has the same color of the erythrocytes.

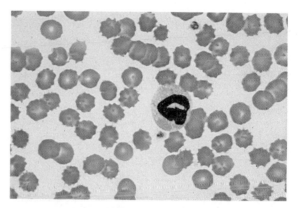

Color Plate 1E Canine distemper. There is a neutrophil with a large gray inclusion body along the cell margin.

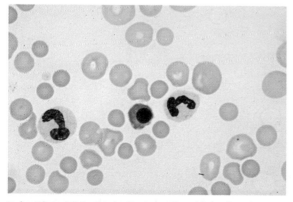

Color Plate 1C Canine immune-mediated hemolytic anemia. About 12 of the erythrocytes are spherocytes, which are distinctly smaller and darker than the other erythrocytes. One metarubricyte and two neutrophils and two polychromatophilic erythrocytes are present.

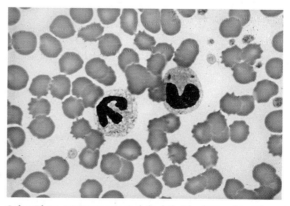

Color Plate 1F Canine toxic left shift. The bean-shaped metamyelocyte has two Döhle bodies in the bluish cytoplasm opposite the poles of the nucleus. The segmented neutrophil has the foamy cytoplasm of toxic vacuolation.

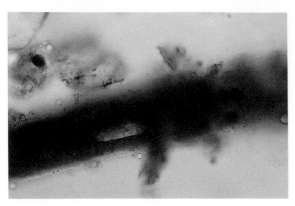

Color Plate 2A Antifreeze poisoning, impression smear of canine kidney. This renal tubule has a calcium oxalate monohydrate crystal in it.

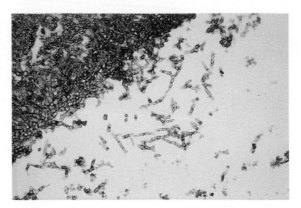

Color Plate 2D Nasal mycosis. A colony of the uniform, septate hyphae of *Aspergillus* is demonstrated. This was from a cytologic smear of nasal exudate with only one colony of fungus.

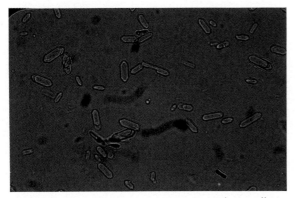

Color Plate 2B Antifreeze poisoning, urine with crystalluria. Many elongated six-sided calcium oxalate monohydrate crystals are present.

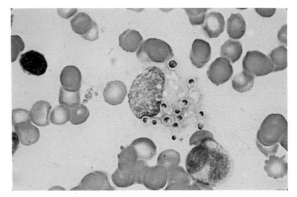

Color Plate 2E Canine histoplasmosis. A partially lysed macrophage from the bone marrow has several oval yeast with distinct cell walls.

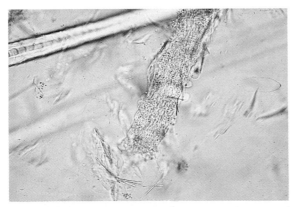

Color Plate 2C Canine ringworm skin scraping. One normal and one swollen fragment hair shaft are present. The damaged shaft is full of small, round *Microsporum canis* arthrospores.

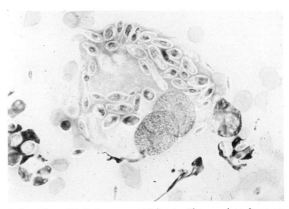

Color Plate 2F Feline sporotrichosis. The exudate from an infected declawed site had this macrophage filled with the pleomorphic yeast.

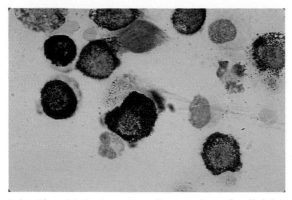

Color Plate 3A Canine mast cell tumor. Several well-differentiated mast cells are filled with uniform granules. Some other partially damaged cells included eosinophils and connective tissue cells.

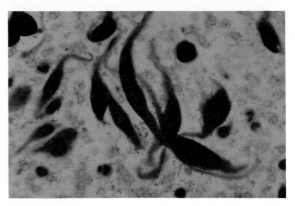

Color Plate 3D Canine sarcoma. The spindle shapes of the cells indicate a connective tissue origin.

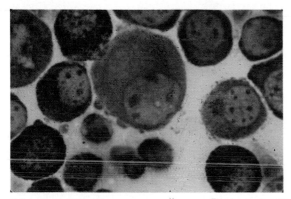

Color Plate 3B Malignant mast cell tumor. These mast cells are very large and variable with large nuclei and multiple nucleoli. The granules are variable in number, with some polarization to one side of the cell.

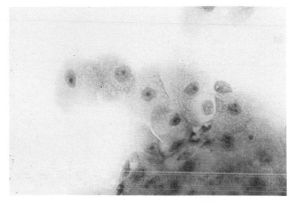

Color Plate 3E Perianal gland adenoma. This common canine tumor can be recognized by the characteristic abundant granular cytoplasm. The resemblance to hepatic cells gives the name *hepatoid tumor*.

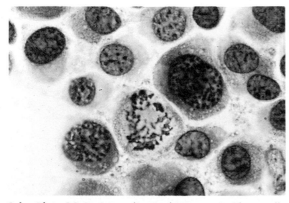

Color Plate 3C Canine malignant histiocytosis. These cells appear very malignant based on the great variation in chromatin patterns in the nuclei, which are very large and variable in size. One cell is in mitosis.

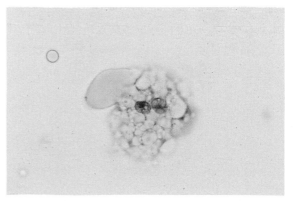

Color Plate 3F Feline fatty liver. This hepatocyte was stained with new methylene blue for cell detail and Sudan stain to illustrate the neutral fats in the hepatocyte's vacuoles and outside the cell. Hepatocytes may normally be binucleated.

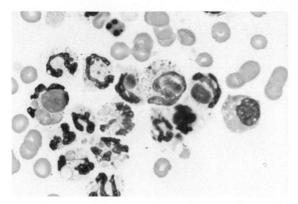

Color Plate 4A Canine lupus arthritis. This area of a synovial fluid smear has one large LE cell and two additional less obvious LE cells. Many other neutrophils have multiple bluish inclusions and are termed *ragocytes*.

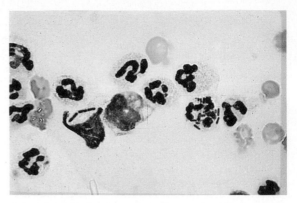

Color Plate 4D Septic exudate. Two neutrophils in this canine abdominal fluid contained rod-shaped bacteria. Note that these neutrophils do not appear degenerate even though the exudate was septic. Do not consider the lysed neutrophil to be a degenerate neutrophil.

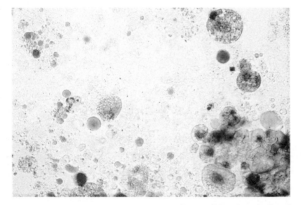

Color Plate 4B Chylothorax. A simple combination stain of new methylene blue and a neutral fat stain (e.g., Sudan stain) demonstrates the chylomicrons in the form of lipid globules in phagocytes and free in the thoracic fluid.

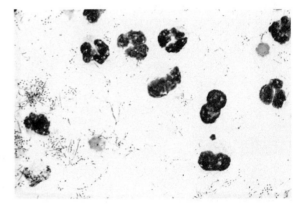

Color Plate 4E Degenerate neutrophils. The degenerate neutrophils in this thoracic fluid have karyolytic (swollen) nuclei as evidence of degeneration caused by the bacterial sepsis about them. The branching filamentous bacterium was *Actinomyces*.

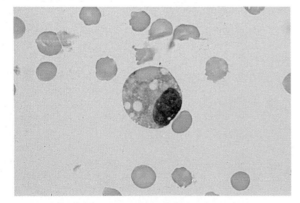

Color Plate 4C Pathologic hemorrhage. Erythrophagocytosis in a macrophage is present. This or hemosiderin in macrophages is evidence that blood present in a fluid was caused by preexisting disease and not the needle used to collect the sample.

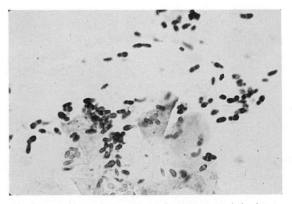

Color Plate 4F Canine yeast otitis. The ear swab had some thin squames and many small budding yeast to indicate a yeast otitis with *Pityrosporum* (*Malassezia*).

oratories usually do not participate in these expensive programs but do use inexpensive testing programs from companies producing control reagents. The laboratories in these programs receive test samples from the company, analyze the samples, and report their results. The performance of each laboratory in the testing program is compared with that of others using the same test method. This outside testing validates the laboratory's accuracy.

One can test the quality of a referral laboratory's results by submitting duplicate samples to that laboratory to test precision or by submitting duplicate samples to two or more laboratories to test accuracy. Share your results with the laboratory's director, who will be happy to discover problems that can be corrected.

SERUM CHEMISTRY ANALYSIS

Inexpensive and simple screening tests of a few parameters are available for in-office laboratories to provide approximate values to guide initial diagnosis and treatment. These cost-effective kits include the Urograph (General Diagnostics*), the S/Pecial Chem CO_2 Apparatus Set, and the Chemstrip bG (Scientific Products, Baxter†). A clinically useful estimate of the BUN can be available in about 1 hour, including preparation of serum and a 30-minute incubation period of the Urograph. The cost is about $0.42 for each chemistry strip used. The S/Pecial Chem CO_2 Apparatus determines the total carbon dioxide of serum, which is about 95% HCO_3. The cost is about $9.00 per test with purchase of the 50-test kit, but using bulk replacement reagents and vials is cheaper. Blood glucose level is estimated for about $0.66 with the Chemstrip bG, which requires one large drop of whole blood and a 1-minute incubation period.

In-Office Chemistry Units ● Accurate and consistent serum chemistry results for the various tests needed in practice require use of a chemistry instrument. Most chemistry units can provide accurate results, but one cannot assign various untrained lay help to the instrument and expect consistent or accurate results. A person knowledgeable in clinical chemistry and QC and a person willing to monitor results over weeks and months should get accurate perform-

ances from most instruments. Instruments vary in ease of operation, the available variety of tests, and how much calibration and QC are required. Many veterinarians purchase in-office chemistry units only to find that without frequent calibration and the consistent use of controls, the results are not trustworthy. Over the years, different manufacturers promote various popular systems that disappear (along with reagents) a few years later. This is evidence to alert veterinarians not to expect too much from these units.

The simplicity, consistency, and accuracy of new dry chemistry units (e.g., Kodak* Ektachem DT60, Vet Test 8008†, and Ames Seralyzer‡) have made it more convenient for certain practices to perform many serum chemistry procedures accurately. Manual manipulations (e.g., pipette use) are simpler than "wet" chemistry systems of varying complexity and cost that use test tubes of liquid reagents and a colorimeter. The manufacturers of wet chemistry units have continued to improve simplicity and consistency to remain competitive with the increasingly popular dry chemistry units. The dry chemistry units are office user-friendly but are more expensive than the basic colorimeters, since one pays for the improved ease of operation and modern technology (Toffaletti, 1986). The companies are developing a wider range of tests and improved reagent stability. Calibration and QC procedures still must be performed. The Kodak Ektachem DT60 should be calibrated every 3 months, and the Ames Seralyzer every 2 weeks (Shull, 1985).

Cost Comparison: Two In-Office Chemistry Units ● There are many hidden costs that may not be considered during the initial purchase of an in-office chemistry instrument. In low test volume situations, the cost of the QC testing, calibration, instrument depreciation, labor, lost interest, and hospital overhead is divided among fewer patients. This can greatly increase the cost of each patient's test results. Will clients be willing to pay this fee, or must the clinic absorb the cost in order to practice the quality of medicine desired?

The cost of performing in-office chemistry procedures at different test volumes is presented in Figures 1–1 and 1–2 and Tables 1–1

---

*General Diagnostics, Division of Warner-Lambert Co., Morris Plains, NJ 07950.

†Baxter Scientific Products, 30500 Cypress, Romulus, MI 48174.

*Eastman Kodak Co., 343 State Street, Rochester, NY 14650.

†Burns Veterinary Supply, 2019 McKenzie, Suite 109, Carrollton, TX 75006 (1-800-527-7421).

‡Ames Division, Miles Laboratories, Inc., Elkhart, IN 46515.

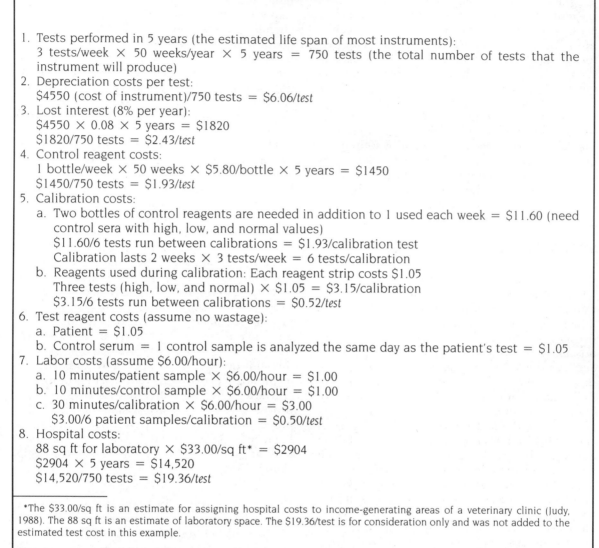

Estimates

1. Tests performed in 5 years (the estimated life span of most instruments):
   3 tests/week × 50 weeks/year × 5 years = 750 tests (the total number of tests that the instrument will produce)
2. Depreciation costs per test:
   $4550 (cost of instrument)/750 tests = $6.06/*test*
3. Lost interest (8% per year):
   $4550 × 0.08 × 5 years = $1820
   $1820/750 tests = $2.43/*test*
4. Control reagent costs:
   1 bottle/week × 50 weeks × $5.80/bottle × 5 years = $1450
   $1450/750 tests = $1.93/*test*
5. Calibration costs:
   a. Two bottles of control reagents are needed in addition to 1 used each week = $11.60 (need control sera with high, low, and normal values)
      $11.60/6 tests run between calibrations = $1.93/calibration test
      Calibration lasts 2 weeks × 3 tests/week = 6 tests/calibration
   b. Reagents used during calibration: Each reagent strip costs $1.05
      Three tests (high, low, and normal) × $1.05 = $3.15/calibration
      $3.15/6 tests run between calibrations = $0.52/*test*
6. Test reagent costs (assume no wastage):
   a. Patient = $1.05
   b. Control serum = 1 control sample is analyzed the same day as the patient's test = $1.05
7. Labor costs (assume $6.00/hour):
   a. 10 minutes/patient sample × $6.00/hour = $1.00
   b. 10 minutes/control sample × $6.00/hour = $1.00
   c. 30 minutes/calibration × $6.00/hour = $3.00
      $3.00/6 patient samples/calibration = $0.50/*test*
8. Hospital costs:
   88 sq ft for laboratory × $33.00/sq ft* = $2904
   $2904 × 5 years = $14,520
   $14,520/750 tests = $19.36/*test*

---

*The $33.00/sq ft is an estimate for assigning hospital costs to income-generating areas of a veterinary clinic (Judy, 1988). The 88 sq ft is an estimate of laboratory space. The $19.36/test is for consideration only and was not added to the estimated test cost in this example.

Figure 1–1 Worksheet for estimating the costs to perform an average chemistry test in a veterinary hospital with a low test volume. Hospital A performs a test (e.g., serum glucose) on three patients per work week with an Ames Seralyzer as its in-office chemistry instrument. The sum of the costs is used to determine a projected cost of an average test. Figure 1–2 illustrates a similar worksheet for a higher volume laboratory.

and 1–2. Readers should work through the figures and tables in sequence to understand some sources of test costs. The calculations are meant to stimulate consideration of several factors for discussion purposes only. The estimated cost in these contrived situations is based on prices that rapidly change and assumptions that will not be universally accepted. Consider the approach, but do not accept the dollar figures for one's own situation. The chemistry units in the examples are the Ames Seralyzer and Kodak DT60.

The initial purchase prices of the analyzers and reagents used in these examples are summarized in Table 1–1. The fabricated practices (Hospitals A and B in Figs. 1–1 and 1–2, respectively) perform few or many tests per week (i.e., levels A and B). Initially the costs are analyzed in two worksheets (Figs. 1–1 and 1–2) using only one instrument (i.e., Ames Seralyzer); cost estimates from Figures 1–1 and 1–2 are then summarized in Table 1–2. The initial costs used for the cost analysis were obtained from Shull

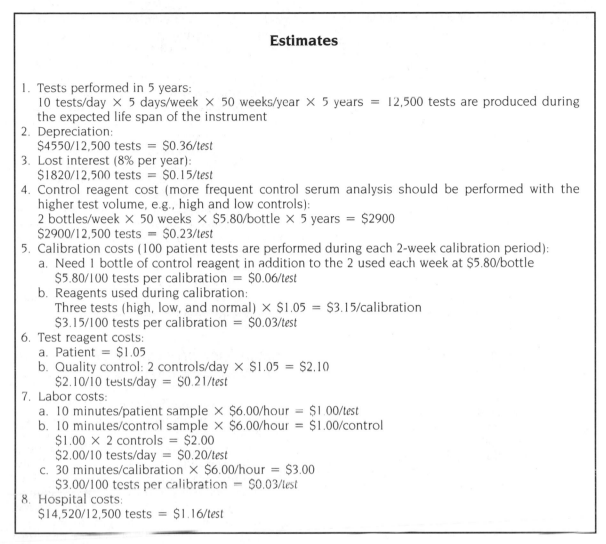

Estimates

1. Tests performed in 5 years:
   10 tests/day × 5 days/week × 50 weeks/year × 5 years = 12,500 tests are produced during the expected life span of the instrument
2. Depreciation:
   $4550/12,500 tests = $0.36/*test*
3. Lost interest (8% per year):
   $1820/12,500 tests = $0.15/*test*
4. Control reagent cost (more frequent control serum analysis should be performed with the higher test volume, e.g., high and low controls):
   2 bottles/week × 50 weeks × $5.80/bottle × 5 years = $2900
   $2900/12,500 tests = $0.23/*test*
5. Calibration costs (100 patient tests are performed during each 2-week calibration period):
   a. Need 1 bottle of control reagent in addition to the 2 used each week at $5.80/bottle
      $5.80/100 tests per calibration = $0.06/*test*
   b. Reagents used during calibration:
      Three tests (high, low, and normal) × $1.05 = $3.15/calibration
      $3.15/100 tests per calibration = $0.03/*test*
6. Test reagent costs:
   a. Patient = $1.05
   b. Quality control: 2 controls/day × $1.05 = $2.10
      $2.10/10 tests/day = $0.21/*test*
7. Labor costs:
   a. 10 minutes/patient sample × $6.00/hour = $1.00/*test*
   b. 10 minutes/control sample × $6.00/hour = $1.00/control
      $1.00 × 2 controls = $2.00
      $2.00/10 tests/day = $0.20/*test*
   c. 30 minutes/calibration × $6.00/hour = $3.00
      $3.00/100 tests per calibration = $0.03/*test*
8. Hospital costs:
   $14,520/12,500 tests = $1.16/*test*

Figure 1–2 Hospital B performs 10 tests (BUN or glucose) per day with an Ames Seralyzer. The higher test volume than in Figure 1–1 greatly reduces the average test's cost. The estimated costs for Hospitals A and B are summarized in Table 1–2 for easier comparison.

(1985) and Baxter Scientific Products catalogs (1984–1985 and 1991–1992).

Based on these hypothetical examples, the minimum cost of an in-office laboratory test is about $3. In a low volume situation and using an expensive chemistry unit, an individual test could potentially cost more than $25. This does not include an overhead charge assigned to hospital space for a laboratory. Compare this with an average cost of $0.75 per test in a profile by a private human medicine laboratory. The $15 serum chemistry profile included alkaline phosphatase, calcium, phosphorus, total bilirubin, total protein, albumin, BUN, creatinine, glucose, lactate dehydrogenase, creatine phosphokinase, serum glutamic-pyruvic transaminase (ALT), serum glutamic-oxaloacetic transaminase (AST), sodium, potassium, total CO_2, chloride, triglyceride, cholesterol, uric acid, and the indirectly calculated globulin and anion gap. If a referral laboratory is available, it is economically wise to use it. The QC practices at large laboratories should ensure more accurate and consistent results. Profile fees are low because of high test volume. Individually analyzed tests are more expensive because the time and labor expense to do a batch of 10 to 15 tests is often little more than for one or two tests. The ALT and sodium evaluations at the same commercial laboratory cost $5 each, and blood gas analysis (always done as an individual test) costs $39.

Referral laboratories often phone results to clients to make their service almost as rapid as an in-office procedure. Many also offer conven-

Table 1–1 INITIAL COSTS OF CHEMISTRY ANALYZERS

	Ames Seralyzer	Kodak DT60
Analyzer		
Main unit	$4495	$ 5500
ALT enzyme module	55	3200
Electrolyte module	NA	3300
Total	4550	12,000
BUN Reagents		
Kit cost	25	40
Tests/kit	25	25
Cost/test	1.00	1.60
Glucose Reagents		
Kit cost	52.50	40
Tests/kit	50	25
Cost/test	1.05	1.60
Potassium Reagents		
Kit cost	72.50	43.75
Tests/kit	50	25
Cost/test	1.45	1.75

Cost sources from Shull (1985); Baxter Scientific Products catalogs, 1984–1985 and 1991–1992; and Kodak price list, March 1, 1992.

ient courier service to pick up samples and return computer-printed reports for patients' records.

The variety of tests a veterinary clinic may offer is also limited by test volume. Offering a wider variety of tests means more reagent storage and increased likelihood that reagents will be outdated before they are used. Never use outdated reagents, since erroneous results will someday cost more than any tiny savings earned by this practice.

HEMATOLOGIC ANALYSIS

Most of the testing needed for basic hematologic conclusions in private practice may be made with minimal equipment. The severity of anemia may be determined by a microhematocrit procedure (see Chapter 2). Quantitation of leukocytes and platelets may be done with Unopette containers and a hemocytometer or estimated from blood smears (see Chapter 2). The plasma protein value is easily obtained with a refractometer. This provides a simple complete blood count (CBC).

Automated hematology cell counters provide a broad profile of hematologic data (CBC) that is more precise, accurate, and rapid and gives more extensive information than is obtained by manual techniques. Most of these instruments are too expensive for most veterinary clinics to afford (see Chapter 2), but referral laboratories maintain the high test volume of hematologic samples required to afford these cell counters. Veterinarians should use these extensive, accurate, and relatively inexpensive CBCs containing abundant information when available.

COMMUNICATIONS WITH REFERRAL LABORATORIES

The basic key to efficient use of referral laboratories is good communications. Laboratory personnel are very willing to discuss how to submit samples properly and prefer this communication to receiving an improper sample. When an unsatisfactory sample is received by a busy laboratory, someone must either try to contact a busy veterinarian, who may not be available, or arbitrarily decide what to do with the specimen. It is very important not to waste the effort to obtain the sample or lose a diagnostic opportunity that may not be available later. Many lab-

Table 1–2 COST SUMMARY WITH AMES SERALYZER

Cost (Tests/5 years)	Hospital A (750)	Hospital B (12,500)
Instrument depreciation/test	$ 6.06	$0.36
Lost interest/test	2.43	0.15
Control reagent costs		
Daily control/test	1.93	0.23
Calibration/test	1.93	0.06
Test reagent costs		
for patient serum/test	1.05	1.05
for control serum/test	1.05	0.21
for calibration/test	0.52	0.03
Labor costs		
for patient sample/test	1.00	1.00
for control sample/test	1.00	0.20
for calibration/test	0.50	0.03
Total costs per test	$17.47	$3.32
Hospital overhead costs per test	$19.36	$1.16

*Cost estimates calculated in Figures 1–1 and 1–2 are summarized in a form that facilitates comparison.

oratories have prepared written information on submission procedures and reference values pertaining to their laboratories (see a listing of referral laboratories in Appendix I). Questions about sample submission and routine charges should be directed to the medical technologist, clerk, or secretary who answers them daily. Use the pathologist's time for questions that are interpretive, diagnostic, or of a policy nature.

Determine the main purpose of the laboratory to understand its attitude toward performing service work for private practitioners. With a commercial laboratory, one should expect excellent service and continued cooperation to maintain test volume and profits. Laboratories with a large veterinary caseload should have a consulting veterinary clinical pathologist, who may periodically speak to local veterinary groups or prepare mailings to inform veterinary clients about the use of new and old tests offered by the laboratory.

University laboratories vary from research laboratories with little service commitment to laboratories funded by a state to primarily provide diagnostic service to the public. Many samples mailed in from veterinarians lack the information needed to make the results useful for prospective and retrospective studies for teaching or research, so mail-in samples may be given a secondary priority. If private diagnostic support is unavailable, then one can work with university administrators to obtain the needed laboratory support by setting a higher priority on service for private practitioners. State veterinary associations have liaison committees that strengthen the university's commitment to service for private practitioners and improve the university's rewards to faculty concentrating on service instead of research. The Ohio Veterinary Medical Association gives a Referral Clinician's Award.

Pure research laboratories tend to have a minimal service commitment. Their funding is based on finishing specific research projects, and diagnostic service usually diverts effort from the research project. Providing additional information about your case or additional samples may stimulate interest in naturally occurring disease and help obtain the specialized test a practitioner needs.

REFERENCE VALUES

Reference values are needed to judge whether a test result is normal or abnormal, but sources of "normal values" are often less than optimal. When one considers the number of species involved, the variety of breed characteristics, the effect of age, sex, and other factors, and the number (more than 120) of "normal" animals that should optimally be used in each of these categories to establish reference values, the expense in terms of time and money is obvious. In human medicine, insurance companies pay for laboratory testing of large numbers of normal people as part of routine physical examinations. This creates a large normal data pool not readily available in veterinary medicine. One attempt to establish hematology reference values at Michigan State University used blood from microfilaria-negative samples for heartworm tests. This sample pool, however, had several dogs with strong eosinophilia, so it was not considered to be representative.

New reference values should be established every time a laboratory changes instruments or the type of reagents, but the expense may be cost prohibitive. For example, it cost $11,000 and much of the time of three people for 4 months to establish new hematology reference values with a new hematology instrument for four laboratory animal species. This included obtaining at least 100 animals per species or temporary access to them, bleeding them, analyzing the blood samples with the instrument, and then statistically evaluating the data and reporting the data in a usable form. The data included only adult values and usually for only one breed per species, so many variables such as age, sex, environment, and breed were not evaluated. One can extrapolate the amount of time and effort needed to maintain current reference values for even one species such as the dog if each breed and the effect of age are considered.

Literature values are often used on a practical basis for many tests and situations, rather than each laboratory's creating its own. Basic hematologic results are more consistent among different laboratories and techniques than are chemistry values (especially enzymes), so hematologic reference values established by one laboratory are commonly accepted by others. A hematology reference text has reference values for a wide variety of age, breed, and sex factors that are useful for interpreting data from pups, kittens, or breeds with unique characteristics (Jain, 1986). Laboratories should develop reference values for their most frequently requested tests and species, but test volume in some species (e.g., pet birds) might be too low to justify establishing one's own reference values. Feline reference values are sometimes neglected, since it is often more difficult to perform a venipuncture on a cat.

Table 1-3 REFERENCE HEMATOLOGIC VALUES FOR 365 SELECTED DOGS

	Units	Mean	SD	Reference Interval
WBC count	1000/μl	10.46	2.66	6.4–15.90
RBC count	10⁶/μl	6.69	0.62	5.57–7.98
Hemoglobin	g/dl	16.44	2.26	13.3–19.2
Hematocrit	%	45.34	4.39	36.8–54.4
MCV	fl	67.7	4.15	59.9–75.2
MCH	pg	24.45	1.60	21.5–27.2
MCHC	g/dl	36.07	1.55	33.6–38.3
Platelets	×10³	344.95	101.2	186–547
MPV	fl	7.31	0.86	5.8–9.2
RDW	%	13.53	1.09	11.9–16.0
HDW	g/dl	1.94	0.33	1.55–2.69
LI		2.46	0.32	1.88–3.15
MPXI		−12.9	4.09	−19 to −7
Neutrophils*	%	70.94	11.49	43–88
Lymphocytes*	%	15.22	8.37	2.8–36.4
Monocytes*	%	5.01	2.42	1.7–10.8
Eosinophils*	%	4.42	5.11	0.0–17.1
Basophils*	%	0.26	0.25	0.1–0.26
LUC*	%	4.17	1.96	1.7–9.2

*Automated differential leukocyte counts.
MCV, mean corpuscular volume; MCH, mean corpuscular hemoglobin; MCHC, mean corpuscular hemoglobin concentration; MPV, mean platelet volume; RDW, red cell distribution width; HDW, hemoglobin distribution width; LI, lobularity index; MPXI, mean peroxidase index; LUC, large unstained cell.

An alternative to obtaining many well-defined normal animals for establishing reference values is to manipulate hospital patient data mathematically to obtain reference values. These values are not from animals proven to be normal but are an inexpensive, readily available source of a data pool large enough to represent the variety in the laboratory's patient population. Statistical manipulations produce cost-efficient reference ranges representing the hospital's population and the laboratory's current instrumentation. The reference ranges in Tables 1–3 and 1–4 were derived from a manipulation of patient values. These reference values included new hematologic parameters (e.g., hemoglobin distribution width, mean platelet volume) that were not available in the literature. New reference values were needed as soon as possible for clinicians to interpret these parameters, until apparently normal animals could be obtained for a more traditional reference range (Appendix II). CBC data from patients were considered acceptable for determining the new reference values if the total leukocyte count, hematocrit, and platelet count were within previously reported reference ranges (Jain, 1986). The assumption was that if a patient's CBC had normal leukocyte counts, hematocrits, and platelet

Table 1-4 REFERENCE HEMATOLOGIC VALUES FOR 33 SELECTED CATS

	Units	Mean	SD	Reference Interval
WBC count	1000/μl	10.88	3.64	6.62–18.05
RBC count	10⁶/μl	7.50	1.18	5.28–9.97
Hemoglobin	g/dl	12.27	1.86	8.9–15.3
Hematocrit	%	36.28	5.96	25.8–48.1
MCV	fl	48.36	2.67	43.4–52.8
MCH	pg	16.3	1.32	14.1–18.6
MCHC	g/dl	33.95	1.92	30.6–35.8
Platelets	×10³	404.27	91.7	300–631
MPV	fl	10.55	1.62	8.5–13.2
RDW	%	15.82	1.41	14.0–18.1
HDW	g/dl	2.30	0.57	1.89–2.73
LI		2.12	0.41	1.3–2.68
MPXI		−31.42	14.75	−47 to −16

MCV, mean corpuscular volume; MCH, mean corpuscular hemoglobin; MCHC, mean corpuscular hemoglobin concentration; MPV, mean platelet volume; RDW, red cell distribution width; HDW, hemoglobin distribution width; LI, lobularity index, MPXI, mean peroxidase index.

counts, then other hematologic parameters (including the new parameters) would usually also be normal. A mean and standard deviation were calculated on these subsets of the patient's data. These subsets were further reduced by removing 2.5% of the lowest and highest values to obtain a 95% reference interval or range. The canine reference values were from 365 samples selected from a total of 737 canine CBCs. Feline reference values were based on 33 feline samples derived from 159 feline hospital samples. Most of the 159 feline samples were removed based on a platelet count below the reference range, which reflects the problem with automated feline platelet counts often being low owing to platelet clumping on routinely collected blood samples and large platelet size.

Laboratory users should request the source of the laboratory's reference values. If needed, one can offer to submit a batch of samples from well-defined normal animals to improve the quality of the reference values. Most laboratory directors are happy to improve their reference values when help is available to obtain samples. If one uses an in-office chemistry unit, then one should establish reference values for the instrument. If reference values are reported for the unit, one can analyze a small number of normal animals (e.g., 40) to ensure that this instrument's results reflect the published reference values.

PROFILES VERSUS INDIVIDUAL TEST SELECTION

There are advantages and disadvantages to individual test selection or use of a profile of tests. The choice is affected by the availability of tests, cost, turnaround time, and the problem to be evaluated. A well-designed profile should, for a minimal fee and minimal redundancy, have a high probability of detecting the common diseases for the particular situation. A CBC is a profile that screens for anemia, inflammatory disease, stress, thrombocytopenia, heartworms, and various other problems. The urinalysis is a profile of tests designed not only to reveal hemorrhagic, inflammatory, or functional deficits in the urogenital tract but also to detect diabetes mellitus, hepatic disease, massive acute muscle injury, or intravascular hemolysis. A hemostatic profile for bleeding animals is discussed in Chapter 5. Serum chemistry profiles have variable numbers and types of tests included, although the "basic profile" includes the same or similar tests in most laboratories. Some criticize profiles for being a "shotgun approach" or a

nonspecific "fishing trip." Profiles instead should be considered cost-effective screens for a large number of common problems.

One must ask as specific a question as possible and know enough about the interpretation of the laboratory test results to know if an answer is possible. Compare "Is the animal anemic?" with "What is wrong with the animal?" A microhematocrit procedure along with a knowledge of the animal's hydration state should answer the first question, but a serum chemistry profile, CBC, urinalysis, and fecal examination may or may not answer the second question. Before requesting a test, ask yourself, "What will a high, low, or normal test result specifically mean in terms of a change in treatment or diagnosis?" If the answer is meaningful, then the test is worth paying for. Normal laboratory results to rule out certain possibilities are as valuable as an abnormal result that identifies a problem.

Individual test selection becomes important if one must perform each test oneself or if certain tests are not offered in an inexpensive profile. Some tests (e.g., lipase or endocrinologic) are not cost-effective enough to have in a profile. Tests that infrequently have abnormal results or are expensive are requested when additional information about the patient indicates a certain problem that justifies the use of these tests. If a certain disease such as diabetes has been diagnosed, then only one test such as urinary glucose may be needed to monitor the treatment process.

STAT TESTS

Rapid turnaround time between sample collection and the availability of results is important in some "stat" situations, such as determining fluid therapy to correct acid-base and electrolyte abnormalities. Some instruments analyze plasma or whole blood, which saves the approximately 30 minutes required for blood to clot and for centrifugation for separation of serum. The large investment in an electrolyte system and blood gas analyzer for a stat laboratory is not cost-effective except for large practices or emergency hospitals. An alternative is to have the owner deliver the sample to a referral laboratory if there is a stat submission arrangement. Either way is expensive, since stat tests are analyzed individually and not as cost-efficient batches (see cost analysis section). Stat tests require laboratory personnel to interrupt their routine work to perform the single test. In-office screening tests for BUN, total CO_2, and glucose provide limited stat testing and were discussed earlier.

INTERNATIONAL SYSTEM OF UNITS

Laboratory data in the literature or from certain laboratories may be in units different from commonly used units. This is especially true of serum enzyme activity, since many enzyme procedures have results reported in units named after the author of the procedure instead of international units per liter. An international system of units is intended to standardize reporting of data in the same units for improved comparison of results. A frequent question is how to convert a result from units one is unaccustomed to (e.g., mmol/L) into familiar units (e.g., mg/dl). See Appendix II for conversion factors, but note that one must also consider other variables (e.g., variations in technique, like the temperature at which the test was performed) while interpreting data from other laboratories.

Bibliography

Belford CJ, Lumsden JH: Assessment of a reflectance photometer in a veterinary laboratory. Can Vet J 1984;24:243–245.

Jain NC: Schalm's Veterinary Hematology. 4th ed. Philadelphia, Lea and Febiger, 1986.

Judy J: Personal communication, 1988.

Kaneko JJ: Clinical Biochemistry of Domestic Animals. 3rd ed. New York, Academic Press, 1980, pp 785–791.

Lehmann HP, Henry JB: SI units. *In* Henry JB (ed): Clinical Diagnosis and Management by Laboratory Methods. 17th ed. Philadelphia, WB Saunders, 1984, pp 1428–1450.

Miale JB: Laboratory Medicine Hematology. 5th ed. St Louis, CV Mosby, 1977, p 439.

Shull RM: Evaluation of four office chemistry systems for veterinary practice. AAHA Trends 1985;1:22–26.

Toffaletti J: Small chemistry analyzers for physician's office testing: A survey. Lab Manage 1986;24:37–41.

2 The Complete Blood Count and Bone Marrow Examination: General Comments and Selected Techniques

The complete blood count (CBC) is a profile of tests performed on blood and plasma. The choice of tests used to describe the quantity and quality of the cellular elements in blood and a few substances in plasma varies with the laboratory. The CBC is a cost-effective screen for many abnormalities. The bone marrow examination is used in selected instances to answer questions the CBC cannot answer.

The conclusions derived from information in the CBC and bone marrow examination, in addition to selected hematologic techniques, follow. Explanations about conclusions are brief, since detailed discussions about the use of diagnostic tests for erythrocytes (red blood cells [RBCs]), leukocytes (white blood cells [WBCs]), and platelets are in Chapters 3, 4, and 5. Technical comments are restricted to commonly needed tests, although a few technically advanced procedures are included.

COMPLETE BLOOD COUNT CONCLUSIONS

Conclusions are the interpretive decisions made from the available evidence; definitions are simply terms used to describe a situation. A diagnosis is a conclusion made by a veterinarian. Definitions like anemia or leukocytosis may be made by technicians performing a laboratory test. Some hematologic definitions from the CBC are listed in Table 2–1.

A list of hematologic conclusions is presented in Table 2–2. Laboratory conclusions are rarely etiologic diagnoses like *Haemobartonella felis* or heartworms but more commonly are general pathologic diagnoses like inflammation, hemolytic anemia, or stress.

The steps in the decision-making process, which are often too rapid to appreciate or understand, should include a series of intermediate conclusions. In learning situations, an early statement of the final diagnosis inhibits the understanding of how to make that diagnosis. It is helpful to trace back the sequence of decisions to aid diagnosis of more complex problems in the future. For example, one may nonspecifically conclude from a CBC that inflammation, stress, and lipemia are present in a dog. The inflammation could be anywhere in the body. Various metabolic problems lead to accumulation of lipid in the plasma. When these conclusions are added to a history of vomiting and a painful abdomen, pancreatitis becomes a likely differential diagnosis. This evidence demonstrates a need to perform serum amylase and lipase tests to prove the presence of pancreatitis.

The etiologic diagnosis will likely come from a combination of more basic laboratory and clinical conclusions and definitions.

Frequency of Abnormalities

A comprehensive profile should frequently detect abnormalities that suggest various common problems in an animal. Numerous hematologic abnormalities are detected by a CBC, and this inexpensive test is an excellent screening tool. Knowing the frequency of laboratory abnormalities gives the perspective needed to establish a diagnosis and prognosis and to understand the significance of the common changes discussed in later chapters. The data in Table 2–3 are from two unpublished surveys of CBC results from consecutive patients at Michigan State University. The larger survey was a computer search of quantitative values. The smaller survey was a manual search of records that included subjective observations. These are of variable sample size (30–737 animals per species) and from only one laboratory, so the values (%) should be considered approximations.

Anemia was moderately frequent (10–29%) and was often regenerative (polychromasia) in dogs. Abnormalities in RBC size and shape were quite common (53% of feline CBCs) but were often mild and insignificant (e.g., 1+ anisocytosis). Anisocytosis indicates variation in RBC size, and 1+ is the smallest amount subjectively noted on a 0 to 4+ scale. Findings like distemper inclusion bodies or 2 to 4+ spherocytes are less common but very diagnostic when identified.

The combination of lymphopenia (43% of feline CBCs) and eosinopenia (33% of feline CBCs) was common. These frequently occur in animals undergoing stress or glucocorticoid therapy. Inflammation was moderately frequent in dogs and cats, as demonstrated by a left shift (5–10%) and leukocytosis (13–19%). Many stimuli for inflammation also cause toxic change, which was also moderate in amount (4–23%). The more frequent toxic change of feline neutrophils (23%) is due to the tendency of cats to form Döhle bodies in even mildly toxic situations. Immune stimulation was indicated by the occasional lymphocytosis (2–3%) and the more common (7%) reactive (i.e., immune-stimulated) lymphocytes. The frequent hyperproteinemia (47% of feline CBCs) was likely secondary to inflammation with increased amounts of immunoglobulin and other proteins in acute phase inflammation or dehydration. Eosino-

Table 2-1 DEFINITIONS OF SELECTED HEMATOLOGIC CHANGES

Hematologic Change	Definition
Anemia	Decreased RBC mass, clinically noted by decreased packed cell volume (PCV)
Polycythemia	Increased RBC mass in body (increased PCV)
Polychromasia	Increased number of polychromatophils (immature RBCs-reticulocytes)
Poikilocytosis	Increased variation in RBC shapes
Anisocytosis	Increased variation in RBC size
Microcytosis	Increased number of small RBCs
Macrocytosis	Increased number of large RBCs
Normocytic	RBCs are of normal size
Hypochromic	RBCs have lower hemoglobin concentration (lower MCHC)
Normochromic	RBCs have normal MCHC
Spherocytosis	Increased number of smaller, spherical RBCs
Echinocytosis	Increased number of RBCs with many spiny projections
Acanthocytosis	Increased number of RBCs with a few elongated, rounded projections
RBC fragmentation	Increased number of small RBC fragments and/or RBCs with extensions ready to break off
Rouleaux	Aggregation of RBCs into linear formations resembling stacks of poker chips
Autoagglutination	Aggregation of RBCs into grapelike clusters
Thrombocytopenia	Decreased number of platelets
Thrombocytosis	Increased number of platelets
Leukocytosis	Increased number of WBCs
Leukopenia	Decreased number of WBCs
Neutrophilia	Increased number of neutrophils
Neutropenia	Decreased number of neutrophils
Left shift	Increased number of immature neutrophils (N-segs)
Right shift	Increased number of hypermature neutrophils (hypersegmentation)
Toxic neutrophils	Neutrophils with certain morphologic changes
Reactive lymphs	Lymphocytes with certain morphologic changes
Monocytosis	Increased number of monocytes
Monocytopenia	Decreased number of monocytes
Lymphocytosis	Increased number of lymphocytes
Lymphopenia	Decreased number of lymphocytes
Eosinophilia	Increased number of eosinophils
Eosinopenia	Decreased number of eosinophils
Basophilia	Increased number of basophils
Basopenia	Decreased number of basophils
Bicytopenia	Decrease in two cell lines (RBCs, WBCs, or platelets)
Pancytopenia	Decrease in three cell lines (RBCs, WBCs, and platelets)

Table 2-2 HEMATOLOGIC CONCLUSIONS THAT MAY BE MADE BASED ON DATA FROM A COMPLETE BLOOD COUNT

Hematologic Conclusion	Typical Evidence
Regenerative anemia	Appropriate degree of increased reticulocytes or polychromasia for severity of the anemia
Nonregenerative anemia	Insufficient increase in reticulocytes for the severity and duration of the anemia
Hemolytic anemia	Strongly regenerative anemia with additional evidence like hemoglobinuria, normal to high plasma protein, and one of the causes of hemolysis
Blood loss anemia	Regenerative anemia with decreased plasma protein, evidence of iron deficiency, or proof of blood loss
Iron deficiency	Microcytic-hypochromic anemia with variable regeneration
Inflammation	Leukocytosis, neutrophilia, and left shift
Stress/steroids	Lymphopenia and eosinopenia; often neutrophilia, and occasionally monocytosis
Excitement/epinephrine	Lymphocytosis, leukocytosis, neutrophilia, and perhaps polycythemia; especially in cats
Toxemia	Significant number of very toxic neutrophils
Leukemia	Significant number of immature hematopoietic blast cells in bone marrow and blood
Bone marrow disease	Pancytopenia or bicytopenia in blood; histologic and cytologic changes in bone marrow samples

Table 2-3 FREQUENCY (%) OF SELECTED ABNORMALITIES IN TWO SURVEYS OF COMPLETE BLOOD COUNTS PERFORMED AT MICHIGAN STATE UNIVERSITY

Abnormality	Dogs (n = 100)	Dogs (n = 737)	Cats (n = 30)	Cats (n = 159)
Anemia (PCV)	23	29	10	20
Anemia (Hgb)	13	29	10	21
Polychromasia	10		0	
Abnormal RBC morphology	38		53	
Microcytic (based on MCV)		3		7
Hypochromic (based on MCHC)		6		9
Macrocytic (based on MCV)		5		7
Hyperchromic (based on MCHC)		1		8
Polycythemia	5	3	7	9
Hypoproteinemia	9		7	
Hyperproteinemia	24		47	
Hemolysis	4		3	
Lipemia	5		3	
Leukocytosis	16	28	13	19
Leukopenia		6		22
Left shift	5		10	
Lymphopenia	27		43	
Lymphocytosis	2		3	
Monocytosis	14		13	
Monocytopenia	0		4	
Eosinophilia	17		10	
WBC toxicity	4		23	
Reactive lymphs	7		7	
Thrombocytopenia	5	15	7	60
Thrombocytosis	5	11	7	6
Clumped platelets	6		23	

philic inflammation was moderately common in cats and dogs (10–17%).

The frequency (5–60%) of thrombocytosis and thrombocytopenia was quite variable. Thrombocytopenia, common in feline samples (60%), was most likely due to a technical problem rather than a disease. Feline platelets tend to clump and so are not counted. Platelet clumping was noted on about 23% of the samples in the small survey of feline CBCs, and platelet counts should not be trusted in those cats.

Magnitude of the Hematologic Abnormalities

Magnitude of a change is a diagnostic variable that should be evaluated. Anemia in ill animals is often mild. About 16% of the 29% of anemic canine samples (see Table 2–3) had a packed cell volume (PCV) >30%. Mild anemias are often secondary to a primary disease (e.g., anemia of chronic inflammation or hepatic failure) and so are not given much attention until the more severe problems are corrected. Use an adjective on processes to denote their severity.

QUANTITATION TECHNIQUES

Submission

Anticoagulated blood is required for cell counts. Properly filling an EDTA blood collection tube avoids an excessive concentration of EDTA (e.g., such as when one obtains only 0.25 ml of blood in a 3-ml tube), which causes RBC shrinkage and a decrease in the PCV (Perman and Schall, 1983). If not analyzed in 2 to 3 hours, the blood should be refrigerated at 4°C, because RBC swelling after 6 to 24 hours of storage raises the hematocrit and mean corpuscular volume (MCV) and lowers the mean corpuscular hemoglobin concentration (MCHC). The RBC, hemoglobin (Hgb), hematocrit (Hct), and RBC indices (MCV, mean corpuscular hemoglobin [MCH], and MCHC) are unchanged if blood is refrigerated for 24 hours (Nelson and Morris, 1984).

Blood smears should be made immediately to avoid artifacts caused by cell exposure to anticoagulants and cell deterioration during storage and shipment. EDTA is the best anticoagulant to use to preserve cell detail. Heparin produces poor staining with a generally blue background. Formalin causes poor staining of Wright's-stained blood smears, resulting in a blue background. One must keep formalin away from blood and cytology smears, both in the laboratory and in packages sent to referral laboratories. Formalin fumes can affect smears without direct contact.

Do not mail slides in the thin, two-slide mail cards that fit into envelopes that are machine processed by the post office. Even with "Hand Cancel" written on these envelopes, they are often machine canceled, which crushes the slides. Mail the slides in a container (e.g., box) too bulky to be machine canceled.

Microhematocrit

The microhematocrit method for determining the PCV (Hct) is routinely used by veterinarians to estimate erythroid mass. It is more consistent and technically easier than a manual RBC count. The microhematocrit provides more useful information than does either the RBC count or Hgb concentration. Gross examination of the plasma in the microhematocrit tube detects icterus, hemolysis, or lipemia. The microhematocrit procedure is also a screening test for heartworm disease in dogs, since microfilariae are concentrated in the plasma just above the buffy coat. The plasma protein concentration can be quantitated with a refractometer on the plasma obtained from one or two microhematocrit tubes.

The PCV is determined by centrifuging anticoagulated blood in a small capillary tube to separate the cells from plasma. The RBCs are packed at the bottom; the WBCs and platelets appear as a thin white line (i.e., buffy coat) between the RBCs and plasma (Fig. 2–1). To calculate the PCV, the length of packed RBCs is divided by the total length of the tube containing packed RBCs, buffy coat, and plasma. Do not include the clay plugging the bottom of the tube. Various microhematocrit reading devices are available.

Error is minimal but usually related to centrif-

ugation. Centrifuge for 5 minutes. When the PCV is >50%, the packing of RBCs by the centrifuge is less complete (i.e., less tight). This causes an exaggeration of the PCV and a slight overestimation of the amount of RBCs in the blood sample compared with the Hgb concentration or the RBC count in electronic counters (Perman and Schall, 1983). The tube should be spun an additional 5 minutes to enhance packing. If the microhematocrit tubes are filled to more than two thirds to three fourths of their volume, the cell packing is also less complete. When the blood is dilute (i.e., PCV <25%), the packing of RBCs is tighter. This exaggerates the decrease in the PCV and makes the animal seem slightly more anemic. Special microhematocrit centrifuges attain high speeds (e.g., 11,500–15,000 rpm), which ensures the proper centrifugal force to pack cells. The speed should be checked periodically, since the poorer cell packing of centrifuges with slower speeds cannot be compensated for by longer periods of centrifugation. Multipurpose centrifuges used to centrifuge larger volumes of fluid may not rotate fast enough to pack cells properly. Check the centrifuge's brushes three to four times per year and replace if worn. Even the small microhematocrit tubes should be evenly balanced in the centrifuge's head to prevent unequal weight distribution. If the head is not properly balanced at high speeds, there is uneven wear on the motor, eventually causing the head to vibrate. Do not use the brake when the head is still rotating at high speeds, since this also causes wear on the motor.

Hemoglobin Concentration

The Hgb concentration is essentially equivalent to the PCV in estimating the erythroid mass. Hgb is obtained as part of the CBC performed by automated hematology instruments, which routinely include a Hgb photometer. Hgb may be more accurate than PCV if cell shrinkage, cell swelling, or cell fragility is pres-

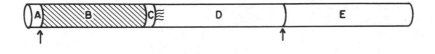

MICROHEMATOCRIT TUBE

Figure 2–1 Microhematocrit tube. Arrows indicate the length of tube that contains blood. The packed cell volume (PCV) = B ÷ (B + C + D). The plasma area (D) adjacent to the buffy coat is where to check for microfilaria. (A, clay seal; B, packed erythrocytes; C, packed leukocytes and platelets (buffy coat); D, plasma; E, empty space in the top of the tube.)

ent. Hgb is measured inaccurately if the plasma is lipemic enough to interfere with light transmission for the photometric analysis. Feline blood may have enough Heinz bodies in the lysed blood suspension to erroneously increase optical density and thus increase apparent Hgb concentration.

Techniques are available to analyze the amount of Hgb in its various normal and diseased forms. If Hgb has iron in the oxidized (i.e., ferric) state (methemoglobin: Hi), it is nonfunctional and cannot carry oxygen (see Chapter 3). Sulfhemoglobin (SHb) is another oxidized form of Hgb that has irreversible denaturation to Heinz bodies. SHb is usually due to some oxidative toxin (see Heinz Body Anemia in Chapter 3). Carboxyhemoglobin (HbCO) has strong binding of carbon monoxide to Hgb, decreasing oxygen-carrying capacity.

Manual Cell Counts/Hemocytometer

Manually counting cells in an inexpensive hemocytometer is the preferable method when test volume is too low to justify an automated cell counter. A hemocytometer is a transparent glass chamber that holds a cell suspension beneath a microscope for counting. The hemocytometer is 0.1 mm deep and has a well-defined space of known volume. The volume is divided into subunits by a grid with a precise surface area (i.e., 3 mm × 3 mm) engraved at the base on each side of the counting chamber. Depending on the surface area of the grid used in a procedure and thus the volume of the hemocytometer, one can mathematically determine the cells in a cubic millimeter (mm³), the traditional unit for reporting blood cell concentrations (Fig. 2–2). In the United States, hematologic cell concentrations are reported as cells/

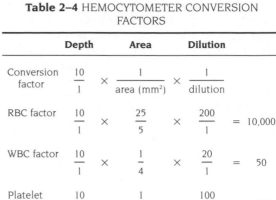

Table 2–4 HEMOCYTOMETER CONVERSION FACTORS

	Depth		Area		Dilution	
Conversion factor	$\dfrac{10}{1}$	×	$\dfrac{1}{\text{area (mm}^2)}$	×	$\dfrac{1}{\text{dilution}}$	
RBC factor	$\dfrac{10}{1}$	×	$\dfrac{25}{5}$	×	$\dfrac{200}{1}$	= 10,000
WBC factor	$\dfrac{10}{1}$	×	$\dfrac{1}{4}$	×	$\dfrac{20}{1}$	= 50
Platelet factor	$\dfrac{10}{1}$	×	$\dfrac{1}{2}$	×	$\dfrac{100}{1}$	= 500

μl, which equals cells/mm³. All other countries (e.g., Canada) report hematologic cell concentrations in cells × 10^9/L. There are 10^6 μl in a liter, so a liter would have a million times more cells (see International System of Units in Chapter 1).

Because blood cells are concentrated, blood is first diluted with Unopette containers (see Chapter 1). The amount of dilution varies with the type of cell counted. The goal is to obtain a cell concentration to use in the hemocytometer that is neither too dense to consistently count each cell in a microscopic field nor too dilute to count enough cells to be accurate. For RBC counts, the blood is diluted 1:200. Since there are fewer WBCs than RBCs in blood, the WBC dilution is usually only 1:20. Platelets are diluted 1:100 by a combined WBC/platelet Unopette. The reciprocal of the dilution (i.e., 1/dilution) is used in calculation of the final conversion factor. Other dilutions are chosen for cytologic samples, so conversion factors must be calculated.

The conversion factors are determined by for-

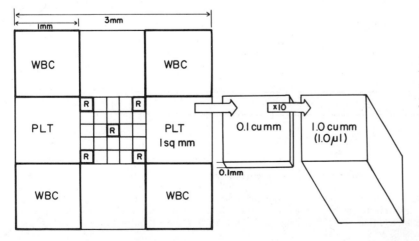

Figure 2–2 Dimensions of a hemocytometer. The hemocytometer grid consists of 9 mm². The central 1 mm² is additionally divided into 25 squares. The areas usually used for erythrocyte, leukocyte, and platelet counts are indicated by R, WBC, and PLT, respectively. Since the hemocytometer is 0.1 mm deep, the cells counted over 1 mm² are in the volume of 0.1 mm³. Multiply by 10 to determine the cells in 1 mm³, which is 1 μl.

mulas as in Table 2–4. If instructions are not available for the method used, calculate the conversion factor (or validate the one used) by the initial formula in Table 2–4. The WBC factor of 50 is based on adjustments for the depth of the hemocytometer (0.1 mm), the dilution factor (1:20), and the area counted (4 mm²). This mathematically converts to 1 µl of undiluted blood.

The volume of the hemocytometer counted varies with the cell's concentration. Since the RBC count is so high, only ⅕ of a square millimeter (0.2 mm²) is counted. The grid is divided into 9 mm², and the central 1 mm² is subdivided into 25 squares (see Fig. 2–2). Five of these 25 subdivisions are counted. For WBC counts, the outer 4 mm² are counted. For platelets, 1 mm² on each side of the central 1 mm² is counted, for a total of 2 mm². The reciprocal of the area is used in calculating the final conversion factor. Since the hemocytometer is only 0.1 mm deep, a figure of 10 is included in the final conversion factor.

The cells in the hemocytometer are counted in duplicate by counting cells over the grids on both sides of the hemocytometer. The number of cells counted from each grid should vary by only 10% for WBC counts and 20% for RBC counts. If the cell suspension was not evenly distributed, as indicated by greater variation, the test should be repeated. If the two cell counts are consistent, the average of the two grids is multiplied by a conversion factor to obtain the cell count per microliter.

Manual counts with a hemocytometer have significant error (e.g., ±20% error may occur with WBC counts). Consider this magnitude of error when interpreting whether a total WBC count has truly changed. A count of 2100 WBCs/µl varies too little from a count of 1900 WBCs/µl the previous day to be considered an improvement. The change could be due to technical variation.

Corrected WBC Count

Since nucleated RBCs (NRBCs) are counted in manual and automated total WBC counts, it is necessary to reduce this WBC count (actually a nucleated cell count) to a corrected WBC count that accurately indicates the WBC count. The correction is done if more than 5 NRBCs are noted while counting 100 WBCs in a WBC differential count. The ratio of NRBCs to WBCs (NRBCs/100 WBCs) is determined. A proportion is used to mathematically adjust the nucleated cell count as follows:

$$\frac{NRBC + 100\ WBC}{100\ WBC} = \frac{\text{nucleated cell count}}{\text{corrected WBC count}}$$

or

Corrected WBC count
$$= \frac{100}{NRBC + 100} \times \text{nucleated cell count}$$

Absolute NRBC Count

The absolute NRBC count is the difference between the nucleated cell count and the corrected WBC count. Reporting NRBCs/100 WBCs can be misleading if the WBC count is very high or low. In these cases, the absolute NRBC count per microliter is better.

Erythrocyte Indices

The indices may be calculated from directly determined measurements (i.e., PCV, RBC count, and Hgb) by the following equations. Automated cell counters may directly measure MCV or MCHC.

Mean corpuscular volume (MCV)
$$= \frac{PCV \times 10}{RBC\ (10^6)}\ \text{(femtoliters)}$$

Mean corpuscular hemoglobin (MCH)
$$= \frac{Hgb \times 10}{RBC\ (10^6)}\ \text{(picograms)}$$

Mean corpuscular hemoglobin concentration
$$(MCHC) = \frac{Hgb \times 100}{PCV}\ \text{(g/dl)}$$

The MCV indicates the average size of the RBCs. An increased, normal, or decreased MCV morphologically describes RBCs as macrocytic, normocytic, or microcytic. The MCH indicates the Hgb per average RBC, and the MCHC indicates the average concentration of Hgb in RBCs. A normal or decreased MCHC morphologically defines the RBCs as normochromic or hypochromic. The MCH is affected by both the size of RBCs (i.e., MCV) and the average Hgb concentration in RBCs.

Automated Hematology Cell Counters

QBC V ● The QBC V (Becton-Dickinson*), for "quantitative buffy coat" analysis, is an in-office hematology analyzer that has been recommended for veterinary clinics (Hart, 1987). The initial costs were about $8000 for the instrument and about $2 per tube used for the test. Consider other costs and the CBC test volume of your practice for the economic impact of purchasing a hematology instrument (see Chapter 1, Serum Chemistry Analysis).

The QBC V analysis is much more rapid (i.e., 7 minutes) than are manual counts. Based on correlation to reference methods in dogs and cats, the accuracy was excellent (r = 0.93–0.99) for Hct, total WBC count, and granulocyte count; good for nongranulocyte count (r = 0.81–0.93); and fair for platelets (r = 0.59–0.78) (Levine et al., 1986; Brown and Barsanti, 1988). Perfect correlation is indicated by an r value of 1.0, and >0.80 is acceptable for a laboratory test. The precision of the QBC V based on the coefficient of variation (CV) was better than that of manual methods and worse than that of impedance (Coulter) counters (Brown and Barsanti, 1988).

The main technical problem was indistinct separation of the RBC and granulocyte layers in 17% of canine samples and 30% of canine samples with a leukocytosis (Brown and Barsanti, 1988). Cell counts in the QBC V are determined from the width of various layers of different cell types, so boundaries of the layers must be distinct. Reasonable estimates of band width were possible in more than half of the samples with the indistinct band separation. Improved QBC tubes had fewer samples with indistinct band separation.

The QBC V determines a two-part WBC differential count. Automated differentials provide useful information but are not an alternative to blood smear evaluation. The cell counter in the author's practice (Technicon H-1) determines an automated five-part differential, but the smear is still microscopically evaluated for RBC abnormalities, toxicity of neutrophils, a left shift, and the presence of platelets and platelet clumps and other alterations. The quantitative data, when combined with the blood smear evaluation, allow more complete and powerful conclusions. The manual screen and automated procedure are relatively quick.

Coulter Counters ● The most common electronic counters have been made by Coulter.* Coulter counters determine cell numbers, cell size (MCV), and Hgb concentration and mathematically calculate the PCV, MCHC, and MCH for a CBC. Newer models provide additional information. The Coulter counting principle is that cells (i.e., RBCs, WBCs, platelets, or other particles) are diluted in an electrolyte solution and drawn through an aperture. The electrical resistance across the aperture varies owing to the size and number of cells passing through it. The frequency of the changing resistance indicates the cell numbers, and the magnitude of the change indicates cell size. (See Fig. 3–4 for a demonstration of macrocytosis in a dog with stomatocytosis.) In-office cell counters of this type (i.e., impedance principle) have been used by veterinarians.

The Coulter counters must be electronically adjusted to count different-sized cells by electronic thresholds established for each species. Canine blood cells are similar enough to human blood cells that few problems occur. Feline blood has smaller RBCs and frequent platelet clumping, causing more concern. Quality control is maintained by routine use of control blood samples, examining cell histograms and electronic flags by the instrument for possible errors.

In Coulter counters, the Hct is calculated, not determined by packing RBCs in a centrifuge, so it should not precisely be called PCV. The MCV is directly measured, and the Hct is calculated by the following equation:

$$Hct = \frac{MCV \times RBC}{10}$$

The PCV (and related values) determined by the microhematocrit method and the Hct of an electronic cell counter often vary slightly. If the variation in PCV between the two methods is >3% to 5%, one should determine the technical reason.

Laser Cell Counters ● Another class of automated hematology analyzers uses an electronic-optical (i.e., laser) detection system to measure the size and internal complexity of cells based on light scatter at different angles. Newer hematologic instruments (e.g., Technicon H-1†)

---

*QBC V Hematology System, Becton-Dickinson, Clay Adams Division, 299 Webro Rd., Parsippany, NJ 07054.

*Coulter Electronics, Inc., 98 Mayfield Ave., P.O. Box 4060, Edison, NJ 08818–4060 (1–800–526–7698).

†Technicon H-1, Technicon Instruments Corp., 953 N. Larch Ave., Elmhurst, IL 60126.

provide greatly expanded information about each cell type. For RBCs, an H-1 report includes the RBC count, Hgb concentration, PCV, RBC distribution width (RDW), Hgb distribution width (HDW), two histograms to visualize the RDW and HDW in graphic form, and an RBC cytogram to illustrate the RBC population and subpopulations based on cell size (MCV) and Hgb concentration (MCHC) (Figs. 2–3 and 2–4). A cytogram illustrating each RBC counted is possible because the instrument determines the size and Hgb concentration of each RBC. The entire population and subpopulations of cells may be considered instead of one average value (e.g., MCV). When restricted to only the average size of all RBCs, one could not appreciate hidden subpopulations of cells. The RDW describes the variability in the size of the RBCs; the HDW describes the variability in Hgb concentration among cells. (See Chapter 3 for clinical use of these parameters.)

The H-1 evaluation of WBCs includes an automated canine differential WBC count. The various subpopulations of WBCs (neutrophils,

eosinophils) are displayed in two cytograms (Figs. 2–5 and 2–6). The peroxidase cytogram is based on the size of the WBCs and their peroxidase content. The neutrophils and eosinophils have the greatest peroxidase content. The monocytes have less peroxidase and merge into the neutrophil cluster (see Fig. 2–5). The basophil cytogram is based on the size and density of the leukocytic nuclei after the cytoplasm is removed by a "basophil" reagent. The basophil reagent strips the cytoplasm off all normal WBCs except basophils. Since human basophils retain their cytoplasm, they appear largest and are thus counted as basophils for the automated WBC differential count. Patterns of the basophil cytogram are useful in detecting blast cells of leukemia, nucleated RBCs, eosinophilia, and left shifts and toxic changes in neutrophils.

The H-1 reports the platelet count and flags various potential errors (e.g., clumped platelets). The mean platelet volume and platelet histogram (Fig. 2–7), which illustrates the distribution of platelets in the population based on size, may be used to judge size variations.

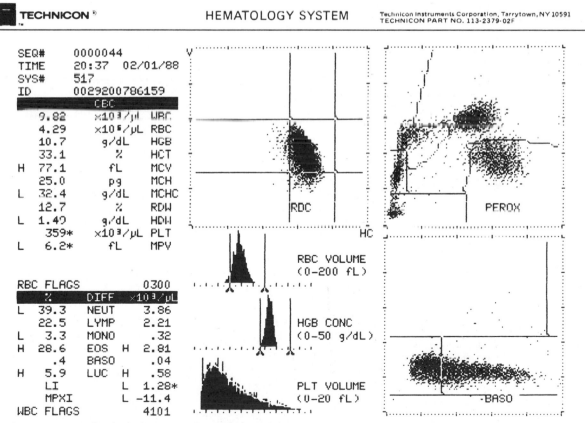

Figure 2–3 Example of a Technicon H-1 hematology analyzer report. This is an example of the extent of information currently available for a canine complete blood count (CBC). The numerical data on the left side include an automated leukocyte differential count at the bottom and 11 other hematologic parameters at the top. Cytograms and histograms are detailed in Figures 2–4 to 2–7.

Normocytic Normochromic

Macrocytic Hypochromic

Microcytic Hypochromic

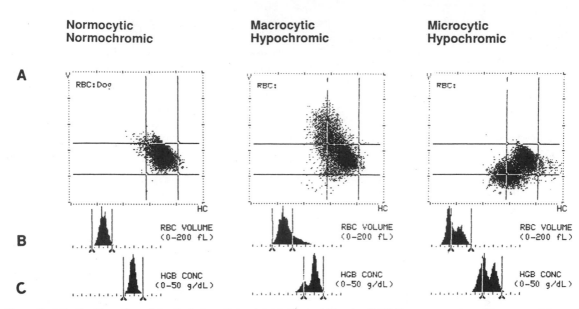

Figure 2–4 Erythroid portion of the Technicon H-1 printout. The red blood cell (RBC) cytograms (row A) are on a 9-box grid dividing the RBCs into normal (e.g., normocytic normochromic), macrocytic hypochromic, microcytic hypochromic, and the other possibilities. The normal canine RBC cytogram on the left has the normocytic normochromic cells in the central box. The cytogram in the center has macrocytic hypochromic cells, mainly reticulocytes, extending toward the upper left from the normocytic normochromic cells. The cytogram on the right from a dog with iron deficiency anemia has a second population of microcytic hypochromic cells adjacent to and to the lower left of the normal RBCs. The RBC volume histogram (row B) illustrates the distribution of RBCs based on volume. The RBC histogram in the center, with reticulocytosis, has a small to medium-sized tail of macrocytic cells extending to the right. The volume histogram of the dog with iron deficiency anemia to the right has a tall peak of microcytic RBCs to the left of the normocytic RBCs. The hemoglobin concentration histogram (row C) illustrates the distribution of RBCs based on individual cells' hemoglobin concentration. The hemoglobin histograms in the center and on the far right have distinct peaks of hypochromic cells to the left of the normochromic RBCs. The histograms allow estimation of the approximate magnitude of the abnormal cell population compared with normal RBCs.

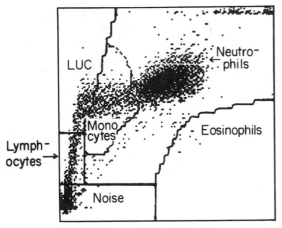

PEROXIDASE ACTIVITY

Figure 2–5 Peroxidase cytogram for the Technicon H-1. The vertical axis is cell size, and the peroxidase content of the cells is on the horizontal axis. The cell types in the various areas are labeled. A more obvious eosinophil cluster is shown in Figure 2–3. The eosinophils and neutrophils have abundant peroxidase, so they are located to the right. Lymphocytes lack peroxidase and are on the left. Large unstained cells (LUC) are on the upper left. The LUC box may contain large lymphocytes, monocytes, and blast cells. The monocytes have a little peroxidase and are located between the neutrophils and lymphocytes or LUC. (Noise is small debris.)

BLOOD SMEAR ANALYSIS

The evaluation of the blood smear is a rapid source of abundant information and so should be a routine part of a clinic's laboratory. Platelet and WBC estimates quickly detect clinically significant changes. RBC estimates are inconsistent, so the microhematocrit should be determined for a quick quantitation of the RBCs. Several qualitative morphologic observations of the WBCs, RBCs, and platelets permit clinically useful conclusions. The section on cytologic smears in Chapter 16 has additional information on preparation and evaluation of smears.

Making the Smear

The smear must have a reasonably large thin area where a monolayer of cells will have optimal morphologic detail and reasonable distribution (Fig. 2–8). The cells in the monolayer should infrequently touch another cell and should not be distorted by various physical forces. In this area, the WBCs flatten out over a

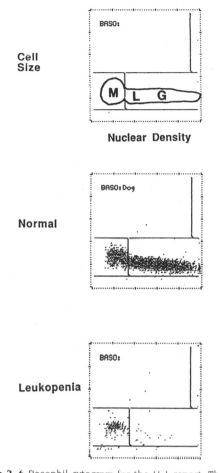

Figure 2–6 Basophil cytogram for the H-1 report. The cytogram has cell size on the vertical axis and nuclear complexity on the horizontal axis. The cytoplasm is stripped from most cells, so mainly nuclei are evaluated. The cytogram is shaped like a worm. The head of the worm (M) contains the nuclei of mononuclear cells like lymphocytes and monocytes. Granulocytes (G), mainly neutrophils, have complex lobulated nuclei, and these appear as the body of the worm. If a left shift (L) with nonsegmented or toxic neutrophils is present, then their nuclei are located at the neck of the worm as a thickened area or the whole cytogram may contract into a ball shape. The cytogram at the bottom was from a dog with parvovirus enteritis and severe leukopenia/neutropenia, with mainly lymphocytes (>90%) remaining.

or damaged areas even if some rule states you must perform a differential count in a certain pattern. A differential cannot be accurate if unidentifiable or questionable cells are included. All smears have some damaged cells with distorted shapes and staining characteristics. It is important to recognize damaged cells (see Fig. 16–2), since cell swelling may make the cell resemble another cell type.

The technique of making a smear should be well learned to allow one to read the smears or to submit readable slides to a consultant. Air-dried blood smears must be made when the blood is collected to avoid cell deterioration. They should be mailed with the EDTA blood to a referral laboratory for a CBC. A common mistake is to make a smear that extends to the end of the glass slide, causing the monolayer area to be lost (see Fig. 2–8). Long smears are caused by using too large a drop of blood to make the smear. When a small drop of blood is applied to the slide, the smear extends only to the middle or distal two thirds of the slide, and the

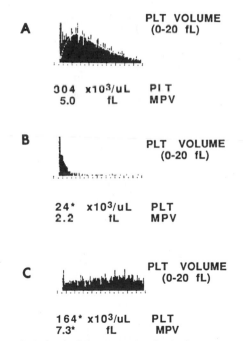

Figure 2–7 Platelet histogram. The platelet histogram for the Technicon H-1 report illustrates the distribution of platelets of various sizes. **A** represents a normal canine platelet histogram. The middle histogram (**B**) is small, indicating thrombocytopenia, and the far left location of the peak indicates a predominance of smaller platelets. This is also reflected by the low MPV of 2.2 fl. This finding in dogs with thrombocytopenia has been associated with immune-mediated thrombocytopenia. The histogram in **C** extends greatly to the right, indicating the presence of large platelets, associated with active thrombopoiesis. The increased MPV of 7.3 fl also reflects the larger platelet volume.

wide area and expose a large surface area for viewing (see Fig. 16–2). The cells in the monolayer are properly stained, allowing good evaluation of cytoplasmic and nuclear detail.

The thin monolayer is the only place where cell evaluation should be performed. Two common errors in reading blood and cytologic smears are to try to identify cells in thick areas of the smear and to try to identify damaged cells. In thick areas, the cells are suspended more upright, so when viewed from above, the cell has a smaller diameter and stains too darkly for proper evaluation. Do not look at thick areas

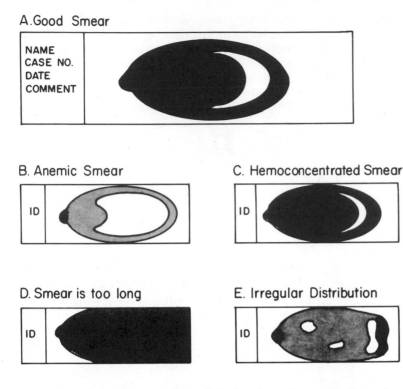

A. Good Smear

NAME
CASE NO.
DATE
COMMENT

B. Anemic Smear

ID

C. Hemoconcentrated Smear

ID

D. Smear is too long

ID

E. Irregular Distribution

ID

Figure 2–8 Examples of blood smears. A good blood smear (**A**) is properly labeled with the animal's identification, date, and other information needed to attribute any abnormality to the correct patient and sample. The smear should include an evenly distributed thin area near the end of the smear. This thin monolayer is illustrated by a clear elliptic area to the right of the smear. The more distal end of the smear has physical distortion and crowding of cells. Smears of anemic blood (**B**) are thin over much of the smear. The thin monolayer (illustrated in **B** by a large clear area) extends back toward the site where the drop was applied, as on the left end of the drawing. In smears of hemoconcentrated blood (**C**), the thin monolayer is only a narrow area near the distal end of the smear or may be absent. If too large a drop of blood is used for the smear, the smear (**D**) extends off the slide, leaving no monolayer region for cellular evaluation. Smears with uneven distribution (**E**) are caused by use of poor quality glass slides or by not making a smooth push while streaking the slide.

monolayer is in an area of the slide that is easily stained and examined. The size of the drop can be easily regulated if it is applied with a microhematocrit tube. To prevent an irregular smear (see Fig. 2–8), avoid using cheaper glass slides that have rough edges and a greasy surface.

Stains

See Chapter 16.

Evaluating Blood Smears

Establish a set routine to consistently evaluate and describe blood smears. Evaluate all three cell types (WBCs, RBCs, and platelets) for both quantity and morphologic characteristics. The evaluation of platelets is frequently forgotten.

Platelet Estimation • Platelet numbers are estimated reasonably accurately (see Fig. 5–10), but the numerical estimate should be only approximate (e.g., very low, low, normal, high, very high) rather than a specific concentration (e.g., 50,000/μl).

Platelet Morphology • Platelet clumping and large platelets are observations of practical use. If the platelets are clumped, they are not evenly distributed, and an estimate or actual platelet count cannot be trusted. Platelet clumping is usually attributed to routine venipuncture trauma to tissues and is more common in cats. Since platelet clumps are large, they tend to be found at the distal end of the smear. Larger than normal platelets (e.g., as large as RBCs) are considered young platelets, suggesting an increased production by megakaryocytes in the bone marrow.

Leukocyte Estimation • Estimation of the WBC count from a blood smear has had few guidelines. One method is to scan the smear using the 10× microscope objective and to estimate subjectively whether the number of WBCs distributed throughout the smear and WBCs pushed to the end of the smear are more or less than normal. Appropriate adjectives (i.e., slightly, moderately, or greatly) are added to an estimated leukocytosis or leukopenia. Another method is to count the number of WBCs in several 10× objective fields in the thin areas of the smear where the platelet estimate and WBC differential are performed. In our laboratory, between 18 and 51 WBCs/10× objective field indicates a normal WBC count for canine blood smears. The correlation of the WBCs/10× field and the actual WBC count was good, as indicated by an r value of 0.87 (Tvedten et al., 1988). Correlation between two tests is acceptable when the r value ≥0.80. Because accuracy deteriorates when the WBC/10× field is >60 (too numerous to count accurately), stop counting at 60 WBCs/10× field and do not expect to differentiate the magnitude of a leukocytosis.

Leukocyte Aggregation • Rare dogs and cats have strong aggregation of WBCs in EDTA blood tubes. Collection of canine blood in heparin sometimes prevents the aggregation and allows accurate total WBC counts. In a cat with large WBC aggregates the WBC count was 36,920/μl in EDTA but 64,650/μl when blood was collected in heparin and immediately put into a hematology analyzer. The cat's WBC count in heparin also aggregated in 15 to 30 minutes, so speed in analyzing the sample was important.

Leukocyte Differential Count • The consistent and rapid way to describe the WBCs is by the absolute (cells/μl) and relative (%) WBC differential counts. The relative differential count is determined by counting 100 to 200 or more WBCs and determining the percentage of each type of WBC. The percentage of each type (e.g., 18% eosinophils) is multiplied by the total WBC count/μl to obtain the absolute count of each WBC (e.g., 1300 eosinophils/μl).

Leukocyte Morphology
Left Shift • The differential WBC count describes neutrophil maturity. Neutrophils younger than segmented neutrophils include bands, metamyelocytes, myelocytes, promyelocytes, and myeloblasts. Some people simply include all immature neutrophils as nonsegmented neutrophils (N-segs). An increase in N-segs is termed a *left shift* and indicates an inflammatory process. Most or all of the N-segs in blood are bands, since the bone marrow tends to preferentially release the most mature form of neutrophils. If the left shift includes N-segs younger than bands, then these metamyelocytes and myelocytes or younger neutrophils should be described in some manner to reflect a more severe inflammatory process. Each developmental stage of neutrophils may be reported (percentage and cells/μl). Neutrophils younger than bands are often simply described in a subjective comment (e.g., "a few metamyelocytes were present") on the CBC report.

Laboratory personnel are often inconsistent in the determination of the maturity of neutrophils and the presence or absence of a left shift. Since a left shift is proof that an animal has an inflammatory disease, one must be accurate and consistent in identifying N-segs. Just as no one criterion consistently identifies a person as mature, no one criterion consistently delineates the transition of a band into a segmented neutrophil. Segmented neutrophils acquire various morphologic markers of maturity to distinguish them from a band, such as

1. Shape: focal narrowing (indentation) of the nucleus (lobe formation) with loss of parallel sides
2. Thinner nucleus
3. Longer nucleus
4. Coarse clumping of nuclear chromatin
5. Rough nuclear margin (where chromatin clumps protrude)

When in doubt (e.g., the nucleus has folded over on itself), identify cells "by the company they keep," which usually means "if unsure, call it a segmented neutrophil, since they are more common than bands." If the animal is toxic, as often is the case in inflammatory diseases, the neutrophils develop abnormally, making consistent identification of various stages of maturation difficult to impossible.

Toxic Neutrophils • Toxic change in blood smear neutrophils (Color Plate 1F) indicates toxemia. When toxic changes are severe, toxemia is usually clinically apparent. The most severe toxic changes are due to bacterial toxins, often related to enteric disease (e.g., parvoviral diarrhea), but other toxins can also cause toxic changes. Toxic change should be reported both by the number of cells affected and by the severity in order to judge if it is significant. When toxicity is mild or few neutrophils are affected, there may be no clinical evidence of toxemia. The following guidelines are used in our laboratory for uniformity in reporting (note that 0–4% toxic neutrophils is insignificant): few, 5% to 10%; moderate, 11% to 30%; and many, >30%.

Severity of toxicity is subjective. Döhle bodies in cats appear so frequently that such neutrophils may not be considered toxic. Mildly toxic canine neutrophils only have Döhle bodies. One may ignore a few 1+ toxic neutrophils with only occasional Döhle bodies. More severe toxicity (e.g., many 2+ to 4+ toxic neutrophils) usually reflects clinical toxemia. Severely toxic neutrophils have characteristics listed in Table 2–5 and in Chapter 4. Because Döhle bodies may be present in neutrophils identified to be severely toxic by other criteria, one must classify the toxicity by the most severe change. Simple subjective criteria are listed in Table 2–5, with 4+ being most severe.

Table 2–5 CHARACTERISTICS OF TOXIC NEUTROPHILS AND A SUGGESTED GRADING SCHEME

Severity	Morphologic Characteristics of Toxicity
1+	Only Döhle bodies are present
2+ or 3+	Variable intensity of cytoplasmic basophilia, foaminess, and/or toxic granulation
4+	Cells too toxic to differentiate from reactive lymphocytes or reactive monocytes; they may appear aged and lytic

Reactive Lymphocytes ● Occasional reactive lymphocytes are commonly found in blood smears of ill and apparently normal animals. Relatively frequent reactive lymphocytes in ill animals suggest strong antigenic stimulation. Identification of reactive change in lymphocytes is based mainly on finding prominent, dark blue, hyaline cytoplasm due to increased protein synthesis (e.g., antibodies). The nucleus may undergo blast transformation or may have a convoluted shape.

Leukemia ● Leukemia is suggested by a marked leukocytosis and more specifically by many blast cells with large nuclei, prominent nucleoli, and fine immature chromatin (see Chapter 4). These cells should be simply categorized as "blasts" or "other cells" when performing a differential WBC count if identification is difficult. Excessive myeloblasts and progranulocytes denote a granulocytic leukemia. Numerous lymphoblasts indicate lymphoblastic leukemia. Increased numbers of blast-transformed reactive lymphocytes may be confused with lymphoid leukemia (see Chapter 4).

Erythrocyte Estimation ● Estimating RBC numbers from a blood smear is not precise owing to variability in the thickness of manually prepared blood smears. Scan the smear at $10\times$ in the thin monolayer, where the WBC differential and other morphologic observations should be made to note the amount of plasma space between RBCs. In anemia, there is wide separation of the RBCs compared with close packing of the RBCs if the blood is hemoconcentrated. Severity of anemia is also indicated by the width of the monolayer. Normally the thin monolayer where the RBCs are separated is a small to moderate elliptical area just behind the distal edge of the smear (see Fig. 2–8). In smears of very anemic blood, the monolayer area extends farther back even to where the drop of blood was initially applied (see Fig. 2–8). In hemoconcentrated blood (e.g., dehydration), the monolayer area is thin or absent. The gross staining intensity of the smear judged against a white background can give an initial impression of erythrocytic

density. Very anemic blood smears grossly appear pale, whereas blood smears from patients with a normal PCV appear red-orange.

Erythrocyte Morphology ● Many RBC morphologic changes are described with both Latin and English names. Some shape changes are diagnostically useful, such as polychromasia (i.e., reticulocytes), microcytic-hypochromic cells, spherocytes, autoagglutination, rouleaux, Heinz bodies, blood parasites, and acanthocytes (Fig. 2–9). Other RBC morphologic changes that may be found but that are of less clinical significance include anisocytosis, poikilocytosis, echinocytes, elliptocytes, codocytes, and leptocytes (see Chapter 3 for the significance of each).

Note that abnormal RBCs may be found in low numbers in normal blood smears. The frequency of the morphologic change in the RBC population must be known for interpretation of its significance. Polychromasia of Wright's (i.e., Romanowsky-type)–stained blood indicates increased numbers of larger than normal, bluish RBCs (i.e., polychromatophils). Polychromatophils represent canine reticulocytes and feline aggregate reticulocytes that are seen on new methylene blue (NMB)–stained smears. Polychromasia indicates increased bone marrow release of erythroid cells. On NMB-stained smears, reticulocytes have dark granular precipitates in a linear pattern (see Chapter 3). Relative guidelines to quantitate reticulocytes and polychromatophils are as follows: in dogs, normal ≤1%, slight increase 1% to 4%, moderate increase 5% to 20%, and marked increase 21% to 50%; and for cats, normal ≤0.4%, slight increase 0.5% to 2%, moderate increase 3% to 4%, and marked increase 5% (Perman and Schall, 1983). The amount of polychromasia should be recorded. The lack of polychromasia in nonregenerative anemia indicates no evidence of active bone marrow erythropoiesis. If polychromasia or lack thereof is not reported, one will later wonder whether polychromasia was absent or simply not evaluated. Thus, lack of polychromasia should be reported in anemic dogs and cats.

Blood smear analysis is an important test in regenerative anemias (i.e., increased polychro-

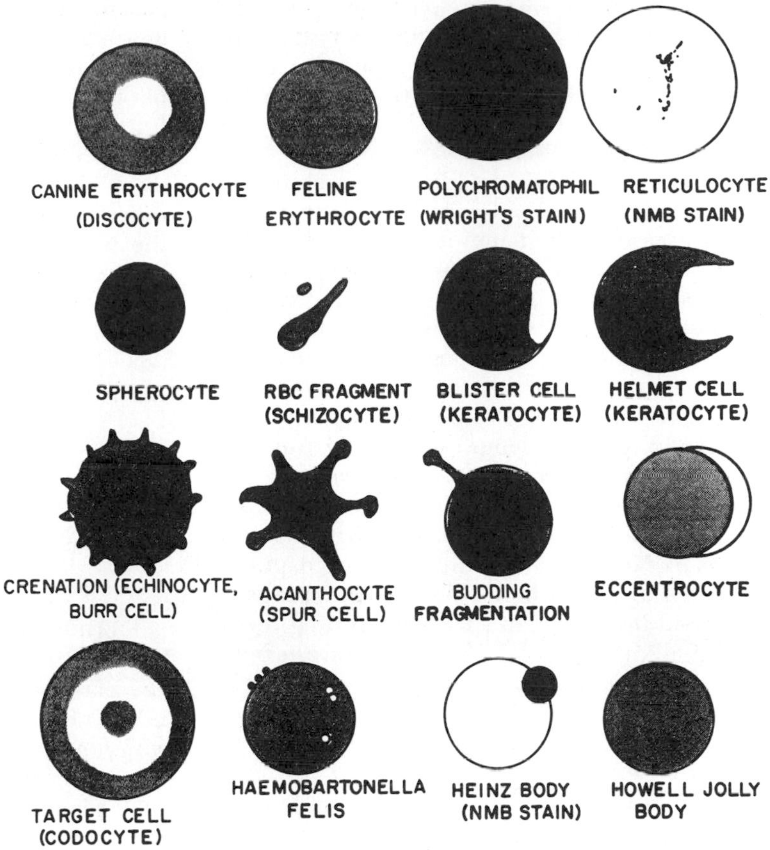

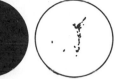
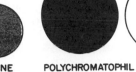

| CANINE ERYTHROCYTE (DISCOCYTE) | FELINE ERYTHROCYTE | POLYCHROMATOPHIL (WRIGHT'S STAIN) | RETICULOCYTE (NMB STAIN) |

SPHEROCYTE   RBC FRAGMENT (SCHIZOCYTE)   BLISTER CELL (KERATOCYTE)   HELMET CELL (KERATOCYTE)

CRENATION (ECHINOCYTE, BURR CELL)   ACANTHOCYTE (SPUR CELL)   BUDDING FRAGMENTATION   ECCENTROCYTE

TARGET CELL (CODOCYTE)   HAEMOBARTONELLA FELIS   HEINZ BODY (NMB STAIN)   HOWELL JOLLY BODY

Figure 2–9 Selected erythrocyte terminology. Some common terms and synonyms are given beneath a drawing of selected morphologic alterations of red blood cells. These are illustrated as they appear on Wright's-stained blood smears except for reticulocytes and Heinz bodies, which are preferentially stained by new methylene blue stain. Two normal erythrocytes are shown first for comparison. (See text for descriptions and diagnostic significance.)

masia), since several morphologic changes in RBCs are specific for certain problems (see Chapter 3). For example, immune-mediated hemolytic anemia is indicated by moderate to abundant spherocytes or the less common autoagglutination. To identify spherocytes in canine blood smears, examine the monolayer area where normal RBCs lie flat and exhibit normal central pallor (see Fig. 2–9). By comparison, the spherocytes are distinctly smaller, are darker, and lack central pallor (Color Plate 1C). Caution is advised, since in thick areas of blood smears, normal canine RBCs lack central pallor and mimic spherocytes. Some blood smears may lack a thin area where the RBCs have optimal morphologic detail and central pallor. Feline RBCs normally lack central pallor, so evaluation for spherocytes is quite difficult.

Autoagglutination is the aggregation of RBCs into grapelike clusters. Autoagglutination may also be noted grossly in the test tube, in which clumps of RBCs flow like sand on the beach. Rouleaux formation is the linking of RBCs into chains resembling stacks of coins. Rouleaux are normal in dogs and more so in cats. An increased prominence of rouleaux in the thin monolayer area of canine blood smears denotes inflammation or other changes in plasma proteins such as gammopathies in lymphoid neoplasms.

Other diagnostic RBC observations in regenerative anemias are blood parasites or Heinz bodies. Hypochromic cells and marked poikilocytosis are noted in iron deficiency anemia (see Chapter 3). Anisocytosis (variable RBC size) alone is not diagnostic, but anisocytosis may be prominent if the blood has many large polychromatophils and small spherocytes mixed with normal RBCs.

Poikilocytosis (variable RBC shapes), if prominent, can reflect systemic illness but is usually nonspecific or represents artifacts of technique. Echinocytes (e.g., crenation), which are often artifacts of slide preparation, can be reduced by more rapid drying of the smear to obtain truer morphologic detail. Echinocytes probably are more numerous in some metabolic diseases. Some abnormal RBCs have irregular spiny shapes that are difficult to distinguish from artifactitious crenation. Echinocytes have numerous, uniform, usually pointed or occasionally rounded projections from the RBC surface.

These projections, when viewed from above the cell, resemble dots and tiny letter *o*'s that mimic *Haemobartonella*. Canine distemper inclusion bodies are rarely seen in RBCs and WBCs (Color Plates 1D and 1E) but are diagnostic for the infection when seen.

Acanthocytes and budding fragmentation suggest abnormal lipid metabolism (e.g., hepatic disease or hemangiosarcoma). Acanthocytes have a few irregular projections with rounded ends often forming a bud. Budding fragmentation has one thin-based projection with a small bud at the surface. Some RBCs resemble a combination of acanthocytes and echinocytes in having sharp-pointed projections that are irregular in length and few in number, which have been termed *echinoacanthocytes*.

RBC fragmentation may be due to metabolic disorders or intravascular trauma. Vascular disorders like disseminated intravascular coagulopathy or a focal thrombus have fibrin strands in the blood flow that can split RBCs hitting them. The small, irregular RBC fragments are termed *schizocytes, keratocytes,* or *helmet cells* (see Fig. 2–9).

Leptocytes are flexible RBCs with seemingly excessive membrane. When they lie flat on the slide, an enlarged area of central pallor is seen. This wider area of central pallor of leptocytes is differentiated from the hypochromasia of iron deficiency by the thickness and color of the rim of Hgb and by RBC indices. Leptocytes have a dark rim of Hgb, whereas iron-deficient cells have a thin, faint rim of Hgb (Color Plate 1A). A common form of leptocyte is the codocyte (target cell), which has a small circle of Hgb in the middle of the area of central pallor (see Fig. 2–9). Leptocytes and codocytes are nonspecific findings occurring in hepatic disease, anemias, and other disorders.

Dacryocytes are teardrop-shaped RBCs. Many other RBC shapes have descriptive names, like *elliptocyte* (oval RBC or ovalocyte). If RBCs have abnormal shapes that do not easily fit the common classifications, then simply report the presence of poikilocytosis and quantitate it from 0 to 4 +. Poikilocytosis need not be diagnostically pursued if more specific indicators of various diseases are present (e.g., increased alanine aminotransferase, serum alkaline phosphatase, or bile acids indicating hepatic disease).

OTHER DETERMINATIONS

Plasma Protein Determination

Plasma protein (i.e., plasma total solids, serum protein) can be determined from the plasma in the top of a centrifuged microhematocrit tube. The tube is scored with a file just above the buffy coat and broken, and the plasma is placed into a refractometer. Most refractometers have an internal scale for plasma total protein and a scale for urine specific gravity. If the scale is graduated for only refractive index, a conversion chart is necessary to convert the index to the protein concentration. Since both the plasma protein and PCV are affected by the hydration status, it is helpful to determine both the plasma protein and PCV to evaluate anemia, polycythemia, or protein disorders.

Fibrinogen and Acute Phase Proteins

Fibrinogen elevations during inflammatory disease can be estimated by a modification of the plasma protein and microhematocrit methods. The plasma fibrinogen is estimated by the difference in the plasma protein concentration readings between two microhematocrit tubes. One reading is a plasma protein concentration from a routinely prepared microhematocrit tube. The second reading is the "plasma" protein concentration on the altered plasma from a microhematocrit tube that was heated at 56° to 58°C for 3 minutes. Fibrinogen is precipitated by heating and then removed by centrifugation. The difference in refractometer readings is the lost fibrinogen. Fibrinogen estimation is most often used in cattle and horses but can be used to identify inflammation in dogs and cats.

A diagnostically useful pattern of changes during acute inflammation includes increased fibrinogen and other acute phase proteins like C-reactive protein (CRP). Prominent increases in serum CRP are used in people to monitor inflammatory disease. Serum CRP also increases in dogs during inflammation. Increased rouleaux on blood smears are caused by the protein changes and may suggest inflammation. Rouleaux cause RBCs to sediment more rapidly. RBC sedimentation may be measured by the erythrocyte sedimentation rate (ESR) to monitor inflammation or occasionally be noted in tubes of EDTA blood. The zetacrit and zeta sedimentation ratio (ZSR) are rapid tests proposed to replace the slow, cumbersome ESR for screening dogs in high volume settings such as laboratory animal care centers at research centers (Martin et al., 1985).

Table 2–6 BASIC BONE MARROW CONCLUSIONS

Bone Marrow Conclusion	Definition
Erythroid hyperplasia	Increased proliferation of erythroid cells (RBC precursors)
Erythroid hypoplasia	Decreased erythroid cell proliferation
Myeloid hyperplasia	Increased myeloid cell proliferation (neutrophils, eosinophils, monocytes, and basophils)
Myeloid hypoplasia	Decreased myeloid cell proliferation
Megakaryocytic hyperplasia	Increased megakaryocyte proliferation
Megakaryocytic hypoplasia	Decreased megakaryocyte proliferation
Aplastic pancytopenia	Absence of erythroid, myeloid, and megakaryocytic cells
Lymphoid hyperplasia	Increased proliferation of lymphocytes and plasma cells

Lipemia, Hemolysis, and Icterus

Lipemia, hemolysis, and icterus are grossly noted in the plasma of the microhematocrit tube. Persistent lipemia not associated with eating suggests certain diseases and causes some artifacts in the hematologic results. Lipemia occurs with recent ingestion of a fatty meal, pancreatitis, diabetic ketoacidosis, hypothyroidism, hepatic disease, and primary lipid disorders as seen in schnauzers (see Chapter 8). The refractometer reading of lipemic plasma for plasma protein will be erroneous owing to the turbidity, which causes an altered refractive index. RBCs are more fragile in lipemic plasma and tend to lyse *in vitro*, so hemolysis often accompanies lipemia. The Hgb concentration is also invalid because of the increased optical density of turbid, lipemic plasma. RBCs appear fuzzy on blood smears, and the background appears blue and foamy.

Hemolysis is more commonly an artifact of collection and handling than an indicator of intravascular hemolysis. Anemias so acute and massive as to have hemolyzed plasma *in vivo* are rare and should be associated with hemoglobinuria. Artifactitious hemolysis should decrease the PCV and MCV and increase the MCHC. Hyperchromasia (i.e., increased MCHC) does not occur normally unless free hemoglobin due to hemolysis is present.

Icterus suggests either a hemolytic anemia or a hepatic problem (see Chapter 9). Some laboratories perform an icterus index on plasma to roughly quantitate the icterus.

Color of Blood

Abnormal color of blood can be seen grossly or by putting a drop on white filter paper. Brown blood suggests methemoglobinemia. In cyanide poisoning blood may be cherry-red, and in carbon monoxide poisoning blood should be bright red.

BONE MARROW EXAMINATION

Conclusions from Bone Marrow Examination

The bone marrow is examined to answer certain questions, usually originating from evaluation of the CBC. Persistent or unexplained decreases in blood cells in blood are appropriately evaluated by a bone marrow aspirate and biopsy. A brief summary of general bone marrow conclusions is in Table 2–6. For more specific details on diagnostic approaches in certain disorders of RBCs, WBCs, and platelets, see Chapters 3, 4, and 5.

The conclusions obtained from a bone marrow aspirate and biopsy are quantitative and qualitative. The quantity of various cell types is determined. In thrombocytopenic animals, the bone marrow examination should indicate whether the number of megakaryocytes is normal, increased, or decreased. This usually answers the question of whether bone marrow production is the cause of the thrombocytopenia. Similar answers should be provided by a bone marrow examination to evaluate other cytopenias identified with the CBC.

The quantitative conclusions include megakaryocytic hyperplasia or hypoplasia, erythroid hyperplasia or hypoplasia, myeloid hyperplasia or hypoplasia, and lymphoid hyperplasia. An adjective to indicate the magnitude of the change (i.e., mild to marked) should accompany the conclusion. The cell production of bone marrow can be properly evaluated only with access to a current CBC.

Hyperplasia/Neoplasia • An increased proliferation of one or more cell types in the bone marrow may be a normal response to anemia, leukopenia, or thrombocytopenia or may be an abnormal neoplastic or dysplastic process. In hemolytic or blood loss anemias, the bone marrow should develop erythroid hyperplasia with adequate time. Consumption of WBCs during inflammatory disease should produce myeloid hyperplasia. Consumption of platelets by immune-mediated thrombocytopenia or disseminated intravascular coagulopathy should provoke a megakaryocytic hyperplasia. A systemic immune response may include lymphocytic-plasmacytic hyperplasia. Excessive immaturity of the proliferating cells (e.g., excessive blast cells), excessive numbers of cells, or morphologic abnormality of the cells in the marrow allows the diagnosis of leukemia or dysplasia (i.e., abnormal development) (see Chapter 4).

Hypoplasia/Aplasia • The marrow may have decreased numbers of (hypoplasia) or totally lack (aplasia) one or more cell types. Repeated sampling may be needed to differentiate hypoplasia from temporary depletion due to increased release and use in the body (e.g., decreased marrow neutrophils in peracute inflammation). Hypoplasia or aplasia indicates that a cytopenia is due to insufficient marrow production of that cell type. Specific causes of marrow hypoplasia and aplasia are described in the appropriate chapters.

Ineffective Hematopoiesis • In certain situations (see Chapters 3 and 4), the marrow may have normal to increased numbers of the precursor cells for the cytopenic cell type. This pattern, if consistent over time, suggests that the proliferation is not effective; the produced cells are not released into the peripheral blood, or they may be dying in the marrow before release.

Abnormal Morphology • Morphologic abnormalities that identify a qualitative defect are usually subtle except for overt anaplastic changes in leukemias. Several abnormalities may be noted, like multinucleation or abnormal nuclear:cytoplasmic (N:C) ratios. For example, feline leukemia virus infection may induce dysplastic erythroid precursors including megaloblastic rubricytes that have excessive amounts of cytoplasm (see discussion of B_{12}/folate deficiency in Chapter 3). The opposite N:C ratio occurs in iron deficiency, in which the late rubricytes and metarubricytes may have slower Hgb production compared with nuclear maturation (see Chapter 3).

Disorderly maturation of a cell line in the marrow is noted if each successively more mature stage does not exceed the abundance of the previous stage. The mature cells of each cell line should predominate. The predominance of very immature hematopoietic precursors usually suggests leukemia (see Chapter 4). One exception is a rare form of immune-mediated hemolytic anemia that destroys not only mature RBCs but also earlier stages. The immune removal of the older cells presents the appearance of a maturation arrest at one stage of development. The lack of polychromasia and reticulocytes gives the unusual pattern of a nonregenerative Coombs'-positive hemolytic anemia.

Myelofibrosis/Necrosis • Myelofibrosis is bone marrow replacement by fibrous connective tissue. This is analogous to chronic interstitial nephritis, in which the kidneys are already scarred when the clinical signs are noted but the original injury to the kidneys is not known. Myelofibrosis is an end-stage marrow. Bone marrow aspirates from a fibrotic marrow are often acellular and not diagnostic, so a biopsy for histopathologic evaluation is required for diagnosis.

Necrosis or degeneration of the marrow may be caused by various chemicals (e.g., chemotherapeutic drugs or estrogen) and by infectious agents (e.g., panleukopenia virus). It is less frequently diagnosed than necrosis of other tissues, perhaps because the marrow is "hidden" in bone. Marrow necrosis is most often diagnosed in acute toxicity studies on new drugs or chemicals at pharmaceutical or chemical companies by toxicologic pathologists. Necrosis of marrow tissue may be followed by scarring (i.e., myelofibrosis).

Fatty Marrow • Fat is the tissue occupying the space in the marrow devoid of hematopoietic cells. A fatty marrow (i.e., white marrow) in an area of bone that should contain hematopoietic cells (i.e., red marrow) suggests a hypoplasia or complete aplasia of all cell types. Like myelofibrosis, it is another form of an end-stage bone marrow, except that the marrow is replaced by fat rather than scar tissue.

BONE MARROW BIOPSY AND ASPIRATE

The collection techniques are well described and photographically illustrated elsewhere (Lewis and Rebar, 1979). For best evaluation, a current CBC, a bone marrow aspirate, and a

Table 2–7 DIFFERENT INFORMATION PROVIDED BY THREE TESTS USED IN BONE MARROW EXAMINATION

Test	Information Provided
CBC	Relatively quantitative information on all three cell types in peripheral blood
	Excellent morphology of peripheral blood cells
Bone marrow aspirate	Excellent morphology of individual marrow cells
	Best determination of ratios of cell types (e.g., M:E ratio)
Bone marrow biopsy	Best quantitation of cell numbers and iron stores in a defined volume of marrow
	Architectural patterns
	Identification of cells that do not exfoliate (e.g., myelofibrosis)

bone marrow biopsy all are needed. The separate types of evidence from the three procedures are summarized in Table 2–7.

Evaluation of Bone Marrow Aspiration Smears

A consistent pattern for describing the quantity and qualitative aspects of the cells present should be followed to make bone marrow smear examination relatively simple and consistent. With a systematic routine, the time and effort required become as minimal as for blood smear analysis.

Cell Quantitation • Initially determine if the smears have an adequate number of hematopoietic cells to represent the bone marrow and then if the cellularity of the smears indicates an increased, normal, or decreased number of developing hematopoietic cells in the marrow. Aspirates from a normally cellular marrow should have many more individual nucleated cells than

Table 2–8 EXPECTED PERCENTAGE OF DIFFERENT CELL TYPES IN CANINE AND FELINE BONE MARROW

Cell Type	Dogs	Cats
Rubriblasts	0.2	0.2
Prorubricytes	3.9	1.0
Rubricytes	27	21.6*
Metarubricytes	15.3	5.6
Total erythroid	46.4	28.7
Myeloblasts	0.0	0.8
Progranulocytes	1.3	1.7
Myelocytes†	9.0	5.0
Metamyelocytes†	9.9	10.6
Bands†	14.5	14.9
Granulocytes (mainly segs)	18.7	13.5
Total myeloid	53.4	45.9
M:E ratio	1.15:1.0	1.6:1.0

*Rubricytes include basophilic and polychromic forms.

†Neutrophilic and eosinophilic forms are combined for myelocytes, metamyelocytes, and band forms.

(Information modified from Jain NC: Schalm's Veterinary Hematology. 4th ed. Philadelphia, Lea and Febiger, 1986.)

are usually seen in blood and include immature forms. Hemodilution of a poorly cellular aspiration sample may be misleading (e.g., increased M:E ratio) because peripheral blood includes WBCs. Aspirates often contain intact tissue fragments of marrow sucked free with the fluid. These marrow particles have some of the value of histologic samples, since they retain some architectural arrangement of the hematopoietic cells and fat cells in a defined space. This is excellent for estimating the cell density in the marrow. For example, if only fragments of fat are present and one is certain the marrow cavity was sampled, then bone marrow aplasia (i.e., fatty marrow) with low hematopoietic cell numbers is suggested. A fatty marrow or myelofibrosis would be more confidently diagnosed with histopathologic evaluation of a bone marrow biopsy specimen.

Include an estimate of the number of megakaryocytes. These are large enough to see while scanning the smear and are often in the marrow particles. At least a few should be seen, but the number expected will vary with the cellularity of the sample.

Myeloid:Erythroid Ratio • The M:E ratio is akin to the differential WBC count for the CBC. Both the relative percentage of each cell type and the total number of cells in the bone marrow are needed to determine whether an absolute increase or decrease is present. The number of cells necessary for an accurate M:E is 500 to 1000 nucleated cells in a bone marrow aspirate. In practice, usually only 100 to 200 intact, well-stained cells are counted to calculate the M:E ratio and percentage of lymphoid cells. For clinical use, one need not determine the percentage of every cell type listed in Table 2–8. Group the cells into three categories (myeloid, erythroid, and lymphoid cell lines). This avoids the long and difficult task of differentiating each cell type (e.g., rubriblasts from prorubricytes, or metamyelocytes from bands). Erythroid cells have coarse nuclear chromatin and dark blue converting to orange-colored cytoplasm. Myeloid cells have nuclei with fine chromatin and gray cytoplasm with various granules and the polymorphonuclear-shaped nuclei in mature cells. Lymphocytes are similar to those in blood. Plasma cells have dark blue cytoplasm with eccentric placement of the nucleus. Include plasma cells with the lymphocyte percentage (usually about 4–5%). Divide the percentage of myeloid cells by the percentage of erythroid cells for the M:E ratio.

Qualitative Observations • Morphologic changes are variable, and many are best discussed with certain problems. Always determine whether the three cell lines have an orderly maturation as expected (see Table 2–8). Hemosiderin in macrophages appears as blue-green granules. The presence and amount of hemosiderin should be indicated, since its absence can suggest iron deficiency anemia. Anemia of chronic inflammation has excessive hemosiderin. Infectious agents such as *Histoplasma* are rarely found. Inflammatory processes like purulent osteomyelitis (e.g., abscess) occur. Neoplastic processes besides leukemias may invade the marrow (see Chapter 16).

Summary of Bone Marrow Smear Evaluation Procedure
1. Quantitate cellularity of the smear(s).
   a. Total nucleated cells
   b. Density of nucleated cells in marrow particles
   c. Number of megakaryocytes
2. Determine a three-cell differential count (myeloid, erythroid, and lymphoid).
3. Calculate M:E ratio.
4. Verify that maturation of each cell line is orderly and complete.
5. Estimate iron (i.e., hemosiderin) stores.
6. Identify morphologic abnormalities like neoplasia, dysplasia, infections, and inflammation.
7. Summarize information into conclusion(s).

Bibliography

Brown SA, Barsanti JA: Quantitative buffy coat analysis for hematologic measurements of canine, feline, and equine blood samples and for detection of microfilaremia in dogs. Am J Vet Res 1988;49:321–324.
Hart AH: Quantitative buffy coat analysis. Proceedings, 22nd Annual Meeting, American Society for Veterinary Clinical Pathology, Monterey, CA, November 9, 1987.
Jain NC: Schalm's Veterinary Hematology. 4th ed. Philadelphia, Lea and Febiger, 1986.
Levine RA, Hart AH, Wardlaw SC: Quantitative buffy coat analysis of blood collected from dogs, cats, and horses. JAVMA 1986;189:670–673.
Lewis HB, Rebar AH: Bone Marrow Evaluation in the Veterinary Practice. St Louis, Ralston Purina, 1979.
Martin DG, Hall JE, Patrick DH: Evaluation of the zetacrit and zeta sedimentation ratio in dogs. Am J Vet Res 1985;46:1326–1329.
Nelson DA, Morris MW: Basic methodology. In Henry JB (ed): Clinical Diagnosis and Management by Laboratory Methods. 17th ed. Philadelphia, WB Saunders, 1984, pp 578–602.
Perman V, Schall WD: Diseases of the red blood cells. In Ettinger SJ (ed): Textbook of Veterinary Internal Medicine: Diseases of the Dog and Cat. 2nd ed, vol II. Philadelphia, WB Saunders, 1983, pp 1948–1952.
Tvedten H, Grabski S, Frame L: Estimating platelets and WBC's on canine blood smears. Vet Clin Pathol 1988;17:4–6.

Harold Tvedten

3 Erythrocyte Disorders

ANEMIA

Anemia is the most common erythrocyte (red blood cell [RBC]) disorder. Anemia can cause various clinical signs (e.g., weakness, lethargy, heart murmur, pica) or may be subclinical and detected only as part of a general diagnostic workup. A brief summary of a diagnostic ap-

proach follows and is outlined in Figure 3–1. A detailed description follows in later sections. The approach simply considers the vascular system as a container with input from the bone marrow. If the marrow can produce RBCs at an expected rate for the severity of the anemia, then the cause of the anemia is not a bone marrow disorder. The two basic causes of ane-

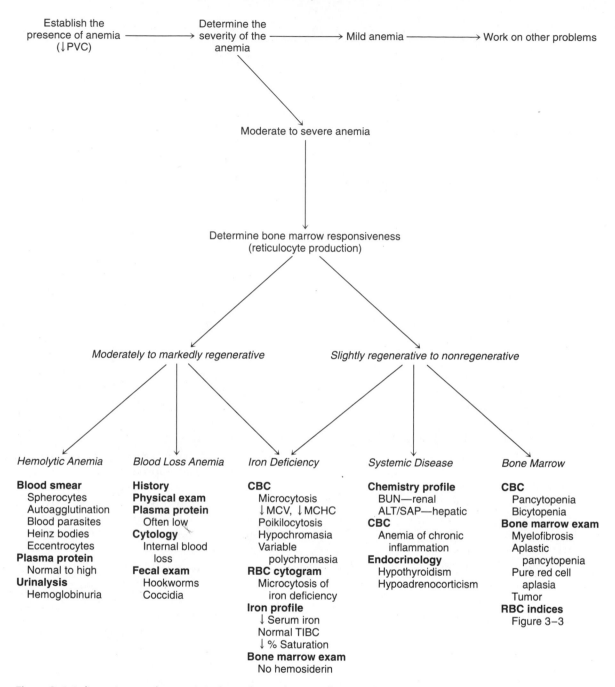

Figure 3–1 A *diagnostic approach to anemia in dogs and cats* relies initially on grading the severity of the anemia and quantitating the regenerative response of the bone marrow to the anemia. After classifying the regenerative response, the basic processes responsible for the anemia are listed and *italicized*. Under each of these categories, the laboratory tests to obtain positive evidence for that anemia are listed in **bold,** and beneath each test are the possible results. (See text for details.)

mia, other than reduced bone marrow production, are loss from the body (i.e., blood loss or external hemorrhage) and destruction in the body (i.e., hemolysis or internal hemorrhage). The spleen complicates this simplistic approach, since contraction causes rapid changes in distri-

bution by releasing a concentrated bolus of stored RBCs; or, to a lesser extent, the spleen can relax to store RBCs, removing them from circulation. It is like a contractile sponge connected to the RBC container. Another consideration is that many poorly regenerative anemias are caused by a combination of effects, such as decreased effective RBC production and a variably shortened RBC life span.

The initial effort should be to document the presence of anemia by the packed cell volume (PCV; see Chapter 2). The hemoglobin concentration and RBC count may be used similarly to document the decrease in the circulating RBC mass, but for simplicity, only the PCV is used in the following discussions. An animal's hydration status must be normal before the PCV properly reflects the degree of anemia.

Hydration status is usually evaluated by considering the plasma protein (PP) concentration and PCV in combination. The PP is a clinically useful, albeit crude, indicator of hydration in the absence of other factors affecting PP, such as protein loss in hemorrhage, intestinal disease, or glomerular disease. PP determination is not a very sensitive test of dehydration but is easily performed and commonly available. Severe dehydration is expected to increase the PP until the animal is rehydrated. When the animal is properly rehydrated, the PCV should reflect the presence and severity of the anemia.

The severity of an anemia must be considered during interpretation of CBC results. Mild anemias are often secondary to other problems and considered only after the problems are addressed, because these anemias (e.g., anemia of chronic inflammation, renal, hepatic, or endocrine) resolve with correction of the primary problem(3). The moderate to severe anemias require diagnostic and therapeutic attention. In dogs, the severity of the anemia is arbitrarily indicated by the following PCV ranges: mild, 30% to 37%; moderate, 20% to 29%; severe, 13% to 19%; and very severe, <13%. In cats, arbitrary classifications are mild, 20% to 26%; moderate, 14% to 19%; severe, 10% to 13%; and very severe, <10%.

Transfusions are usually necessary when the PCV is <11% in cats and <13% in dogs (Jain, 1986), if no contraindications are present. Transfusion reactions become more likely after the first transfusion, so it is best to use blood transfusions only when the anemia is severe. If a factor (e.g., immune-mediated hemolysis) is likely to lyse the transfused cells rapidly, then the transfusion may worsen the situation by stimulating disseminated intravascular coagulation (DIC), immune response to foreign antigen, or an anaphylactic response, or simply by adding the burden of removing RBC debris. Blood should be crossmatched to find blood donors less likely to cause transfusion reactions.

After documenting the presence of anemia and grading its severity, determine the bone marrow's erythroid production by the reticulocyte response (discussed next). Moderately to markedly regenerative anemias should be due to blood loss or hemolysis (see Fig. 3–1) and not poor marrow production. A slight or absent reticulocyte response by 3 to 5 days after onset of the anemia in a moderate to severe anemia indicates inadequate marrow production (i.e., nonregenerative anemias). Iron deficiency anemia is marked by variable bone marrow regeneration. In adults, it is usually caused by chronic external blood loss, which is initially a regenerative anemia but with time and increasing severity of iron depletion becomes nonregenerative. Each of the various types of anemia can be investigated by certain tests (see Fig. 3–1) that provide evidence for concluding that that type is present. Most evidence is initially from the complete blood count (CBC).

Reticulocyte Evaluation

Reticulocyte quantitation is the easiest and most consistent way to evaluate bone marrow erythropoiesis in dogs and cats and usually obviates bone marrow biopsy and aspiration. Reticulocytes are immature RBC precursors. Their life span in canine blood is usually about 1 day before they mature into RBCs, so reticulocyte numbers in peripheral blood reflect recent bone marrow release of erythroid cells. A CBC should routinely include reticulocyte data when the PCV is <30% in dogs and 20% in cats. Different measurements include absolute reticulocyte numbers per microliter, reticulocyte index (RI), reticulocyte percentage, corrected reticulocyte percentage, and estimated polychromasia on blood smears. The techniques, advantages, and disadvantages are described in the following sections. Any may be used effectively if potential errors are known. The expected time course of reticulocyte responses in dogs and cats is discussed with external blood loss.

Reticulocyte Techniques • An equal amount of blood is incubated with 0.5% new methylene blue for 15 to 20 minutes. An air-dried smear of the mixture is prepared, and 1000 RBCs and reticulocytes are counted to calculate what percentage of the nonnucleated erythroid cells are reticulocytes. The reticulocytes are nonnucleated RBCs in which the stain has precipitated out a dye-RNA-protein complex. Nucleated RBCs like metarubricytes and rubricytes are not reticulocytes and should not be included in the

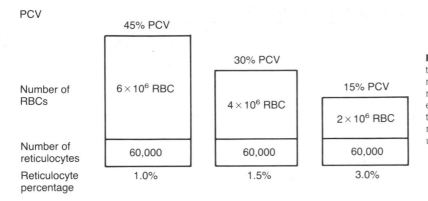

Figure 3–2 Increasing the severity of the anemia and thus decreasing the number of mature RBCs increases the relative percentage of reticulocytes even when the absolute number of reticulocytes per volume of blood remains constant. (PCV, packed cell volume.)

reticulocyte count. Mature RBCs lack RNA and a reticulum. The absolute number of reticulocytes per microliter is determined by multiplying the reticulocyte percentage by the RBC count.

The reticulocytes may be reported as simply a percentage, but this can be misleading since it is a ratio of reticulocytes to mature cells. In anemia, the mature cells are variably reduced, thus exaggerating the reticulocyte percentage (Fig. 3–2). Some guidelines from Perman and Schall (1983) assess the degree of activity of the bone marrow based on the percentage of reticulocytes (Table 3–1). This was modified in our laboratory to provide absolute reticulocyte number guidelines to judge the magnitude of bone marrow regeneration (Table 3–2). The absolute reticulocyte count is a more consistent indicator of bone marrow production of RBCs despite various degrees of anemic severity.

Reticulocyte Index • Without the RBC count, one cannot calculate the absolute reticulocyte count, and determining the RBC count requires a tedious, somewhat inaccurate manual count or having access to an automated cell counter. Since the microhematocrit test is simple, easy, and more universally available than is the RBC

count, the RI is suggested as an alternative reticulocyte production indicator; the RI is a consistent indicator of bone marrow production of RBCs, since it is adjusted for the degree of anemia (Table 3–3). The RI may also be adjusted for the likely life span in days of the canine reticulocyte in peripheral blood, which can artifactually exaggerate the reticulocyte percentage. The RI is also called the *reticulocyte production index* (Jain, 1986). Note that the corrected reticulocyte percentage is considered by many to be sufficient for interpretation without the life span adjustment to the RI.

In dogs, an RI ≥3 is a marked regenerative response that suggests a hemolytic anemia more than an external blood loss of some duration. Hemolytic anemias tend to be more regenerative than are external blood loss anemias, since the various nutrients for erythropoiesis remain in the body. Very recent blood loss (e.g., 4–5 days ago, which is the time of peak response) or internal blood loss may also be markedly regenerative. An RI >1 indicates a regenerative anemia, so the RI of 1 in Table 3–3 denotes inadequate regeneration despite an initial reticulocyte percentage of 4%.

Feline Reticulocytes • Feline reticulocytes differ from canine reticulocytes in that all do not rap-

Table 3–1 DEGREE OF ERYTHROID REGENERATION IN ANEMIA

Degree of Stimulation	Percentage of Reticulocytes	
	Dogs	Cats
Normal	1	0–0.4
Sight	1–4	0.5–2
Moderate	5–20	3–4
Marked	21–50	5+

(From Perman V, Schall WB: Diseases of the red blood cells. In Ettinger SJ (ed): Textbook of Veterinary Internal Medicine: Diseases of the Dog and Cat. 2nd ed, vol 2. Philadelphia, WB Saunders, 1983.)

Table 3–2 RETICULOCYTE GUIDELINES*

Degree of Regeneration	Canine Reticulocytes/μl	Feline Aggregate Reticulocytes (II, III)/μl	Feline Punctate Reticulocytes/μl
None	60,000	<15,000	<200,000
Slight	150,000	50,000	500,000
Moderate	300,000	100,000	1,000,000
Marked	>500,000	>200,000	1,500,000

*Used at Michigan State University as modified by Dr. D. J. Weiss.

Table 3–3 STEPS IN CALCULATION OF THE RETICULOCYTE INDEX

Step 1 Corrected reticulocyte percentage (CRP)

$$CRP = \text{reticulocyte } \% \times \frac{\text{patient's hematocrit}}{\text{normal hematocrit}}$$

Example Dog with PCV of 22.5% and 4% reticulocytes

$$CRP = 4\% \times \frac{22.5\%}{45\%} = 2\%$$

Step 2 Dogs are similar to people in releasing reticulocytes from their bone marrow earlier than normal when they are anemic. These "shift" reticulocytes live longer than the usual 1 day, as seen below. This exaggerates the reticulocyte percentage, so the CRP is further adjusted by dividing it by the expected maturation time in days, which varies with the severity of the anemia:

$$RI = \frac{CRP}{\text{life span of reticulocytes}}$$

Hematocrit	Expected Reticulocyte Life Span (days)
45	1.0
35	1.5
25	2.0
15	2.5

The reticulocytes in the example should live about 2 days when the PCV = 22.5%; thus, remaining in circulation twice as long will double the percentage of reticulocytes without the bone marrow production of reticulocytes being doubled. The reticulocyte index (RI) is adjusted for this to more truly reflect marrow release by dividing by 2.

$$RI = \frac{2\%}{2 \text{ days}} = 1$$

idly mature in 1 day to mature RBCs and a total reticulocyte count may not reflect recent marrow release. The slowly maturing reticulocytes should be subdivided into punctate and aggregate (Cramer and Lewis, 1972) to reflect significant differences in stages of maturation and life span in blood (Fig. 3–3). Punctate reticulocytes are more mature reticulocytes with relatively long life spans in blood. Aggregate reticulocytes mature into punctate reticulocytes. Normally there are 1.4% to 10.8% punctate reticulocytes but only 0.4% to 0.9% aggregate reticulocytes.

RETICULOCYTES

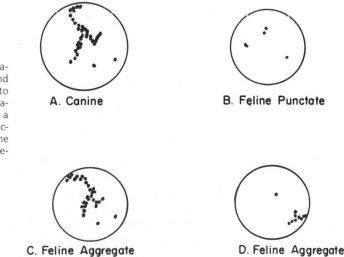

Figure 3–3 Reticulocytes in the dog and cat. The canine reticulocyte (**A**) is typical in appearance and therefore interpretation. The feline reticulocytes (**B** to **D**) vary in appearance and in subsequent interpretation. The feline punctate reticulocyte (**B**) has only a few "dots" of reticulum, no linear aggregates of reticulum, and a relatively long life span in blood. The aggregate reticulocytes (**C** and **D**) have linear aggregates and a short life span in blood.

A. Canine

B. Feline Punctate

C. Feline Aggregate

D. Feline Aggregate

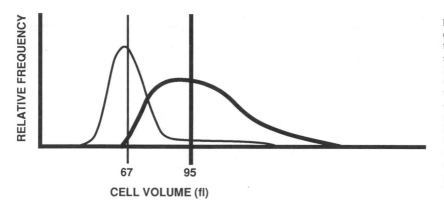

Figure 3–4 Erythrocyte volume distribution histogram of a miniature schnauzer-beagle dog with stomatocytosis and macrocytosis. Normal canine red blood cells (RBCs) with a mean corpuscular volume of 67 fl are indicated by the curve to the left. The abnormal macrocytic RBCs are represented by the curve to the right. There was no increase in reticulocytes. (Courtesy of Brown et al: Erythrocyte indices and volume distribution in a dog with stomatocytosis. Vet Pathol 1994; 31:247–250, 1994.)

The type of reticulocyte must be indicated because there can be great variation between an aggregate reticulocyte value and a total (aggregate + punctate) value, which can greatly alter the interpretation.

In persistent hemorrhage or a hemolytic process with a large and prolonged RBC turnover, the combined punctate and aggregate reticulocyte count may approach 100%. This makes the technical performance of the reticulocyte differential count tedious. Flow cytometric analysis of feline blood in which the RNA of reticulocytes was stained with fluorochrome thiazole orange was an accurate automated method to determine the aggregate reticulocyte count, but the punctate reticulocytes failed to stain positively for RNA (Regan et al., 1992).

The life span of the feline reticulocyte is difficult to define, since the aggregate and punctate are a continuum; therefore, a feline RI is not interpretable. The feline corrected reticulocyte percentage (see CRP in Table 3–3) may be used to compensate for various degrees of anemia and thus more consistently reflects marrow activity. Dogs have occasional reticulocytes resembling punctate reticulocytes, but their numbers are too few to cause confusion and they need not be counted separately.

Polychromasia • Polychromasia is an increased number of polychromatophils noted on Wright's-stained canine blood smears. These larger, slightly blue RBCs are the same as reticulocytes seen on new methylene blue–stained smears. The feline aggregate reticulocyte appears as a polychromatophil, but the punctate reticulocytes do not (Alsaker et al., 1977). Thus, polychromasia on feline CBC reports reflects the aggregate reticulocyte numbers, whereas polychromasia on canine blood smears reflects total reticulocyte numbers. Polychromasia in both species denotes current or active bone marrow erythropoiesis.

Macrocytosis • The presence of larger than normal RBCs can be documented by the mean corpuscular volume (MCV), but automated instruments have more sensitive methods of demonstrating macrocytic RBCs. Reticulocytosis is a common cause of macrocytosis, but young RBCs that have lost their ribosomes may also be increased during active erythropoiesis. Macrocytosis may be a more sensitive or consistent sign of erythropoiesis. Other causes of macrocytosis are swelling of RBCs in EDTA tubes during prolonged storage, transfused blood, breed-associated macrocytosis (e.g., poodles), and feline leukemia virus (FeLV) infections in cats (see stomatocytosis, Fig. 3–4).

Nucleated RBCs; Basophilic Stippling • Other hematologic findings expected in regenerative anemias include anisocytosis, Howell-Jolly bodies, nucleated RBCs (NRBCs; metarubricytosis), and basophilic stippling. These are observed on blood smears but are neither as quantitative nor as specific an indicator of regenerative ability as are reticulocyte numbers.

Circulating NRBCs should not be the major criteria to quantitate bone marrow erythropoiesis in dogs and cats that have strong reticulocyte responses. NRBC release into blood also occurs independently of increased erythropoiesis in splenic disease, extramedullary hematopoiesis, lead poisoning, hyperadrenocorticism, leukemias, and other bone marrow diseases.

Basophilic stippling is neither a specific nor a sensitive method for diagnosing lead poisoning. Lead poisoning should be diagnosed on the basis of toxicology findings (Appendix I). Basophilic stippling occurs more commonly in regenerative anemias in dogs than it does in lead poisoning. However, observing the pattern of "basophilic stippling and circulating NRBCs in the absence of reticulocytosis" is a reasonable indication to determine the blood lead concentrations in dogs that have a history and clinical signs consistent with lead poisoning. Circulating NRBCs and basophilic stippling are abnormal findings in the absence of a regenerative anemia.

Siderocytes/Sideroblasts • Siderocytes are abnormal RBCs with basophilic granules (i.e., Pappenheimer's bodies) that may resemble basophilic stippling in Wright's-stained blood. Pappenheimer's bodies are uncommon and differ from basophilic stippling in being iron positive on Prussian blue–stained smears and usually being larger, darker, and more focal in distribution than basophilic stippling. Sideroblasts are nucleated erythroid cells in bone marrow with iron-positive granules. Abnormal sideroblasts have more numerous and larger granules. Siderocytes and abnormal sideroblasts indicate abnormal erythropoiesis (i.e., dyserythropoiesis). One reported cause is chloramphenicol therapy in a dog (Harvey et al., 1985).

Classification Based on MCV and MCHC

Morphologic classification of anemias has been based on the RBC indices. The MCV and the mean corpuscular hemoglobin concentration (MCHC) can also be used to differentiate regenerative and nonregenerative anemias, but the morphologic classification does not quantitate the marrow response as well as the reticulocyte data. On a practical basis, the three common categories to consider in dogs are macrocytic-hypochromic, normocytic-normochromic, and microcytic-hypochromic anemias.

Macrocytic-hypochromic anemias are typically regenerative anemias with increased numbers of reticulocytes that are relatively larger (i.e., increased MCV) than mature RBCs. Reticulocytes are hypochromic (i.e., decreased MCHC), since they have not finished hemoglobin synthesis and the hemoglobin present is in a larger cellular volume.

Normocytic-normochromic anemias are nonregenerative anemias with primarily mature RBCs remaining in circulation with too few reticulocytes to increase the MCV or decrease the MCHC. Anemias that are due to hemorrhage or hemolysis and that are of such recent onset (e.g., 1–2 days) as to preclude a regenerative bone marrow response are normocytic-normochromic and are termed *preregenerative*.

Microcytic-hypochromic anemias are almost always due to iron deficiency, preventing an ad-

equate production of hemoglobin. The RBCs are small (i.e., low MCV) and insufficiently hemoglobinized (i.e., low MCHC). Note that the Japanese Akita breed normally has microcytic RBCs (i.e., MCV of about 60 fl).

An infrequent morphologic classification is macrocytic-normochromic anemia. Macrocytic-normochromic RBCs occur rarely in dogs owing to a deficiency of vitamin B_{12} (e.g., malabsorption). Macrocytic anemia that was responsive to folic acid treatment has been associated with phenytoin and methotrexate (i.e., folate antagonist) use. Macrocytic RBCs (i.e., MCV >80 fl) may occur in some poodles without any anemia. Macrocytic-normochromic RBCs are most common in FeLV-related myeloproliferative disorders in cats (especially erythremic myelosis; see later section on FeLV). Macrocytosis in cats without reticulocytosis is suggestive of FeLV infection.

Regenerative Anemias

Adult animals with anemias due only to RBC destruction (i.e., hemolysis) or blood loss should have normal bone marrow able to respond in a full and strong manner to the anemia. Greater than 500,000 reticulocytes/µl often occur in dogs with hemolytic anemias, internal hemorrhage, or recent external blood loss (see Table 3–2). Many anemias, however, are neither markedly regenerative nor completely nonregenerative. Finer degrees of interpretation are needed with more subtle changes. The slight to moderate regenerative states (see Fig. 3–1) must be interpreted in terms of duration of the anemia, severity of the anemia, and potential for multiple causes. A mild anemia (e.g., canine PCV 30–35%) may not stimulate much reticulocytosis, since the mildly stimulated bone marrow would slowly respond with mainly mature RBCs; so a mild anemia from blood loss or hemolysis could be classified as nonregenerative. If one does not consider the magnitude of the anemia and mindlessly adheres to a diagnostic scheme, then mild blood loss or hemolysis may not be considered if reticulocyte response is not noted.

An intestinal neoplasm is an example of multiple etiologic factors contributing to an anemia. If the mass is bleeding, this external blood loss should initially stimulate good regeneration; but persistent bleeding may lead to iron and protein deficiency. Neoplasms are often inflamed, and anemia of chronic inflammation interferes with iron utilization for erythropoiesis. Lymphosarcoma of the intestine may also involve the bone marrow. Thus, the degree of regeneration could be quite variable and less than expected. Many anemias do not have precise onsets or short durations. Bleeding episodes may vary in intensity and frequency to give an irregular pattern unlike the predicted pattern after one episode of blood loss (see Fig. 3–5).

Blood Loss Anemia

That a regenerative anemia is due to blood loss is often obvious from the history or physical examination. External blood loss into the gastrointestinal tract or internal blood loss into a body cavity, however, may be occult. Gastrointestinal bleeding is indicated by a dark, tarry stool or fresh red blood in the stool. Tests for occult blood in the stool are of questionable value, since myoglobin in the usual meat diet of dogs and cats gives frequent false positives. Fluid cytology can document bleeding into body cavities, and the amount of hemorrhage is indicated by gross color and turbidity and by determining the PCV of the fluid.

The expected pattern of hematologic results in blood loss varies greatly with how many days have passed since the onset of the hemorrhage, severity of blood loss, whether the bleeding was one acute episode or persistent, whether the hemorrhage was into the body or external blood loss, and species variation. Time-related changes and species variations are illustrated in Figure 3–5 and in following discussions.

External Blood Loss ● The PCV in an adult dog will not immediately reflect the severity of acute blood loss anemia for 1 to 3 days, until the fluid volume of the vascular space is replaced and the remaining RBCs and PPs are diluted. Availability of fluids should be considered in an animal's ability to rapidly replenish the vascular volume. Splenic contraction in the first few hours releases stored, concentrated RBCs and may mask the severity of the anemia. Release of reticulocytes should be noticed by 3 days after hemorrhage, and peak reticulocytosis should be noted about 5 days after hemorrhage (see Fig. 3–5) (Perman and Schall, 1983). Fairly rapid improvement in the PCV occurs over the first 2 weeks until the PCV reaches the low-normal reference range. Later there is less hypoxia to stimulate strong erythropoietin production, so this is followed by a slower elevation in erythroid mass that may take a month after hemorrhage to return to the dog's original PCV.

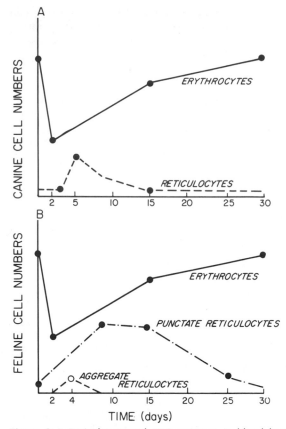

Figure 3–5 Reticulocyte and RBC response in blood loss anemia. The reestablishment of the erythroid mass as indicated by the packed cell volume or RBC count is similar in both species after one episode of blood loss. It is most rapid in the first 2 weeks and is slower during the next 2 weeks. The reticulocyte responses in the dog and cat are most different (Perman and Schall, 1983). The feline aggregate reticulocyte response is lower in magnitude than the canine reticulocyte response but fairly similar in onset and duration. The feline punctate reticulocyte response is uniquely long and of great magnitude.

In adults, chronic hemorrhage over days to weeks causes iron deficiency (Color Plate 1A) and a negative protein balance, which impairs erythropoiesis and causes inadequate regenerative responses. Thus, blood loss anemia would initially (e.g., first 1–2 days) appear nonregenerative, quickly cause marked bone marrow responsiveness, and then, with time and sufficient blood loss, have the degree of regeneration gradually decrease to poor. In pups and kittens with little reserves and preexisting maximum erythropoiesis to match growth rate, this depletion occurs quickly.

A low or low-normal PP value is useful in regenerative anemias to indicate external blood loss, since PPs are lost with the blood. In hemolytic anemias and internal blood loss, the PP concentration tends to be normal to slightly high, since no protein is lost from the body and some immune stimulation and production of acute phase proteins are likely. The PPs are replaced by the liver and lymphoid tissues more quickly than the bone marrow can replace RBCs, so hypoproteinemia less consistently reflects the degree or severity of external hemorrhage than does the PCV. The degree of hypoproteinemia is also affected by hepatic disease, immune stimulation, and other factors that may accompany the hemorrhagic disease.

The feline PCV response to blood loss somewhat parallels the canine response for the first 2 weeks. This is the period of most rapid improvement in the circulating RBC volume. The feline aggregate reticulocyte response reaches a peak about 4 days after hemorrhage (see Fig. 3–5) (Perman and Schall, 1983). The feline aggregate reticulocytes do not become as numerous as the canine reticulocytes. The feline punctate reticulocyte response reaches a later peak about 1 week after hemorrhage and may remain elevated for 3 weeks or more. The punctate reticulocytes may still be at a high level while the PCV has returned to the low-normal range, so the punctate reticulocyte response does not reflect active bone marrow erythropoiesis.

Feline punctate reticulocytes can help time the onset of an anemia. Moderate to markedly increased aggregate reticulocytes with few punctate reticulocytes could suggest a recent anemia (e.g., 2–4 days). Mainly punctate reticulocytes suggest an anemia that began 1 to 3 weeks earlier, or an anemia too mild to stimulate an aggregate reticulocyte response. Aggregate reticulocytes may not be released in significant numbers into the peripheral blood in mild to moderate anemias in cats but are expected in severe anemias.

The ability of a young animal to respond to blood loss is less than that of an adult. Puppies and kittens already have high rates of bone marrow erythropoietic activity to match the growth rate. When the bone marrow is already at a high rate of erythropoiesis, one cannot expect as great an increase in erythropoiesis in regenerative anemias as in an adult that normally has a low-level, steady-state production of RBCs. Also, while kittens are fed a milk diet, they often have a subclinical iron deficiency that limits erythropoiesis.

Age-related changes in puppies must be considered. The PCV in 2- to 6-week-old puppies may normally be around 28%, and the PP normally may be less than 6 g/dl. Puppies have around 3% to 7% reticulocytes at 2 months of age or younger, with the highest percentage (7%) occurring at 0 to 2 weeks of age. Adult dogs usually have <1% reticulocytes. Using adult values, one would incorrectly conclude that young animals have anemia, reticulocytosis, and hypoproteinemia, which signify external blood loss. Therefore, use age-related reference values (Jain, 1986), and do not expect the same magnitude of increased erythropoiesis during anemia in puppies and kittens that occurs in adults.

Internal Blood Loss • The hematologic pattern is similar to hemolytic anemia, since the RBCs lost into tissues are destroyed and their constituents conserved to allow maximal bone marrow response. Some RBCs lost into the body cavities may be recirculated intact via the lymphatics.

Hemolytic Anemias

Hemolytic anemias are usually diagnosed by finding a markedly regenerative anemia that lacks hypoproteinemia or other evidence of blood loss. Careful evaluation of the blood smear is essential to identify the positive evidence for specific causes of hemolytic anemias, such as blood parasites, Heinz bodies, or an immune-mediated hemolytic process. Rarely is there hemoglobinuria and hemoglobinemia to prove hemolysis.

A common classification of hemolytic diseases is to identify the site of hemolysis as intravascular versus extravascular. Extravascular hemolysis occurs in macrophages in the spleen, liver, and bone marrow. Intravascular hemolysis is often a more acute, severe process than is purely extravascular hemolysis. Complement-mediated damage may injure RBCs, allowing them to lyse in blood vessels in the less frequent but severe IgM forms of immune-mediated hemolytic anemia. Heinz body anemias may have RBCs so fragile that they lyse intravascularly. RBC "ghosts" (i.e., empty RBC membranes) may sometimes be seen in blood smears from animals with intravascular hemolysis due to Heinz body anemia. The combination of hemoglobinemia and hemoglobinuria is proof of intravascular hemolysis (see Chapter 7).

Extravascular hemolysis is much more common and consists of slower removal of RBCs by macrophages in the spleen, liver, and bone marrow. Splenomegaly and hepatomegaly are evidence for extravascular hemolysis. Extravascular hemolysis may also be antibody and complement mediated.

Icterus can occur in both forms of hemolysis

because extravascular hemolysis occurs in animals with intravascular hemolysis in addition to RBCs lysing in vessels. The increased rate of bilirubin production from damaged RBCs in macrophages temporarily exceeds the capacity of the liver to remove it. In severe anemias, the liver may also have hypoxic or toxic damage to contribute to the icterus. Intravascular hemolysis usually has a more rapid rate of hemolysis and thus more frequent and greater icterus. Serum bilirubin determinations (i.e., total and conjugated) are of limited use to differentiate anemias because many exceptions to the expected patterns occur.

Immune-Mediated Anemias • Immune-mediated hemolytic anemias (IHAs) are common. RBCs with sufficient antibody or complement on them are destroyed in macrophages or blood. The term *autoimmune hemolytic anemia* should be avoided since the antigen to which the immune response is occurring is rarely identified. *Autoimmune* indicates that the immune reaction is to the animal's own antigens. If the animal has a blood parasite like *Haemobartonella* or a virus like FeLV, or if the anemia chronologically matches the use of a drug, the anemia is not likely autoimmune but probably directly or indirectly due to a foreign antigen. The removal of transfused RBCs is an immune-mediated hemolytic process but not an autoimmune process.

The diagnosis of IHA is strongly supported by use of the Coombs' (i.e., direct antiglobulin) test, but the diagnosis can confidently be made in dogs despite a negative Coombs' test or when a Coombs' test is not available. About 30% of canine immune-mediated hemolytic anemia cases are Coombs' negative. The CBC pattern in canine IHA is usually consistent and diagnostic. The components of the pattern are a moderate to severe anemia (e.g., PCV = 16%), marked reticulocytosis (e.g., 625,000/µl), polychromasia (e.g., 3+ or 4+), normal to slightly increased PP (e.g., 7.2 g/dl), marked leukocytosis (e.g., 54,000/µl), significant spherocytosis (e.g., 2+ or more) in most (e.g., 82%) dogs, and occasional autoagglutination and occasional thrombocytopenia (e.g., 29%). Much of this basically indicates a hemolytic anemia. The RI is usually >3, suggesting a hemolytic anemia. The mean RI in one study of IHA was 4.8. Spherocytes, when definite and numerous, are a major differentiating feature, as is autoagglutination. Also diagnostically useful is the lack of evidence of other causes of hemolytic anemia such as Heinz bodies. Thrombocytopenia, when concurrently present with IHA, may be immune

mediated or due to disseminated intravascular coagulation.

Spherocytosis • Spherocytosis is a subjective morphologic observation from blood smears. One must have confidence in the person examining the smear, since errors in identifying spherocytes are common; however, spherocytes can be consistently identified by experienced observers using a well-made canine blood smear (see Chapter 2 for blood smear evaluation). Feline RBCs routinely lack central pallor, making it difficult or impossible to identify spherocytes. Therefore, spherocytes are rarely identified with confidence and should not be used as a primary diagnostic feature of IHA in cats.

Spherocytes must be quantitated, since any normal blood smear has an occasional abnormal cell (including spherocytes), and other fragmentation processes also cause spherocytosis. A significant number of spherocytes is required to diagnose immune-mediated anemia (Color Plate 1C). Weiss (1984) suggested that spherocytes be quantitated on the basis of the number per microscope field when using the 100× oil immersion objective (i.e., 1000× magnification). These fields should contain about 250 canine RBCs and be in the thin monolayer area where cell morphology can be evaluated (see Chapter 2). Since the number of RBCs per field may vary with the severity of the anemia, a corresponding percentage estimate is added in parentheses by the author to amplify Weiss's recommendations. The scale is 1+ to 4+, in which 1+ equals 5 to 10 spherocytes per 1000× field (2–4%); 2+, 11 to 50 (4.4–20%); 3+, 51 to 150 (20.4–60%); and 4+, more than 150 spherocytes per field. Note that <2% spherocytes is not reported.

Autoagglutination • Autoagglutination is essentially diagnostic for IHA. Since the end point of the Coombs' test is agglutination of the RBCs, autoagglutination of an unaltered blood sample is the equivalent of a positive polyvalent Coombs' test. Antibodies occurring *in vivo* coat the RBCs, causing autoagglutination. Antibodies causing RBC agglutination without the need for the Coombs' reagent are called *complete antibodies* and are usually IgM.

Care should be taken to avoid mistaking rouleaux for autoagglutination. Rouleaux microscopically resemble linear stacks of coins and should be dispersed by mixing blood with an equal amount of saline before making a wet mount (i.e., drop of the mixture on a glass slide under a coverslip) for microscopic evaluation.

Autoagglutination on a direct wet mount should resemble grapelike clusters. Note that both may be present simultaneously.

Feline Immune-Mediated Hemolytic Anemia • IHA in cats is harder to diagnose than in dogs. Spherocytosis and marked leukocytosis that strongly suggest canine IHA are not typical in cats. In feline hemolytic anemias, the Coombs' test is the major test for IHA. Other considerations in cats include the concurrent presence of *Haemobartonella felis* and FeLV infections. *H. felis* induces a Coombs'-positive IHA, and the organism may not be consistently found on a single blood smear analysis. The blood parasite and other causes of an IHA should be regenerative, but concurrent FeLV infection may inhibit a proper bone marrow response. FeLV is commonly associated with *H. felis* infection in cats, so all three conditions may coexist and should be tested for.

Coombs' Test • The Coombs' test identifies antibody or complement on RBCs. The usual test is a "polyvalent direct antiglobulin test" in which a polyvalent Coombs' reagent is mixed with the patient's RBCs. The polyvalent Coombs' reagent contains species-specific antibodies against various classes of antibodies and complement. If the patient's RBCs have enough antibody or complement to be detected and if the ratio of these antibodies and the antiglobulin is proper, then gross or microscopic hemagglutination occurs (i.e., a positive reaction).

The sensitivity of the Coombs' test is reasonable, being positive in about 60% to 70% of canine IHA cases. Possible reasons for false negatives include insufficient quantity of antibody on RBCs, temperature at which the test was performed, improper antigen:antibody ratio, or other technical problems. The storage life of an EDTA blood sample for a Coombs' test is unknown. With time, the antibody and complement should elute off the RBC. Alsever's solution has been used in laboratories to preserve antibody-coated sheep RBCs for a month and to preserve positive control blood samples for Coombs' testing. How necessary Alsever's solution might be for submission of a Coombs' sample by mail is not known. Alsever's solution is not commonly available. The effect of steroid treatment *in vivo* is not predictable. Dogs have remained Coombs' positive for variable lengths of time during corticosteroid treatment of IHA.

The specificity of the Coombs' test for IHA is considered good, but positive reactions also occur during strong immune reactions (e.g., generalized demodectic mange or ehrlichiosis) when excessive quantities of antibodies or complement in plasma coat the RBCs. This is a fairly frequent event. Of 134 Coombs'-positive anemias in dogs, half were positive for the third component of complement (C3), but there was infrequent evidence of intravascular or extravascular hemolytic anemia in these patients (Slappendale, 1979). A Coombs' test is usually not requested in the absence of a regenerative anemia, but diagnosticians need to be aware of false positives and negatives.

EDTA-anticoagulated blood is required because the EDTA prevents *in vitro* binding of complement, which would cause a false-positive polyvalent Coombs' reaction (Jain, 1986). C3 coats normal RBCs if clotted blood is left in the refrigerator. Other positive reactions occur in various infectious, inflammatory, neoplastic, and immune-mediated diseases in the absence of IHA.

Specific Coombs' testing involves using reagents that are specific for one type of antibody class (i.e., IgG). Different temperatures may be used to further define the characteristics of the antibody on a patient's RBCs. The goal is to better predict the probable behavior of the IHA when a dog is initially evaluated. IgG is less likely to bind complement, so an IgG-type IHA is unlikely to cause intravascular hemolysis. Experimentally IgG-mediated IHA responds best to glucocorticoid treatment (Jain, 1986). IgM is a large antibody that is more likely to link RBCs and cause autoagglutination. IgM tends to bind complement and is more likely than IgG to cause intravascular hemolysis, hemoglobinuria, and a more severe disease.

Results of specific antibody-type Coombs' testing in dogs in our hospital have not been consistent with literature reports, so the expense of Coombs' testing beyond the polyvalent direct antiglobulin test has not currently proved justified for routine patient care.

Cold Hemagglutinin Disease • Rarely, antibodies are produced that preferentially bind to RBCs in blood colder than normal body temperature, such as can occur in peripheral capillary beds (i.e., of the ears or paws) in cold weather. If these antibodies cause enough agglutination of RBCs to occlude capillaries, poor blood flow through the peripheral tissues and ischemic necrosis ensue. Cold agglutinin disease may or may not be associated with a hemolytic anemia.

The antibody expected in cold agglutinin disease is IgM. It is incorrect to call all IgM antibodies cold antibodies, however, since not all IgM antibodies preferentially act in cold temperatures. Similarly, not all cases of IgM binding to RBCs cause intravascular hemolysis or autoagglutination.

Test results for cold hemagglutinin disease should be interpreted with caution. The disease occurs infrequently enough that most laboratories are not experienced in its evaluation. Techniques are more involved than just refrigerating the sample. Antibodies that act in cold temperatures (i.e, cold agglutinins) are normally found in dogs and people. In people, the titer should be >1:64 to be considered abnormal. A proven cutoff value to indicate significance in dogs and cats is not available. One cat with cold agglutinin disease had a cold agglutinin titer of 1:52,000 (Schrader and Hurvitz, 1983). The RBC agglutination that occurs after incubation at refrigerator temperature (4° C) is dispersed as the blood warms to body temperature.

Heinz Body Anemia • Various oxidative toxins damage hemoglobin, causing it to precipitate and form Heinz bodies. Heinz bodies may be detected on routine Wright's-stained blood smears and are prominent on new methylene blue–stained smears using the same method as for reticulocyte smears (see Fig. 2–9). The diagnosis is uncomplicated and relatively easy in dogs, since Heinz bodies are normally absent; any Heinz bodies found in canine RBCs during hemolytic anemia are diagnostic. Additional evidence would be a history of exposure to a toxin (i.e., eating onions or being treated with benzocaine, vitamin K_3, or methylene blue).

An eccentrocyte is a RBC shape change suggesting exposure to some of the oxidative toxins that also cause Heinz body anemia. Eccentrocytes have an eccentric rim of a water-clear area. Eccentrocytes have been mistaken for spherocytes, as have pyknocytes, which may accompany eccentrocytes.

Normal and ill cats frequently have Heinz bodies, since feline hemoglobin seems more susceptible to oxidative damage and the feline spleen is inefficient in removing Heinz bodies. One must consider the size and number of the Heinz bodies, the PCV, the reticulocyte response, and exposure to a likely toxin to determine their significance. Increased numbers of Heinz bodies may be found in nonanemic cats eating semimoist cat foods containing propylene glycol and a salmon-based diet. Increased numbers of Heinz bodies have been found in cats with diabetes mellitus, hyperthyroidism, and lymphosarcoma (Christopher, 1989). The number of Heinz bodies in feline blood may be ranked as occasional if <10%, moderate if 10% to 50%, and marked if >50% of RBCs have

Heinz bodies. The frequency of Heinz bodies must be combined with large size and other supporting evidence. Abnormally large size is demonstrated when the Heinz body bulges noticeably from the RBCs' normal shape (Color Plate 1B). Heinz bodies in normal cats are usually small.

In a hemolytic-type anemia, the presence of large and numerous Heinz bodies is good evidence of an oxidative toxin. Concurrent exposure to known causes of Heinz body anemias like acetaminophen (i.e., Tylenol), methylene blue, or phenazopyridine is adequate proof. Methylene blue was used as a urinary tract antiseptic but may be ingested by cats drinking water out of fish aquariums treated with it.

Methemoglobinemia • Diagnosis and quantitation of the severity of methemoglobinemia are accomplished by specific testing for methemoglobin, which is usually available from human referral laboratories. The gross appearance of blood is often the first sign of methemoglobinemia. Blood with methemoglobinemia is darker and browner than normal and may not turn red when exposed to air. Placing a drop of blood on white filter paper allows one to see a brown color more easily. The animal's mucous membranes may appear darker than normal or cyanotic if more than 30% of the hemoglobin is affected. Methemoglobinemia is also suggested by the concurrent presence of a Heinz body anemia.

Methemoglobin is a nonfunctional form of hemoglobin formed by oxidative damage, which makes the animal hypoxic despite a normal PCV. Unless considered, the true lack of oxygen-carrying capacity of blood in combined Heinz body anemia and methemoglobinemia would be underestimated by the PCV or the usual cyanmethemoglobin procedure for determining the hemoglobin concentration. The oxyhemoglobin method for hemoglobin concentration measures only oxyhemoglobin (oxygenated form of hemoglobin), whereas the cyanmethemoglobin method measures all types of hemoglobin, including methemoglobin.

Oxidative toxins that cause Heinz body anemia often also cause concurrent methemoglobin formation, but methemoglobinemia or Heinz body anemia may exist as a separate disorder (Jain, 1986). Ketamine anesthesia in cats has been associated with methemoglobinemia. Acetaminophen in cats can cause both methemoglobinemia and Heinz body anemia. Benzocaine in dogs causes both methemoglobinemia and Heinz body anemia, but benzocaine in cats apparently just causes methemoglobinemia.

Methylene blue in cats also causes methemoglobinemia without Heinz bodies.

Oxidation of the iron in hemoglobin to the ferric state is the process in methemoglobin formation. This is reversible, unlike the formation of sulfhemoglobin (i.e., the denatured form of hemoglobin in Heinz bodies). Methemoglobin accumulation is normally prevented by methemoglobin reductase. Rarely, this enzyme may be deficient in dogs, causing significant methemoglobinemia and cyanosis. Just the routine oxidative damage to hemoglobin from carrying oxygen converts about 1% of total hemoglobin to methemoglobin in normal dogs. Without the methemoglobin reductase to convert the methemoglobin to normal, methemoglobin accumulates to toxic levels.

Blood Parasites • *H. felis* (e.g., feline infectious anemia) is routinely diagnosed by blood smear evaluation. Since stain precipitate is coccoid in shape and about the same size as the organism, one should find at least two distinct ring forms on RBCs to be sure that *H. felis* and not stain precipitate is present. Ring forms are like small letter *o*'s with a dark outer ring and a pale interior (see Fig. 2–9). Ring forms are at the minimum size limits of what one can distinguish with a good microscope. Finding the small coccoid forms on RBCs is suspicious, but the ring forms are needed for confident diagnosis. The acridine orange stain and fluorescent-labeled antibody stains are more sensitive in finding the organism on blood smears than are routine Wright's-type stains.

Parasitemic episodes, when one can find *H. felis* on blood smears, are often present for relatively short periods (i.e., 1–2 days) separated by periods when few or no organisms can be seen on the smear. It is therefore recommended that smears be evaluated on several consecutive days to improve the likelihood of diagnosis. Obtaining capillary blood by pricking the ear with a lancet is suggested, because it will contain a higher concentration of parasitized RBCs. Splenomegaly occurs with extravascular hemolysis as macrophages remove the damaged cells and organisms as in other hemolytic anemias.

Haemobartonella canis principally causes anemia in splenectomized dogs. It may occur in carrier dogs after they are splenectomized or in previously splenectomized dogs after they contract the infection from blood transfusions or ticks. Glucocorticoid therapy may produce a functional splenectomy. *H. canis* appears as distinct chains of cocci on RBCs. The uniformly arranged cocci must be differentiated from stain precipitate that randomly falls on cells and

intercellular areas. Stain precipitate on the glass slide away from the blood smear may be used for comparison since it is definitely an artifact there.

Babesia canis can produce severe anemia in dogs. Intravascular hemolysis is demonstrated by hemoglobinuria. Extravascular hemolysis is indicated by splenomegaly. Transmitted by ticks, it is often accompanied by *Ehrlichia canis* and other organisms and may be more common in racing greyhound dogs. The diagnosis may be made by demonstrating the intraerythrocytic piriform (i.e., pear-shaped or teardrop-shaped) organisms on blood smears, particularly capillary blood, or by serology. *Babesia gibsoni* is smaller.

Cytauxzoon felis is a tick-transmitted fatal disease of cats. It is diagnosed most consistently at necropsy by histologic evidence of large schizonts in the endothelial cells of the lungs, liver, spleen, and lymph nodes. Endemic areas include Missouri, Oklahoma, Arkansas, Mississippi, Georgia, Florida, and Louisiana. The presence of small piriform or safety pin–shaped organisms in RBCs on blood smears is found in <50% of affected cats (Glen and Stair, 1984). The organism "signet ring" bodies measure 1 to 5 μm and have a small, peripherally located nucleus. The cats are icteric, have small hemorrhages at necropsy, and have the typical "sick cat" clinical signs of depression, anorexia, fever, and dehydration.

Other Hemolytic Anemias • Zinc-induced hemolytic anemia is uniquely diagnosed by an abdominal radiograph. A common cause of zinc poisoning is ingestion of zinc nuts from portable kennels or pennies. These objects are found in the stomach by radiographic examination. Dogs may have intravascular hemolysis with hemolyzed serum, hemoglobinuria, icterus, severe anemia, and increased serum zinc levels (normal canine serum zinc = 0.7–1.1 mg/kg). If serum zinc is to be measured, first contact the laboratory to obtain the proper type of collection tube lest the serum zinc be artificially increased by contamination from the tube.

Hypophosphatemia is most commonly associated with postparturient hemoglobinuria in cattle but also has been associated with hemolytic anemia in dogs and cats. In dogs and cats, hemolysis may occur when serum phosphorus level is <1.0 mg/dl. Hypophosphatemia in dogs and cats may be a complication of diabetes mellitus (Willard et al., 1987).

Hypersplenism is a historical diagnosis made before splenomegaly was shown to be a result of RBC alteration and destruction rather than a cause. Splenomegaly is expected in hemolytic anemias owing to the proliferation of macrophages to meet this need. "Hypersplenism" is usually, if not always, a compensatory response to a hemolytic process and should not be considered a disease process or syndrome. The primary goal should be to identify the primary cause of the RBC insult.

Splenectomy may temporarily slow a hemolytic or thrombocytopenic process but also removes an important blood filter and site of extramedullary hematopoiesis. Splenectomy contributed to deterioration in the PCV and reticulocyte count in a poodle with familial hemolytic anemia, since splenectomy removed much of the dog's source of extramedullary hematopoiesis (Randolph et al., 1986).

Pyruvate Kinase Deficiency ● Pyruvate kinase (PK) deficiency in basenji dogs is an autosomal recessive genetic disease causing severe and persistent extravascular hemolysis. Characteristic features include a moderate to severe anemia (i.e., PCV = 18–25%) with marked reticulocytosis (i.e., 25–45%) and splenomegaly in young basenji, West Highland white terrier, or beagle dogs.

If the PK activity is measured for a definitive diagnosis, adjustments in PK referenced values must be made, since reticulocytes have higher enzyme activities than do mature RBCs. The PK-deficient RBCs have inefficient energy production and thus have a short half-life. Myelofibrosis and osteosclerosis in PK deficiency are perhaps related to the chronic, massive bone marrow production of RBCs.

Other Hereditary Hemolytic Anemias ● Phosphofructokinase deficiency may occur in English springer spaniels. Hemoglobinuria is a common presenting complaint, and splenomegaly and/or icterus may be noted. Diagnosis is by analysis of RBC enzyme activity after ruling out more common causes of hemolytic anemia. Hyperventilation-induced hemolysis was identified in an English springer spaniel that had RBCs that were sensitive to *in vivo* increases in the blood's pH (Harvey and Giger, 1984). Hyperventilation during stress or exercise caused enough of a respiratory alkalosis to induce intravascular hemolysis with hemoglobinuria and hemoglobinemia.

Familial nonspherocytic hemolytic anemia has been described in a family of poodles (Randolph et al., 1986). The cause was not determined despite extensive evaluation. PK activity in the patient's RBCs was not decreased. Bone marrow regeneration characterized by 6.8% to 9.8% reticulocytes and a reticulocyte index <2 despite a PCV of 13% to 21% indicated slight to moderate RBC release by the bone marrow. It was fatal as early as 3 years of age. The dogs had widespread hemosiderosis indicating extravascular hemolysis in macrophages in various sites. Myelofibrosis and osteosclerosis were noted at necropsy, as in dogs with PK deficiency. A hereditary nonspherocytic hemolytic anemia in beagles also was studied extensively without identifying a cause (Maggio-Price et al., 1988). The anemia in beagles was not as severe, was not fatal, and lacked hemosiderosis, myelofibrosis, and osteosclerosis.

Dwarfism in Alaskan malamutes has been associated with stomatocytosis (Fletch et al., 1973). Stomatocytes are RBCs that morphologically appear to have mouthlike central pallor. The MCHC was consistently <30 g/dl. Compared with age-matched normal Alaskan malamutes, the dwarfs were not anemic.

Miniature schnauzers may have stomatocytosis as an autosomal recessive trait without clinical signs. A miniature schnauzer-beagle cross with inherited stomatocytosis and prominent macrocytosis did not appear anemic (PCV = 48%) but had a mild reduction in RBCs (5.01 × 10^6/μl) and hemoglobin (12.5 g/dl) (Brown, 1992). This macrocytosis was demonstrated by the Coulter RBC volume distribution histogram in Figure 3–4. Stomatocytosis also occurs in Drentse patrijshond breed familial stomatocytosis-hypertrophic gastritis.

Nonregenerative Anemias

Nonregenerative anemias are less well understood than the regenerative anemias, since the mechanisms of the various nonregenerative anemias are usually complex. The CBC pattern is usually a normocytic-normochromic anemia without diagnostic morphologic changes in RBCs. Many nonregenerative anemias are secondary problems too mild to pursue diagnostically. The diagnostic effort is more productively spent on primary diseases such as neoplasia, renal or hepatic disease, or chronic inflammation.

Diagnostic Approach ● A diagnostic approach is summarized in Figure 3–6. The number of depleted cell lines in the CBC report makes the first differentiation (Weiss and Armstrong, 1984). A pancytopenia (i.e., decreased RBCs, leukocytes, and platelets) or bicytopenia (i.e.,

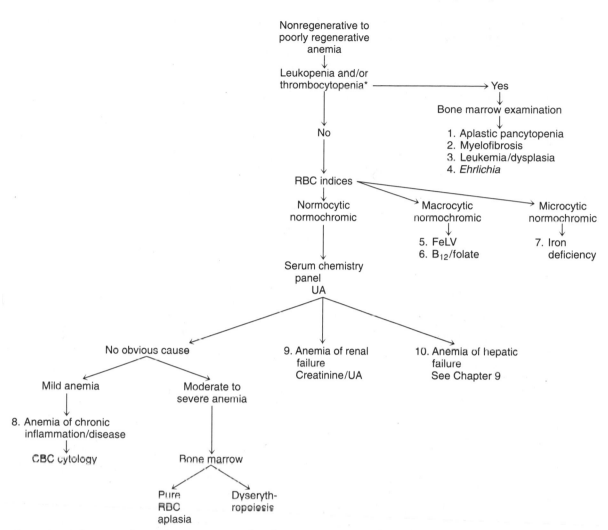

Figure 3-6 *Laboratory evaluation of nonregenerative and poorly regenerative anemia.* A bicytopenia or pancytopenia (*) found on the complete blood count (CBC) indicates a bone marrow biopsy, and an aspirate should be performed to make diagnoses 1 to 3. The RBC indices may suggest causes 5 to 7. A normocytic-normochromic anemia may be evaluated by bone marrow examination or further tests for diagnoses 8 to 10. UA, urinalysis.

two of the three cell types) usually indicates bone marrow disease, which is best diagnosed by a bone marrow biopsy and aspirate.

If RBCs are the only cell type decreased, the RBC indices and blood smear evaluation usually identifies one of three types of nonregenerative anemias (i.e., microcytic-hypochromic anemia, macrocytic-normochromic anemia, or normocytic-normochromic anemia). Microcytic-hypochromic anemia is usually due to iron deficiency. Macrocytic-normochromic anemia without reticulocytosis in cats is often associated with FeLV-induced myeloproliferative disorders (i.e., dysplastic to neoplastic diseases). Macrocytic-normochromic anemia occurs uncommonly in dogs taking certain medications or having malabsorption problems and may be attributed to a deficiency of vitamin B_{12} or folate. Hypersegmentation of neutrophils and other myelodysplastic changes also suggest a cobala-min (B_{12}) or folate problem. Familial macrocytosis in poodles and selective cobalamin malabsorption in giant schnauzers are associated with these changes.

Normocytic-normochromic anemias are the most common nonregenerative anemias; if persistent and severe enough, they may be further evaluated by bone marrow aspiration and biopsy. One striking, albeit infrequent, bone marrow diagnosis is termed *pure red cell aplasia* (PRCA), which is a marked to total deficiency of only erythroid cells. The more common bone marrow pattern in normocytic-normochromic anemias is mild suppression of erythropoiesis in which erythroid precursors are seemingly adequate in number. The following common causes of normocytic-normochromic anemias must then be differentiated by additional evidence available from the serum chemistry profile, urinalysis, CBC, and special tests: (1) anemia of chronic inflammation, (2) anemia of renal disease, (3) anemia of hepatic disease, and (4) anemia of decreased endocrine function.

Anemia of chronic inflammation is probably the most common cause of nonregenerative anemia and is diagnosed when a mild to moderate anemia is present in an animal with an inflammatory disease. There is usually proof of inflammation, but the anemia is not usually proved to be anemia of chronic inflammation, since more severe problems are present and the anemia is usually too mild and cost ineffective to pursue.

During inflammation, macrophages release interleukin-1 (i.e., IL-1 or leukocyte endogenous pyrogen), which initiates several processes including fever. IL-1 causes iron to be "sequestered" in macrophages in a less available form and thus reduces serum iron and restricts the availability of iron to developing rubricytes. The pathogenesis of the anemia is more complex than a relative iron deficiency. Anemia of chronic inflammation may be differentiated from iron deficiency anemia by a serum iron profile, if necessary (Table 3–4).

Anemia of chronic renal disease is diagnosed by the presence of a nonregenerative anemia plus evidence of renal failure (see Chapter 7, azotemia and isosthenuria). The mechanism of the anemia is more complex than a relative deficiency of erythropoietin. Ineffective erythropoiesis, a shortened RBC life span, and blood loss may contribute to the anemia (Weiss and Armstrong, 1984).

The nonregenerative anemia of chronic hepatic disease is supported by data from serum chemistry profiles (see Chapter 9). RBC morphologic changes (i.e., acanthocytes and budding fragmentation) support hepatic disease as the cause. Anemia of hepatic disease is due to

Table 3–4 COMPARISON OF SELECTED PARAMETERS IN ANEMIA OF CHRONIC INFLAMMATION AND IRON DEFICIENCY ANEMIA

	Anemia of Chronic Inflammation	Iron Deficiency Anemia
RBC indices	Normocytic-normochromic	Microcytic-hypochromic
Serum iron	Low	Low
Total iron binding capacity	Usually decreased	Usually normal
Bone marrow iron	High	Low
Serum ferritin	High	Low
Inflammation	Present	Need not be present

various factors. Abnormal lipid metabolism is believed to cause the altered RBC shapes and a shortened RBC life span (e.g., mild, slow hemolysis). Coagulation defects from reduced hepatic synthesis of coagulation and anticoagulant factors may cause hemorrhage. Anemia of chronic inflammation may coexist with hepatitis. Decreased hepatic function can lead to deficiencies of nutrients needed for hematopoiesis (Weiss and Armstrong, 1984).

Mild anemias can be due to hypothyroidism or hypoadrenocorticism. These animals would present primarily for other problems (e.g., endocrine dermatosis or weight loss) rather than anemia. Specific diagnosis is by hormone assay (see Chapter 8). The anemia is usually clinically insignificant.

Aplastic Pancytopenia and Myelofibrosis ● The CBC usually provides the first suggestion of aplastic pancytopenia (e.g., pancytopenia or bicytopenia reflecting poor marrow production of two or three cell lines). Diagnosis of aplastic pancytopenia and myelofibrosis is proved by histopathologic examination of a bone marrow core biopsy. Bone marrow aspirates in aplastic pancytopenia are poorly cellular, perhaps only retrieving fat, so the aspirate may simply seem to be a poor sample. A good cortex-to-cortex bone marrow biopsy includes the fatty or fibrotic marrow for definitive diagnosis.

After some bone marrow insults, all that may remain is scar tissue or fat. The histologic diagnosis of a scarred fibrotic marrow is myelofibrosis. A fatty marrow is termed *aplastic pancytopenia*. The more common term, *aplastic anemia*, is incorrect and misleading, since myeloid and megakaryocytic cells are usually also depleted. If only erythroid cells are absent in a marrow, then PRCA is most descriptive. Myelofibrosis and a fatty marrow should be thought of in terms similar to end-stage kidneys or hepatic cirrhosis. As in an end-stage kidney, there is usually no morphologic evidence for the cause of the damage. Aplastic pancytopenia is often idiopathic.

Possible causes include estrogens, phenylbutazone, meclofenamic acid, quinidine, griseofulvin, thiacetarsamide, *E. canis*, viruses, and immune-mediated processes. Some drugs like chloramphenicol in cats or sulfadiazine, mainly in Doberman pinschers, cause transient leukopenia or other cytopenias while the drug is given, but these effects are reversible after the drug is discontinued. Aplastic anemia due to quinidine, griseofulvin, and thiacetarsamide is reversible (Weiss, 1992). One can determine a titer for *E. canis* in dogs with nonregenerative anemia and thrombocytopenia in endemic areas. In areas with few cases of *E. canis* (e.g., Michigan), one would initially check for estrogen toxicity due to an estrogen-secreting Sertoli cell tumor of a retained testis or an estrogen treatment (e.g., unwanted pregnancy or to decrease the size of the prostate or perianal gland). Various treatments have the potential to induce aplastic anemia, including cancer chemotherapy or irradiation. One common problem with many drugs that keeps them off the market is myelotoxicity. Nonsteroidal anti-inflammatory drugs (e.g., phenylbutazone or ibuprofen) may cause marrow aplasia. Viruses like feline panleukopenia, FeLV, and canine parvovirus may attack rapidly developing marrow cells.

Estrogen Toxicity • Canine estrogen toxicity may cause bone marrow destruction, leaving a fatty marrow and an aplastic pancytopenia, especially after some time (e.g., 1–3 weeks); but early in some cases, a leukemoid reaction of >100,000 WBCs/μl occurs. The leukocytosis may delay or mislead the diagnostician, since it indicates strong bone marrow production of at least one cell line, which seems unlikely during bone marrow toxicity. A bicytopenia consisting of a nonregenerative anemia and thrombocytopenia may exist, with a total WBC count varying from very high to very low, depending on individual animal variation.

An estrogen-induced leukemoid response is illustrated in Figure 3–7. The WBC count peaked at 120,000/μl 15 days after the estradiol. It had a thrombocytopenia between 8 and 12 days after estradiol, but the thrombocyte count rapidly returned to normal. The lowest platelet count was 14,000/μl when the dog had intestinal bleeding. A nonregenerative anemia was most severe (i.e., PCV = 19%) 20 days after the estradiol. Despite the severe hematologic changes, the dog returned to normal by a month after the estradiol toxicity.

Testicular tumors may cause pancytopenia or bicytopenia. The testicular neoplasms are usually Sertoli cell tumors, but this is not universal, nor can one consistently document an increased serum estradiol level. Sertoli cell tumors are the type expected to secrete estrogen or estrogen-like substances and cause feminization. The PCVs in anemias associated with testicular tumors have ranged from 6% to 38%. The reticulocytes were decreased in number or only trivially increased. Thrombocytopenia has varied from 3000 to 93,000/μl, and the severity may permit bleeding.

Another form of endogenous estrogen toxicity that causes aplastic pancytopenia is protracted estrus in pet ferrets. Females remain in estrus for months if not bred. The anemia was severe (i.e., PCV = 5–10%; normal, 41–46%) in five ferrets (Kociba and Caputo, 1981). The anemia was nonregenerative with 0 to 15,750 reticulocytes/μl (normal, 78,000–470,000). Leukopenia was severe at 800 to 2400 WBCs/μl (normal, 5300–10,200). Thrombocytopenia was present in all ferrets and severe enough (7000 platelets/μl in one ferret) to cause petechial and ecchymotic hemorrhages. The marrow was fatty, with reduced hematopoietic cells. Ovariohysterectomy is protective in these pets.

Ehrlichia canis • Acute canine ehrlichiosis commonly (90%) causes anemia. The anemias are usually (i.e., 21 of 24 dogs) nonregenerative (i.e., RI <1). The PCV varies widely from normal to 5%. Thrombocytopenia is usually present (see Chapter 5) (Troy et al., 1980). Nonregenerative anemia (± thrombocytopenia and/or leukopenia) may also be caused by bone marrow suppression due to chronic ehrlichiosis.

Feline Leukemia Virus • FeLV-infected cats frequently (i.e., 90%) have altered erythroid parameters (Weiser and Kociba, 1983). FeLV is associated with most cases of feline nonregen-

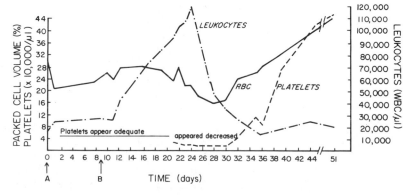

Figure 3–7 Estrogen toxicity in a dog. The transient, time-related hematologic changes in a dog with an excessive dose of estradiol included a bicytopenia consisting of thrombocytopenia and nonregenerative anemia and a profound leukemoid response: At A, a bleeding episode occurred; at B, estradiol was given.

erative anemia. One pattern suggestive of FeLV infection is a macrocytosis (MCV > 52 fl) without increased reticulocytes. Regenerative anemias with release of large reticulocytes should have a macrocytosis, but nonregenerative anemias should be normocytic; a nonregenerative anemia with macrocytosis is unusual. The normal cats had an MCV of about 43 fl. The cats with regenerative anemias (increased reticulocytes) but without FeLV had an MCV similar to that of the cats with nonregenerative anemias and FeLV (i.e., 60–62 fl). The cats with both regenerative anemias and FeLV had a high mean MCV of 67 fl.

Feline Immunodeficiency Virus ● FIV-infected cats often develop nonregenerative anemia. Neutropenia may be seen concurrently in some of these patients (Fleming et al., 1991). Rarely, hemolytic anemia, apparently due to the virus and not secondary infection with *Haemobartonella,* may be seen (Willard MD: Personal observation).

Feline Panleukopenia Virus ● Infectious panleukopenia causes a severe, absolute granulopenia and lymphopenia. Anemia is mild and may not be detected, since the PCV may not decrease below the reference range and the cats may be dehydrated from diarrhea and anorexia, causing a relative polycythemia. The anemia is usually nonregenerative, but an increase in reticulocytes may be noted during the recovery period.

Pure Red Blood Cell Aplasia ● PRCA is a severe nonregenerative anemia characterized by bone marrow that has few or no erythroid precursors yet normal-appearing myeloid and megakaryocytic lines. The cause of the absence of erythroid cells is not clear but may be immune mediated. Weiss (1985) reported evidence of immune destruction of erythroid precursor cells in four of eight dogs with PRCA. The Coombs' test did not accurately detect which dogs had the immune response. Glucocorticoid therapy has been effective in some cases. Parvovirus infection has been associated with PRCA. Other viruses such as equine infectious anemia damage erythroid cells indirectly through immune-mediated damage, so parvovirus-induced PRCA may also be immune mediated.

Dyserythropoiesis ● In several nonregenerative anemias, the bone marrow seems to have adequate to increased numbers of erythroid precursors, yet reticulocytes are not released into the blood in adequate numbers. The cause is not apparent. Ineffective erythropoiesis may unexpectedly decrease the myeloid:erythroid (M:E) ratio on a bone marrow report of an animal with a nonregenerative anemia. If myeloid hyperplasia is present because of concurrent inflammation, the M:E will be variable.

Iron Deficiency Anemia ● Iron deficiency anemia (Color Plate 1A) was previously considered uncommon in dogs and cats; however, iron deficiency occurred in 11% of anemic dogs in Florida (Harvey et al., 1982). The presenting problem is usually persistent blood loss from hookworms, fleas, or bleeding intestinal neoplasms. The PCV may range from 7% to 36%. Hypoproteinemia may be present if external bleeding is recent enough and of great enough magnitude to exceed the body's compensatory mechanisms. Note that puppies normally have lower PP concentrations than do adult dogs, so use age-matched reference values when evaluating anemic puppies. A reactive thrombocytosis (i.e., >500,000 platelets/μl) commonly occurs. The degree of reticulocytosis and polychromasia is variable. Blood loss anemias start as strongly regenerative anemias but become nonregenerative with developing iron deficiency.

The CBC is the usual way of diagnosing iron deficiency anemia. Microcytosis (i.e., MCV <60 fl) and hypochromasia (i.e., MCHC <32 g/dl) in dogs are reasonably diagnostic. Newer automated hematology cell counters are more sensitive than is the MCV in identifying iron deficiency–induced RBC microcytosis (see Chapter 2, Laser Cell Counters).

Iron deficiency anemia is surprisingly common (i.e., 70%) in 5-week-old kittens (Weiser and Kociba, 1983). Kittens at this age had the highest frequency of microcytosis. By 7 weeks of age, the kittens stopped producing microcytic cells. The age-related changes implicated the all-milk diet in rapidly growing animals as the cause. The microcytosis in kittens was detected with RBC size distribution curves. This was a more sensitive detector of microcytosis than the MCV (i.e., only 35% of the affected kittens had MCV <37 fl). The microcytic cell population due to iron deficiency may be too small to lower the average for all RBCs, or there may be another subpopulation of larger cells such as reticulocytes to offset the effect of the microcytic cells. MCV is an average value of all RBCs. The MCHC was not a useful indicator of iron deficiency in the kittens. The occurrence and severity of the iron deficiency anemia in kittens were variable to severe (i.e., PCV 12–30%). Kittens at

5 weeks of age should have a PCV of 23% to 29%.

RBC fragmentation and abnormal RBC shapes are common on blood smears of dogs and cats with iron deficiency anemia. This poikilocytosis has caused confusion in the past, but if recognized as part of the pattern of iron deficiency anemia, it should not cause confusion.

The serum iron profile is most conclusive but is usually not necessary or cost-effective. Periodically obtaining an iron profile during the long treatment period of weeks to months, however, can provide confidence and understanding, since the owner and veterinarian may often be discouraged at how slowly the PCV returns to normal. Expected iron profile values in iron deficiency (Table 3–5) are compared with iron values in dogs with anemia of chronic inflammation (Schalm, 1978; Feldman et al., 1981), which also causes decreased serum iron. The decrease in the total iron binding capacity (TIBC) in anemia of chronic inflammation is due to the effect of inflammatory mediators on altering hepatic protein synthesis. Some proteins like transferrin and albumin have decreased rates of synthesis, whereas other proteins (i.e., acute phase proteins) like fibrinogen have increased synthesis.

A brief review of the techniques involved in the iron profile is helpful to understand what the terms mean and how the numbers are derived. TIBC is a measure of transferrin, the serum protein that binds iron. Free or ionic iron is toxic, so circulating iron must be protein bound. A colorimetric procedure for serum iron directly measures the iron bound to transferrin. The other direct measurement is the unsaturated iron binding capacity (UIBC). This measures the additional amount of iron that the serum transferrin will bind. TIBC is calculated by adding the serum iron plus the UIBC. This is basically adding the amount of iron on the transferrin (TIBC) plus the additional amount of iron it will accept. The percentage of saturation is the serum iron divided by the TIBC. Saturation near 100% is dangerous, since any additional iron may be in the free (i.e., toxic) form.

POLYCYTHEMIA

Polycythemia is usually defined by an increase in the PCV, hemoglobin concentration, or RBC count of a blood sample above the reference range. Only the PCV is used for these discussions, but recall that the hemoglobin or RBC counts are essentially equivalent. Polycythemia (i.e., increased PCV) of the blood sample does not automatically imply that the absolute erythroid mass in the body is increased. Polycythemia is categorized into absolute polycythemia (i.e., increased bone marrow production has increased the body's mass of RBCs) and relative polycythemia (i.e., the increased PCV is due to decreased plasma volume or results from splenic contraction without increased marrow production).

Critical cardiovascular problems are caused by the hyperviscosity of hemoconcentrated blood in polycythemia and the low blood volume of severe, relative polycythemia. An exponential-type increase in viscosity of blood occurs as the PCV becomes >60%. Neurologic signs such as seizures and collapse may be noted, probably related to poor perfusion of the brain.

If a patient is not anemic and its normal PCV is known, the volume of fluids for therapy may be estimated (Rose, 1984). In dehydration, the deficit may be estimated as follows:

$$\text{Extracellular fluid deficit} = 0.2 \times \text{body weight} \times \left(\frac{\text{PCV}}{\text{normal PCV}} - 1 \right)$$

Relative Polycythemia

Polycythemia is usually relative and due to increased RBC concentration secondary to de-

Table 3–5 IRON PROFILE VALUES IN DOGS WITH IRON DEFICIENCY ANEMIA AND ANEMIA OF CHRONIC INFLAMMATION

	Iron-Deficient Mean (Range)	Normal* Mean (Range)	ACI Mean ± SD	Normal† Mean ± SD
Serum iron (μl/dl)	30 (8–60)	149 (84–233)	62 ± 14	113 ± 8
TIBC (μl/dl)	387 (234–659)	391 (284–572)	193 ± 28	309 ± 36
UIBC (μl/dl)	357 (216–633)	243 (142–393)		
Saturation (%)	8 (2–19)	39 (20–59)		

*Harvey et al. (1982).
†Feldman et al. (1981).
TIBC, total iron binding capacity; UIBC, unbound iron binding capacity; ACI, anemia of chronic inflammation.

creased fluid in the vascular system (i.e., dehydration, hemoconcentration, or hypovolemia). Another cause is splenic contraction. This is not an absolute increase in the RBC mass in the body but only a distribution shift of a concentrated bolus of RBCs out of their splenic storage site. The spleen is part of the vascular system. These types are termed *relative polycythemia*.

A practical way to diagnose relative polycythemia due to hemoconcentration or dehydration is to note a return of the PCV to normal after fluid therapy replaces any plasma volume deficit (Fig. 3–8). Hemoconcentration would also be characterized by a concurrent increase in PP, detection of a clinical syndrome expected to cause fluid loss (e.g., diarrhea or vomiting), and other clinical evidence of hypovolemia. There are laboratory tests to determine the plasma volume, such as injecting Evans blue dye (T-1824) intravenously to label the PPs, but this type of test is primarily for experimental use.

The relative polycythemia of splenic contraction may be more difficult to diagnose, since one cannot consistently predict the degree of splenic contraction or relaxation. Splenic contraction would be expected after exercise or a fearful situation. Splenic relaxation occurs with some anesthetics. One may repeat the PCV when the animal seems calm to check for a return of the PCV toward normal. However, the animal may still have an epinephrine release causing splenic contraction.

Absolute Polycythemia

Absolute polycythemia is subdivided into primary and secondary conditions. Do not confuse the terms *secondary* and *relative* polycythemia. Primary absolute polycythemia is polycythemia vera, which is a rare myeloproliferative disorder. It is essentially diagnosed by ruling out all other causes of polycythemia. The PCV usually remains at 70% to 80% despite fluid therapy. Erythropoietin is not found to be increased, if one has access to such an assay. Primary polycythemia is treated by bloodletting (i.e., phlebotomy) to avoid the hyperviscosity that occurs at PCV values of ≥60%.

Secondary polycythemia is divided into appropriate and inappropriate forms. Appropriate secondary polycythemia is caused by increased production of erythropoietin due to hypoxia (e.g., pulmonary or cardiac disease or living at a high altitude). An arterial blood gas analysis and the partial pressure of oxygen should document the hypoxia.

Rarely, polycythemia may be due to renal diseases (e.g., neoplasia such as renal carcinomas) in which inappropriate and excessive erythro-

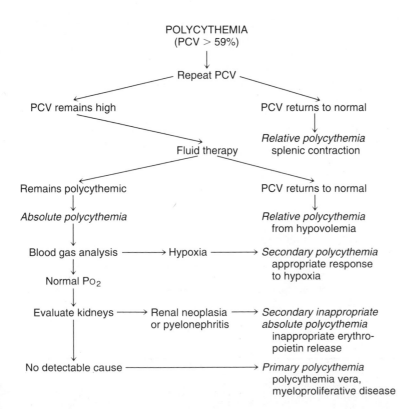

Figure 3–8 Diagnostic approach to polycythemia. The italicized common conclusions are made using the various procedures listed. Primary polycythemia is diagnosed by exclusion when splenic contraction is unlikely; the hydration status is normal; no hypoxia is found from pulmonary, cardiac, or hemoglobin disorders; and the kidneys are normal.

poietin secretion occurs. Inappropriate secondary absolute polycythemia has been reported in dogs with renal cell carcinoma, renal lymphosarcoma, and chronic pyelonephritis. The PCVs vary from 64% to 81%. Serum erythropoietin, which is normally not detectable in dogs, is increased (i.e., ≥0.1–0.3 IU/ml). After removal of the diseased kidney, the PCV and erythropoietin values should return to normal.

Bibliography

Alsaker RD, Laber J, Stevens J, Perman V: A comparison of polychromasia and reticulocyte counts in assessing erythrocytic regenerative response in the cat. JAVMA 1977; 170:39–41.

Brown DE, Weiser MG, Thrall MA, Giger U: Inherited stomatocytosis with macrocytosis in a dog. Proceedings, Annual Meeting, American Society for Veterinary Clinical Pathology. San Diego, CA, November 16, 1992.

Christopher MM: Relation of endogenous Heinz bodies to disease and anemia in cats: 120 cases (1978–1987). JAVMA 1989;194:1089–1095.

Cramer DV, Lewis RM: Reticulocyte response in the cat. JAVMA 1972;160:61–67.

Duncan JR, Prasse KW: Veterinary Laboratory Medicine: Clinical Pathology. 2nd ed. Ames, Iowa State University Press, 1986, pp 128–131.

Feldman BF, Kaneko JJ, Farver TB: Anemia of inflammatory disease in the dog. Ferrokinetics of adjuvant-induced anemia. Am J Vet Res 1981;42:583.

Flemming FJ, McCaw DL, Smith JA, et al: Clinical, hematologic, and survival data from cats infected with feline immunodeficiency virus: 42 cases (1983–1988). JAVMA 1991;199:913–916.

Fletch SM, Smart ME, Pennock PW, Subden RE: Clinical and pathologic features of chondrodysplasia (dwarfism) in the Alaskan malamute. JAVMA 1973;162:357–361.

Glen BL, Stair EL: Cytauxzoonosis in domestic cats: Reports of two cases in Oklahoma with a review and discussion of the disease. JAVMA 1984;184:822–825.

Harvey JW, Giger U: Hyperventilation-induced hemolysis in a dog associated with alkaline-sensitive erythrocytes. Vet Clin Pathol 1984;13:33.

Harvey JW, French TW, Meyer DJ: Chronic iron deficiency anemia in dogs. JAAHA 1982;18:946–960.

Harvey JW, Wolfsheimer KJ, Simpson CF, French TW: Pathologic sideroblasts and siderocytes associated with chloramphenicol therapy in a dog. Vet Clin Pathol 1985;14:36–42.

Jain NC: Schalm's Veterinary Hematology. 4th ed. Philadelphia, Lea and Febiger, 1986.

Kociba GJ, Caputo CA: Aplastic anemia associated with estrus in pet ferrets. JAVMA 1981;178:1293–1294.

Maggio-Price L, Emerson CL, Hinds TR, et al: Hereditary nonspherocytic hemolytic anemia in beagles. Am J Vet Res 1988;49:1020–1025.

Perman V, Schall WB: Diseases of the red blood cells. In Ettinger SJ (ed): Textbook of Veterinary Internal Medicine: Diseases of the Dog and Cat. 2nd ed, vol 2. Philadelphia, WB Saunders, 1983.

Randolph JF, Center SA, Kallfelz FA, et al: Familial nonspherocytic hemolytic anemia in poodles. Am J Vet Res 1986;47:687–695.

Reagan WJ, Vap LM, Weiser MG: Flow cytometric analysis of feline reticulocytes. Vet Pathol 1992;29:503–508.

Rose BD: Clinical Physiology of Acid-Base and Electrolyte Disorders. 2nd ed. New York, McGraw-Hill, 1984, p 300.

Schalm OW: Morphologic classification of anemias. Vet Clin Pathol 1978;7:6–8.

Schrader LA, Hurvitz AI: Cold agglutinin disease in a cat. JAVMA 1983;183:121–122.

Slappendale RJ: The diagnostic significance of the direct antiglobulin test (DAT) in anemic dogs. Vet Immunol Immunopathol 1979;1:49–59.

Troy GC, Vulgamott JC, Turnwald GH: Canine ehrlichiosis: A retrospective study of 30 naturally occurring cases. JAAHA 1980;16:181–187.

Weiser MG, Kociba GJ: Sequential changes in erythrocyte volume distribution and microcytosis associated with iron deficiency in kittens. Vet Pathol 1983;20:1–12.

Weiss DJ: Uniform evaluation and semiquantitative reporting of hematologic data in veterinary laboratories. Vet Clin Pathol 1984;13:27–31.

Weiss DJ: Canine pure red cell aplasia: Identification of antibody-mediated suppression in 2 of 5 cases. Proc ASVCP 1985:18.

Weiss DJ, Armstrong PJ: Non-regenerative anemias in the dog. Comp Cont Ed 1984;6:452–459.

Weiss DJ: Aplastic anemia. In Kirk RW, Bonagura JD (eds): Current Veterinary Therapy XI: Small Animal Practice. Philadelphia, WB Saunders, 1992.

Werner LL: Coombs' positive anemias in the dog and cat. Comp Cont Ed 1980;96:96–101.

Willard MD, Zevbe CA, Schall WD, et al: Severe hypophosphatemia associated with diabetes mellitus in six dogs and one cat. JAVMA 1987;190:1007.

Harold Tvedten

4 Leukocyte Disorders

○ **Miscellaneous Leukocyte Disorders**
    Feline Leukemia Virus
    Feline Immunodeficiency Virus
    Pelger-Huet Anomaly
    Chediak-Higashi Syndrome
    Canine Leukocyte Function Defects

    Cyclic Hematopoiesis
    Storage Diseases
    Canine Parvovirus
    Feline Panleukopenia

BASIC LEUKOCYTE CONCEPTS

The interpretation of specific abnormalities of the leukogram (e.g., neutrophilia or lymphopenia) and the diagnostic characteristics of most hematopoietic neoplasms are described in this chapter. Technical aspects affecting small clinical laboratories and general comments on complete blood count (CBC) conclusions are in Chapter 2. Certain basic leukocyte (white blood cell [WBC]) concepts must be reviewed to avoid common errors in interpretation and to aid understanding of the mechanisms of certain WBC changes.

Absolute Versus Relative Leukocyte Values

For initial evaluation of the leukogram (i.e., the WBC data on a CBC), each type of WBC should be individually interpreted by its absolute values. The leukogram can then be summarized by a few terms. For example, mature neutrophilia, lymphopenia, and monocytosis indicate, in a few words, that the CBC had an increase in the number of mature, segmented neutrophils with no increase in the number of immature nonsegmented neutrophils (N-segs), the lymphocyte count was decreased, and the monocyte count was increased. The interpretation of increases or decreases of each cell type is made as described later.

The use of absolute WBC data allows more consistent evaluation of various patients than the relative percentage values do. The relative WBC count in per cent is obtained from the WBC differential count from a blood smear examination. The absolute values are derived by multiplying the percentage of each cell type by the total WBC count. For example, 65% segmented neutrophils (segs) with a 10,000/µl WBC count is equal to 6500 segs/µl. Question: Is 6500 segs/µl always normal? Yes. Is 65% segs always normal? No. If the WBC count is 1000/µl, then that dog would have a neutropenia with only 650 segs/µl. If the WBC count is 50,000/µl, then there is a neutrophilia of 32,500 segs/µl (see Fig. 4–1 for a comparison of the absolute and relative numbers of N-segs).

Leukocyte Pathways/Leukocyte Pools

In order to interpret a concentration, one must consider where the sample was collected and what compartment the data represent (e.g., a high creatinine concentration is normal for urine but abnormal for serum). Depending on where the sample is obtained, the number and

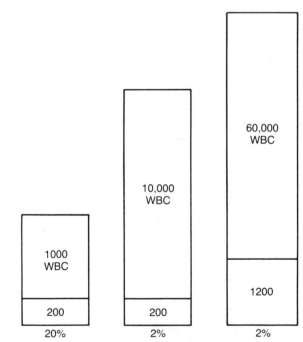

Figure 4–1 Relative and absolute leukocyte counts. The bottom chamber of each bar indicates the absolute number of nonsegmented neutrophils (N-segs), and the percentage below the bars indicates the relative number of N-segs. The relative change between the first and second bar (i.e., 20% to 2%) seems great, yet there was no change in the absolute number of N-segs in the blood (i.e., 200 N-segs/µl). The relative percentage of N-segs between the second and third bar seems identical, yet there is a normal number of N-segs in a dog with 200 N-segs/µl and a true increase with 1200 N-segs/µl in the third bar.

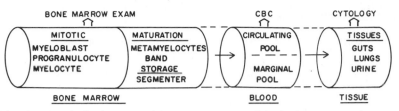

Figure 4–2 Neutrophil pathway in the body. Neutrophils in various areas of the body are grouped into pools for evaluation. The bone marrow cells are divided into the mitotic, maturation, and storage pools (see text). Neutrophils in blood are either in the circulating pool, which is sampled by a complete blood count (CBC), or the marginal pool, hidden from the CBC. Neutrophils move in one direction into the tissues, where they are evaluated by cytology or histopathology. (Modified after Boggs DR, Winkelstein A: White Cell Manual. 3rd ed. Philadelphia, FA Davis, 1975; and Prasse, 1983.)

types of WBCs mean different things. A bone marrow aspirate and biopsy allows conclusions about the degree of marrow activity (e.g., myeloid hyperplasia or hypoplasia) and qualitative observations on morphologic alterations. The CBC allows quantitative and qualitative observations about WBCs freely circulating in the peripheral blood. The leukogram of a CBC represents the current balance of bone marrow production, tissue demand, and distribution of WBCs in the vascular system (Figs. 4–2 to 4–4). Cytologic preparations like lymph node aspirates evaluate WBCs in tissues in terms of numbers, degree of degeneration, and possible identification of an etiologic agent.

Pools are used to conceptualize where WBCs

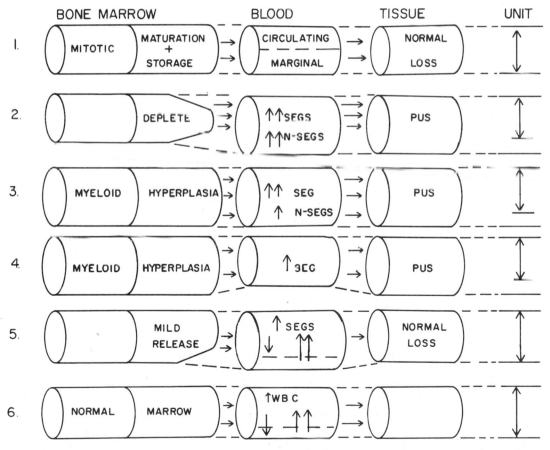

Figure 4–3 Illustrations to visualize cell movements in neutrophilia and leukocytosis. Examples are (1) normal, (2) inflammation of recent onset, (3) inflammation of a few days' duration, (4) chronic inflammation, (5) stress/steroid reaction, and (6) exercise/epinephrine response. (See text for descriptions of the processes.) The unit at the far right illustrates the increased migration of neutrophils into inflamed tissues in 2, 3, and 4. A normal migration of neutrophils into tissues is expected in 1, 5, and 6. The double arrows in blood of 5 and 6 indicate increased movement out of the marginal pools into the circulating pools due to the effect of glucocorticoids (5) or epinephrine (6).

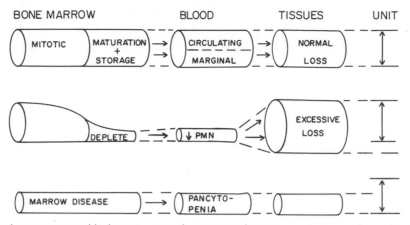

Figure 4–4 Causes of neutropenia and leukopenia. Examples are normal (top), excessive tissue demand (middle), and primary bone marrow disease (bottom). (See text for descriptions.) Neutropenia of severe inflammatory disease (middle) is characterized by rapid migration of neutrophils into inflamed tissues in excess of normal (i.e., exceeds unit arrow that represents normal) and in excess of bone marrow production capacity. This depletes the storage and maturation pools and even draws on the mitotic pool of the marrow (i.e., myelocytes and earlier forms are released into blood). Neutropenia/leukopenia of primary marrow disease is often characterized by pancytopenia or bicytopenia. A lack of neutrophils for migration into tissues predisposes the animal to infections.

are in various compartments along the WBC pathways. The pool concept, when understood, can simplify interpretation of data. The bone marrow is usually divided into two or three pools. The earliest compartment is the mitotic pool of myeloblasts, promyelocytes, and myelocytes. The maturation pool is young neutrophils (i.e., metamyelocytes and bands) that lack mitotic ability. The storage pool includes the segs being stored for a sudden tissue demand. The maturation and storage pools are combined in Figure 4–2 for simplicity.

The WBCs described by the leukogram are those collected from the circulating pool. The marginal pool is a "hidden" population of neutrophils that marginate along vascular linings in capillaries of the lungs and elsewhere. In dogs, the circulating and marginal pools are about equal. A cat has a marginal pool two to three times its circulating pool. This is important in the interpretation of neutrophil and total WBC count changes, since certain mediators in the body (i.e., epinephrine, endotoxin, and mediators of anaphylaxis) cause rapid shifts in the distribution of cells within the vascular system and alteration in the leukogram.

Neutrophils normally spend only about 10 hours in the vascular system, then migrate into the respiratory, digestive, and urinary tracts at a low rate in response to bacteria and debris. The cells may be seen in respiratory cytologic samples and urine but are quickly lysed in the septic environment of the stool. During inflammatory disease, the neutrophils may collect as visible pus. In diseases like enteritis, the neutrophils in

the tissue phase may be hidden from cytologic or gross observation but are reflected in the leukogram.

QUANTITATIVE LEUKOCYTE CHANGES

Neutrophil/Leukocyte Changes

Neutrophilia/Leukocytosis • Leukocytosis is usually synonymous with a neutrophilia. In 232 CBCs with a leukocytosis of >17,000 WBCs/μl, 226 (97.4%) had a neutrophilia. Other cell types had minor effects on the WBC count. Only 88 (37.9%) had a mild monocytosis, 11 (4.7%) had an eosinophilia, and 10 (4.2%) had a lymphocytosis.

Neutrophilia and leukocytosis have four main causes or diagnostic considerations: (1) inflammation, (2) stress/steroids, (3) exercise/epinephrine, and (4) leukemia. Leukemia is discussed later. Keys to differentiate the first three are summarized in Figure 4–5. Inflammation is most specifically demonstrated by the presence of a left shift (i.e., an absolute increase in N-segs). Inflammation may also be suggested by a magnitude of leukocytosis usually not reached by the other two processes. In the absence of these indicators, the absolute lymphocyte count is useful. A lymphopenia usually indicates an endogenous (i.e., stress) or exogenous glucocorticoid effect. A transient leukocytosis accompanied by a lymphocytosis implies an epinephrine or exercise effect. Combinations are

Figure 4–5 Evaluation of leukocytosis and neutrophilia. The common causes of neutrophilia and subsequent leukocytosis may usually be differentiated on the basis of the immaturity of the neutrophils, the magnitude of the neutrophilia in the absence of leukemia, and the tendency of the lymphocytes to increase or decrease. Granulocytic leukemia is rare and not considered here. When the laboratory finding is present (i.e., yes), the conclusion to the right is made. When the laboratory finding is absent (i.e., no), one moves down to the next differentiating feature. Note that inflammation may be responsible for total WBC counts less than 30,000–40,000/μl that are associated with lymphopenia due to concurrent stress. Note also some leukograms lack features to clearly indicate the causes(s).

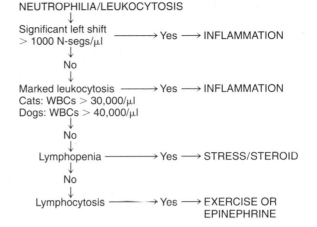

common (e.g., inflammation and stress). When mild changes are present (e.g., chronic inflammation with small leukocytosis and little or no left shift), a specific cause of the leukocytosis is hard to determine.

Inflammation • Inflammation is a common and important laboratory diagnosis. Most inflammatory processes involve neutrophils, so the major consideration in a neutrophilia/leukocytosis is active inflammation (see preceding for differential diagnosis). Neutrophils predominate in suppurative or exudative diseases, but other WBCs (e.g., eosinophils, monocytes/macrophages, and lymphocytes) are involved in other forms of inflammation and are a minor or variable component of suppurative diseases (see following sections on these other WBCs). Bacterial infections are a common cause, but fungal, protozoal, and viral infections may also be responsible. However, many inflammatory processes are not septic in origin, so inflammation does not mean infection. Nonseptic causes of inflammation include necrosis (e.g., pancreatitis, pansteatitis), chemicals (e.g., turpentine is an experimental method of abscess formation), immune-mediated diseases (e.g., lupus, immune-mediated hemolytic anemia), and toxins (e.g., endotoxin). Neoplasms may be responsible for inflammatory leukograms by either (1) allowing secondary bacterial infections, (2) damaging normal tissue, (3) outgrowing their blood supply and necrosing, or (4) producing a paraneoplastic effect. The CBC is indicated to document the presence of an inflammatory disease, to suggest the current prognosis, and to monitor recovery. The CBC will not normally document sepsis or specific etiologic agents or pinpoint the location of the inflammation but may justify additional testing (e.g., cytology, culture, serum chemistries, radiographs, ultrasonography, or serology) to identify the cause and/or the location of the disease.

The leukogram is not always abnormal when an animal has an inflammatory disease. This is especially true if the inflammation is mild, chronic, or not invading tissues (e.g., surface inflammation like cystitis). Other means to document inflammation include cytology and urinalysis. The finding of increased rouleaux in canine blood smears supports the conclusion of inflammation. Fibrinogen and other acute phase proteins are not commonly measured in dogs and cats but are additional indicators of inflammation.

The severity of the left shift is indicated by the absolute number of N-segs and how immature the neutrophil population became. Forms of N-segs seen in the blood include bands (i.e., stabs), metamyelocytes, myelocytes, and even promyelocytes (Color Plate 1F). Bands usually compose most of the left shift, since the most mature neutrophils tend to leave the bone marrow first. Neutrophils younger than bands indicate a more severe left shift, and the severity of the left shift reflects the severity of the inflammatory process. Prasse (1983) recommends a cutoff of 1000 N-segs/μl as a minimum to indicate a purulent-exudative process of some intensity. Milder left shifts of 300 to 1000/μl occur in nonsuppurative diseases (e.g., hemorrhagic, catarrhal, or nonsuppurative granulomatous diseases).

Laboratories vary in how left shifts are reported. Often, all immature neutrophils are included in an N-seg category. If there are many myelocytes and metamyelocytes, then the severity of the left shift is hidden, since one expects that the N-segs are band neutrophils. If the bands are becoming depleted and metamyelo-

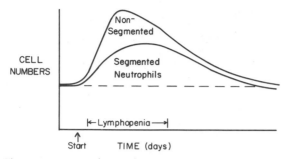

Figure 4–6 Expected WBC changes with resolving inflammation. The greatest leukocytosis and left shift are expected early in the acute stages of inflammation. This period is also accompanied by the lymphopenia of stress. During later phases of inflammation, a more mature neutrophilia is expected, since bone marrow hyperplasia and marrow production of neutrophils should be adequate to allow maturation of neutrophils before release into blood. Tissue demand for neutrophils also tends to decrease during recovery.

cytes and myelocytes are being released, there must be great tissue demand and consumption of neutrophils. If the percentage and absolute number of metamyelocytes, myelocytes, and promyelocytes are reported, one can better judge the severity. Excessive numbers of blast cells or irregular maturation patterns may suggest a granulocytic leukemia.

Time-Related Changes ● Expected changes in the leukogram through a typical inflammatory process are illustrated in Figures 4–3 and 4–6. A poorer prognosis is implied by variations from the expected response. The greatest left shift would be expected in the early stages of the disease process (see Fig. 4–6). The storage pool of segs in the marrow is depleted, followed by release of bands and metamyelocytes in the maturation pool (Fig. 4–3, part 2). Over days, myeloid hyperplasia in the bone marrow should provide adequate rate of production of neutrophils to allow more maturation of neutrophils to occur before their release into blood and thus a lessening of the severity of the left shift (Fig. 4–3, part 3). As the tissue inflammation decreases, the marrow should reach a production rate sufficient for most cells to mature be-

fore release into the blood. Thus, chronic stages of the process may have little to no left shift, and the magnitude of the leukocytosis may be minimal to absent (Fig. 4–3, part 4). This chronic phase is the hardest to identify as an inflammatory process from the CBC data without other information (e.g., exudate found by cytology). Individual animals vary from this pattern owing to treatments or variations in the disease intensity.

Prognosis ● The magnitude of the neutrophilia/leukocytosis or neutropenia/leukopenia in inflammation reflects the balance of bone marrow production and tissue demand (see Figs. 4–3 and 4–4). Leukocytosis, neutrophilia, and left shift of a magnitude of change that is typical for the species suggest a reasonable balance between bone marrow production and tissue demand. This is CBC evidence of a favorable prognosis. Obviously, other factors not derived from the CBC data, such as the particular tissue inflamed (e.g., subcutaneous abscess versus acute pancreatitis) and the cause of the inflammation, are also critical in the prognosis.

What is a typical magnitude of leukocytosis? Canine leukocytosis is usually <40,000 WBCs/μl. In 182 canine CBCs with a leukocytosis, 151 (83%) were from 17,500 to 39,990 WBCs/μl. About 12% were moderate to marked increases (i.e., 40,000–60,360/μl), and 5% had a marked to extreme leukocytosis of 61,050 to 127,500/μl. Of 30 feline CBCs with a leukocytosis, 21 were <30,000 WBCs/μl, whereas six were from 30,000 to 50,000/μl and three were >50,000/μl. The magnitude of feline leukocytosis is usually less than in dogs, with some from the 30,000 to 50,000 WBC/μl range but rarely >75,000/μl (Jain, 1986).

Four criteria suggesting a poor prognosis are summarized in Table 4–1. Causes are discussed with leukopenia/neutropenia. If the bone marrow is responding to an inflammatory process as seen by a left shift, then dogs and cats should have a leukocytosis unless the inflammation is unusually severe. A degenerative left shift is a left shift without increased neutrophils. This is

Table 4–1 LEUKOGRAM FINDINGS CONSIDERED POOR PROGNOSTIC INDICATORS

Finding	Reason for Poor Prognosis
Degenerative left shift	Tissue demand exceeds the bone marrow's production
Leukopenia	Tissue demand exceeds the bone marrow's production
Nonsegmented neutrophils exceed segmented ones	Bone marrow's release of neutrophils is at a rate too high to allow maturation of neutrophils
Leukemoid reaction	Tissue demand is marked, and the excessive neutrophilia seems ineffective

the classic WBC pattern taught to portend a poor prognosis, but it is often misused. Be careful to understand the principle and not be locked to a definition.

One must consider the magnitude of the leukocytosis and left shift. The reference ranges of normal WBC and neutrophil counts are broad. If the left shift is mild and the WBC or neutrophil count is in the normal to high-normal range, one could inappropriately apply the definition of a degenerative left shift. However, this is inappropriate, since this pattern simply signifies a mild inflammatory response and there is not the poor prognosis suggested by "degenerative left shift." The greater the leukopenia/neutropenia or the more the left shift is >1000/μl, the poorer the prognosis.

Leukopenia may be too severe (e.g., <600 WBCs/μl) to note an increased absolute number of immature neutrophils, so there is no left shift and thus no degenerative left shift. Leukopenia and neutropenia are unfavorable prognostic signs by themselves. Either the bone marrow production is insufficient or the use of neutrophils in the tissues is too strong or both. Leukopenia/neutropenia during acute stages of canine parvovirus infection is from marked loss of neutrophils into the gut, combined with a virus that may interfere with granulopoiesis.

Finding more immature neutrophils than segs in the blood suggests that the marrow cannot produce neutrophils at a rate sufficient for them to mature properly. Even if a leukocytosis exists, this third pattern indicates excessive tissue demand and a poorer prognosis.

A leukemoid reaction is so marked a leukocytosis (i.e., >50,000–100,000 WBCs/μl) that it resembles a granulocytic leukemia (see Granulocytic Leukemia for differentiating features). A poor prognosis is indicated, since the magnitude of the stimulus on the bone marrow suggests a serious problem. Despite numerous neutrophils, the disease is not corrected. For example, a cat with pyometra may have abundant uterine pus, yet without proper drainage, the exudative process is not curative. Besides anatomic problems, there are functional defects like leukocyte adhesion protein deficiency (canine granulocytopathic syndrome) in Irish setter dogs, in which the WBCs are unable to ingest organisms (Trowald-Wigh et al., 1992). The lack of adhesion proteins CD11b and CD causes severe recurrent infections. Of 12 affected puppies, 8 had leukemoid reactions ranging from 49.4 to 107.5 × 10^9 WBCs/L, and all had a leukocytosis. Some common causes of a leukemoid reaction include pyometra, abscesses, and estrogen toxicity.

Toxic Neutrophils • Toxic changes in circulating neutrophils (see Chapter 2) indicate toxemia. Toxemia suggests the presence of inflammation. Bacterial toxins stimulate the most severe toxic changes in neutrophils, but nonbacterial toxins may also be responsible. The significance of and confidence in the conclusion of toxemia are based on the number of neutrophils altered (e.g., percentage or few-moderate-many) and severity of toxicity (e.g., 1+ to 4+). A few 1+ toxic neutrophils are usually ignored, whereas many 4+ toxic neutrophils are an unfavorable prognostic sign (Color Plate 1F). The numerical values on a CBC may be normal, yet the subjective observation of toxic changes may indicate disease (see Chapter 2, Blood Smear Analysis). An example was a cat with a crushed paw that had been infested with maggots. Grossly necrotic tissue should have stimulated an inflammatory leukogram, but the WBC count and differential were normal; the only change on the cat's CBC was toxic neutrophils. Severely toxic neutrophils in a young dog with diarrhea are strongly suggestive of parvovirus infection. Abundant bacterial toxins are absorbed from the damaged bowel to cause the toxic change in neutrophils.

Leukopenia/Neutropenia • Neutropenia and leukopenia occur infrequently in dogs and cats. The two most likely causes are excessive tissue consumption in an inflammatory process and primary bone marrow disease (see Fig. 4–1 and Table 4–9). A third cause of neutropenia/leukopenia usually seen only in experimental settings is a temporary shift of neutrophils into the marginal pool and thus "out of sight" of the CBC. Endotoxin and mediators of anaphylaxis can cause this "pseudoneutropenia" of decreased total WBC and neutrophil counts without really changing the number of cells in the total blood granulocyte pool.

Neutropenias of excessive tissue consumption (see Fig. 4–4) are severe diseases in which very immature neutrophils are drawn from the marrow, even from the mitotic pool (e.g., myelocytes and progranulocytes). An inflammatory process involving large surface areas (e.g., peritonitis from a ruptured bowel) or septicemia is likely to cause such a leukopenia. Infections with gram-negative bacteria are frequently associated with a consumptive neutropenia. When a severe left shift, marked toxicity, and a decreasing or low WBC count are present, then a gram-negative bacterial infection should be suspected. In contrast, localized suppurative processes like an abscess or pyometra with pyogenic bacteria are likely to cause a leukocytosis.

Table 4–2 BASIC CAUSES OF NEUTROPENIA TO BE CONSIDERED IN DOGS AND CATS

	Animals Affected
Consumption of Neutrophils	
Overwhelming sepsis/endotoxemia (e.g., peritonitis from intestinal perforation)	Dogs/Cats
Salmonellosis	Dogs/Cats
Immune-mediated destruction	Dogs
Bone-Marrow Suppression	
FeLV	Cats
FIV	Cats
Parvovirus	Dogs/Cats
Ehrlichiosis	Dogs
Bone marrow toxicity	Dogs/Cats
Estrogen (endogenous/ exogenous)	
Phenylbutazone	
Other drugs	
Bone marrow neoplasia	Dogs/Cats
Myelophthisis/myelonecrosis	Dogs/Cats
Immune-mediated destruction of precursors	Dogs/Cats

Courtesy of Dr M.D. Willard.

To differentiate leukopenia of overwhelming infection from leukopenia of bone marrow disease, use the CBC to check the status of other cell lines. A pancytopenia or bicytopenia including a nonregenerative anemia or thrombocytopenia is strong evidence of bone marrow disease and indicates a bone marrow aspirate and biopsy. Primary bone marrow disease is often characterized by decreased production of all cell lines. Neutrophils have a short life span in blood, so they may be decreased before erythrocytes (red blood cells [RBCs]) and platelets. Consider the time course in differentiating these two causes of neutropenia. Bone marrow–related leukopenias tend to be slowly developing, persistent problems, whereas diseases causing a consumptive leukopenia/neutropenia are acute, with rapid changes for the better or worse. Toxic changes in neutrophils, rouleaux, and immature neutrophils suggest leukopenia due to severe inflammation/infection.

Neutropenia/leukopenia of marrow toxicity occurs during anticancer chemotherapy, and some guidelines are available to anticipate sepsis from the neutropenia (Couto, 1986). Neutrophil counts are often lowest 5 to 7 days after initiation of treatment, and <2000 neutrophils/μl requires monitoring the patient for sepsis. Sepsis (probably from enteric bacteria) is assumed if a patient has <500 neutrophils/μl and is febrile. Chemotherapy with myelosuppressive agents should usually be discontinued if the neutrophil count is <2500/μl or the platelet count is <50,000/μl.

Myeloid Hypoplasia/Myeloid Hyperplasia ● A bone marrow examination is required if the neutropenia/leukopenia is persistent and unexplained. Possible morphologic conclusions include myelofibrosis, a fatty marrow, myeloid hypoplasia, or ineffective granulopoiesis (see Chapter 2). An etiologic diagnosis (e.g., estrogen or phenylbutazone toxicity) is not usually obtained from the marrow aspirate and biopsy.

Ineffective granulopoiesis is suggested when developing myeloid cells are present in the marrow in adequate numbers but for some reason are not effective in releasing mature neutrophils into circulation. It is an example of a dysplastic change in the absence of a leukemic process. Ineffective granulopoiesis occurs in feline leukemia virus (FeLV) infections. About half of the neutropenic cats that were infected with FeLV had marked granulocytic hyperplasia in one study (Prasse, 1983). Myeloid hypoplasia in the other half of the FeLV-infected cats is more expected with a virus killing the marrow cells and causing a neutropenia. Neutropenia with normal to increased myeloid cells in the marrow indicates ineffective granulopoiesis if one proves tissue consumption of neutrophils is not the cause of the neutropenia.

Leukopenia/neutropenia, in the absence of tissue consumption of neutrophils, is usually due to damage or depletion of developing myeloid cells (i.e., myeloid hypoplasia). Other causes of myeloid hypoplasia include feline panleukopenia virus, canine parvovirus, endogenous and exogenous estrogen toxicity in dogs, *Ehrlichia canis*, cancer chemotherapy, and other drugs like phenylbutazone or trimethoprim-sulfadiazine (see Chapter 3, Aplastic Pancytopenia). If these causes of a neutropenia have been ruled out, then glucocorticosteroid treatment for immune-mediated removal of neutrophils may be attempted, since steroid-responsive neutropenia has occurred in dogs and cats. Falsely low total WBC counts may occur from WBC clumping in EDTA *in vitro* (see Chapter 2).

Myeloid hyperplasia of the bone marrow is expected with inflammation of >2 to 3 days' duration. The leukocytosis and left shift in the CBC prove it, so the expense and effort of a bone marrow biopsy are redundant. Myeloid hyperplasia as a bone marrow examination diagnosis is usually secondary to investigation of another problem, such as nonregenerative anemia, thrombocytopenia, or leukemia, that has a concurrent inflammatory response.

Stress/Steroid Pattern ● Stress and steroids are common causes of neutrophilia. The classic CBC pattern is a mature neutrophilia, moderate leukocytosis, lymphopenia, eosinopenia, and, especially in dogs, monocytosis. The mature neutrophilia may have a right shift, which is an increased number of more mature, hypersegmented neutrophils. Stress reaction mediated by glucocorticoids and steroid therapy (e.g., prednisolone, dexamethasone) are common. The initial leukocytosis of steroid treatment in dogs may reach 30,000 to 40,000 WBCs/μl, mainly due to neutrophilia. The typical response is 15,000 to 25,000 WBCs/μl (Duncan and Prasse, 1986). The blood changes occur over 4 to 12 hours and return to normal in 24 hours, so one may miss the initial change depending on when the sample is taken. In people, the initial hematologic response is not dose dependent nor affected by the pharmacologic half-life of the glucocorticoid. In cats, the leukocytosis is usually not quite as high and a monocytosis may not be present. The hematologic pattern from hyperadrenocorticism and probably long-term steroid treatment is mainly eosinopenia and lymphopenia without neutrophilia, leukocytosis, or monocytosis.

A stressed or steroid-treated animal with a concurrent process stimulating an eosinophilia may have a variable eosinophil count, depending on which has the stronger effect.

Age affects the expected lymphocyte count, with younger animals having greater numbers. Jain (1986) uses the following as minimal numbers for lymphocytes of dogs in different age categories: 3 to 6 months, 2000/μl; 8 to 24 months, 1500/μl; and over 24 months, 1000/μl. Lower lymphocyte numbers are considered lymphopenia.

Not all the expected stress/steroid WBC changes may be present in each case, even after a known injection of a glucocorticoid. Thus, use a "best fit" approach to classify a leukogram. For example, Table 4–3 lists hematologic data from a normal dog treated repeatedly with dexamethasone. One day after treatment (i.e., Saturday), five of the expected steroid/stress changes were present (i.e., leukocytosis, neutro-

philia, no left shift, eosinopenia, and monocytosis). Lymphopenia was not present, even though this is usually the most consistent change. On day 3 (i.e., Monday), a lymphocytosis, monocytosis, and eosinophilia best resembled a physiologic leukocytosis. Only on day 5 (i.e., Wednesday) was the classic steroid/stress pattern present. This illustrates the variability and the need to fit the pattern to the most consistent conclusion even when the cause is known.

A left shift is not expected in animals with only stress or steroid treatment. A right shift with hypersegmented neutrophils is more likely, since steroids decrease emigration of neutrophils from the vascular system. This increases the half-life of neutrophils in blood and allows them to continue to mature and increase the number of lobes in the nucleus. A hypersegmented neutrophil has five or more lobes. Steroids also increase marrow release of neutrophils, but this effect is usually too mild to stimulate release of bands and metamyelocytes. The storage pool of mature segs should be adequate to prevent a left shift during a stress/steroid response unless something like an inflammatory process has depleted it before the steroid effect. Mature neutrophils are preferentially released from the marrow. More than 1000 N-segs/μl, and probably 500 N-segs/μl, indicates an inflammatory disease. A lymphopenia indicates concurrent stress or steroid treatment.

The effects of steroid treatment on canine WBCs are better understood by considering Tables 4–4 and 4–5. Figure 4–3, part 5, illustrates the neutrophil changes in steroid/stress neutrophilia. The neutrophils in blood are increased with a shift of cells to the circulating pool. There is slower emigration of neutrophils into tissues, but this is not likely a major factor. The mild bone marrow release is mainly from the storage pool of segs.

Exercise/Epinephrine Pattern • A transient physiologic leukocytosis occurs in animals dur-

Table 4–3 LEUKOCYTE CHANGES IN A DOG TREATED WITH DEXAMETHASONE

	Friday	Saturday	Monday	Tuesday	Wednesday
WBCs/μl	12,200	22,200	19,600	31,100	29,300
Segs/μl	9525	18,648	10,976	26,433	25,491
N-segs/μl	0	0	196	0	0
Lymphs/μl	1905	1998	5096	1866	879
Monos/μl	635	1554	2156	2799	3132
Eosins/μl	635	0	1176	0	0

Hematologic data are from an apparently normal dog treated daily with dexamethasone except on Sunday to create the steroid/stress leukogram for illustrative purposes. Data for Friday, the first day before treatment, should be used as the reference values.

Table 4–4 EFFECTS OF CORTISONE ON CANINE GRANULOCYTES

	Granulocyte Count (cells/μl)	TBGP (×10⁷/kg)	T½ (hours)	Granulocyte Turnover Rate (×10⁷ cells/kg/day)
Control	5600 (3.0–8.4 × 10³)	88 (53–112)	5.3 (3.8–6.3)	301 (157–468)
Treated	13,800 (8.7–30.1 × 10³)	162 (67–269)	7.6 (6.0–10.2)	352 (136–438)

Values are given as mean (range). A neutrophilia in the cortisone-treated dogs is reflected in an increased granulocyte count, which is approximately the absolute neutrophil count. The total blood granulocyte pool (TBGP) is the total number of granulocytes (mainly neutrophils) in the body and is based on body weight. It illustrates a true increase in the neutrophils in the blood of dogs treated with glucocorticoids. The half-life (T½) of neutrophils illustrates a longer life span of neutrophils in the vascular system. The granulocyte turnover rate documents an increased release of neutrophils from the marrow. (From Boggs DR, Winkelstein A: White Cell Manual. 3rd ed. Philadelphia, FA Davis, 1975.)

ing exercise and epinephrine release as a result of fear. There is no real increase in the total blood neutrophil pool (TBNP), but only a shift of cells into the circulating pool, where they are "seen" by the CBC. There is no increase in release of neutrophils from the marrow or any significant decrease in the emigration of neutrophils out of the vascular system. It is difficult to recognize a physiologic leukocytosis in dogs except in research settings, since the changes are mild and often stay within the reference range. Physiologic leukocytosis in cats is greater in magnitude since cats have a marginal neutrophil pool almost three times as large as the circulating pool (see Table 4–5). Distribution shifts into the circulating pool are significant in cats. In young healthy cats, the WBC count often reaches 20,000/μl, with 6000 to 15,000 lymphocytes/μl (Duncan and Prasse, 1986). Dogs have nearly equal marginal and circulating neutrophil pools.

Monocytosis/Monocytopenia

Monocytes are the immature blood stage of macrophages in the tissues. More specific indi-

Table 4–5 TOTAL BLOOD NEUTROPHIL POOL, CIRCULATING NEUTROPHIL POOL, AND MARGINAL NEUTROPHIL POOL IN DOGS AND CATS

	Dog	Cat
TBNP × 10⁸/kg	10.2	28.9
CNP × 10⁸/kg	5.4	7.8
MNP × 10⁸/kg	4.8	21.0

The total blood neutrophil pool (TBNP) in cats is larger than in dogs mainly owing to a very large marginal neutrophil pool. The relatively large feline marginal neutrophil pool (MNP) compared with the dog allows a larger potential shift of neutrophils into the circulating neutrophil pool (CNP) and a noticeable leukocytosis during fear and excitement. (Data from Prasse KW: White blood cell disorders. In Ettinger SJ (ed): Textbook of Veterinary Internal Medicine. Diseases of the Dog and Cat. 2nd ed, vol 2. Philadelphia, WB Saunders, 1983.)

cators (e.g., enzyme content and functional ability) define when a monocyte matures into a macrophage, but it is convenient to consider the monocytes of blood and bone marrow as immature and the macrophages in tissue as the mature form of the same cell. Tissue macrophages include hepatic Kupffer's cells, alveolar macrophages, epithelioid cells, giant cells, and histiocytes.

Macrophages remove large substances like necrotic debris, certain organisms like fungi, foreign bodies, abnormal RBCs, and neoplastic cells. A monocytosis is expected during diseases likely to have a persistently high need for macrophages. In immune-mediated hemolytic anemia, for example, the RBCs with antibody or complement on them are continuously being destroyed, and the necrotic cell debris must be removed. Macrophages are a later component of all inflammatory processes. Monocytosis occurs with suppurative, pyogranulomatous, granulomatous, necrotic, malignant, hemolytic, hemorrhagic, or immune-mediated diseases (Prasse, 1983).

The differential diagnosis of monocytosis includes the stress/steroid response especially in dogs, disorders requiring macrophages, and chronic inflammatory diseases. Both acute stressful and chronic disorders are similarly associated with a monocytosis. Monocytosis occurred in 30% of 760 (i.e., 228) dogs. Chronic disorders were present in 135 cases, and acute stressful disorders in 97. In 225 cats, 11% had a monocytosis. Eleven had acute stressful problems, and 16 had chronic disorders. Thus, when monocytosis occurs, first check the CBC for evidence of the stress/steroid pattern. If lymphopenia and eosinopenia are not present, then evaluate the animal for chronic inflammation and processes with cell destruction. A monocytosis without other information (e.g., history or histopathology) is insufficient to conclude that a chronic disease process is present.

Monocytopenia is not a significant finding in cats or dogs. Low numbers are normally present. Monocytes are not evenly distributed on a blood smear; they may be missed on a differential count.

Lymphocytosis

Persistent lymphocytosis usually signifies strong immune stimulus of some duration from a chronic infection, viremia, or immune-mediated disease. Supportive laboratory evidence in addition to history and physical findings could include hyperproteinemia with a polyclonal gammopathy, reactive lymphocytes, CBC evidence of an inflammatory process, and cytologic/histologic samples from the affected tissues (see Chronic Lymphocytic Leukemia and Acute Lymphoblastic Leukemia for diagnosis of leukemia). Nondisease causes of lymphocytosis include physiologic leukocytosis in healthy cats. This would be a transient process associated with exercise or excitement. Both puppies and kittens normally have higher lymphocyte counts than adults, and age-related reference values should be consulted.

Circulating lymphocyte numbers need not represent the mass of lymphoid tissue in the body. Lymphocytes migrate into and out of blood from the lymphoid tissues, in contrast to the unidirectional movement of neutrophils from the marrow to the tissues. Changes in distribution may significantly affect the blood's lymphocyte count yet be unrepresentative of lymphoid hyperplasia or atrophy.

Reactive Lymphocytes

Reactive lymphocytes are immune-stimulated lymphocytes with darkly basophilic cytoplasm, larger size, and occasionally irregular shape of the nucleus. Blast-transformed lymphocytes are essentially the same, except with a blast-type nucleus (i.e., large, light chromatin and the presence of a nucleolus). Rare reactive lymphocytes may be in normal blood smears, and a few to several may be in blood smears of animals ill with various diseases. These are not of special diagnostic significance. The numbers of reactive lymphocytes do not consistently reflect the degree of immune stimulation, nor are they specific for any disease. They can lead to misdiagnosis of lymphosarcoma and acute lymphoblastic leukemia (see those sections).

Lymphopenia/Eosinopenia

Lymphopenia and eosinopenia are usually due to stress or exogenous glucocorticoid treatment (see the earlier discussion of stress/steroid changes under Neutrophilia/Leukocytosis). Lymphopenia is expected in acute severe disease, and the return of the lymphocytes into the normal range is a good prognostic sign of decreasing stress. Additional causes of lymphopenia to consider include loss of lymph in protein-losing enteropathy of lymphangiectasia in dogs, chylothorax in dogs and cats, destruction of the lymphatic circulation by diseases like lymphosarcoma, and granulomatous diseases interfering with recirculation of lymphocytes (Prasse, 1983).

Lymphopenia occurs in some viral diseases by direct viral damage to the lymphoid tissue and through stress. Viral diseases of dogs associated with lymphopenia include distemper, infectious canine hepatitis, parvovirus, and coronavirus enteritis. Similarly, cats with panleukopenia and FeLV may have lymphopenia.

One should not speculate that the presence of a lymphopenia reflects mainly a T-cell effect. Depending on the technique to classify circulating lymphocytes in dogs and cats, as few as 13% to 21% may be T cells (Jain, 1986). This is unlike in people, in whom most peripheral blood lymphocytes are T cells.

Eosinopenia usually supports a diagnosis of stress/steroid effect. Eosinophils may normally be absent on a feline differential WBC count and may compose only 2% of a normal canine differential WBC count. An eosinopenia in a normal animal may be due to missing the infrequent eosinophils on a differential count of 100 WBCs. An eosinopenia may be the most consistent finding in chronic stress/steroid situations but is not as convincing a laboratory sign by itself compared with lymphopenia. Eosinopenia in greyhounds and other dogs may be from not identifying "vacuolated or gray" eosinophils in which the granules do not stain orange. These are often misidentified as vacuolated neutrophils or monocytes.

Eosinophilia

General Comments ● Eosinophilia suggests an eosinophilic inflammatory process somewhere in the body. The inflammation may be helpful in cleansing the body of something, or it may be harmful in damaging various tissues. Specific diagnostic suggestions to locate the inflammation and identify the cause follow, but this section summarizes the common functions of eosinophils, their interactions with lymphocytes and mast cells (or basophils), and how they are regulated. This helps one understand when and why eosinophils may be elevated in the blood.

Eosinophils kill parasites and regulate the intensity of hypersensitivity reactions mediated by IgE antibodies (Fig. 4–7). Eosinophils are attracted to inflamed tissue by mast cell products and lymphokines. Mast cells and lymphocytes recognize the presence of an allergen or parasite in the tissues, the former acting as a sentry just below body surfaces to detect and respond to the presence of a parasite or allergen. The mast cells are specifically targeted to a parasite or allergen by IgE or IgG from B lymphocytes. Eosinophils regulate the mast cells' effect by phagocytizing mast cell granules, inhibiting degranulation, and counteracting mediators.

Eosinophils kill parasites by attaching to them and forming a digestive vacuole between the eosinophil and parasite. The parasiticidal substances in the eosinophil granules damage the wall of the parasite or ova. For a strong eosinophilic response to occur, the parasite must be in the animal's tissues. Parasites that do not invade tissue (e.g., *Giardia* or tapeworms) are not expected to cause an eosinophilia, whereas migrat-

ing lung flukes like *Paragonimus kellicotti* should. Some parasites may not stimulate an eosinophilia until they die and expose previously hidden antigens. The inflammatory response to certain allergens is similar to that for tissue-invasive parasites. Lymphocytes respond to the allergen or parasites by producing an IgE-type immune response.

Thus, in both parasitic and allergic processes, there is extensive interaction of different lymphocytes, mast cells, basophils, and eosinophils. Mediators of each cell type act locally or at the bone marrow to regulate the numbers and activities of other cells. T lymphocytes and mast cells produce eosinophilopoietins, which act on the bone marrow to increase eosinophil production. Consider this team of cells when evaluating an eosinophilia (see Fig. 4–7).

Note that most inflammatory processes include a mixture of inflammatory cells responding to various concurrent stimuli. The classification of the inflammation is based on the predominant cell type. Mast cells are also important in the initiation of neutrophilic inflammation, and eosinophils may be a variable component of any inflammatory process.

Diagnostic Approach • Comprehensive surveys of patients with eosinophilia produce long lists

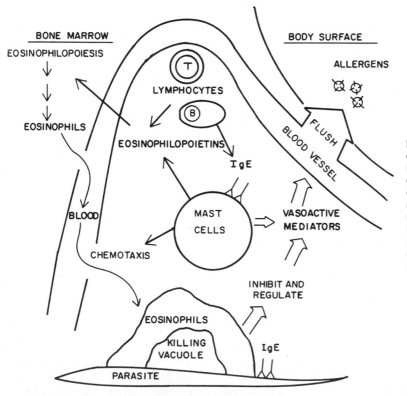

Figure 4–7 Eosinophil functions and cell interactions. Mast cells primed with immunoglobulin like IgE act through degranulation of mediators to attract eosinophils to sites of allergic and parasitic problems and to act on blood vessels to flush away allergens. Eosinophils kill parasites and regulate hypersensitivity reactions. Lymphocytes prime the reaction and stimulate eosinopoiesis. (See text for details.)

of diseases. Many of the diseases have no obvious link to the generalizations made about eosinophils, mast cells, and IgE. Parasitic and allergic processes should be considered first, but fungal, viral, protozoan, and bacterial infections are often associated with eosinophilia, as are inflammatory diseases of various tissues and toxic reactions.

Certain diseases are more likely when an eosinophilia is present, yet the converse is not true. An eosinophilia may be infrequent in these diseases. Food hypersensitivity, for example, was accompanied by an eosinophilia (i.e., >1000 eosinophils/μl) in only two of seven dogs (White, 1986). However, food allergy is a consideration in an animal with an unexplained eosinophilia. Cats with food hypersensitivity may have a marked eosinophilia, but a lack of eosinophilia does not rule out food allergy.

Since mast cells are numerous at the surface of the skin, the digestive tract, and the respiratory tract, it is useful to organize one's approach by those systems (Figs. 4–8 and 4–9). An approach in cats is discussed first. First, carefully examine the skin for evidence of a skin reaction to fleas, possible food hypersensitivity, or other causes of dermatitis. Eosinophilic plaque and linear granuloma may cause an eosinophilia.

The respiratory tract may be evaluated cytologically by using swabs, material left on tracheal tubes, washes, or bronchial brush preparations.

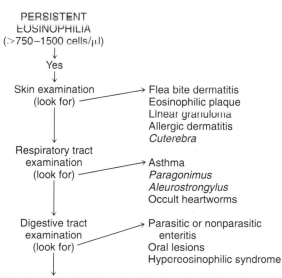

Then look for other disorders like hematopoietic and nonhematopoietic neoplasms, a variety of inflammatory and infectious diseases, or idiopathic changes.

Figure 4–8 Evaluation of feline eosinophilia. This is one suggested approach to consider most of the common causes of eosinophilia in cats. Develop a routine system of checking body surfaces for the most likely to the least likely causes of eosinophilia.

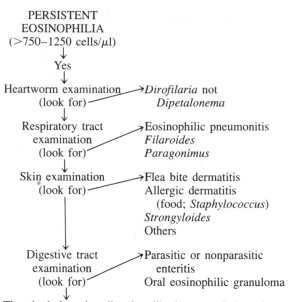

Then look for other disorders like hematopoietic and nonhematopoietic neoplasms, a variety of inflammatory and infectious diseases, estrus, or idiopathic changes.

Figure 4–9 Evaluation of canine eosinophilia. This is one suggested approach in the consideration of most of the common causes of persistent eosinophilia in dogs. Check first for heartworms, and then check the various body surfaces in order of the most likely to the least likely causes.

Eosinophilic pulmonary inflammation suggests feline asthma in the absence of evidence of parasites (e.g., *Paragonimus, Aleurostrongylus,* or *Dirofilaria*). Check the upper respiratory tract for *Cuterebra* or other lesions.

Next the digestive tract is evaluated, primarily by fecal examination. The presence of an endo- or ectoparasite does not imply that it caused the eosinophilia, especially if the eosinophilia was marked or persisted after anthelmintic treatment. Tapeworms, ascarids, and hookworms were not associated with an eosinophil count higher than controls in 35 cats (Prasse, 1983). Nonparasitic inflammatory disease of the digestive tract may stimulate eosinophilia.

Hypereosinophilic syndrome is an unexplained idiopathic disease process in which many tissues like the intestines may be infiltrated and damaged by eosinophils. In some cats, this includes eosinophilic enteritis and eosinophilic leukemia. The division between hyperplasia and neoplasia of eosinophils may not be obvious in this syndrome.

Consider finally the presence of a hidden neoplasm that can release the mediators of eosinophilopoiesis in some odd, unexplained eosinophilias. For example, T lymphocytes produce substances to stimulate eosinopoiesis in the marrow. Two cats with intestinal lymphosarcoma had >60,000 eosinophils/μl in their blood. Mast cells produce substances that stimulate eosinophilopoiesis or release of stored eosinophils from the bone marrow. Mast cell tumors should be considered as a potential cause, especially in dogs. Eosinophilia was not observed in 14 cats with cutaneous mast cell tumors (Buerger and Scott, 1987).

A diagnostic approach to a persistent eosinophilia in dogs is similar (see Fig. 4–9). The frequency of heartworm disease with eosinophilia makes a microfilaria test a reasonable starting point, even in dogs with disease in other organ systems. Radiographs and an occult heartworm test may be better. A transtracheal wash may provide cytologic evidence of eosinophilic inflammation due to eosinophilic pneumonitis or may identify a specific etiologic parasite (e.g., *Paragonimus* or *Filaroides*).

Digestive tract examination includes physical examination of the oral cavity. Eosinophilic granuloma in the oral cavity of Siberian husky dogs has caused eosinophilia. It is diagnosed by histopathology or cytology and morphologically resembles the disease of cats. Hypersensitivity-type skin diseases should be considered (i.e., fleas or food allergy). Intestinal parasites seem more likely to cause eosinophilia in dogs than in cats, but a positive fecal examination should not halt consideration of other causes of eosinophilia. Estrus in dogs occasionally causes eosinophilia.

Canine mast cell neoplasms more consistently have eosinophilic infiltration than a peripheral blood eosinophilia. Only 2 of 16 dogs with systemic mastocytosis had eosinophilia (O'Keefe et al., 1987). Lymphosarcomas rarely have an eosinophilic infiltrate or produce eosinophilia. The lack of an eosinophilia in various neoplastic and nonneoplastic diseases with a tissue eosinophilia might be explained by the short half-life of eosinophils in the peripheral blood (i.e., approximately 30 minutes in dogs).

Basophilia

Basophilia has two common diagnostic considerations. It is caused by the same processes causing an eosinophilia or is associated with lipemia. Eosinophilia usually accompanies a basophilia as part of the IgE, eosinophil, and basophil/mast cell process. Basophil granules contain substances similar to mast cell granules. Basophilias of up to 4275 cells/μl have been reported in canine respiratory disease and up to 1280 basophils/μl in canine skin disease (Jain, 1986). The cats in the study had milder basophilia (i.e., <600 cells/μl). This association with body surfaces is like that of eosinophils. Basophils may aid in resistance to ectoparasites. Basophilia of the blood and skin has been noted in the immune reaction to ticks in cattle and guinea pigs. Basophil degranulation was associated with release of the ticks.

Basophilia in the absence of an eosinophilia in some dogs has been associated with altered lipid metabolism. Basophils and mast cells are the major source of heparin in the body. Heparin enhances the activity of lipoprotein lipase along blood vessels in clearing fat from the blood. Basophilia occurred in 5 of 16 dogs with systemic mastocytosis (O'Keefe et al., 1987).

Basophilia may not be recognized, since feline and canine basophils are easy to misidentify. Feline basophil granules are large, fill the cytoplasm, are a light lavender color, and may be mistaken for eosinophils with faded granules. The large, round basophil granule, however, is different from the rod-shaped eosinophil granule. The basophil granules may also include some dark-staining granules. Canine basophils have few granules, which may not stain well and are most often misidentified as canine monocytes. Characteristic features of the canine basophils include a long polymorphonuclear-shaped nucleus that is longer than a neutrophil nucleus and thinner than most monocyte nuclei. The cytoplasm has a lavender hue, and the cell may be easier to observe by scanning under low power. Basophils of cats and dogs are rare, a factor that contributes to the lack of confidence in identification.

Mastocytemia

Mastocytemia varies in importance from an incidental finding to an indication of malignant, disseminated mast cell neoplasia. The number of mast cells is a major consideration in determining the significance. Atypical cell morphology may also denote malignancy. Mastocytemia has been reported in dogs with acute inflammatory disorders, including 8 of 58 dogs with parvoviral enteritis (Stockham et al., 1984). This mastocytemia was mild (e.g., 2–9 mast cells per blood smear), but up to 30 to 90 mast cells per smear were found. Mastocytemia occurred in 1 of 52 randomly selected blood smears. An occasional error in identifying mastocytemia is that degenerating cells (neutrophils?) may become darkly granular and mimic mast cells, especially in old samples. When in doubt, confirm mastocytemia with a fresh blood sample.

Buffy coat preparations of peripheral blood

are often evaluated for the presence of mast cells in patients with mast cell neoplasms. However, finding mast cells in peripheral blood in numbers so low that concentration techniques are required has not been proved to consistently diagnose systemic involvement of mast cell neoplasia. In 11 cats with cutaneous mast cell tumors, the buffy coat analysis identified 1 cat with mastocytemia. This cat lived another 5 years, so its mastocytemia seemed insignificant.

Systemic mastocytosis has been diagnosed in 16 dogs with hemolymphatic involvement (O'Keefe et al., 1987). The four criteria for hemolymphatic involvement were (1) mast cells on peripheral blood or bone marrow smears, (2) >10 mast cells/1000 nucleated cells in bone marrow smears (normal canine marrow has 0–1 mast cells/1000 nucleated cells), (3) involvement of spleen or liver, and (4) involvement of lymph nodes distant from the primary neoplasm. All 16 dogs had at least two of these criteria, and 88% died or were euthanatized because of the neoplasm. Mastocytemia occurred in 10% to 38% of canine cases of systemic mastocytosis.

The number of mast cells in blood should improve one's confidence in concluding systemic involvement. Four of six dogs with systemic mastocytosis had prominent mastocytemia (i.e., mean 1625 mast cells/μl; range 800–4100) Two dogs with mast cell leukemia had 3441 to 14,337 mast cells/μl in their CBCs (Jain, 1986). Two cats with malignant splenic mastocytosis had 2% to 11% mast cells (769 mast cells/μl in one instance) observed on a WBC differential from routine blood smears (Confer and Langloss, 1978). Buffy coat preparations should contain more than two or three mast cells (Macy, 1986).

To confirm disseminated mast cell neoplasia, use histology or cytology to prove invasion of the spleen, bone marrow, liver, or distant lymph nodes. Bone marrow examination for mast cell infiltration is more sensitive in documenting systemic mastocytosis and has fewer false-positive results (see Chapter 16 for histologic and cytologic grading of mast cell neoplasms).

LEUKEMIA

General Comments

Leukemia is suspected when WBC numbers are high or when WBCs appear abnormal on blood smear evaluation or CBC reports. Leukemia is most readily diagnosed by an abundance of hematopoietic blast cells in blood or bone marrow. Little experience is required to recognize hematopoietic blast cells with large nuclear size, fine and well-dispersed chromatin patterns, and the presence of a nucleolus. A rare mitotic figure does not suggest leukemia, since cells capable of mitosis (e.g., rubricytes, myelocytes, monocytes, and reactive lymphocytes) are frequently encountered in nonleukemic animals. Diagnosis of specific leukemias is made with criteria that follow. It is not expected that most veterinarians will make final diagnoses of specific leukemias, but since diagnostic classification systems vary, certain criteria are listed for reference. Diagnostic criteria of pathologists should be understood to compare similar diagnoses and to know how to provide appropriate samples.

Several well-prepared, unstained smears of fresh blood should be sent to an experienced veterinary hematologist for diagnosis. The smears usually are of blood collected in EDTA for convenient handling, but some hematologists prefer smears made from blood without anticoagulant. Some of the smears can be used for cytochemical stains, although special fixation may be preferred. A tube of EDTA blood is needed to obtain various cell counts. Bone marrow smears and a core biopsy sample are usually needed but are not usually part of the initial evaluation.

WBC alterations include hyperplasia, dysplasia, and neoplasia. This range of processes occurs in other tissues (e.g., stratified squamous epithelium) There are hyperplastic changes like acanthosis and hyperkeratosis plus highly reactive cellular changes (e.g., at the edge of an ulcer). Dysplastic changes are mild cellular transformations that may be due to various irritants. Neoplastic changes may be benign (e.g., papillomas-warts) or malignant (e.g., squamous cell carcinoma). These terms are generally well accepted and comfortable to veterinarians in the context of epithelial tissue proliferation, but they seem to cause more confusion when applied to hematopoietic tissue.

There are mixed opinions on the value of specific diagnosis and treatment of certain leukemias and confusion over the different diagnostic schemes. Veterinary understanding of leukemias is still incomplete and in a stage of rapid growth. Prognosis and treatment protocols for an animal vary with the diagnosis. The prognosis for most leukemias is poor, but some forms (e.g., chronic lymphocytic leukemia) have a reasonably good prognosis, some patients surviving for years. Solid tissue neoplasms of lymphoid cells are treatable. Thymoma can

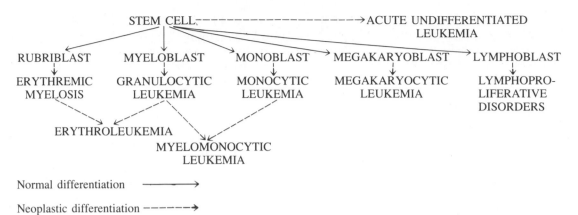

Figure 4–10 Simple scheme depicting hematopoiesis and origin of the most common neoplastic disorders of hematopoietic cells. (Modified after Jain NC. Schalm's Veterinary Hematology. 4th ed. Philadelphia, Lea and Febiger, 1986.)

frequently be cured by surgery. A solitary cutaneous lymphosarcoma mass was cured by surgery (McKeever et al., 1982). Clinical staging of canine lymphosarcoma reflected prognosis (Carter et al., 1986).

The classification schemes for hematopoietic neoplasms are primarily based on the type of cell affected. Recall the differentiation of the various cell types in the marrow and their derivation from a stem cell (Fig. 4–10). The initial separation of hematopoietic neoplasms is into lymphoproliferative and myeloproliferative disorders. The lymphoproliferative disorders involve forms of the lymphocyte; myeloproliferative disorders include one or more of the other hematopoietic cell types. The myeloproliferative disorders are generally less responsive to treatment than are the lymphoproliferative disorders. A study group of 10 veterinary clinical pathologists of the American Society for Veterinary Clinical Pathology (ASVCP) evaluated criteria to classify acute myeloid leukemias in dogs and cats (Jain, 1991). Modifications of the French-American-British (FAB) classification system for acute leukemias in people (Table 4–6) were used for a canine and feline scheme (Fig. 4–11). Both the FAB and the ASVCP systems rely on differential counts of well-prepared blood or bone marrow smears with percentages of blasts or certain cell types to classify the process. A cell count of >30% blast cells without orderly maturation indicates acute myeloid leukemia (AML), acute undifferentiated leukemia (AUL), or erythroleukemia (M6). Less than 30% blast cells indicates myelodysplastic syndrome (MDS), chronic myeloid leukemias, or even leukemoid reactions.

Various systems are used to diagnose lymphoid neoplasms. Criteria include size of the lymphoid cell, cleavage of the nucleus, other nuclear and cytoplasmic characteristics, and histologic pattern (i.e., diffuse, follicular, and nodular). The National Cancer Institute's system of histologic grading (Table 4–7) had demonstrated prognostic significance. Communicate with the pathologist to clarify the type of classification used.

Lymphoproliferative disorders (lymphosarcoma [LSA], malignant lymphoma) usually form solid masses. Cytology or histopathology is

Table 4–6 CLASSIFICATION OF HUMAN ACUTE LEUKEMIAS: FRENCH-AMERICAN-BRITISH SYSTEM

L1 Small cells up to twice the size of small lymphocytes with regular nuclear shape and little cytoplasm.*
L2 Most cells are twice as big as small lymphocytes, heterogeneity is prominent, and nucleoli are large and variable in size and number.*
L3 Cells are large with moderately abundant, basophilic, often vacuolated cytoplasm that completely surrounds the nucleus; mitotic index is high (5%), and nucleoli are prominent.
M1 Acute myeloblastic leukemia without maturation.
M2 Acute myeloblastic leukemia with partial maturation.
M3 Hypergranular promyelocytic leukemia; microgranular variant.
M4 Myelomonocytic leukemia.
M5 Monocytic leukemia.
M6 Erythroleukemia
M7 Megakaryoblastic leukemia.

*A scoring system is used to help differentiate the L1 and L2 acute lymphoid leukemias.

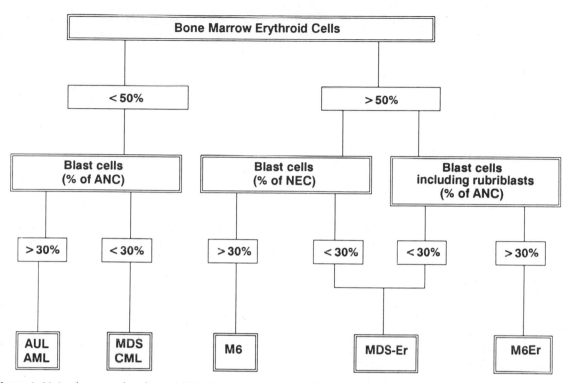

Figure 4–11 A scheme to classify myeloid leukemias and myelodysplastic syndromes in dogs and cats. ANC = all nucleated cells; NEC = nucleated erythroid cells. (From Jain NC, et al: Proposed criteria for classification of acute myeloid leukemia in dogs and cats. Vet Clin Pathol 1991;20:63–82. Reprinted with permission of Veterinary Clinical Pathology.)

usually diagnostic. Myeloproliferative disorders (MPDs) are more variable, since one or more cell types may be abnormal and one type may evolve to another. These are characteristically leukemic and rarely form solid masses called *chloromas*. Blood and bone marrow evaluation is thus most diagnostic for MPDs. The anemia in MPDs tends to be more severe than in lymphoproliferative disorders.

Leukemia ● Leukemia (literally "white blood") specifically means a hematopoietic neoplasm that originated in the bone marrow. Leukemia need not involve the peripheral blood, so some confusing terms are *aleukemic leukemia* (i.e., no circulating neoplastic cells) and *subleukemic leukemia* (i.e., few circulating neoplastic cells). If neoplastic cells in blood are derived from solid tissue masses of LSA without involvement of the bone marrow, this is uniquely termed *lymphosarcoma cell leukemia* (rare terminology in veterinary medicine).

A common division of leukemias is acute versus chronic. Acute leukemias have abundant immaturity including blast cells, whereas chronic leukemias have a well-differentiated population (e.g., acute lymphoblastic [ALL] versus chronic lymphocytic leukemia [CLL]). This division is significant, with the chronic leukemias generally having a more favorable prognosis than the acute leukemias.

Various combinations of anemia, thrombocytopenia, and leukopenia are expected with leukemic involvement of the bone marrow. Although not diagnostic for a leukemia, they may be the initial problem that leads to the diagnosis. These cytopenias may be detected on a physical examination (e.g., petechial hemorrhages

Table 4–7 CLASSIFICATION SYSTEM FOR HUMAN NON-HODGKIN'S LYMPHOMA: NATIONAL CANCER INSTITUTE'S WORKING FORMULATION

Malignancy Grade	Cell Morphology
Low	Diffuse small lymphocytic (DSL)
	Follicular small cleaved (FSC)
	Follicular mixed cleaved (FM)
Intermediate	Diffuse large (DL)
	Follicular large (FL)
	Diffuse small cleaved (DSC)
	Diffuse mixed (DM)
High	Lymphoblastic (LB)
	Small noncleaved (SNC)
	Immunoblastic (IB)

in thrombocytopenia, or pale mucous membranes in anemia).

Dysplasia and Preleukemia ● Dysplastic changes may be observed in hematopoietic cells with or without neoplasia. One common dysplastic change is megaloblastic erythroid precursors that have an excessive amount of cytoplasm compared with the nucleus. This is termed *asynchronous maturation,* in which the maturity of the nucleus (i.e., size and chromatin pattern) may differ from that of the cytoplasm (i.e., color and granule development). Other alterations include irregularities in the size, shape, or number of nuclei. Possible causes include FeLV, nutritional deficiencies (e.g., cobalamin and folate), exogenous drugs or toxins, preleukemic changes, leukemia, or idiopathic changes.

Preleukemic changes include cytopenias of one or more cell types in peripheral blood and morphologic evidence of dysplasia. It takes courage (or foolishness) to forecast or diagnose a neoplastic process with only dysplasia and cytopenia(s). It is safer to wait and see the course of the disease. If the changes were preleukemic, then ample evidence of leukemia will be forthcoming. One must not treat, except with supportive care, until the diagnosis is clear.

Canine Hematopoietic Neoplasms/Leukemias

Canine Lymphoproliferative Disorders ● Lymphoid neoplasia in dogs includes LSA, ALL, CLL, plasma cell myeloma, cutaneous LSA (and mycosis fungoides), and thymoma. The diagnostic approach to these varies with the presenting signs. Generalized lymphadenopathy in a dog is evaluated initially with cytologic or histologic examination of several nodes. LSA may involve other or additional tissues (e.g., gut, skin), so if the presenting problem suggests a particular tissue, then that area is best evaluated cytologically or histologically. Hypercalcemia (i.e., >12 mg/dl) occurred in 20.5% of dogs with LSA (Madewell, 1985), so it is a useful clue to initiate a search for LSA or other neoplasia (see Chapter 8). Localized edema suggests LSA or other diseases of the lymphatics that may block lymph flow (see Chapter 10). LSA-induced immune suppression can be suggested by cryptococcosis or other infections.

Lymphosarcoma ● The most common canine hematopoietic neoplasm is LSA. Dogs with LSA responded to therapy for a mean of 161 days

Table 4–8 CLASSIFICATION OF LYMPHOMA BY CLINICAL INVOLVEMENT: WORLD HEALTH ORGANIZATION STAGING SYSTEM

Clinical Stage	Criteria
I	Only one lymph node or lymphoid tissue in one organ except bone marrow
II	Several lymph nodes in one region are involved
III	Generalized involvement of the lymph nodes
IV	Involvement of liver and/or spleen
V	Manifestations in blood with involvement of bone marrow and/or other organ systems

(0–523 days) (Carter et al., 1986). Survival of the dogs in clinical stage III (Table 4–8) was significantly better (mean 305 days) than in stages II, IV, or V. LSA in these dogs was usually classified as high-grade malignancy by the NCI system (see Table 4–7). The dogs with high-grade LSA more often went into complete remission with treatment but did not survive longer than dogs with LSA of intermediate-grade malignancy.

Cytologic and/or histologic evaluation of enlarged lymph nodes is the usual diagnostic method, since the multicentric form is the most common presentation. The multicentric form is an anatomic classification describing neoplastic involvement of the peripheral lymph nodes, spleen, liver, and other organs (Table 4–9). Several lymph nodes frequently must be evaluated, since the cells may be necrotic and the sample nondiagnostic. Not all dogs with LSA have lymph node involvement, although lymph nodes are usually neoplastic. If one or more lymph nodes are hyperplastic or reactive, do not conclude that LSA is absent in the patient. If LSA is still suspected, histologic or cytologic sampling of likely sites (e.g., spleen, liver, and gut) may be useful, especially if suggested by clinical signs (e.g., diarrhea or splenohepatomegaly).

Table 4–9 CLASSIFICATION SYSTEM FOR CANINE LYMPHOSARCOMA BY ANATOMIC SITE

Classification	Criteria
Multicentric	Peripheral lymph nodes and other organs involved
Thymic	Mass in anterior ventral thorax
Alimentary	Mass in ileum, mesenteric lymph nodes, liver, kidney, and/or spleen
Unclassified	Involvement of skin, eye, and/or central nervous system

(From Jain NC: Schalm's Veterinary Hematology. 4th ed. Philadelphia, Lea and Febiger, 1986.)

Few dogs with LSA have overt leukemia with a significant number of lymphoblasts in peripheral blood. Two leukemic forms of lymphoid neoplasia discussed later are ALL and CLL. Of 72 dogs with LSA, only 21% had a lymphocytosis whereas 25% had a lymphopenia (Jain, 1986). The CBC is not sensitive in identifying canine LSA.

Bone marrow involvement is used in staging LSA (see Table 4–8) and determining treatment. Bone marrow evaluation is needed since CBC results may not reflect marrow involvement and vice versa. Of 75 dogs with multicentric LSA, 27 had excessive lymphocytes in bone marrow (i.e., >20%), whereas only eight had a circulating lymphocytosis (Madewell, 1985). Of the 27 dogs with excessive marrow lymphocytes, 23 had a cytopenia of one or more cells in the peripheral blood. Core biopsies of the marrow were most sensitive in identifying leukemic involvement of the marrow (Raskin and Krehbiel, 1989). Of 53 dogs with multicentric LSA, the combination of peripheral blood, bone marrow aspirates, and bone marrow biopsy samples identified 30 (57%) as having leukemic involvement of bone marrow and blood. Cytopenias included anemia (packed cell volume [PCV] <37%) in 32%, thrombocytopenia (<200,000 platelets/µl) in 49%, and leukopenia (<6000 WBCs/µl) in 9% of the 75 dogs. Megaloblastic rubricytes may be noted in LSA.

Lymph node cytology should be learned in order to diagnose LSA. Be cautious and restrict diagnosis to obvious cases (see Chapter 16). LSA of the gut or other sites may be diagnosed cytologically, but sites other than lymph nodes are best diagnosed by histopathologic evaluations.

Acute Lymphoblastic Leukemia ● Diagnosis of ALL in dogs is by evaluation of blood and bone marrow smears. CBC alterations are the usual method of diagnosis. However, bone marrow is more consistently abnormal, with a dense infiltration by lymphoblasts. Treatment prolongs survival, so accurate diagnosis is indicated. Mean survival in 21 dogs with ALL was 68 days (range 2–241 days), whereas three untreated dogs survived 1, 5, and 13 days (Matus et al., 1983). Four dogs (19%) had complete remissions, defined as eliminating circulating lymphocytes and having less than 12% lymphocytes and no atypical lymphoblasts in the bone marrow.

A diagnosis of ALL requires a large number of atypical lymphoid cells. Lymphoblasts in blood exceeded 5000/µl in 76% of dogs with ALL. This abundance of immature lymphoblasts

allows a confident diagnosis. The diagnosis of ALL or other leukemias may be confused by reactive or blast-transformed lymphoid cells on blood smears if numbers are not considered. In many nonneoplastic diseases or other processes (e.g., vaccination of young animals), one can find a few atypical lymphocytes on a blood smear. These large blue lymphoid cells due to immune stimulation may have prominent nucleoli or irregular nuclear shapes and resemble malignant lymphoblasts. A few (i.e., one to five?) lymphoblasts seen during a short blood smear examination need not indicate leukemia even in dogs with cytologic evidence of LSA in lymph nodes. Of 75 dogs with multicentric LSA, 49 had atypical or immature lymphoid cells in the blood but only eight had a lymphocytosis (Madewell, 1985). The use of buffy coat preparations to concentrate the WBCs to find a few lymphoblasts is not advised. Buffy coat preparations for lupus erythematosus cell identification (i.e., LE preparations in dogs without ALL) often have several blast-transformed lymphoid cells. Blast cells may be present in low numbers in nonleukemic animals, and manipulations of blood samples may stimulate blast formation.

Secondary effects on other cell types in ALL included anemia in 87% and <100,000 platelets/µl in 46% of dogs. Splenomegaly is commonly present (i.e., 73%), but lymphadenopathy occurred in about 50% of the ALL cases. Thus, the leukemic form of lymphoid malignancy may be present with minimal or no tissue involvement; therefore, lymph node cytology may not be helpful. Hypercalcemia was not detected. ALL in five dogs classified by the FAB system was always L2 (i.e., with nucleoli, nuclear clefting and indentation, and heterogeneous) (Couto, 1985).

Chronic Lymphocytic Leukemia ● CLL must be differentiated from LSA or ALL and usually has a relatively favorable prognosis. Of 17 dogs studied, 53% were alive 1 year and 29% were alive 2 years after diagnosis (Leifer and Matus, 1986). Differentiation of CLL from ALL or lymphoblastic LSA is based on the relatively normal morphology of the lymphocytes compared with the lymphoblasts of ALL or the common form of LSA.

The initial diagnosis of CLL is usually made by the magnitude of the lymphocytosis. The mean lymphocyte count in 22 dogs with CLL was 39,400 lymphocytes/µl (6000 to >100,000/µl). An important question is, At what point is lymphocytosis too great for nonneoplastic processes? Perhaps a figure of 15,000 to 20,000 lymphocytes/µl is the break point. One's confidence in the diagnosis of CLL increases proportionally to the increase in the lymphocyte count. Lymphocyte counts >50,000 to 100,000/µl are diagnostic of a neoplastic process even with normal lymphocyte morphology.

Additional diagnostic proof is provided by histologic patterns in bone marrow, spleen, and lymph nodes. Histopathology often reveals a solid infiltrative mass of lymphocytes with loss of normal architecture of the organ. The bone marrow in CLL has been consistently infiltrated with small well-differentiated lymphocytes, so bone marrow aspirates and biopsy specimens must be included.

The percentage of lymphoid cells on a bone marrow aspirate that suggests CLL is not well defined. The cellularity of the smear, particles, or a biopsy sample is needed to interpret a relative figure like the percentage of lymphocytes. Dogs normally have <15% and routinely have a mean of 4% to 5% lymphocytes and plasma cells on a bone marrow aspirate cell differential. Cats normally have more lymphocytes in the marrow (e.g., 10–15%) (Jain, 1986). One dog with CLL had 64% to 77.5% lymphoid cells in the marrow (Harvey et al., 1981). One expects an increase of lymphocytes and plasma cells in the marrow of animals with a systemic immune response.

Anemia occurred in 19 of 22 dogs with CLL. The anemia was mild to moderate, with a PCV of 19% to 34%. A clinically insignificant thrombocytopenia (i.e., 110,000–193,000 platelets/µl) was reported in 10 dogs. Hypercalcemia was not noted. CLL progressed to LSA in two dogs.

Monoclonal gammopathy occurred in 15 of the 22 dogs. Bence Jones proteins were found in the urine of 6 of 13 dogs with monoclonal gammopathy. The monoclonal gammopathies were mainly IgM or IgA. These large antibodies increase the viscosity of serum. Of nine dogs examined, six had increased viscosity of 4.4 to 8 seconds compared with water (normal, <1.8 seconds). Only one or two of the dogs had clinical signs of hyperviscosity syndrome. The severity of hyperviscosity is greatly increased by dehydration. Hemolytic anemia and decreased resistance to infection and other neoplasms are complicating factors in CLL.

Plasma Cell Myeloma ● Plasma cell myeloma is a lymphoproliferative disorder of plasma cells in the bone marrow; plasmacytoma is a neoplasm of plasma cells in soft tissue (i.e., liver and kidney). Bone marrow evaluation is usually needed for diagnosis. Histologic evaluation of the lytic area of bone or soft tissue masses is most conclusive when biopsy of the organ is possible. Significant numbers of plasma cells and atypical mor-

phologic features are needed on marrow aspirates for diagnosis. More than 15% to 20% plasma cells are expected in the bone marrow aspirates of people with multiple myeloma. This or a higher cutoff might be appropriate in dogs. If the number of plasma cells is only mildly to moderately increased and the plasma cells are fairly well differentiated, then a diagnosis of plasma cell myeloma is equivocal and should be proved by histopathologic examination.

Normal plasma cells may occasionally be binucleated. Plasma cells frequently have prominent vacuolation called *Russell's bodies* or *Mott's cells* during immune stimulation. Cytologic evidence of a neoplastic rather than a reactive plasma cell proliferation should include irregular nuclear shapes and/or nuclear immaturity indicated by large size and light-dispersed chromatin patterns. Neoplastic plasma cells retain the characteristic eccentric position of the nucleus and cytoplasmic pattern.

Serum protein changes such as hyperviscosity are discussed in Chapter 12. Radiographic evidence of lytic bone lesions is supportive. Hypercalcemia may occur. Plasma cell leukemia is rare in dogs.

Cutaneous Lymphosarcoma and Mycosis Fungoides ● Cutaneous lymphoproliferative disorders represent about 8% of LSA cases (McKeever et al., 1982). These usually begin in the skin and proceed to lymphadenopathy. Histopathologic examination is used to diagnose the type of lymphoproliferative disorder and rule out various other skin disorders. Mycosis fungoides has unique histologic features of focal accumulation of lymphoid cells in the epidermis, called *Pautrier's microabscesses,* and the lymphoid cells have markedly convoluted nuclei.

Thymoma ● Thymomas present as a cranial mediastinal mass with various signs (e.g., coughing, dyspnea, or chylothorax). Thymoma must be differentiated from LSA invading the mediastinal lymph nodes or thymus. Canine thymomas are often benign and treatable, whereas LSA is uniformly malignant and ultimately fatal. In cats, 10 of 11 thymomas were benign (Carpenter and Holzworth, 1982); and in dogs, 12 of 22 were benign (Bellah et al., 1983). Histopathology and to a lesser extent cytology are the most diagnostic tests. Cytologically, thymomas have small, well-differentiated lymphocytes and possibly epithelial cells, whereas LSA has large lymphoblasts. Two thymoma cases showed a mature lymphocytosis in excess of 25,000 lymphocytes/µl. This could be confused with CLL.

Canine Myeloproliferative Disorders • MPDs must be differentiated from lymphoproliferative disorders or nonneoplastic proliferations of hematopoietic cells (e.g., leukemoid reaction). MPDs are severe diseases, essentially nonresponsive to treatment compared with some lymphoproliferative disorders. Treatment protocols (if the owner is willing) vary with the type of leukemia. Leukemoid reactions to inflammatory diseases must be differentiated from leukemia to select the right treatments (e.g., remove pyometra) and give a comparatively good prognosis.

Canine MPDs involve a neoplastic proliferation in blood or bone marrow of one or more of the nonlymphoid hematopoietic cells (see Fig. 4–10 or Table 4–6 for illustrations of the classifications). Although the MPDs usually fail to form distinct masses, they often infiltrate and enlarge the spleen, liver, and lymph nodes.

The initial sign may be anemia, thrombocytopenia, or even leukopenia. The leukemia may be identified during hematologic screening if numerous blasts are present. Blast cells of MPD are distinguished from lymphoblasts if sequential differentiation into more mature forms is established. Cytochemical staining of blood and bone marrow has become more standard in classification of leukemias (Table 4–10) to aid in the differentiation of cell types on blood smears and bone marrow. Cytoplasmic contents specific to certain cell lines are stained if the cells are differentiated well enough to form them.

Bone marrow smears and sections are needed to diagnose the leukemia according to the FAB classification and because the marrow population is often more immature than are the cells in blood. In some MPD cases, relatively mature cells are released from the marrow so the blood smear does not appear overtly malignant yet the marrow population is obviously leukemic. Histologic sections of bone marrow and other organs support blood and marrow smear evaluation but must be properly fixed, processed, and cut to provide the nuclear and cytoplasmic detail needed for proper cell identification.

Selective characteristics of various canine MPDs follow. Since anemia and thrombocytopenia are common to all, they are not discussed, nor is the frequency of hepatosplenomegaly and lymphadenopathy.

Granulocytic Leukemia • Neutrophils are most commonly involved, but basophilic leukemia and eosinophilic leukemia occur. Granulocytic leukemia usually has extreme leukocytosis (i.e., average of 119,900 WBCs/μl in 22 canine cases) (Grindem et al., 1985a). However, WBC counts ranged from 10,800 to 467,000, and blast cells in blood ranged from 0% to 81%. AML (i.e., granulocytic leukemia) should have a significant

Table 4–10 SELECTED CYTOCHEMICAL STAINS FOR IDENTIFICATION OF CELL TYPES IN CANINE AND FELINE LEUKEMIAS

Stain	Cells That Stain
Peroxidase	
Dog	Young and especially mature neutrophils; slight monocyte staining
Cat	Mature and especially young neutrophils; slight monocyte staining
Sudan black B	
Dog	Mature neutrophils; slight staining of eosinophils and monocytes
Cat	Young and mature neutrophils
Leukocyte alkaline phosphatase	
Dog	Mild staining of young myeloid cells, basophils, and eosinophils; strong staining of leukemic myeloblasts; variable staining of leukemic lymphoblasts
Cat	Young and mature eosinophils
Alpha-naphthyl butyrate esterase (ANBE)	
Dog	Monocytes, lymphocytes, megakaryocytes
Cat	Monocytes, focal staining of lymphocytes
ANBE + fluoride*	
Dog	Lymphocytes; mild staining of megakaryocytes
Periodic acid-Schiff	
Dog	Young and especially mature neutrophils, lymphocytes, megakaryocytes; mild staining of eosinophils and monocytes
Cat	Young and especially mature neutrophils; mild staining of monocytes and megakaryocytes

*Inhibition of ANBE with fluoride is used to inhibit or reduce the staining of monocytes.
(Modified from Grindem CB, Stevens JB, Perman V: Cytochemical reactions in cells from leukemic dogs. Vet Pathol 1986;23:103–109; Facklam NR, Kociba GJ: Cytochemical characterization of feline leukemic cells. Vet Pathol 1986;23:155–161.)

increase in myeloblasts in the bone marrow or blood. A positive alkaline phosphatase cytochemical reaction reflects leukemia in dogs.

Leukemoid (leukemia-like) reactions in inflammatory diseases may be difficult or temporarily impossible to differentiate from myelogenous leukemia. More than 100,000 neutrophils/μl may be due to an inflammatory process (e.g., pyometra or abscess) or estrogen toxicity. Eosinophilia >60,000/μl in two cats with intestinal LSA was a leukemoid reaction, not eosinophilic leukemia. Thus, unlike lymphocytosis in CLL, magnitude alone does not indicate granulocytic leukemia. If the leukocytosis is mainly segs and bands, then it is probably leukemoid. Toxic change in neutrophils and clinical evidence of an inflammatory/infectious disease, plus response to antibiotics, also support a diagnosis of leukemoid reaction.

Blasts, progranulocytes, and atypical cells denote acute granulocytic leukemia. A disorderly maturation sequence may suggest a neoplastic process. In blood and bone marrow, one expects an orderly maturation of the granulocytes, with the more mature stages outnumbering younger stages. An exception is during repopulation of the bone marrow after depletion due to a toxin or infectious agent (e.g., feline panleukopenia virus). Repopulation begins with a wave of immature cells (e.g., myeloblasts, progranulocytes, and myelocytes) without the expected predominance of mature bands and segs. This may resemble leukemia on a percentage basis but matures with time until a normal marrow population exists.

Chronic Granulocytic (Myelogenous) Leukemia (CGL or CML) ● CGL differs from acute granulocytic leukemia in having well-differentiated granulocytes, mainly neutrophils. The diagnosis of CGL has been made on a clinical basis by a marked, persistent leukocytosis in the absence of a demonstrable infectious or inflammatory cause (Leifer et al., 1983). Thus, diagnosis was by duration and exclusion. Since CGL is rare and without specific hematologic criteria, the diagnosis should be made with caution. CGL was not diagnosed by magnitude of leukocytosis or morphologic atypia or an irregular maturation sequence. Only one of seven dogs with CGL had a younger stage outnumbering a more mature stage (i.e., 33,800 metamyelocytes/μl exceeded 30,420 bands/μl) in the blood. The left shift usually went back only to metamyelocytes. The bone marrow had myeloid hyperplasia (i.e., myeloid:erythroid ratio of 3.5:1 to 24:1) but had orderly myeloid maturation. CGL seemed treat-

able until blast crisis occurred. Four of the seven dogs developed a blast crisis.

Refractory Anemia with Excess Blasts (RAEB) ● RAEB is considered a dysmyelopoietic syndrome or preleukemia in the FAB system. Anemia and often neutropenia are associated with a hypercellular bone marrow with 5% to 20% myeloblasts. If blasts exceed 30%, then granulocytic leukemia (AML) is suggested. What had been previously considered subleukemic granulocytic leukemia in FeLV-infected cats may be RAEB, which may progress to acute granulocytic leukemia, predispose to infections, or remain a debilitating process (Prasse, 1983).

Monocytic Leukemia ● Leukemias involving monocytes may be more common than previously believed. Cytochemical staining probably accounts for the improved accuracy preventing misdiagnosis of ALL. The WBC count averaged 125,700/μl (range 16,800–800,000) in nine dogs (Grindem et al., 1985a). Blast cells averaged 8% (range 0–60.5%), and monocytes averaged 52% (range 9–97%) in the blood. The bone marrow is almost completely replaced by leukemic cells, so it is a more consistent indicator than is the CBC.

Myelomonocytic Leukemia ● Acute myelomonocytic leukemia was the most common leukemia in one survey (Grindem et al., 1985a). The blasts in blood averaged 42% (range 0–98%) and the WBC count averaged 106,000/μl (range 1100–422,400) in 12 dogs.

Megakaryoblastic Leukemia (Megakaryocytic Myelosis) ● MPDs involving megakaryocytes and platelets are rare, and their classification is not well established. Abnormalities vary from hyperplastic and dysplastic changes to megakaryoblastic leukemia. Megaloblastic leukemia in a dog had very abnormal, obviously malignant megakaryocytic and megakaryoblastic cells in the bone marrow, in the spleen, and on buffy coat preparation of blood (Shull et al., 1986). A more well-differentiated leukemia of megakaryocytes is primary thrombocythemia. Nonleukemic changes in megakaryocytes include increases in the number of differentiated but dysplastic megakaryocytes in the marrow or large numbers of normal or atypical platelets in the blood. It is often unclear how to classify and treat animals with dysplastic or excessive numbers of megakaryocytes and platelets. The term *MPD with megakaryocytic predominance* was used to describe the illness in a dog with unclassified malignant cells plus concurrent bizarre mega-karyocytic hyperplasia mainly in the bone marrow and a thrombocytosis of 1.5 to 2.0 $\times$ 10^6 platelets/μl (Harvey et al., 1982).

Erythroleukemia • Erythroleukemia involves proliferation of immature and atypical erythroid and myeloid cells. The blood was not overtly leukemic in six dogs with a mean WBC count of 12,900/μl (range 3500–19,900) and a mean of 2% blast cells (range 0.5–3.5) (Grindem et al., 1985a). These dogs averaged as many nucleated RBCs (NRBCs) in blood as WBCs (e.g., 106 NRBCs/100 WBCs; range 1–298) and had a severe anemia (i.e., PCV 8–14%) without reticulocytes. Leukoerythroblastic reaction is a condition that may mimic erythroleukemia. Leukoerythroblastic reaction occurs when immature erythroid and granulocytic cells appear in the blood of dogs and cats with nonneoplastic severe diseases (e.g., hemolytic or blood loss anemia and hemangiosarcoma) or MPD. A malignant proliferation of only immature erythroid cells is erythremic myelosis.

Polycythemia Vera • (see Chapter 3)

Mast Cell Leukemia • (see Mastocytemia, earlier)

Feline Hematopoietic Neoplasms/Leukemias

Feline Lymphoproliferative Disorders • *Lymphosarcoma* • LSA and lymphoid leukemia are relatively common in cats (e.g., 200 cases/100,000 cats/year) (Essex and Francis, 1976). As in dogs, the leukemic phase of the disease is less common than the solid tissue form. Of 49 cats with LSA, only 6 had overt leukemia with 65,000 to 693,000 WBCs/μl and 19,559 to 693,000 lymphoid cells/μl (Jain, 1986). Half of the cats had lymphopenia. Bone marrow examination is more likely to diagnose LSA than is a CBC. The marrow had lymphocytic infiltration in 12 of 19 cats examined, whereas only 7 of these 19 cats with LSA had lymphoblasts or prolymphocytes in the blood. When an acute leukemia is present, clinicians tend to expect a lymphoid leukemia, but the converse is true. Acute lymphoid leukemia cases (i.e., 57) were less common than acute MPD (i.e., 110) in cats (Grindem et al., 1985b).

The most common anatomic forms of lymphosarcoma in cats, unlike dogs, are the thymic or alimentary, so peripheral lymph node cytology is less rewarding than is cytology or histology of thoracic and abdominal fluid or masses. The primary cytologic criteria are documentation of a lymphoid mass and that the majority of the cells are lymphoblasts or other immature forms as for lymph node cytology. Hyperplastic or reactive lymphoid masses should have a more heterogeneous population composed mainly of well-differentiated cells including plasma cells. FeLV is commonly (i.e., 70%) associated with feline LSA, with most exceptions involving the alimentary or unclassified anatomic forms.

Lymphoid Leukemia • ALL in cats is less common than the solid tissue form of LSA. In a review of 57 cats with ALL, the WBC count had a mean of 48,000/μl (range 1200–693,000), with 0% to 83% blasts (mean 18%) and 6% to 100% lymphoid cells (mean 66%) (Grindem et al., 1985b). The PCV was between 4% and 35%, with a mean of 16%.

Feline Myeloproliferative Disorders • Cats with MPD present with nonspecific signs like inappetence, lethargy, and weakness. If a cat has macrocytic nonregenerative anemia, multiple cytopenias, or a persistent anemia despite regeneration, then bone marrow evaluation should be performed to diagnose two general forms of nonlymphoid hematopoietic neoplasia. If maturation defects in two or three cell lines and increased myeloblasts (i.e., >5%) are present, diagnosis of AML or MDS may be based on the FAB system, which uses the percentage of myeloblasts and nucleated erythroid cells (see Fig. 4–11). Thirty per cent or more myeloblasts reflects AML. Less than 30% myeloblasts indicates MDS. AML is subdivided into five categories (see later descriptions) and erythroleukemia (M6). Erythroleukemia is diagnosed if >50% of the marrow cells are nucleated erythroid cells and the marrow has ≥30% myeloblasts. Of 60 cats, 21 had MDS, 39 had AML, and 6 of the 39 with AML had erythroleukemia (Blue et al., 1988). Myeloblasts were noted in peripheral blood in two thirds of AML cats but in no MDS cats.

The blast cells in blood and bone marrow are often too undifferentiated to classify, so the terms *stem cell leukemia, blast cell leukemia, reticuloendotheliosis,* or *undifferentiated cell leukemia* have been used. If differentiation is present, there may be more than one cell line involved initially or as the disease progresses with time. Thus, MPD is often a sufficient diagnosis, especially since the prognosis is uniformly poor and many cases are euthanatized at this level of diagnosis. Sixty cats classified simply into two broad categories of nonlymphoid neoplasia included 18 cats with MDS and 38 with AML that died or were euthanatized within 1 week of diagnosis (Blue et al., 1988). More specific diagnoses were made for 10 cats with acute feline leukemias. These were fairly evenly distributed through the categories of the FAB system, with the FAB class (and number of cats) being M2 (2), M4 (1), M6 (2), L1 (2), L2 (1), and L3 (1) (Grindem et al., 1985b). All 10 cats died or were euthanatized within 24 days. Prognosis does not seem to be improved by more specific diagnosis.

FeLV viremia is commonly associated with MDS (71%) and AML (90%). Thrombocytopenia (one third to one half of MDS or AML cats) and bleeding (e.g., retinal hemorrhage) occasionally occur. Splenomegaly is common with variable lymphadenopathy and hepatomegaly. Preleukemic changes include nonregenerative anemia with macrocytosis, leukopenia, thrombocytopenia, and combinations of cytopenias.

Dysplastic changes in the three cell lines support the diagnosis of leukemia but do not confirm it. Dysplastic changes vary. The erythroid line may have excessive numbers of rubriblasts and prorubricytes (apparent maturation arrest), megaloblastic rubricytes, nuclei with apparently decreased chromatin, lobulation or multinucleation, and sideroblasts. Normal feline marrow lacks sideroblasts or stainable hemosiderin. The myeloid line may have excessive numbers of myeloblasts (i.e., apparent maturation arrest), abnormal granulation, bizarre hypersegmentation, hyposegmentation (i.e., Pelger-Huet type), giant neutrophils, or monocytoid neutrophils. The megakaryocytic line may have dwarf megakaryocytes, hypolobulated or multiple round nuclei, or hyperlobulated nuclei with blue cytoplasm.

Specific Categories of Feline Myeloproliferative Disorders ●

The following specific classifications of feline MPD may be made. Characteristics of these forms are listed.

Acute Undifferentiated Leukemia ● In a literature review, AUL, previously called *reticuloendotheliosis,* was the most common acute myeloid leukemia (Grindem et al., 1985b). Cytochemical staining was not consistently used in these cases. The mean WBC count was 23,400/μl (range 6800–78,000), with a mean of 24% blasts (range 0–78) in blood. NRBCs/100 WBCs averaged 56.5 (range 0–288), suggesting an erythroid component.

Granulocytic Leukemia ● Granulocytic leukemia in

35 cats, plus 5 with eosinophilic leukemias and 1 with basophilic leukemia, was as common as AUL (i.e., 37 cats). These 78 feline cases composed about 71% of the 110 acute MPD cases reviewed. Leukocytosis in granulocytic leukemia is usually marked, with a mean WBC count of 75,500/μl (range 2700–369,000). Blast cells in blood averaged 20% (range 0–72).

Erythremic Myelosis and Erythroleukemia ● Erythremic myelosis (i.e., neoplasia of just erythroid precursors) had a mean of 187.5 NRBCs/100 WBCs (range 0–964), and erythroleukemia (i.e., neoplasia of erythroid and myeloid precursors) had an average of 82 NRBCs/100 WBCs (range 9–232). Both had a similar number of blasts in blood, with 0% to 28%. Severe anemia occurred in erythroleukemia (mean PCV 10%; range 7–14) and erythremic myelosis (mean PCV 14%; range 8–30). Myeloblasts should exceed 30% of nonerythroid marrow cells in erythroleukemia, and dysplastic megakaryoblasts may be present.

Monocytic Leukemia and Myelomonocytic Leukemia ● These two leukemias had similar CBC results reported. Leukocytosis was marked, with mean WBC counts of 105,200/μl (range 8000–342,000) in monocytic and 114,000/μl (range 35,500–178,400) in myelomonocytic leukemia. Blast cells were common in blood, with means of 26% (range 0–92) in monocytic and 39% (range 8–95) in myelomonocytic leukemia. The average PCV was about 18% in each. Granulocytic cells exceed 20% of nonerythroid bone marrow cells in myelomonocytic leukemia, but granulocytic cells are usually less than 20% in monocytic leukemia.

Megakaryocytic Leukemia ● Megakaryocytic leukemia (megakaryocytic myelosis) has been described in five cats (see comments on the disease in dogs).

MISCELLANEOUS LEUKOCYTE DISORDERS

Feline Leukemia Virus

FeLV frequently does not cause neoplasia. Of 95 cats infected with FeLV, only 18 had LSA or MPD (Prasse, 1983). FeLV viremia was relatively common in apparently normal cats killed by trauma (i.e., 3%) and in 16% of 1095 cats necropsied for any reason (Reinacher and Theilen, 1987). Various diseases have been associated with FeLV, including regenerative, nonregen-erative, and aplastic anemia, pancytopenia, thrombocytopenia, bleeding, panleukopenia-like syndrome, FeLV-associated enteritis, thymic atrophy, lymphatic hyperplasia, immuno-suppression, bacterial infections, feline infectious peritonitis, emaciation, and hepatitis. FeLV viremia is diagnosed mainly by enzyme-linked immunoassay (ELISA) procedures and indirect fluorescent antibody (IFA) tests currently available from many reference laboratories (see Chapter 15 regarding FeLV).

Feline Immunodeficiency Virus

FIV infections may be associated with various hematologic disorders including neutropenia, anemia, and thrombocytopenia (Shelton et al., 1991). Many diseases have been associated with FIV, including various infections, malignancies, lymphadenopathy, colitis, and central nervous system disorders. FIV is diagnosed by ELISA and Western blot procedures available at various laboratories (see Chapter 15).

Pelger-Huet Anomaly

This condition should be remembered since it presents as a complete left shift in the granulocytes but does not denote inflammation. This hereditary hyposegmentation of granulocyte nuclei is essentially an incidental finding in occasional dogs. Almost all neutrophils appear to be bands or younger, and thus the differential appears as a severe left shift. The great increase of N-segs compared with segs mistakenly suggests a poor prognosis. A dog with femoral fractures and Pelger-Huet anomaly had 31,000 WBCs/μl, 30,167 N-segs/μl, and only 311 segs/μl; these findings looked like an overwhelming left shift. Pelger-Huet anomaly is considered innocuous except for the confusion caused on a WBC differential count.

Pelger-Huet anomaly is diagnosed by the characteristic appearance of neutrophils and eosinophils with bean-shaped to round nuclei. The nuclear chromatin pattern has a coarse, clumped, mature pattern. The cytoplasm has a clear, mature, and nontoxic appearance. Normal bands and metamyelocytes of the same shape have finer chromatin patterns and a bluer, more immature-appearing cytoplasm. Despite almost all of the neutrophils appearing to be bands or younger based on nuclear shape, there is no inflammation and the disorder lasts the life of the animal. Some decreased neutrophil migration has been demonstrated in the laboratory, but neutrophil function is essentially normal.

Pseudo–Pelger-Huet anomaly may occur as a process of transient duration. One dog probably acquired it as a result of various treatments including sulfadiazine-trimethoprim (Shull and Powell, 1979). Another case was in a dog with hyperadrenocorticism (Prasse KW: Personal communication, 1980).

Chediak-Higashi Syndrome

Chediak-Higashi syndrome occurs in Persian cats with yellow eyes and blue smoke-colored hair (Kramer et al., 1975). It should be recognized since the cats have clinical problems and the owners may need genetic counseling. The autosomal recessive disease affects the size of cytoplasmic granules, causing characteristic large inclusions in neutrophils. A similar effect on melanin granules is associated with the color dilution of hair and eyes. Diagnosis is by blood smear analysis and the cat's gross appearance. The neutrophil inclusions are peroxidase and Sudan positive. The cats are photophobic and tend to develop cataracts. Feline Chediak-Higashi syndrome is associated with increased bleeding time and platelet dysfunction. No increased susceptibility to infections has been noted in cats, unlike this syndrome in other species.

Canine Leukocyte Function Defects

Neutrophil function defects are suspected in animals with recurrent or persistent infections. Diagnosis of neutrophil dysfunction requires ruling out other causes of decreased resistance to infection and special tests (e.g., a WBC bactericidal assay). These tests are currently research tools of a few specialists to whom the animal must be referred for diagnosis. Contact the closest university veterinary clinic. A defect termed *canine granulocytopathy syndrome* was identified in a 5-month-old Irish setter with recurrent bacterial infections starting soon after birth (Renshaw et al., 1975). A persistent leukemoid reaction of 71,400 to 200,000 WBCs/μl and a fairly mature neutrophilia suggested that even an excess of neutrophils could not resolve the infections. This is likely the WBC adhesion protein defect of Irish setter dogs (Trowald-Wigh et al., 1992). The neutrophils totally lack adhesion proteins CD11b and CD18, cannot phagocytize C3b-opsonized particles, and have diminished adherence. Twelve puppies from six litters in Sweden were 10 to 20 weeks of age. Eight of 12 had leukemoid responses yet relatively mild left shifts. Eight of 12 had lymphocytosis (5200–13,262/μl), as expected in chronic persistent infections.

A bactericidal defect occurred in eight closely related Doberman pinschers with chronic rhinitis and pneumonia (Breitschwerdt et al., 1987). Neutrophils could phagocytize but not kill bacteria. Immunoglobulin concentrations, complement concentrations, and mitogen-stimulated lymphocyte transformation responded as expected. Half of the Dobermans had an eosinophilia but often not a leukocytosis.

Cyclic Hematopoiesis

Canine cyclic hematopoiesis (i.e., gray collie syndrome or cyclic neutropenia) is an autosomal recessive disease diagnosed by cyclic neutropenia (i.e., 0–400 neutrophils/μl) occurring at 11- to 12-day cycles in silver-gray collie pups. This should be suspected when recurrent infections occur at a young age. A stem cell defect also causes cyclic decreases in hematopoiesis of platelets, other WBCs, and RBCs, but because of a longer half-life of these cells in blood, the change is less obvious. In addition to the neutropenia, a bactericidal defect predisposes the dogs to frequently lethal infections. A similar disorder has been seen in a Labrador puppy. All the littermates died within months of birth, and this puppy had erratic cycles of neutropenia that spontaneously resolved (Willard MD: Personal communication, 1993).

Cyclic hematopoiesis also occurs in occasional FeLV-infected cats (Swenson et al., 1987). Oscillations of neutrophils, other WBCs, reticulocytes, and platelets occur at 8- to 16-day intervals. Hemograms at 2- to 3-day intervals should document the cyclic neutropenia, but daily CBCs may be required to document cycling of other cells. Oral ulceration occurred during neutropenia. Waves of myelopoiesis in the bone marrow resembled that found in gray collies. Also similar was increased hematopoiesis of one cell line, while another was decreased (penic). For example, reticulocytosis occurred during neutropenia.

Storage Diseases

Certain rare inherited enzyme defects result in the accumulation of enzyme substrates in various cells. These diseases are often suggested by severe problems in the central nervous system or skeleton but may be identified on a CBC by inclusions in circulating WBCs. Mucopolysaccharidosis occurs in cats and dachshunds. The characteristic purple granules can be differentiated from toxic granulation since the rest of the cytoplasm is clear and nontoxic. Additionally, toxic granulation is not common in dogs and cats.

Canine Parvovirus

The pattern of neutropenia, lymphopenia, severe neutrophil toxic change, plus diarrhea and/or vomiting is strongly suggestive of acute canine parvovirus enteritis. Damage to the gut's epithelium with absorption of bacterial toxins probably accounts for the severe toxic change. Leukopenia is not a consistent feature of canine parvovirus, with only 11 of 31 dogs having <6000 WBCs/μl when examined (Stann et al., 1984). It seems leukopenia is likely early in the disease, but the WBC count becomes normal to increased with time. A leukopenic episode may easily be missed. Diagnosis of parvovirus enteritis is by detection of virus in feces (see Chapter 9) or by intestinal histopathology.

Feline Panleukopenia

Feline parvovirus infection causes a profound neutropenia and leukopenia. The WBC count often drops to <1000/μl. An absolute lymphopenia occurs, but lymphocytes may be 70% to 80% of a differential WBC count (Jain, 1986). As the bone marrow repopulates, the prominence of immature myeloid precursors may resemble a myeloid leukemia. Neutrophils first released into the blood include giant forms and atypical nuclear patterns. The nonleukemic nature of the hematologic changes becomes evident over a few days.

Bibliography

Baxter JD, Rousseau GG: Glucocorticoid Hormone Action. New York, Springer-Verlag, 1979, pp 449–465.

Bellah JR, Stiff ME, Russell RG: Thymoma in the dog: Two case reports and review of 20 additional cases. JAVMA 1983;183:306–311.

Bennett JM, Catovsky D, Daniel MT, et al: Proposals for the classification of the acute leukaemias. Br J Haematol 1976;33:451–458.

Bennett JM, Catovsky D, Daniel MT, et al: Proposed revised

criteria for the classification of acute myeloid leukemia. Ann Intern Med 1985;103:620–625.

Blue JT, French TW, Kranz JS: Non-lymphoid hematopoietic neoplasia in cats: A retrospective study of 60 cases. Cornell Vet 1988;78:21–42.

Boggs DR, Winkelstein A: White Cell Manual. 3rd ed. Philadelphia, FA Davis, 1975, pp 21–31.

Bowles CA, Alsaker RD, Wolfle TL: Studies of the Pelger-Huet anomaly in foxhounds. Am J Pathol 1979;96:237–245.

Breitschwerdt EB, Brow TT, DeBuysscher EV, et al: Rhinitis, pneumonia, and defective neutrophil function in the Doberman Pinscher. Am J Vet Res 1987;48:1054–1062.

Buerger RG, Scott DW: Cutaneous mast cell neoplasia in cats: 14 cases (1975–1985). JAVMA 1987;190:1440–1444.

Carpenter JL, Holzworth J: Thymoma in 11 cats. JAVMA 1982;181:248–251.

Carter RF, Harris CK, Withrow SJ, et al: Chemotherapy of canine lymphoma with histopathological correlation: Doxorubicin alone compared to COP as first treatment regimen. JAAHA 1986;23:587–596.

Confer AW, Langloss JM: Long-term survival of two cats with mastocytosis. JAVMA 1978;172:160–161.

Couto CG: Clinocopathologic aspects of acute leukemias in the dog. JAVMA 1985;186:681–685.

Couto CG: Toxicity of anticancer chemotherapy. Proceedings, 10th Annual Kal Kan Symposium for the Treatment of Small Animal Diseases. Kal Kan Foods, October 1986 at The Ohio State University, Columbus, Ohio. Published by Kal Kan Foods, Inc, Vernon, CA, pp 37–46.

Duncan JR, Prasse KW: Veterinary Laboratory Medicine. 2nd ed. Ames, IA, Iowa State University Press, 1986.

Essex M, Francis D: The risk to humans from malignant diseases of their pets: An unsettled issue. JAAHA 1976;12:386.

Facklam NR, Kociba GJ: Cytochemical characterization of leukemic cells from 20 dogs. Vet Pathol 1985;23:155–161.

Facklam NR, Kociba GJ: Cytochemical characterization of feline leukemic cells. Vet Pathol 1986;23:155–161.

Grindem CB, Perman V, Stevens JB: Morphological classification and pathologic characteristics of spontaneous leukemia in 17 dogs. JAAHA 1985a;21:219–226.

Grindem CB, Perman V, Stevens JB: Morphological classification and pathologic characteristics of spontaneous leukemia in 10 cats. JAAHA 1985b;21:227–236.

Grindem CB, Stevens JB, Perman V: Cytochemical reactions in cells from leukemic dogs. Vet Pathol 1986;23:103–109.

Harvey JW, Terrell TG, Hyde DM, Jackson RI: Well-differentiated lymphocytic leukemia in a dog: Long-term survival without therapy. Vet Pathol 1981;18:37–47.

Harvey JW, Henderson CW, French TW, Meyer DJ: Myeloproliferative disease with megakaryocytic predominance in a dog with occult dirofilariasis. Vet Clin Pathol 1982;11:5–10.

Jain NC: Schalm's Veterinary Hematology. 4th ed. Philadelphia, Lea and Febiger, 1986.

Jain NC, Blue JT, Grindem CB, et al: Proposed criteria for classification of acute myeloid leukemia in dogs and cats. Vet Clin Pathol 1991;20:63–82.

Kramer JW, Davis WC, Prieur DJ, et al: An inherited disorder of Persian cats with intracytoplasmic inclusions in neutrophils. JAVMA 1975;166:1103–1104.

Leifer CE, Matus RE: Chronic lymphocytic leukemia in the dog: 22 cases (1974–1984). JAVMA 1986;189:214–217.

Leifer CE, Matus RE, Patnaik AK, Mackwen EG: Chronic myelogenous leukemia in the dog. JAVMA 1983;183:686–689.

Macy DW: Canine and feline mast cell tumors. Proceedings, 10th Annual Kal Kan Symposium for the Treatment of Small Animal Diseases. Kal Kan Foods, October 1986, Ohio State University, pp 101–111.

Madewell BR: Hematological and bone marrow cytological abnormalities in 75 dogs with malignant lymphoma. JAAHA 1985;22:235–240.

Matus RE, Leifer CE, MacEwen G: Acute lymphoblastic leukemia in the dog: A review of 30 cases. JAVMA 1983;183:859–862.

McKeever PJ, Grindem CB, Stevens JB, Osborne CA: Canine cutaneous lymphoma. JAVMA 1982;180:531–536.

Medleau L, Latimer KS, Duncan JR: Food hypersensitivity in a cat. JAVMA 1986;189:692–693.

O'Keefe DA, Couto CG, Burke-Schwartz C, Jacobs RM: Systemic mastocytosis in 16 dogs. J Vet Intern Med 1987;1:75–80.

Prasse KW: White blood cell disorders. In Ettinger SJ (ed): Textbook of Veterinary Internal Medicine. Diseases of the Dog and Cat. 2nd ed, vol 2. Philadelphia, WB Saunders, 1983.

Raskin RE, Krehbiel JD: Incidence of leukemic blood and bone marrow in dogs with multicentric lymphoma. JAVMA 1989;194:1427–1429.

Reinacher M, Theilen G: Frequency and significance of feline leukemia virus infection in necropsied cats. Am J Vet Res 1987;48:939–945.

Renshaw HW, Chatburn C, Bryan GM, et al: Canine granulocytopathy syndrome: Neutrophil dysfunction in a dog with recurrent infections. JAVMA 1975;166:443–446.

Rosenberg SA, Berard CW, Brown BW Jr: National Cancer Institute sponsored study of classifications of non-Hodgkin's lymphomas. Cancer 1982;49:2112–2135.

Shelton GH, Linenberger ML, Abkowitz JL: Hematologic abnormalities in cats seropositive for feline immunodeficiency virus. JAVMA 1991;199:1353–1357.

Shull RM, Powell D: Acquired hyposegmentation of granulocytes (pseudo-Pelger-Huet anomaly) in a dog. Cornell Vet 1979;69:241–247.

Shull RM, DeNovo RC, McCracken MD: Megakaryoblastic leukemia in a dog. Vet Pathol 1986;23:533–536.

Stann SE, DiGiacomo RF, Giddens WE Jr, Evermann JF: Clinical and pathologic features of parvoviral diarrhea in pound-source dogs. JAVMA 1984;185:651–655.

Stockham SL, Basel DL, Schmidt DA: Idiopathic mastocytemia in dogs. Vet Clin Pathol 1984;13:33.

Swenson CL, Kociba GJ, O'Keefe DA, et al: Cyclic hematopoiesis associated with feline leukemia virus infection in two cats. JAVMA 1987;191:93–96.

Trowald-Wigh G, Håkansson L, Johannisson A, et al: Leucocyte adhesion protein deficiency in Irish setter dogs. Vet Immunol Immunopathol 1992;32:261–280.

Weiss DJ: Uniform evaluation and semiquantitative reporting of hematologic data in veterinary laboratories. Vet Clin Pathol 1984;13:27–31.

White SD: Food hypersensitivity in 30 dogs. JAVMA 1986;188:695–698.

Harold Tvedten

5 Hemostatic Abnormalities

The laboratory approach to hemostatic abnormalities is considered in this chapter in three main parts. The first section, laboratory tests, discusses what specific interpretations may be made from individual test results; conclusions are then derived from groups of test results, including a profile of hemostatic tests. The second main section addresses selected hemostatic diseases and their diagnosis. Important technical aspects are separated into the third section, since readers are easily distracted and fatigued by detailed technical aspects; this technical information is read as needed.

Evaluation of a bleeding patient or a potentially bleeding patient relies extensively on hemostatic tests. Most of the necessary tests are routinely used in human hospitals; with a little effort in establishing the hospital laboratory's cooperation and appropriate reference values, these tests will be available for most veterinary practices. In the absence of this, a small clinic may be limited to a few tests described in the section on techniques for small practices. The simple diagnostic approach to be described is intended for veterinarians in general practice. The amount of information has been greatly minimized to that which still allows understanding and diagnosis of most bleeding problems. Those readers wishing to flesh out this clinical overview are referred to reference texts (Feldman et al., 1986).

Bleeding problems range from severe, overt problems (e.g., epistaxis) requiring emergency care to a potential problem suspected in the breed (e.g., Doberman pinscher dogs) or laboratory signs (e.g., falling platelet count or hepatic disease). Signs of a bleeding problem include prolonged bleeding due to minor trauma (e.g., venipuncture or loss of deciduous teeth), prolonged bleeding after parturition or estrus, and hemorrhages that vary in severity from bruises to petechial or ecchymotic hemorrhages to large hematomas. Gastrointestinal tract bleeding may appear as fresh red blood or dark tarry stools. Bleeding into joints and other body cavities may be diagnosed from fluid cytology. These and other presenting patterns may require laboratory evaluation to identify the defect quickly.

An organized, simple, and consistent approach for diagnosis of hemostatic defects should be prepared in advance of any bleeding problem (Fig. 5–1). The initial consideration is whether the bleeding is due to defective hemostasis or whether there is adequate reason for the bleeding (e.g., trauma). If there is no explanation for the bleeding or it seems excessive, hemostatic tests are used to document and localize the defect.

LOCALIZATION OF THE DEFECT

Initially the hemostatic defect should be localized to a general area of the hemostatic mechanism, which can simply be considered to have four main areas: the blood vessels, the platelets, the coagulation factors, and the fibrinolytic system (Table 5–1). If damaged, a vessel is initially sealed by a plug of aggregated platelets; this platelet plug is then stabilized by fibrin strands generated through the coagulation system. The fibrinolytic system degrades the clot to reopen the vascular lumen while the vessel heals.

Laboratory test results must be evaluated in light of other information. Clinical signs and physical examination findings are much less specific than are laboratory tests in localizing the defect but initially suggest whether a hemostatic defect is either a platelet or a coagulation

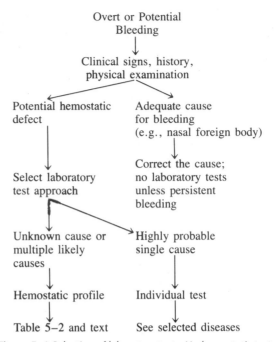

Figure 5–1 Selection of laboratory tests. No hemostatic tests are necessary if there is an adequate explanation for a bleeding process. If a hemostatic defect is likely and either several causes are possible or the cause is uncertain, screen all parts of the hemostatic mechanism for a defect with a profile of laboratory tests. When the evidence suggests only one probable cause, select the most appropriate test to evaluate that defect.

problem. In vascular injury, the platelets in the blood come in contact with collagen beneath the endothelium and begin aggregation to form the platelet plug (Fig. 5–2). The coagulation factors stimulated by the collagen, tissue thromboplastin, and platelets form fibrin strands to stabilize the plug. Small hemorrhages like petechiae and ecchymoses suggest a platelet defect, since the lack of a platelet plug allows a little blood to leak out of the vessel, but before the size of the hemorrhage becomes too large, the normal coagulation factors in contact with collagen around the vessel form a fibrin clot to stop the hemorrhage (see Fig. 5–2). Epistaxis is often associated with platelet defects, perhaps because of the paucity of tissue between the vessels and the open nasal cavity.

In contrast, coagulation defects are characterized by large hemorrhages like hematomas and bleeding into joints. A platelet plug forms in coagulopathies, but since it is not stabilized by fibrin strands, it breaks down, allowing bleeding. The defect or variable deficiency of one or more coagulation factors slows the formation of a clot, which should have formed rapidly after contact with the collagen in the interstitial tissue. During this time, a large amount of hemor-

Table 5-1 HEMOSTATIC MECHANISMS: FUNCTION AND APPROPRIATE LABORATORY TESTS

	Platelets*	Coagulation Factors*	Fibrinolytic System*	Blood Vessel*
Normal function†	Platelet plug	Fibrin clot	Dissolve clot	Retain blood
Means of evaluation‡	**Platelet numbers** Platelet count Platelet estimate	**Factor activity** ACT or APTT PT	**Plasmin activity** FDP	**Vascular integrity** Histopathology
	Thrombocytopenia	*Coagulopathy*	*Consumptive coagulopathy*	*Vascular disease*
	Platelet function Bleeding time			
	Platelet dysfunction			

*Four basic portions of the hemostatic mechanism.
†Basic function of the four portions. Note all portions interact with the others (e.g., the fibrin clot stabilizes the platelet plug, and platelets accelerate the clotting process).
‡The parameter in bold type is evaluated by the tests listed beneath it. Possible abnormality that may be identified from the tests is italicized. Coagulation factor activity is described in the text and Figures 5–4 to 5–8.

rhage can occur before the fibrin clot or pressure of adjacent tissues stops the bleeding (see Fig. 5–2).

A hemostatic profile of five or six tests is recommended whenever possible in the presence of clinically significant bleeding of undetermined cause (see Fig. 5–1) as the primary method to localize the defect. Many hemostatic disorders either are rapidly changing or affect multiple areas of the hemostatic mechanism. Evaluation of the findings of one or two individual tests may miss the full extent of the defect or lead to an incomplete or erroneous conclusion. Certain situations, on the other hand, may require only a single test, such as a factor VIII–related antigen (VIII-Ag) analysis as a presurgical screen for elective surgery on a Doberman dog potentially having von Willebrand's disease (vWD) or a prothrombin time (PT) for a dog that has eaten warfarin (see later discussion of selected diseases for specific diagnostic approaches).

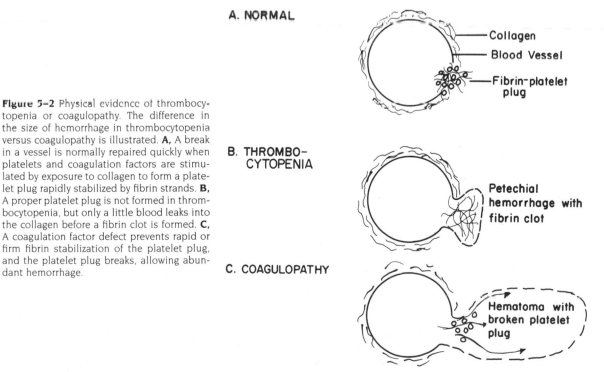

A. NORMAL

— Collagen
— Blood Vessel
— Fibrin-platelet plug

B. THROMBO-CYTOPENIA

Petechial hemorrhage with fibrin clot

C. COAGULOPATHY

Hematoma with broken platelet plug

Figure 5–2 Physical evidence of thrombocytopenia or coagulopathy. The difference in the size of hemorrhage in thrombocytopenia versus coagulopathy is illustrated. **A,** A break in a vessel is normally repaired quickly when platelets and coagulation factors are stimulated by exposure to collagen to form a platelet plug rapidly stabilized by fibrin strands. **B,** A proper platelet plug is not formed in thrombocytopenia, but only a little blood leaks into the collagen before a fibrin clot is formed. **C,** A coagulation factor defect prevents rapid or firm fibrin stabilization of the platelet plug, and the platelet plug breaks, allowing abundant hemorrhage.

The profile includes a platelet count for platelet quantity, a buccal mucosa bleeding time (BMBT) for platelet function, the activated partial thromboplastin time (APTT) for the intrinsic and common pathways, the PT for the extrinsic and common pathways, and fibrin degradation products (FDP) quantitation for evaluation of the rate of clot formation and breakdown (Table 5–2). Alternative tests are substituted as needed. The activated clotting time (ACT) is similar to the APTT in interpretation. A blood smear platelet estimate is often adequate to quantitate platelets. The VIII-Ag test is added for dogs, since vWD is common. This profile should detect most of the hemostatic defects.

History, clinical signs, physical examination findings, breed incidence, and other characteristics of specific diseases of the hemostatic mechanism aid in diagnosis. Disease diagnosis requires pattern recognition, much like bird watching. The more often you identify a bird, the easier it is to recognize it the next time, and the more subtle detail about it becomes apparent.

LABORATORY TESTS

This section includes most of the information needed to decide when to use a few common tests and how to interpret their results. The subsections consider platelet problems, coagulopathies, and fibrinolysis (see Simple Hemostatic Test Procedures for the performance of selected tests).

Platelet Evaluation

Platelet problems are the most common cause of bleeding and should be evaluated first. Thrombocytopenia is commonly due to excessive removal of platelets in disorders such as immune-mediated thrombocytopenia or disseminated intravascular coagulation (DIC), or decreased production of platelets during bone marrow disease. Abnormalities in platelet function may be less obvious but occur as part of vWD, in lymphoproliferative disease with circulating abnormal paraproteins, with drug treatment (e.g., aspirin), and as primary defects (e.g., basset hound thrombopathy).

Platelet Morphology ● Platelet clumping is the most common and meaningful morphologic observation. It is an indication to disregard the platelet count and carefully redraw the sample to obtain blood with even platelet distribution. Platelet clumping in some cats cannot be avoided. When platelet clumps are noted on the smear or detected electronically by automated cell counters, the platelet count is not reported.

Numerous large platelets suggest active thrombopoiesis and an active bone marrow. The assessment of "increased numbers of large platelets" on a blood smear is subjective, but newer automated hematology cell counters give a mean platelet volume, platelet histogram, and platelet count that objectively evaluate changes in platelet size during active platelet production. The larger platelets are more functionally active, a fact that has been used to explain why some dogs with platelet counts <10,000/μl do not bleed (Davenport and Carakostas, 1982). Platelets on a smear occasionally have pseudopods and an irregular shape. This is likely an artifact of the platelets being activated during handling of the sample. Primary platelet disorders like thrombasthenic thrombopathia in otter hounds are too rare to consider in most practices. Those dogs have large and morphologically bizarre platelets.

Platelet Count ● The platelet count is useful to classify the severity of a thrombocytopenia and to monitor the course of the disease and response to treatment. The two alternatives are manual counts with a hemocytometer and automated counts with certain hematology cell counters. Based on ease of operation and better accuracy and precision, the automated platelet count should be used if available. Since hemocytometers are cheap and readily available and

Table 5–2 HEMOSTATIC SCREENING PROFILE

Preferred Test	Alternate Test	Parameter Tested
Platelet count	Blood smear	Platelet quantity
Bleeding time	Clot retraction	Platelet function
APTT	ACT	Coagulation factors
Prothrombin time	None	Coagulation factors
FDP	Protamine SO$_4$	Fibrinolysis
Factor VIII antigen	Coagglutinin cofactor	von Willebrand's disease

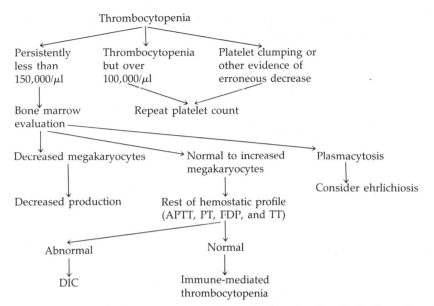

Figure 5-3 Initial diagnostic approach to thrombocytopenia. After establishing that there is significant thrombocytopenia not due to technical error, diagnose one of the three likely causes by a bone marrow evaluation and the rest of the hemostatic profile. A bone marrow disease is diagnosed by decreased megakaryocytes. Disseminated intravascular coagulation (DIC) is proved by abnormalities in the fibrin degradation products (FDP) and by coagulation factor tests, such as activated partial thromboplastin time (APTT) and prothrombin time (PT). An abnormal bleeding time suggests DIC if the thrombocytopenia is mild to moderate (e.g., >40,000/μl) but is expected in severe (e.g., <20,000/μl) thrombocytopenia of any cause. Immune-mediated thrombocytopenia is diagnosed by ruling out the other abnormalities.

most practices have the necessary microscope, veterinarians may prefer to use a manual count. Feline platelets tend to clump, frequently causing inaccurate platelet counts.

Platelet Mass • Platelet mass is reported by some hematology analyzer systems. Mass is the product of platelet number times mean platelet volume (MPV). Platelet mass should be a more physiologic or functional measurement. For example, if a breed has a low platelet count yet large platelets and a high enough MPV to have a platelet mass similar to other breeds, one may expect normal platelet function.

Platelet Estimate • An estimate of platelet numbers from a stained blood smear is quicker than an actual platelet count and is reasonably accurate (Tvedten et al., 1988). The average number of platelets in 10 oil immersion fields on blood smears is counted. Normal dogs have 8 to 29 platelets, and cats have 10 to 29. If a dog has about 20,000 platelets/μl, which is of the severity probably needed to cause bleeding, then one would expect to see only about one platelet per oil immersion field. Scan the smear to ensure that the platelet distribution is even and there is no platelet clumping.

Diagnostic Approach to Thrombocytopenia •

The first step in evaluation of thrombocytopenia is to confirm that it is not an error of collection, sample handling, or the test itself (Fig. 5-3). If one does all of the steps oneself, then the answer is usually apparent. In a team effort, it is important to keep good records, including at least listing potential errors (e.g., "cat resisted venipuncture").

Next, the severity of the thrombocytopenia is classified. Thrombocytopenia is defined as any platelet count less than the appropriate reference range; however, reference ranges vary among laboratories and techniques. Jain (1986) reports a canine platelet reference range of 200,000 to 500,000/μl, whereas our reference range for manual platelet counts is 166,000 to 575,000/μl. One should interpret mild thrombocytopenia (i.e., between 100,000 and 200,000/μl) with caution if one is uncertain of the quality of the venipuncture or if laboratory errors due to platelet clumping or large platelet size are possible. Mild thrombocytopenia may be due to diseases such as ehrlichiosis but are also commonly due to sampling errors. Persistent thrombocytopenia of 100,000 to 175,000 platelets/μl after careful venipuncture and platelet counting technique is significant. A therapeutic trial with doxycycline or an *Ehrlichia* titer is a reasonable plan for such a problem.

Severe thrombocytopenia is defined as

<20,000 platelets/µl, since it is at this level that clinical signs are expected (e.g., petechial and ecchymotic hemorrhages, epistaxis, or gastrointestinal hemorrhage). Exceptions occur; some animals may not bleed with 10,000 platelets/µl, whereas others may bleed at 40,000 to 50,000 platelets/µl. Factors such as platelet size, platelet functional activity, blood vessel/endothelial support, and severity of the challenge to the hemostatic mechanism all may contribute to the presence or absence of bleeding. Linking the severity of change in laboratory data to clinical signs is important. For example, if the platelet count is 80,000/µl and yet clinical bleeding is occurring, then some factor in addition to thrombocytopenia is likely (e.g., DIC).

The three common causes of thrombocytopenia are (1) bone marrow defects limiting adequate platelet production, (2) immune-mediated removal, and (3) consumption of platelets during intravascular coagulation. Evaluation of a bone marrow aspirate and biopsy sample is usually effective in documenting decreased or compensatory increased platelet production by judging megakaryocytic numbers and maturity. No significant bleeding usually occurs as a result of bone marrow aspiration or biopsy, so bone marrow evaluation is the best initial diagnostic procedure in thrombocytopenia (see Fig. 5–3). One can rule out a consumptive coagulopathy (i.e., DIC) by the rest of the hemostatic profile. If no other defects are detected, then the animal has a pure platelet problem.

Immune-mediated thrombocytopenia (IMT) is often diagnosed by ruling out a marrow problem and DIC. It is further confirmed by response to immunosuppressive therapy. More direct diagnostic methods are in a state of change. Antiplatelet antibody tests have been established for research projects (Bloom et al., 1985). New assays are under development and evaluation, and they appear promising. Two indirect indicators of IMT include a low MPV or a platelet count <20,000/µl (Northern and Tvedten, 1992). Of 17 thrombocytopenic dogs with microcytosis (low MPV), 16 had IMT. Of 22 dogs with a platelet count <20,000/µl, 21 had IMT. The platelet count and MPV in IMT became low enough to be near background levels for the H-1 hematology analyzer.

Platelet Function Tests ● *Bleeding Time* ● The bleeding time (BT) is a useful and sensitive test of platelet function. Note that inadequate platelet function causing prolonged BT may be due to significant thrombocytopenia as well as abnormal platelet function with normal platelet numbers. The BT is considered "normal" in coagulation defects like hemophilia, since the bleeding stops initially in the expected time owing to the formation of platelet plugs. Since the platelet plug is not stabilized by fibrin strands, the incision is prone to rebleed if it is traumatized later. A qualifier needs to be added—for example, "normal bleeding time but bleeding recurred later."

The BMBT is a sensitive and specific platelet function test in dogs (Jergens et al., 1987). A spring-loaded disposable device creates a standardized cut in the mucosal surface of the upper lip. The technique is described later. In one study, the BMBT in healthy dogs was 2.61 ± 0.48 minutes and it identified three of three dogs with platelet counts of <20,000/µl, seven of seven Doberman pinscher dogs with vWD, and five of six uremic dogs. The BMBT seems more sensitive than prior BT tests (e.g., the cuticle bleeding time).

Clot Retraction Test ● This is a crude, insensitive test of platelet function used mainly in the past. Platelets are contractile and with time pull the fibrin strands together to form a firm clot. After a tube of blood has clotted, it is kept at 37°C. Inspection after 1 hour should demonstrate some serum squeezed out of the clot and thus visible outside of the clot. At 24 hours, the clot should be maximally retracted. Some laboratories report the relative volume of serum produced from the original volume of blood to make the test more quantitative. It is unlikely that this makes this crude screening test any better than a yes-no answer to whether platelet function is adequate. Also, the clot may be inspected for abnormal lysis (e.g., clot lyses quickly during the 24-hour incubation at 37°C, suggesting increased fibrinolytic activity of DIC).

Diagnostic Approach to Abnormal Platelet Function ● A platelet function defect is identified when adequate numbers of platelets are present yet the bleeding time or other platelet function test result is abnormal. The defect in platelet function is attributed to known causes (Table 5–3) by history of drug administration or the diagnosis of diseases such as vWD. Platelet dysfunction due to a drug is commonly diagnosed by a history of drug administration and a return of normal platelet function 4 to 5 days after stoppage of use of the drug. Lists of drugs that potentially cause platelet dysfunction are available (Davenport and Carakostas, 1982). If neither a drug is implicated nor a disease

Table 5-3 SELECTED CAUSES OF ABNORMAL PLATELET FUNCTION

Cause	Selected Examples
Drugs	Aspirin, ibuprofen, phenylbutazone, indomethacin, corticosteroids
Acquired	Lymphoproliferative disorders, disseminated intravascular coagulation, uremia
Hereditary	von Willebrand's disease and rare disorders in basset hounds, otter hounds, foxhounds, and a Scottish terrier

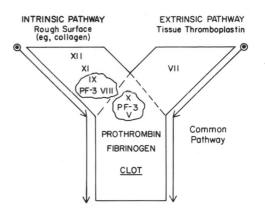

Figure 5-4 A simplified coagulation cascade. Consider the cascade as a letter Y with three portions. The intrinsic pathway includes factors XII, XI, IX, and VIII. The extrinsic pathway contains factor VII. The common pathway includes factors X, V, prothrombin, and fibrinogen. Platelet factor-3 (PF-3) on activated platelets speeds the coagulation process. The intrinsic pathway is initiated by contacting rough surfaces (e.g., collagen) and activates the common pathway by a complex of IX, VIII, and PF-3. The end point of the common pathway is the clot. Tissue thromboplastin from damaged cells and VII in the extrinsic pathway also initiates the common pathway. (Several factors are not included for the purpose of simplicity.)

known to interfere with platelet function, consult a specialist better able to define the dysfunction by more experimental tests such as responses to various stimuli in platelet aggregation tests.

Coagulation Factor Evaluation

Coagulation factors are divided into three areas (intrinsic pathway, extrinsic pathway, or common pathway). This makes a manageable number out of a complex system. A simplified version of the coagulation cascade is diagrammed as a letter Y, not because of equal biochemical significance in coagulation but for simplicity of diagnosis (Fig. 5-4). Factors not likely to cause clinical problems or for which testing is not readily available are not discussed, so coagulation cascade is incomplete.

The intrinsic pathway consists of factors XII, XI, IX, and VIII and is initially activated by plasma contacting a rough surface such as collagen outside a blood vessel. Platelets are important in clot formation since they provide platelet factor 3 (PF-3), which is a lipoprotein exposed on the surface of activated platelets. Without PF-3 (e.g., severe thrombocytopenia), the coagulation process would be much slower. PF-3 acts with factors IX and VIII as a complex at the end of the intrinsic pathway, which starts the common pathway. A complex of factors X, V, and PF-3 is also formed in the common pathway. The common pathway consists of factors X, V, prothrombin, fibrinogen, and other factors. The extrinsic pathway is essentially factor VII, since a deficiency of tissue thromboplastin is unexpected and calcium is never low enough in a living animal to inhibit clotting. The discussion of the APTT, ACT, and PT illustrates how to evaluate these factors and pathways.

Prothrombin Time • The PT evaluates the extrinsic and common pathways (Fig. 5-5). The factors in the common pathway likely to cause clinical problems are X, V, thrombin, and fi-

brinogen. One of the major uses for PT is evaluating vitamin K antagonist poisoning or similar situations in which hepatic synthesis of vitamin K–related coagulation factors is impaired. Of the vitamin K–related factors (II, VII, IX, and X), factor VII has the shortest half-life; if synthesis of these factors is stopped or slowed significantly, then factor VII will be deficient earliest. Since factor VII is in the extrinsic pathway and the PT is the only test evaluating the common pathway, the PT is elevated earliest and has the

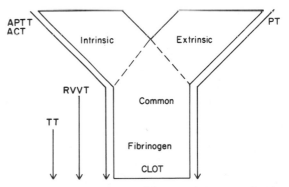

Figure 5-5 Hemostatic tests of the coagulation cascade. The activated partial thromboplastin time (APTT) and the activated coagulation time (ACT) test all factors of the intrinsic and common pathways. The Russell's viper venom time (RVVT) tests all factors of the common pathway. The thrombin time (TT) tests fibrinogen. The prothrombin time (PT) tests factor VII and the factors of the common pathway.

greatest relative increase as a percentage increase above the normal mean.

The PT is used in conjunction with the APTT or ACT, since the PT divides the area evaluated by these two tests into the intrinsic and common pathways (Fig. 5–6).

Activated Partial Thromboplastin Time • This is the most sensitive and specific test of the intrinsic pathway (factors XII, XI, IX, and VIII) plus the common pathway. The APTT tests for all the coagulation factors except factor VII (see Fig. 5–5). It is thus the most useful test to have available to screen for decreased activity of one or more coagulation factors.

Activated Clotting Time • The ACT is used in much the same way as the APTT for defects in the intrinsic or common pathway. It is more crude in having a visual end point of a whole blood clot in a special Vacutainer tube. It is less sensitive in that a factor must be decreased to <5% of normal to prolong the ACT, whereas the APTT will be prolonged at the factor deficiency of <30% of normal (Duncan and Prasse, 1986). Note that a carrier of hemophilia A or B with 40% to 60% of VIII or IX would not be detected by the routine APTT. The ACT is less specific than the APTT in that severe thrombocytopenia may prolong the ACT (e.g., 10 seconds). The APTT is not affected by thrombocytopenia, since phospholipid is present in the reagent to provide a similar function as PF-3.

The major advantage of the ACT is that it is cheap and easy to use, requiring only special Vacutainer tubes and a heating block or water bath to keep the tube at body temperature.

Russell's Viper Venom Time (RVVT) • The amount and quality of factors X, V, thrombin, and fibrinogen are evaluated by the RVVT (see Fig. 5–5), which tests only the common pathway. The RVVT may not be readily available, since it is used less frequently than APTT, PT, ACT, or modified thrombin time (TT).

Thrombin Time • The TT is a test of the amount and activity of fibrinogen (see Fig. 5–5). It should not be confused with the modified TT. The TT may be used to monitor the anticoagulant activity of heparin and FDP. The modified TT has an excess of thrombin added to the reagent, making it insensitive to these anticoagulants. The modified TT is simply a specific and sensitive way to quantitate fibrinogen. The modified TT is more commonly available than is the TT.

Factor VIII–Related Antigen • The VIII-Ag test is specifically used to diagnose vWD. The incidence in some breeds like Doberman dogs is so high (i.e., almost 66%) that any bleeding tendency is a reasonable indication for the VIII-Ag test. The coagglutinin cofactor test is similar in interpretation. See the discussion of vWD for more details. Be sure to measure VIII-Ag before any blood transfusions are administered. Transfusions cause VIII-Ag activity to increase.

Specific Factor Analysis • Specific factor analysis may be used when a problem has been resolved to a likely factor or group of factors (e.g., intrinsic pathway factors). This test would be offered only at unique laboratories possessing plasma with previously identified factor deficiencies available for use as reagents in a modification of the APTT (Appendix I).

Diagnostic Approach to Coagulopathies • The initial consideration is whether a coagulation factor test result is truly elevated. Kociba (1978) recommends considering a 5-second increase in the PT or a 7-second increase in the APTT as being significant in dogs and cats. Lesser elevations are possibly abnormal, but this conclusion must be strengthened with other information or repeated testing.

A defect in the intrinsic pathway (XII, XI, IX, or VIII) would be identified by the combination of a normal PT and prolonged APTT (see Fig. 5–6). A defect in the extrinsic pathway (factor VII) is identified by the combination of a normal APTT and prolonged PT (Fig. 5–7).

A defect in the common pathway (X, V, prothrombin, or fibrinogen) or multiple defects involving the intrinsic, common, and extrinsic

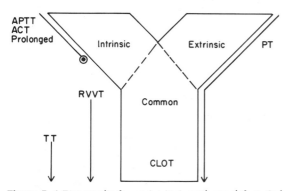

Figure 5–6 Test results for an intrinsic pathway defect. Only the activated partial thromboplastin time (APTT) or activated coagulation time (ACT) results should be abnormal. Identifying a specific factor from factors XII, XI, IX, and VIII is performed by specific factor analysis and consideration of clinical signs, history, and physical findings.

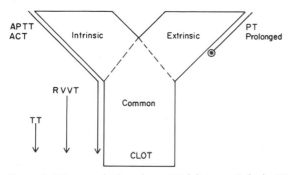

Figure 5-7 Test results for a factor VII deficiency. Only the PT would be abnormal.

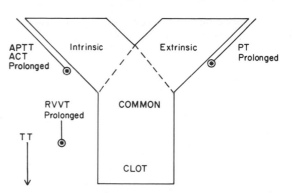

Figure 5-8 Test results for vitamin K antagonist toxicity. Inhibition of the vitamin K–related factors (II, VII, IX, and X) in warfarin poisoning creates defects in all three pathways. The thrombin time (TT) should be normal since fibrinogen is not affected. A factor X deficiency would have the same laboratory test pattern since a defect in the common pathway slows clot formation despite normal intrinsic and extrinsic pathways. Hepatic failure may have a similar pattern unless fibrinogen synthesis is affected.

pathways would prolong the PT and APTT. If available, the RVVT would evaluate just the common pathway and the TT would evaluate just fibrinogen when both the PT and APTT are prolonged. All tests except the TT would have prolonged results in vitamin K antagonist toxicity, since the vitamin K factors (II, VII, IX, and X) would be deficient, creating defects in the intrinsic, extrinsic, and common pathways while the quantity of normal fibrinogen should be adequate (Fig. 5–8). Since the liver synthesizes most factors, severe hepatic failure would cause multiple defects in the coagulation cascade. A defect in the common pathway would prolong both the PT and APTT, since the normal intrinsic and extrinsic pathways must pass through the common pathway to form a clot (Table 5–4).

Other information is usually available to make a good clinical judgment before specific factor analysis. Clinical signs, breed incidence, sex, and other information in addition to the hemostatic profile allow a fairly accurate diagnosis without the need for the RVVT, TT, or specific factor analysis. For example, if you have

a client with a litter of young dogs in which half of the males have severe clinical signs of bleeding including hematomas, and the dogs have a normal PT yet prolonged APTT, then you could be confident that they have a problem with either factor VIII or IX. The APTT and PT combination has localized the defect to the intrinsic pathway. The historical evidence of a sex-linked hereditary problem has implicated factors VIII and IX as the only two sex-linked defects. The severity of the bleeding has ruled out factors XII and XI in the intrinsic pathway, since they have no clinical signs (i.e., factor XII) or mild clinical signs (i.e., factor XI) of bleeding. Factor IX and VIII defects (i.e., hemophilia B and A) both have a similar impact on the owner, and you may have solved the owner's problem as far as he or she desires. The cost:benefit ratio of

Table 5-4 EXPECTED HEMOSTATIC TEST RESULTS IN SELECTED DISEASES

Disease	Hemostatic Profile				
	Bleeding Time	Platelet Count	APTT	PT	FDP
Thrombocytopenia (e.g., ehrlichiosis)	I	D	N	N	N
Platelet dysfunction (e.g., aspirin treatment)	I	N	N	N	N
Intrinsic pathway defect (e.g., hemophilia A or B)	N*	N	I	N	N
Factor VII deficiency	N	N	N	I	N
Multiple factor defects (e.g., vitamin K antagonism)	N*	N	I	I	N
Common pathway defect (e.g., factor X deficiency)	N*	N	I	I	N
Disseminated intravascular coagulation	I	D	I	I	I
von Willebrand's disease	I	N†	N‡	N	N

*Initially stops in normal time period but may start bleeding again.
†Mild thrombocytopenia may occur if concurrently hypothyroid.
‡Usually normal but may be increased.
I, increased; D, decreased; N, normal. See text for details on these diseases and others that may give similar patterns.

more specific testing compared with the economic impact of the diagnosis determines the need for additional tests for a more confident diagnosis.

Fibrin Degradation Products

Quantitation of FDP is primarily used to document an increased breakdown of fibrin clots in the body. This is interpreted to be due to excessive clotting in the body and suggestive of DIC, which is a common acquired disorder secondary to many inflammatory, neoplastic, or necrotic diseases. The commonly used, simple agglutination test* uses antihuman FDP, but cross-reactivity occurs for various animal species (Kociba, 1976). Based on recommended serum dilutions, a concentration of >40 μg/ml is the maximum value measured with the test using a dilution of 1:20. The concentration is 2 μg/ml times the reciprocal of the dilution. Reporting the dilution instead of the concentration may be preferred. Some recommend greater dilutions to assess values >50 μg/ml (1:25 dilution) (Kociba, 1976) or >32 μg/ml (1:16 dilution) (Duncan and Prasse, 1986). Using higher upper values increases the specificity of the test by requiring a higher amount of FDP to denote excessive clot breakdown. The higher specificity reduces the sensitivity. Alternatives to the FDP agglutination test include the protamine sulfate test. The diagnostic and disease characteristics of DIC are discussed later.

Blood Vessel Evaluation

Blood vessels are difficult to evaluate except histologically. A skin biopsy is infrequently performed on a bleeding animal, but in the presence of edema, petechiae, and a normal platelet count, or edema plus DIC, the skin biopsy may document vasculitis. In certain diseases, enough information is available to predict vasculitis or other vascular defect. A vasculitis in horses may occur after *Streptococcus equi* infections. Antigen-antibody complexes occasionally deposit in the vessels, causing an Arthus reaction and a nonthrombocytopenic purpura with petechial hemorrhages and edema. Immune-mediated vasculitis in dogs is uncommon (Randell and Hurvitz, 1983). Other examples of vascular disease in small animals include the rare connective tissue diseases (i.e., Ehlers-Danlos syndrome or feline epitheliogenesis imperfecta). Vascular disease is often diagnosed by ruling out other possibilities or at necropsy.

USE OF THE HEMOSTATIC PROFILE

When a profile of tests is used, one can summarize the status of the hemostatic mechanism on that day. Interpret each test in terms of what it specifically evaluates and list the individual conclusions of what is normal or abnormal. Then, based on the laboratory pattern and clinical evidence, make a disease diagnosis. See Table 5–4 for typical patterns expected in various diseases and refer to it as diseases in the next section are discussed.

SELECTED DISEASE PATTERNS

Disseminated Intravascular Coagulation

DIC is one of the more common hemostatic disorders that occurs secondary to a wide variety of diseases characterized by the formation of necrotic tissue and rough surfaces. The extrinsic system is initiated by tissue thromboplastin from damaged, necrotic cells; the intrinsic system is initiated by rough surfaces such as exposed collagen beneath damaged endothelial cells. Inflammatory diseases create areas of necrosis and exposed collagen, which stimulate clotting; many infections, such as canine infectious hepatitis (Wigton et al., 1976), kill the animal through a DIC-type episode. Neoplasms (e.g., hemangiosarcoma) often have necrotic, inflamed areas, and treatment of neoplasms (e.g., chemotherapy) may create additional necrosis and increase the likelihood of DIC. Hemolytic anemias produce abundant red blood cell (RBC) necrotic debris. Substances such as amniotic fluid strongly induce clotting. Both explain the high incidence of DIC in hemolytic anemia and obstetric disorders. Vasculitis may induce DIC, since the vessels are devoid of endothelial cells. Endothelial cells, besides providing a smooth surface, act to inhibit platelet aggregation. If DIC and edema are concurrently present, a skin biopsy sample may document a vasculitis. For this discussion, DIC is considered to include various situations causing excessive clotting in the vascular system, even if it is localized or chronic and not disseminated and per-

---

*Thrombo-Wellcotest, Wellcome Reagents Limited, Beckenham, England.

acute. *Consumptive coagulopathy* is an alternative term when various factors are consumed in a relatively localized process.

One expects DIC to consume platelets and coagulation factors during formation of excessive clotting. The breakdown of these clots causes increased FDP, which act as anticoagulants to interfere with platelet function and clotting and serve as a key diagnostic feature. Thus, any or all hemostatic test results may be abnormal, but since increased production of coagulation factors and platelets can variably compensate for consumption, no result is always abnormal (Table 5–5). Only three of the five tests in the hemostatic screening profile need to show abnormal results to diagnose DIC (Kociba, 1976). The diagnosis is made with greater confidence when thrombocytopenia and coagulation factor deficiency are concurrently identified. Decreased antithrombin III (AT-3; discussed later in this chapter) is probably one of the most sensitive indicators of DIC (Feldman et al., 1981; Green, 1989); however, hepatic insufficiency and protein-losing states may also decrease it, making it less specific.

von Willebrand's Disease

von Willebrand's disease is common but difficult to understand and diagnose. Unlike hemophilia A, it involves a defect in factor VIII and is associated with abnormal platelet function. Platelet numbers are usually normal, although in some dogs with concurrent hypothyroidism a mild thrombocytopenia exists and the clinical signs of vWD are more severe (Dodds, 1983). Dodds' simple way to visualize this molecular disease is to think of factor VIII as a molecule with two parts (Fig. 5–9). The larger part is antigenically recognized as VIII-Ag and also acts as von Willebrand's factor (vWF) to allow platelets to function normally. The smaller part (factor VIII coagulant activity; VIII-C) can be chem-

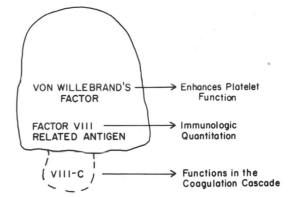

Figure 5–9 Simple visualization of the factor VIII molecular complex. Three methods are used to quantitate the amount or function of the large or small part of the molecule. Platelet function, e.g., buccal mucosa bleeding time (BMBT), is impaired if the large part (i.e., von Willebrand's factor) is deficient or defective. The factor VIII–related antigen is decreased if the large portion is deficient (e.g., von Willebrand's factor). The activated partial thromboplastin time (APTT) is prolonged when the VIII-C cannot participate in the intrinsic pathway (e.g., hemophilia A).

ically separated and still function in the coagulation cascade for clot formation. These three tests evaluate factor VIII in different ways. The APTT measures the activity of VIII-C in the intrinsic system in forming a clot. VIII-Ag immunologically measures the quantity of the larger part of the molecule. Platelet function tests (e.g., BT) measure the functional activity of vWF. Several subtypes of vWD are being identified in people by precise characterization of the molecule, and dogs also have more than one subtype (Johnson et al., 1987).

The clinical signs are often mild and variable. In one study of otoplasty of Doberman pinscher dogs, many of the owners and surgeons were unaware of any bleeding tendency in affected dogs. However, the bleeding tendency was quantitated by the increased number of gauze sponges needed for hemostasis during surgery. The number of sponges was negatively correlated to the concentration of VIII-Ag or coagglutinin cofactor (Johnson et al., 1985). Obscure lameness in Doberman pinscher dogs with vWD has been associated with periosteal ossifications on the pelvis due to hemorrhages. With the exception of VIII-Ag, most of the common hemostatic tests like APTT and ACT fail to identify vWD despite very low levels of immunologically detectable factor VIII.

Before the awareness of the frequency of vWD, many of the more severe cases were misdiagnosed as hemophilia A. The two diseases are most specifically differentiated by VIII-Ag (Table 5–6). When VIII-Ag is <30% of normal,

Table 5–5 FREQUENCY OF LABORATORY ABNORMALITIES IN DISSEMINATED INTRAVASCULAR COAGULATION

Abnormality	Frequency of Abnormal Results	
	Feldman et al. (1981)	Kociba (1978)
Increased FDP	61%	94%
Prolonged APTT	87%	95%
Prolonged PT	80%	72%
Decreased platelet count	80%	48%

Table 5–6 DIFFERENTIATION OF VON WILLEBRAND'S DISEASE AND HEMOPHILIA A

Test	von Willebrand's Disease	Hemophilia A
APTT	Usually normal	Increased
Buccal mucosal bleeding time	Prolonged	"Normal"
Factor VIII antigen	Decreased	Normal to increased

the animal will more likely have bleeding tendencies, although as canine subtypes are identified there will likely be better correlation of laboratory results and clinical signs. VIII-Ag is normal to increased in hemophilia A. The APTT is consistently elevated in hemophilia A, whereas in vWD the APTT is often normal despite the paucity of VIII-Ag. Remember that a transfusion raises VIII-Ag activity.

Ehrlichia canis

Ehrlichiosis can be difficult to recognize, although a positive serologic titer is a sensitive and specific test (see Chapter 15 and Appendix II). The classic pattern was severe thrombocytopenia in a German shepherd dog with epistaxis and ticks, but any dog may be affected, and epistaxis is more infrequent than originally thought. Thrombocytopenia should initiate consideration of *E. canis,* since it is typically found in ehrlichiosis. The platelet count is often >20,000/μl and yet may still be associated with bleeding (e.g., epistaxis, hyphema, petechia). Other hematologic findings suggesting ehrlichiosis include mild to severe nonregenerative anemia (approximately 90% of cases) and leukopenia/neutropenia (approximately 50% of cases). Neutropenia may be severe enough to allow overwhelming sepsis. In some dogs, the bone marrow unexpectedly has normal to increased cellularity despite pancytopenia. Especially in endemic areas (e.g., Arizona, Texas, and Florida), any dog with thrombocytopenia, an unusual anemia, bicytopenia, pancytopenia, or evidence of a chronic infection warrants a titer or empirical treatment with doxycycline for *E. canis.*

The acute phase of the disease resembles other infections with fever, anorexia, weight loss, and lymphadenopathy. The chronic form is more variable, although hyperproteinemia and hypergammaglobulinemia are frequently present; the latter is occasionally severe enough to induce serum hyperviscosity (see Chapters 12

and 15). A polyclonal gammopathy is expected, but occasional electrophoretograms with almost monoclonal peaks may suggest a lymphoid neoplasm (see Chapter 12). Numerous plasma cells in the bone marrow may also mislead one into diagnosing a plasma cell myeloma. The exuberant immune response may lead to an immune-complex glomerular disease and proteinuria.

Vitamin K Antagonist Poisoning

Warfarin and similar rodenticides are common causes of acquired bleeding disorders. The second-generation rodenticides have a long functional half-life (i.e., 15–20 days for diphacinone, compared with 40 hours for warfarin) (Feldman et al., 1986). These rodenticides act in a similar manner by interfering with vitamin K epoxide reductase, which returns vitamin K epoxide to an active form. This inhibition results in a functional vitamin K deficiency and reduced hepatic synthesis of factors II, VII, IX, and X.

The PT is preferred to monitor the toxic effect. When factor synthesis is inhibited, the factor with the shortest half-life becomes deficient earliest. Of the inhibited factors, the half-life of canine VII is only 2 to 4 hours (Green et al., 1978), compared with 14 to 16 hours for factors IX and X and 41 hours for prothrombin (II). Since factor VII is in the extrinsic system, the earliest and greatest relative increase is noted in the PT. Some clinics use the thrombotest or PIVKA (proteins induced by vitamin K absence or antagonism). This test measures precursor coagulation proteins from the liver that accumulate and spill into the circulation when there is vitamin K antagonism (Mount, 1986). After vitamin K_1 therapy, the liver can reach maximum prothrombin synthesis in 9 to 11 hours, and the PT should be back to normal in 1 to 2 days with regular warfarin toxicity.

Antithrombin III and Thrombosis

The frequency of thrombotic disease in people and the availability of funds to investigate those diseases permit complete testing of the hemostatic mechanisms. The quantity and activity of appropriate procoagulant and anticoagulant factors are analyzed in human patients. The balance of procoagulants and anticoagulant factors in veterinary diseases and clinical patients is incompletely understood. AT-3 is an anticoagulant factor that can be analyzed. Heparin inhibits thrombin and other procoagulant factors indirectly by activating AT-3. Since AT-3 is usually decreased in DIC (Feldman et al., 1981), heparin therapy may be ineffective if AT-3 is too low. In people with AT-3 <40% of normal, the response to heparin is poor (Green, 1984). In people, the likelihood of thrombosis is great when AT-3 is <50% of normal. Decreased AT-3 occurs in dogs in hepatic insufficiency owing to decreased synthesis, and deficiency of AT-3 in glomerular disease was attributed to increased loss with proteinuria (Green, 1984). Protein-losing enteropathies may also decrease AT-3.

Availability of the AT-3 assay is variable. Automated assays with chromogenic substrates (e.g., DuPont Automatic Clinical Analyzer: ACA) are used by some veterinary laboratories and allow routine testing. Other tests of AT-3 function may be available only on a research basis. Variation in interpretation of different test methods in domestic animals is not yet well characterized.

Other anticoagulant factors produced in the body include protein C and protein S. Knowledge of their action and amount in various diseases or in specific patients is needed to fully predict the outcome of a thrombotic episode. These tests are available only on a research basis for different species and geographic areas.

SIMPLE HEMOSTATIC TEST PROCEDURES

Blood Smear Platelet Estimate

After routine preparation and staining of a blood smear, determine the average number of platelets in 5 to 10 oil immersion fields to estimate platelet numbers. This should be adequate to rank the count as very low, low, normal, or high (Fig. 5–10). Dogs normally should have 8 to 29 platelets/field, and cats should have 10 to 29/field (Weiss, 1984). Some precautions should be observed. One should count the platelets in 100× oil immersion fields in the thin area where one properly evaluates leukocyte morphology. On most smears, this is where the RBCs infrequently touch each other and central pallor in canine RBC is prominent. In anemic, bleeding animals, there will be fewer RBCs per field in the proper area. An alternative is to consider 1 platelet/100× oil immersion field as approximately equal to 15,000 platelets/μl (Green, 1989). One must also be assured of uniform platelet distribution. If platelet clumps are present, neither the platelet

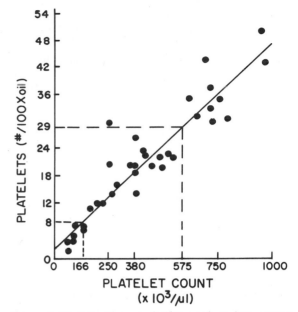

Figure 5–10 Estimation of platelet numbers from canine blood smears. The number of platelets in an average 100 × oil immersion field may be used to estimate the platelet count. Between 8 and 29 platelets/100× oil immersion field represents a normal canine platelet count. A regression line indicates the relationship of the two factors.

count nor the estimate may be trusted. Platelet clumps that are large are usually found at the distal end of the smear and are large enough to be seen at 10× scanning power.

Platelet Count

Details about counting platelets are available in Chapter 2, but a few important points should be noted. The hemocytometer must be clean and free of scratches. Because platelets are the size of dust particles, nicks and scratches in the glass may cause misidentification of dust as platelets. One should keep one very good hemocytometer just for platelet counts. A phase microscope helps to differentiate platelets from other particles. Lowering the condenser on a regular microscope also aids in visualizing the relatively transparent platelets. A platelet stain* improves platelet identification in a hemocytometer but is usually unnecessary.

Collection and handling are especially important. A venipuncture adequate for a routine CBC is often inadequate for an accurate platelet count. A two-syringe or two-Vacutainer technique is recommended. The first blood out of a

*Platelet Stain, Unopette reorder number 5896, Becton-Dickinson, Rutherford, NJ.

needle will contaminate the container with tissue thromboplastin and stimulate platelet clumping. Remove the first syringe or Vacutainer containing the tissue fluids and collect a cleaner sample in a second Vacutainer or syringe. Allowing blood to flow from a bare needle also washes out tissue thromboplastins. EDTA is an adequate anticoagulant, but better accuracy with platelet counts is obtained with 3.8% citrate at a 1:9 ratio with blood (e.g., 0.5 ml sodium citrate plus 4.5 ml blood).

Tardiness in analysis allows platelet clumping and an inaccurate (i.e., lower) platelet count. Various references suggest 1/2 to 6 hours as a maximum tolerable limit, but an unpublished study of 21 dogs suggests clinically accurate platelet counts could be obtained with analysis of EDTA blood up to 2 days old with the Technicon H-1 hematology analyzer (Fig. 5–11). This suggests that EDTA blood sent in the mail for 1 or 2 days still may have platelet count results that can detect marked changes.

Bleeding Time

The canine BMBT is performed on the upper lip. Increased venous pressure is obtained with a gauze muzzle that also serves to hold the upper lip everted for easy access. A sphygmomanometer is used in people to obtain a pressure of 40 mm Hg, but in dogs the pressure is not yet standardized. A device* is used to make a standard cut. Care is taken not to press on or manipulate the wound. As needed, a filter paper is used to absorb the excess blood at 15-second intervals without touching the incision. Anesthesia is usually not needed except for excitable dogs that shake their heads. Some hemostatic control, such as epinephrine on cotton or Gelfoam, should be available for the rare animals with such severe bleeding defects that they fail to stop bleeding on their own. One experimental dog with a platelet function defect required prolonged pressure on the cut with gauze soaked with thrombin reagent to stop the bleeding. Prior aggregation curve analysis demonstrated that the defective platelets would respond to thrombin.

A cuticle bleeding time (CBT) is simply done by clipping the toenails slightly too short and observing when the bleeding stops. It should be within 5 to 6 minutes. The advantage is that this can be a routine part of presurgical preparation of the patient, and clients will appreciate the free nail trim. Clinical experience suggests the CBT is inconsistent (e.g., one dog had a platelet count of 22,000/μl yet a normal CBT).

---

*Simplate-II, Organon Teknika Corp., Organon/General Diagnostics, 100 Akzo Ave., Durham, NC 27704.

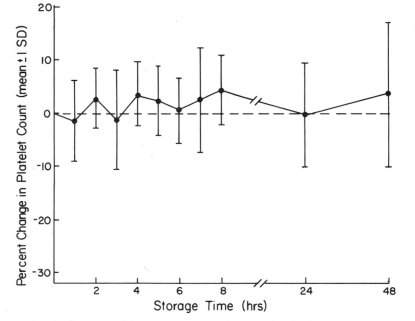

Figure 5–11 Stability of the platelet count. The mean percentage change in the platelet count with time is compared with the initial platelet count for 21 canine EDTA blood samples stored at room temperature for 8 hours and refrigerated for 2 days. The standard deviation is indicated by bars.

Activated Coagulation Time

Special Vacutainer tubes* contain purified siliceous earth to provide abundant surface area for "activating" the intrinsic system. A clot should form in <100 seconds in a dog, compared with 3 to 13 minutes for the Lee-White clotting time. There is less incubation time and labor cost with the ACT than with the Lee-White, especially in coagulopathies. ACT reference values are 60 to 100 seconds for dogs and <60 seconds for cats (Duncan and Prasse, 1986). It is a whole blood procedure obviating the need for using anticoagulants or obtaining plasma. The ACT Vacutainer tubes cost about $70.70 for 100 tubes.

The technique starts with a two-tube collection in which the first tube containing any tissue thromboplastin from the venipuncture is discarded or used for another purpose. A heating block or water bath is used to prewarm the tubes to 37°C and maintain that temperature until the clot forms. The blood is incubated at 37°C for 60 seconds after blood enters the tube. Then at 5-second intervals the tube is inverted until the first visible clot is formed. This is the end point.

Submission of Plasma for Factor Analysis

Mailing plasma to referral laboratories requires special care. Contact the laboratory for the required handling procedure. Green (1989) recommends the following procedure: Use 3.8% citrate as the anticoagulant in a 1:9 ratio (e.g., 0.5 ml Na citrate + 4.5 ml blood). Separate the plasma within 30 minutes of collection by high-speed centrifugation (i.e., 2500–3500 rpm) for 15 minutes. Use plastic pipettes and containers to collect and save the plasma. Rapidly freeze the plasma in 1-ml aliquots with a mixture of alcohol and dry ice. Store or ship the samples at −20°C or less. Mail in Styrofoam containers with 10 to 12 pounds of dry ice.

*Activated Coagulation Time, Becton-Dickinson, Rutherford, NJ.

Bibliography

Bloom JC, Blackmer SA, Bugelski PJ, et al: Gold-induced thrombocytopenia in the dog. Vet Pathol 1985;22:492–499.

Davenport DJ, Carakostas MC: Platelet disorders in the dog and cat. Part I: Physiology and pathogenesis. Comp Cont Ed 1982;4:762–797.

Dodds WJ: Canine von Willebrand's disease. Vet Refer Lab Newsletter 1983;7:1–4.

Duncan JR, Prasse KW: Veterinary Laboratory Medicine: Clinical Pathology. 2nd ed. Ames, IA, Iowa State University Press, 1986.

Feldman BF, Madewell BR, O'Neill MA: Disseminated intravascular coagulation: Antithrombin, plasminogen, and coagulation abnormalities in 41 dogs. JAVMA 1981;179:151–154.

Feldman BF, Carroll EJ, Jain NC: Coagulation and its disorders. In Jain NC (ed): Schalm's Veterinary Hematology. 4th ed. Philadelphia, Lea and Febiger, 1986, pp 388–445.

Green RA: Hemostasis disorders: Coagulopathies and thrombotic disorders. In Ettinger SJ (ed): Textbook of Veterinary Internal Medicine. Diseases of the Dog and Cat. 2nd ed, vol 3. Philadelphia, WB Saunders, 1989, pp 2246–2264.

Green RA: Clinical implications of antithrombin III deficiency in animal diseases. Comp Cont Ed 1984;6:537–545.

Green RA, White F, Osweiler GA: An evaluation of activated coagulation time in warfarin-intoxicated dogs. Vet Clin Pathol 1978;7:9–11.

Jain NC: Schalm's Veterinary Hematology. 4th ed. Philadelphia, Lea and Febiger, 1986.

Jergens AE, Turrentine MA, Kraus K, Johnson GS: A buccal mucosa bleeding time for dogs. Vet Clin Pathol 1987;16:10.

Johnson GS, Schlink GT, Fallon RK, Moore CP: Hemorrhage from the cosmetic otoplasty of Doberman pinschers with von Willebrand's disease. Am J Vet Res 1985;46:1335–1340.

Johnson GS, Turrentine MA, Dodds WJ: Type II von Willebrand's disease in German shorthair pointers. Vet Clin Pathol 1987;16:7.

Kociba GJ: The diagnosis of hemostatic disorders. Vet Clin North Am 1976;6:609–623.

Kociba GJ: Disseminated coagulation. Proceedings, 29th Annual Meeting, American College of Veterinary Pathologists, San Antonio, TX, 1978.

Mount ME: Proteins induced by vitamin K absence or antagonism. In Kirk RW (ed): Current Veterinary Therapy IX. Philadelphia, WB Saunders, 1986, pp 513–515.

Northern J, Tvedten HW: Diagnosis of microthrombocytosis and immune-mediated thrombocytopenia in dogs with thrombocytopenia: 68 cases (1987–1989). JAMA 1992;200:368–372.

Randell MG, Hurvitz AI: Immune-mediated vasculitis in five dogs. JAVMA 1983;183:207–211.

Tvedten HW, Grabski S, Frame L: Estimating platelets and leukocytes on canine blood smears. Vet Clin Pathol 1988;17:4–6.

Weiss DJ: Uniform evaluation and semiquantitative reporting of hematologic data in veterinary laboratories. Vet Clin Pathol 1984;13:27–31.

Wigton DH, Kociba GJ, Hoover EA: Infectious canine hepatitis: Animal model for viral-induced disseminated intravascular coagulation. Blood 1976;47:287.

Stephen P. DiBartola
Robert A. Green
Helio S. Autran de Morais

6 Electrolytes and Acid-Base

○ **Serum Potassium Concentration**
○ **Urinary Fractional Excretion of Potassium**
○ **Serum Sodium Concentration**
   Abnormal Serum Sodium Concentrations
○ **Urinary Fractional Excretion of Sodium**
○ **Serum Chloride Concentration**

○ **Osmolality and Osmolal Gap**
   Osmolality
   Osmolal Gap
○ **Blood Gas Analysis**
○ **Total Carbon Dioxide**
○ **Anion Gap**

Electrolyte and acid-base disorders may result from many different diseases. Timely correction of fluid, electrolyte, and acid-base disturbances often is of more immediate benefit to patients than is a specific diagnosis.

SERUM POTASSIUM CONCENTRATION

Commonly Indicated • Systemic diseases characterized by prolonged anorexia, vomiting, diarrhea, muscle weakness (e.g., cats with cervical ventroflexion), bradycardia, supraventricular arrhythmias, oliguria, anuria, or polyuria are indications for serum potassium determination. Serum potassium concentration should be measured if hypoadrenocorticism, oliguric-anuric renal failure, diabetic ketoacidosis, prolonged vomiting of stomach contents, overzealous use of diuretics (e.g., furosemide, thiazides) or angiotensin-converting enzyme inhibitors (e.g., captopril, enalapril), urethral obstruction, uroabdomen, or postobstructive diuresis is suspected or if there has been prolonged fluid therapy.

Analysis • Serum potassium concentrations are

measured in serum, plasma, or urine by flame photometry (rarely used now), ion-specific potentiometry, and dry reagent methods. Different methods provide comparable results.

Normal Values • Dogs and cats, 3.5 to 5.5 mEq/L.

Danger Values • Levels < 2.5 mEq/L (muscle weakness) or > 7.5 mEq/L (cardiac conduction disturbances) are considered dangerous.

Artifacts • Serum potassium concentrations exceed plasma concentrations because potassium is released from platelets during clotting. This difference is most pronounced in animals with thrombocytosis. Hemolysis causes hyperkalemia only if red blood cells (RBCs) have a high potassium content. Normal canine and feline RBCs contain little potassium; however, an Akita's RBCs have high potassium content (i.e., 70 mEq/L), and hemolysis causes hyperkalemia during storage of blood. These causes are referred to as *pseudohyperkalemia*, because they only occur *in vitro*. Using lithium heparin tubes for collection plus prompt separation of plasma from cells prevents this.

Samples obtained through an improperly cleared intravenous catheter may yield falsely increased or decreased potassium concentrations. When obtaining blood from an intravenous catheter, remove and discard a small volume from the catheter before withdrawing a sample for analysis. Blood samples collected in tubes with potassium EDTA anticoagulant may have increased measured plasma potassium concentration.

Drugs That May Alter Serum Potassium Concentration ● Hypokalemia may be due to administration of furosemide, thiazides, laxatives, exchange resins (e.g., sodium polystyrene sulfonate), mineralocorticoids (e.g., fludrocortisone, deoxycorticosterone pivalate), insulin, sodium bicarbonate, amphotericin B, or potassium-free and glucose-containing crystalloid solutions. Peritoneal dialysis can be responsible if potassium-free dialysate is used for a long time.

Hyperkalemia may be due to heparin solutions containing chlorbutol, massive digitalis overdose, propranolol, angiotensin-converting enzyme inhibitors (e.g., captopril, enalapril), potassium-sparing diuretics (e.g., triamterene, spironolactone, amiloride), and nonsteroidal anti-inflammatory drugs.

Causes of Hypokalemia (Table 6–1 and Fig. 6–1) ● Decreased intake, translocation of potassium from extracellular to intracellular fluid, and increased loss via the kidneys or gastrointestinal tract are the major causes. Dilution of serum potassium concentration by administration of potassium-free fluids, especially those containing glucose, may contribute to hypokalemia. Decreased intake may aggravate existing hypokalemia but is unlikely to cause hypokalemia by itself. Hypokalemia often results from a combination of prolonged anorexia, loss of muscle mass, and ongoing urinary or gastrointestinal losses.

Translocation of potassium from extracellular to intracellular fluid may occur with acute alkalosis or insulin-mediated glucose uptake by cells. Alkalemia as well as insulin causes potassium to enter cells. Both of these situations typically are iatrogenic (e.g., treatment for diabetic ketoacidosis). Hypothermia may cause potassium to enter cells, this effect being reversed when hypothermia is corrected. Hypokalemic periodic paralysis in young Burmese cats causes potassium to enter body cells and is characterized by recurrent episodes of limb muscle weakness and neck ventroflexion, increased creatine kinase concentrations, and hypokalemia.

Table 6–1 CAUSES OF HYPOKALEMIA

Decreased intake
  Unlikely to cause hypokalemia by itself unless diet is
    aberrant
  Administration of potassium-free fluids (e.g., 0.9% NaCl,
    5% dextrose in water)
Translocation (extracellular fluid → intracellular fluid)
  Alkalemia
  Insulin/glucose-containing fluids
  Catecholamines
  Hypothermia?
  Hypokalemic periodic paralysis (Burmese cats)
Increased loss
  Gastrointestinal ($FE_K < 6\%$)
    Vomiting of gastric contents
    Diarrhea
  Urinary ($FE_K > 6\%$)
    Chronic renal failure in cats
    Diet-induced hypokalemic nephropathy in cats
    Distal (type I) RTA
    Proximal (type II) RTA after $NaHCO_3$ treatment
    Postobstructive diuresis
    Dialysis
    Mineralocorticoid excess
      Hyperadrenocorticism
      Primary hyperaldosteronism (adenoma, hyperplasia)
    Drugs
      Loop diuretics (e.g., furosemide, ethacrynic acid)
      Thiazide diuretics (e.g., chlorothiazide,
        hydrochlorothiazide)
      Amphotericin B
      Penicillins

(From DiBartola SP: Fluid Therapy in Small Animal Practice. Philadelphia, WB Saunders, 1992, p 99.)

Excessive gastrointestinal (e.g., vomiting, diarrhea) and urinary (e.g., polyuria) potassium losses commonly cause hypokalemia. Vomiting gastric contents results in loss of potassium as well as chloride, which perpetuates potassium depletion and metabolic alkalosis by enhancing urinary losses of potassium and hydrogen ions. Hypokalemia occurs in approximately 20% to 30% of cats and 10% of dogs with chronic renal failure. Hypokalemia may also occur in distal (type I) renal tubular acidosis (RTA). Hypokalemic nephropathy characterized by tubulointerstitial nephritis may develop in cats fed high-protein diets marginally replete in potassium and containing urinary acidifiers. Hypokalemia commonly occurs during the postobstructive diuresis following relief of feline urethral obstruction. Hypokalemia may occur in canine hyperadrenocorticism owing to the mineralocorticoid effects of endogenous steroids (e.g., corticosterone and deoxycorticosterone) and is more common with adrenal-dependent versus pituitary-dependent disease.

The most common causes of moderate to severe hypokalemia (i.e., < 2.5–3.0 mEq/L) are chronic vomiting of gastric contents, urinary

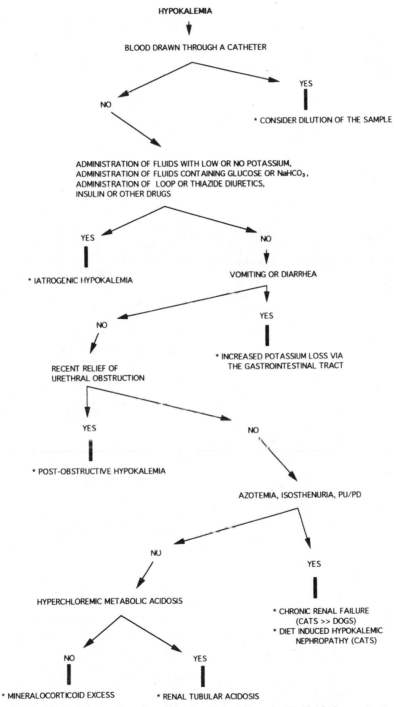

Figure 6–1 Algorithm for the clinical approach to hypokalemia. (From DiBartola SP: Fluid Therapy in Small Animal Practice. Philadelphia, WB Saunders, 1992, p 98.)

losses (e.g., postobstructive diuresis, polyuric chronic renal failure), overzealous use of loop diuretics (especially in anorexic animals), and insulin and sodium bicarbonate therapy during treatment of diabetic ketoacidosis.

Causes of Hyperkalemia (Table 6–2 and Fig. 6–2) ● Increased potassium intake, translocation of potassium from intracellular to extracellular fluid, and decreased urinary potassium excretion are the major causes. Increased intake is rarely the sole cause, unless potassium administration is greatly excessive or if there is concurrent renal or adrenal impairment.

Translocation of potassium from cells to extracellular fluid occurs with acute mineral acidosis (i.e., hyperchloremic or normal anion gap metabolic acidosis), insulin deficiency, and acute tumor lysis syndrome (i.e., potassium released from damaged neoplastic cells during chemotherapy plus decreased urinary potassium excretion due to acute renal failure). Metabolic

acidosis due to mineral acids (e.g., NH_4Cl, HCl) but not organic acids (e.g., lactic acid, keto acids) causes potassium to shift out of cells. The effect of inorganic metabolic acidosis on serum potassium concentration varies, raising potassium 0.17 to 1.67 (mean, 0.75) mEq/L per 0.1-U decrement in pH. Respiratory acidosis has minimal effect on potassium. Insulin deficiency and hyperosmolality contribute to hyperkalemia in diabetic ketoacidosis. Acute tumor lysis syndrome complicated by renal failure and hyperkalemia has occurred after radiation or chemotherapy for lymphoma.

Hyperkalemia occurs uncommonly if renal function is normal. In chronic renal failure, hyperkalemia usually occurs only if oliguria supervenes. The most common causes of decreased urinary potassium excretion are urethral obstruction, ruptured bladder, anuric or oliguric renal failure, and hypoadrenocorticism. Hyperkalemia may occur within 48 hours of feline urethral obstruction, but it does not usually occur for at least 48 hours after urinary bladder rupture. Hyperkalemia, hyponatremia, and Na:K ratios < 27:1 are usually (but not always) found in animals with hypoadrenocorticism. An adrenocorticotropic hormone (ACTH)-stimulation test (see Chapter 8) is necessary to diagnose hypoadrenocorticism because identical electrolyte abnormalities can occur in dogs with trichuriasis, salmonellosis, perforated duodenal ulcer, or pleural or peritoneal effusion.

Hyporeninemic hypoaldosteronism may impair urinary potassium excretion and contribute to hyperkalemia in patients with diabetes mellitus or renal disease. This uncommon cause of hyperkalemia can be ruled out by measuring aldosterone (not cortisol) concentrations before and after ACTH administration. A rare cause of hyperkalemia is hyperkalemic periodic paralysis, which has been reported in only one dog.

The most important causes of serious hyperkalemia (i.e., > 6.0 mEq/L) are oliguric/anuric acute renal failure (e.g., ethylene glycol ingestion), urethral obstruction in male cats, and hypoadrenocorticism. Pseudohyperkalemia should be eliminated first. If serum potassium concentration is > 7.0 mEq/L and the patient is asymptomatic (e.g., normal electrocardiogram), serum potassium concentration should be measured again using lithium heparin plasma. After artifact has been eliminated, the history should be examined for iatrogenic causes. If the hyperkalemia might be iatrogenic, the drug in question should be discontinued and serum potassium rechecked in 1 to 2 days. However,

---

Table 6–2 CAUSES OF HYPERKALEMIA

Pseudohyperkalemia
  Thrombocytosis
  Hemolysis (e.g., Akitas)
Increased intake
  Unlikely to cause hyperkalemia in presence of normal renal/adrenal function unless administration is greatly excessive
Translocation (intracellular fluid → extracellular fluid)
  Acute mineral acidosis (e.g., HCl, NH_4Cl)
  Insulin deficiency (e.g., diabetic ketoacidosis)
  Acute tumor lysis syndrome
  Reperfusion of extremities after aortic thromboembolism in cats with cardiomyopathy
  Hyperkalemic periodic paralysis (one case report in a pit bull)
  Drugs
    Nonspecific beta-blockers (e.g., propranolol)*
Decreased urinary excretion
  Urethral obstruction
  Ruptured bladder
  Anuric or oliguric renal failure
  Hypoadrenocorticism
  Selected gastrointestinal disease (e.g., trichuriasis, salmonellosis, perforated duodenal ulcer)
  Chylothorax with repeated pleural fluid drainage
  Hyporeninemic hypoaldosteronism
  Drugs
    Angiotensin-converting enzyme inhibitors (e.g., captopril, enalapril)*
    Potassium-sparing diuretics (e.g., spironolactone, amiloride, triamterene)*
    Prostaglandin inhibitors*
    Heparin*

---

*Only likely to cause hyperkalemia in conjunction with other contributing factors (e.g., decreased renal function, concurrent administration of potassium supplements).
(From DiBartola SP: Fluid Therapy in Small Animal Practice. Philadelphia, WB Saunders, 1992, p 108.)

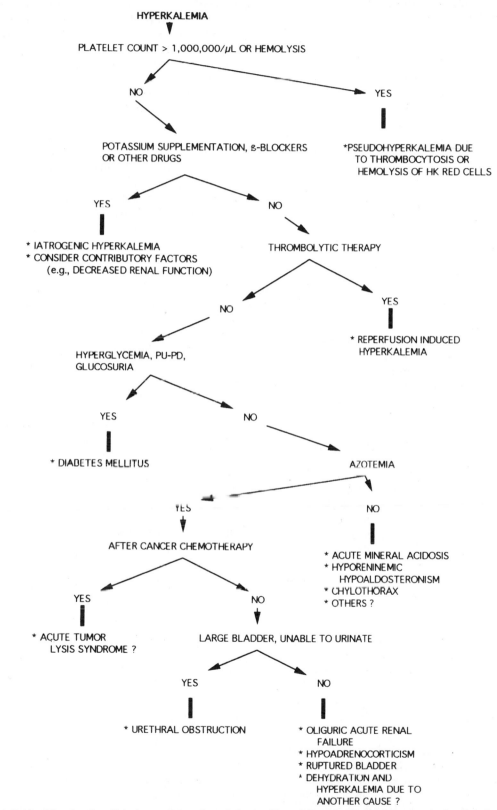

Figure 6–2 Algorithm for the clinical approach to hyperkalemia. (From DiBartola SP: Fluid Therapy in Small Animal Practice. Philadelphia, WB Saunders, 1992, p 107.)

diagnostic evaluation should continue in case another disease is present.

URINARY FRACTIONAL EXCRETION OF POTASSIUM

Purpose • Fractional excretion of potassium (FE_K) may help differentiate renal and nonrenal sources of potassium loss. FE_K can be calculated as follows: $[(U_K/S_K)/(U_{Cr}/S_{Cr})] \times 100$, where

U_K = urine concentration of potassium (mEq/L)

S_K = serum concentration of potassium (mEq/L)

U_{Cr} = urine concentration of creatinine (mg/dl)

S_{Cr} = serum concentration of creatinine (mg/dl)

Normal Values • Dogs and cats, 6% to 20%.

Danger Values • FE_K should be $\leq$ 6% if there are nonrenal sources of potassium loss (e.g., gastrointestinal loss). Values > 6% in hypokalemic patients reflect inappropriate renal potassium loss in animals with normal renal function.

SERUM SODIUM CONCENTRATION

Common Indications • Common indications for serum sodium determination include systemic diseases characterized by vomiting, diarrhea, polydipsia and polyuria, muscle weakness, abnormal behavior, abnormal mentation, seizures, edema, pleural or peritoneal effusion, or dehydration. Serum sodium should be determined whenever adrenal, renal, hepatic, or cardiac failure has been diagnosed or in cases of prolonged fluid or diuretic therapy.

Analysis • Measured in serum, plasma, or urine by flame photometry (rarely used now), ion-specific potentiometry, and dry reagent methods.

Normal Values • Dogs, 140 to 150 mEq/L; cats, 150 to 160 mEq/L.

Danger Values • Clinical signs of hypo- and hypernatremia are more related to the rapidity of onset than to the magnitude of the change and associated plasma hypo- or hyperosmolality. Neurologic signs (e.g., disorientation, ataxia, seizures, coma) may occur at serum sodium concentrations < 120 or > 170 mEq/L in dogs.

Artifacts • Decreased serum sodium concentration (measured by flame photometry or indirect potentiometry) with normal plasma osmolality is called *pseudohyponatremia*. Pseudohyponatremia is due to hyperlipidemia or severe hyperproteinemia and has no clinical significance. Pseudohyponatremia usually does not occur when serum sodium concentration is measured by direct potentiometry. Hyperviscosity of hyperproteinemia can lead to "short samples" (and artifactual hyponatremia) with certain aspiration techniques. Samples obtained through an improperly cleared intravenous catheter may yield falsely increased or decreased sodium concentrations. When obtaining blood from an intravenous catheter, a small volume of blood should be removed and discarded before withdrawing the sample for analysis.

Drugs That May Alter Serum Sodium Concentration • Hyponatremia may develop during thiazide or furosemide therapy. Some drugs cause *syndrome of inappropriate antidiuretic hormone secretion (SIADH)* in people, but drug-induced SIADH has not been documented in dogs or cats. Hypernatremia may develop during administration of desoxycorticosterone acetate or pivalate, fludrocortisone, sodium bicarbonate, or hypertonic saline or with sodium phosphate enema solutions in cats and small dogs.

Abnormal Serum Sodium Concentrations

Serum sodium concentration represents the amount of sodium relative to the amount of water in extracellular fluid and provides no direct information about total body sodium content. Patients with hyponatremia or hypernatremia may have decreased, normal, or increased total body sodium content. An increased serum sodium concentration implies hyperosmolality, whereas a decreased serum sodium concentration usually but not always implies hypo-osmolality.

Causes of Hyponatremia (Table 6–3) • Evaluation of hyponatremia requires knowledge of a patient's plasma osmolality. Hyponatremia with hyperosmolality may be caused by hyperglycemia in diabetes mellitus or by mannitol ad-

Table 6–3 CAUSES OF HYPONATREMIA

With normal plasma osmolality (pseudohyponatremia)
  Hyperlipidemia
  Hyperproteinemia
With high plasma osmolality
  Hyperglycemia
  Mannitol infusion
With low plasma osmolality
  And hypervolemia
    Severe liver disease
    Congestive heart failure
    Nephrotic syndrome
    Advanced renal failure
  And normovolemia
    Psychogenic polydipsia
    Syndrome of inappropriate antidiuretic hormone
      secretion (SIADH)
    Antidiuretic drugs
    Myxedema coma of hypothyroidism
    Hypotonic fluid infusion
  And hypovolemia
    Gastrointestinal loss
      Vomiting
      Diarrhea
    Third space loss
      Pancreatitis
      Peritonitis
      Uroabdomen
      Chylothorax with repeated pleural fluid drainage
    Cutaneous loss
      Burns
    Hypoadrenocorticism
    Diuretic administration
    "Salt-losing" nephropathy

(From DiBartola SP: Fluid Therapy in Small Animal Practice. Philadelphia, WB Saunders, 1992, p 73.)

ministration. However, most hyponatremic patients are hypo-osmolar.

The second step in a hyponatremic patient is to estimate total body sodium and extracellular fluid volume. History may indicate fluid loss. Physical examination evaluates a patient's volume status (e.g., skin turgor, moistness of mucous membranes, capillary refill time, pulse rate and character, appearance of jugular veins, presence or absence of ascites).

Volume-depleted hyponatremic patients have a total body sodium deficit exceeding that of water. They may have lost fluid by nonrenal or renal routes. Gastrointestinal (e.g., vomiting, diarrhea), third space (e.g., pancreatitis, peritonitis, uroabdomen, pleural effusion), and cutaneous losses (e.g., burns) constitute nonrenal routes of fluid and salt loss. Gastrointestinal fluid losses are frequently hypotonic (i.e., more water is lost than sodium). However, impaired water excretion plus replacement of the lost fluids by drinking water dilutes remaining serum sodium. Fluid and salt loss by the renal route may be due to hypoadrenocorticism, diuretics, or renal disease. Hyponatremia also has

been associated with chronic blood loss and hemoabdomen in dogs.

Hyponatremia may occur despite increased total body sodium if the extracellular fluid compartment is expanded (i.e., ascites or edema). Impaired water excretion dilutes serum sodium. Overt signs of hypervolemia usually are not present because the majority of retained water is distributed to the intracellular compartment. Hyponatremia with hypervolemia is primarily observed in congestive heart failure, severe liver disease, and nephrotic syndrome.

Hyponatremia with normovolemia may occur as a result of primary (psychogenic) polydipsia, SIADH, and continued administration of hypotonic fluids or drugs with antidiuretic effects, as well as in severe hypothyroidism (i.e., myxedema coma). Apparent psychogenic polydipsia (see Chapter 7) usually occurs in large breeds of dogs. These dogs have severe polydipsia, polyuria, and hyposthenuria and demonstrate mild plasma hypo-osmolality and hyponatremia. SIADH refers to ADH release in the absence of normal osmotic or nonosmotic stimuli. This syndrome can be due to malignancy, pulmonary disease, or central nervous system disorders. Diagnosis of SIADH requires first ruling out adrenal, renal, cardiac, and hepatic disease (i.e., other causes of hyponatremia) and then finding inappropriately high urine osmolality (> 100 mOsm/kg) despite hypo-osmolality. Drugs that stimulate ADH release or potentiate its renal effects may lead to hyponatremia with normovolemia.

The most common causes of significant hyponatremia (i.e., Na < 135 mEq/L) in dogs and cats include vomiting, advanced congestive heart failure (with or without concomitant diuretic therapy), and hypoadrenocorticism.

Causes of Hypernatremia (Table 6–4) ● Hypernatremia plus extracellular fluid hypertonicity is caused by a pure water deficit, loss of hypotonic fluid, or gain of sodium. The main causes of hypertonicity due to pure water loss are hypodipsia and diabetes insipidus. Hypodipsia, hypernatremia, and hypertonicity due to an abnormal central nervous system thirst mechanism occur in young female miniature schnauzers. Clinical signs include anorexia, lethargy, weakness, disorientation, ataxia, and seizures.

Central diabetes insipidus (see Chapter 7) is due to a partial or complete lack of ADH production and release. Animals with central diabetes insipidus have severe polydipsia and polyuria; hyperosmolality and hypernatremia are common. Nephrogenic diabetes insipidus comprises a group of disorders characterized by

Table 6-4 CAUSES OF HYPERNATREMIA

Pure water deficit
    Primary hypodipsia (e.g., miniature schnauzers)
    Diabetes insipidus
        Central
        Nephrogenic
    High environmental temperature
    Fever
    Inadequate access to water
Hypotonic fluid loss (without adequate replacement)
    Extrarenal
        Gastrointestinal
            Vomiting
            Diarrhea
            Small intestinal obstruction
        Third space loss
            Peritonitis
            Pancreatitis
        Cutaneous
            Burns
    Renal
        Appropriate
            Osmotic diuresis
                Diabetes mellitus
                Mannitol
            Chemical diuretics
        Inappropriate
            Chronic renal failure
            Nonoliguric acute renal failure
            Postobstructive diuresis
Impermeant solute gain
    Salt poisoning
    Hypertonic fluid administration
        Hypertonic saline
        Sodium bicarbonate
        Hyperalimentation fluid
        Sodium phosphate enema
    Hyperaldosteronism
    Hyperadrenocorticism

(From DiBartola SP: Fluid Therapy in Small Animal Practice. Philadelphia, WB Saunders, 1992, p 64.)

istration of hyperosmolar solutions (e.g., hypertonic saline, sodium bicarbonate) during cardiac resuscitation can cause transient hypernatremia. Hyperadrenocorticism and administration of sodium phosphate enemas to cats and small dogs may cause mild hypernatremia. Primary hyperaldosteronism is rare. Clinically significant hypernatremia (i.e., Na > 160 mEq/L in dogs and 170 mEq/L in cats) usually is due to a pure water deficit or loss of hypotonic fluid.

URINARY FRACTIONAL EXCRETION OF SODIUM

Purpose ● Determination of fractional sodium excretion (FE_{Na}) helps differentiate prerenal from primary renal azotemia and renal from extrarenal sodium loss in hypovolemic patients with hypernatremia or hyponatremia. FE_{Na} is calculated by using the equation

$$[(U_{Na}/S_{Na})/(U_{Cr}/S_{Cr})] \times 100, \text{ where}$$

U_{Na} = urine concentration of sodium (mEq/L)

S_{Na} = serum concentration of sodium (mEq/L)

U_{Cr} = urine concentration of creatinine (mg/dl)

S_{Cr} = serum concentration of creatinine (mg/dl)

Normal Values ● Values for FE_{Na} in normal dogs and cats should be < 1%.

Danger Values ● FE_{Na} should be < 1% in animals with prerenal azotemia; > 1% suggests par-

structural or functional renal abnormalities that interfere with urine concentration (Table 6-5).

Hypotonic fluid losses probably are the most common type. They may be extrarenal (e.g., gastrointestinal, third space, and cutaneous) or renal. Gastrointestinal losses include vomiting, diarrhea, and small intestinal obstruction. Third space losses include pancreatitis and peritonitis.

Cutaneous losses are usually not important in dogs and cats. Renal losses may result from osmotically or chemically induced diuresis or defective urinary concentrating ability due to intrinsic renal disease. Note that if a patient replaces these fluid losses by drinking and retaining adequate amounts of water, it may become *hypo*natremic owing to dilution of remaining sodium.

Hypertonicity due to excessive salt ingestion is unlikely if an animal has an intact thirst mechanism and access to water. Therapeutic admin-

Table 6-5 CAUSES OF NEPHROGENIC DIABETES INSIPIDUS

Congenital (primary)
Acquired (secondary)
    Functional
        Drugs
            Glucocorticoids
            Lithium
            Demeclocycline
            Methoxyflurane
            E. coli endotoxin
        Metabolic
            Hypokalemia
            Hypercalcemia
    Structural
        Medullary interstitial amyloidosis
        Chronic pyelonephritis
        Chronic interstitial nephritis

(From DiBartola SP: Fluid Therapy in Small Animal Practice. Philadelphia, WB Saunders, 1992, p 67.)

enchymal renal disease in azotemic animals. Prerenal azotemia with $FE_{Na} > 1\%$ may occur despite normal renal function if the animal is being treated with a diuretic (e.g., furosemide). In hypovolemic patients with hypernatremia or hyponatremia, FE_{Na} values $< 1\%$ suggest non-renal fluid losses (e.g., gastrointestinal, third space) whereas values $> 1\%$ suggest renal fluid losses (e.g., hypoadrenocorticism, diuretic administration, renal disease).

SERUM CHLORIDE CONCENTRATION

Common Indications • Systemic diseases characterized by vomiting, diarrhea, polyuria and polydipsia, and dehydration.

Analysis • Measured in serum, plasma or urine by colorimetric titration, spectrophotometry (autoanalyzers), ion-specific potentiometry, coulometric-amperometric titration, or reflectance photometry in dry reagent systems.

Normal Values • Dogs, 105 to 115 mEq/L; cats, 115 to 125 mEq/L.

Danger Values • Unknown. Muscle twitching or seizures in hypochloremic animals are probably due to metabolic alkalosis and decreased ionized calcium concentration, whereas clinical signs associated with hyperchloremia are probably due to hyperosmolality.

Artifacts • Artifactual hyperchloremia results from decreased plasma water content (i.e., pure water loss, hypotonic fluid loss, pure NaCl gain), whereas artifactual hypochloremia results from increased plasma water content (i.e., congestive heart failure, hypoadrenocorticism, third space accumulation). Serum chloride concentration may be corrected for abnormalities of plasma water content using the following formulas:

$$Dogs: [Cl^-]_{Corr} = [Cl^-] \times 146/[Na^+]$$

$$Cats: [Cl^-]_{Corr} = [Cl^-] \times 156/[Na^+]$$

Normal values for $[Cl^-]_{Corr}$ are 107 to 113 mEq/L for dogs and 117 to 123 mEq/L for cats.

Pseudohypochloremia • Pseudohypochloremia results when chloride is measured in lipemic or markedly hyperproteinemic samples using techniques that are not ion selective. Hyperviscosity

may cause problems in some machines that dilute the sample before analysis. In lipemic samples, chloride concentration is underestimated by some titrimetric methods and overestimated by colorimetric methods. Pseudohyperchloremia may be due to certain pigments (e.g., hemoglobin, bilirubin) when colorimetric methods are used. Ion-specific electrodes and coulometric-amperometric systems are more accurate, but other halides (e.g., bromide, iodide) are measured as chloride, resulting in falsely increased measurements.

Drugs That May Alter Serum Chloride Concentration • Corrected hyperchloremia may be due to excessive gain of chloride relative to sodium (e.g., NH_4Cl, KCl, 0.9% NaCl with or without added KCl, total parenteral nutrition with cationic amino acids such as arginine HCl and lysine HCl, hypertonic saline). Acetazolamide, spironolactone, and amiloride may retain chloride by their effects on renal tubular function. Corrected hypochloremia may be due to disproportionate losses of chloride relative to sodium (e.g., furosemide, thiazides) or to excessive intake of sodium without chloride (e.g., sodium bicarbonate, extremely high doses of sodium penicillin or carbenicillin).

Causes of Corrected Hypochloremia (Table 6–6) • The most common causes of hypochloremia are chronic vomiting of gastric contents and aggressive furosemide or thiazide therapy. Administration of sodium without chloride (e.g., sodium bicarbonate, large doses of sodium penicillin or carbenicillin) may also cause hypochloremia. Hypochloremia due to increased renal chloride excretion is a normal adaptation to chronic respiratory acidosis. Most patients with hypoadrenocorticism have hypochloremia at presentation but on correction for decreased plasma water usually have normal or

Table 6–6 CAUSES OF CORRECTED HYPOCHLOREMIA

Pseudohypochloremia
Excessive loss of chloride relative to sodium
  Vomiting of stomach contents
  Therapy with loop diuretics or thiazides
  Chronic respiratory acidosis
  Hyperadrenocorticism
Therapy with solutions containing high sodium concentrations relative to chloride
  Sodium bicarbonate
  Sodium penicillin or carbenicillin (high doses)

(From deMorais HSA: Chloride ion in small animal practice: The forgotten ion. Vet Emerg Crit Care 1992; 2:21.)

increased serum chloride concentrations. Persistent hypochloremia is an indication to determine serum sodium, potassium, and total carbon dioxide (TcO_2) concentrations ± blood gas analysis.

Causes of Corrected Hyperchloremia (Table 6–7) ● Hyperchloremia results from excessive sodium loss relative to chloride, excessive chloride gain relative to sodium, or renal chloride retention. Small bowel diarrhea causes hyperchloremic metabolic acidosis due to loss of bicarbonate-rich, chloride-poor fluid (i.e., excessive sodium loss). Salt poisoning or therapy with NH_4Cl, KCl, cationic amino acids, hypertonic saline, or 0.9% $NaCl$ with or without added KCl represents excessive chloride gain. (Physiologic saline solution has 154 mEq chloride per liter but contains 174 mEq chloride per liter if supplemented with 20 mEq KCl per liter.)

Corrected hyperchloremia due to renal chloride retention occurs in RTA (e.g., hypoadrenocorticism causing type IV RTA) or may be found in normally hydrated diabetic patients with normal renal function, as well as during the resolution of ketoacidosis. It may also be iatrogenic (e.g., acetazolamide, spironolactone, amiloride). The most common causes of hyperchloremia are dehydration ($[Cl^-]_{Corr}$ may be normal) and hyperchloremic (normal anion gap) metabolic acidosis. Persistent hyperchlore-

Table 6–7 CAUSES OF CORRECTED HYPERCHLOREMIA

Pseudohyperchloremia
  Potassium bromide therapy
Excessive loss of sodium relative to chloride (as compared
  with extracellular fluid composition)
  Diarrhea
Excessive gain of chloride relative to sodium (as compared
  with extracellular fluid composition)
  NH_4Cl
  KCl
  Total parenteral nutrition with solutions containing
    cationic amino acids (e.g., lysine HCl, arginine HCl)
  0.9% NaCl with or without KCl supplementation
  Hypertonic saline
  Salt poisoning
Chloride retention
  Early renal failure
  Renal tubular acidosis (types I and II)
  Hypoadrenocorticism (type IV renal tubular acidosis)
  Diabetes mellitus
  Chronic respiratory alkalosis
  Drug-induced
    Acetazolamide
    Spironolactone
    Amiloride

(From de Morais HSA: Chloride ion in small animal practice: The forgotten ion. Vet Emerg Crit Care 1992; 2:22.)

mia is an indication for determining serum sodium, potassium, and TcO_2 concentrations and blood gas analysis.

OSMOLALITY AND OSMOLAL GAP

Osmolality

A change in *permeant* solutes (e.g., urea) does not cause movement of water because these solutes are distributed equally throughout total body water. A change in *impermeant* solutes (e.g., sodium, glucose) causes movement of water because such solutes do not readily cross cell membranes. *Tonicity* refers to the ability of a solution to initiate water movement and is dependent on impermeant solutes.

Occasional Indications ● Serum or plasma osmolality helps differentiate causes of hyponatremia, aids in the early diagnosis of ethylene glycol intoxication, evaluates hydration status and renal concentrating ability during water deprivation testing, and aids in evaluating patients with diabetic ketoacidosis.

Disadvantages ● Special equipment (e.g., freezing point depression or vapor pressure osmometer) is required.

Analysis ● Osmolality is *measured* in serum, plasma, or urine by freezing point or vapor pressure osmometry. It is estimated (i.e., *calculated*) by several different formulas. In the absence of excessive unmeasured osmoles, the following formula may be used:

$$1.86([Na^+ mEq/L] + [K^+ mEq/L]) + \text{glucose (mg/dl)}/18 + \text{BUN (mg/dl)}/2.8 = \text{osmolality (mOsm/kg)}$$

Tonicity may be estimated as serum or plasma osmolality (mOsm/kg) − blood urea nitrogen (mg/dl)/2.8.

Normal Values ● Serum or plasma osmolality: dogs, 290 to 310 mOsm/kg; cats, 308 to 335 mOsm/kg. Urine osmolality values depend on water balance and vary widely. Ranges in dogs and cats are 50 to 2800 mOsm/kg and 50 to 3000 mOsm/kg, respectively.

Danger Values ● Signs due to hypo-osmolality or hyperosmolality are related more to rapidity rather than to magnitude of change. Neurologic signs (e.g., disorientation, ataxia, seizures, coma) may occur when serum or plasma osmolality is < 250 mOsm/kg or tonicity is > 360 mOsm/kg.

Osmolal Gap

Osmolal gap is defined as the difference between the *measured* and *calculated* serum (or plasma) osmolality: Osmolal gap (mOsm/kg) = measured serum (or plasma) osmolality − calculated serum (or plasma) osmolality. This gap identifies unmeasured osmoles (e.g., ethylene glycol metabolites) and pseudohyponatremia (i.e., normal osmolality plus hyponatremia as measured by flame photometry or instruments that dilute the sample before analysis). Vapor pressure osmometry does not detect volatile solutes (e.g., methanol). If measured osmolality is less than calculated osmolality, there is probably a laboratory error.

Normal Values • Dogs, 10 to 15 mOsm/kg; cats, unknown.

Danger Values • Osmolal gap > 25 mOsm/kg indicates a search for intoxication (e.g., ethylene glycol, methanol, ethanol).

Causes of Serum or Plasma Hypo-Osmolality • Same as described for hyponatremia.

Causes of Serum or Plasma Hyperosmolality • Same as described for hypernatremia, plus hyperglycemia, severe azotemia, and intoxications (e.g., ethylene glycol, ethanol, methanol). The most common causes of serum osmolality > 360 mOsm/kg are diabetic ketoacidosis, uremia, and hypernatremia. Hyperosmolality is an indication for measurement of serum sodium, potassium, urea nitrogen, and glucose concentrations, plus calculating anion and osmolal gaps.

Causes of Increased Osmolal Gap • Pseudohyponatremia and acute intoxications (e.g., ethylene glycol, methanol, ethanol) increase the osmolal gap. If pseudohyponatremia is ruled out, an increased osmolal gap mandates a search for recent exposure to these toxins. The increase in osmolal gap in dogs with ethylene glycol intoxication peaks at 6 hours, persists for at least 12 hours, but may be normal 24 hours after ingestion. If ethylene glycol intoxication is likely, urinalysis looking for calcium oxalate monohydrate or dihydrate crystals, blood gas analysis, anion gap calculation, and appropriate toxicologic analyses are indicated.

BLOOD GAS ANALYSIS

Frequent Indications • Blood gas analysis is useful in any severely ill dog or cat (e.g., severe dehydration, hypovolemia, vomiting, diarrhea, oliguria-anuria, hyperkalemia, dyspnea, or tachypnea). Blood gas analysis is necessary for proper evaluation of gas exchange and alterations of TCO_2 in patients with respiratory disorders. Urine pH cannot substitute for blood gas analysis because of problems like paradoxical aciduria in patients with hypochloremic metabolic alkalosis.

Advantages • It can differentiate types of metabolic and respiratory acid-base disturbances and indicate proper therapy. It can also evaluate pulmonary gas exchange.

Disadvantages • Expensive equipment is necessary. Careful technique is required in obtaining and handling blood specimens to prevent artifacts. The need for rapid analysis prohibits use of remote laboratories.

Analysis • Blood gas analyzers are equipped with specific electrodes to measure pH, carbon dioxide tension (PCO_2), and oxygen tension (PO_2). The concentration of HCO_3^- is calculated. Arterial blood is ideal, but free-flowing jugular blood is acceptable for evaluation of a patient's acid-base status. However, arterial samples are imperative if one wishes to evaluate pulmonary function. In normal resting dogs, venous samples from the pulmonary artery, jugular vein, and cephalic vein have similar blood gas values, whereas arterial blood has a slightly lower [HCO_3^-] (21 mEq/L versus 22–23 mEq/L for venous blood) and considerably lower PCO_2 (37 mm Hg versus 42–43 mm Hg for venous blood). This relationship may not be true in patients with abnormal cardiovascular function.

A 3-ml syringe with a 25-gauge needle is used to collect 0.5 to 1.5 ml of blood. Enough heparin (1000 U/ml) is drawn into the syringe to coat the interior, and then it and all air are expelled, leaving the dead space of the syringe filled with heparin (approximately 0.1–0.2 ml). After the blood is collected, air bubbles must be dislodged and expelled. The needle may be inserted into a rubber stopper, or a tightly fitting cap may be placed over the syringe hub to prevent exposure of the sample to room air. The syringe is rolled between the palms of the hands to mix the sample. The sample then is submitted in the syringe in which it was collected. Analysis should occur within 15 to 30 minutes of collection if stored at 25° C or within 2 hours if immersed in an ice water bath.

Normal Values ● Venous blood: dogs, pH 7.32 to 7.40, P_{CO_2} 33 to 50 mm Hg, $[HCO_3^-]$ 18 to 26 mEq/L; cats, pH 7.28 to 7.41, P_{CO_2} 33 to 45 mm Hg, $[HCO_3^-]$ 18 to 23 mEq/L. Arterial blood: dogs, pH 7.36 to 7.44, P_{CO_2} 36 to 44 mm Hg, $[HCO_3^-]$ 18 to 26 mEq/L; cats, pH 7.36 to 7.44, P_{CO_2} 28 to 32 mm Hg, $[HCO_3^-]$ 17 to 22 mEq/L. Arterial P_{O_2} in normal dogs and cats breathing room air at sea level is approximately 100 mm Hg.

Danger Values ● pH < 7.10 represents severe acidosis, which may cause cardiopulmonary complications (e.g., impaired myocardial contractility); pH > 7.60 denotes severe alkalosis.

Artifacts ● P_{CO_2} decreases and pH and P_{O_2} increase if the sample is exposed to air. Air bubbles in the sample may increase P_{O_2} and decrease P_{CO_2} if they occupy ≥ 10% of the sample volume. P_{CO_2} increases and pH decreases if the analysis is delayed. The rate of change is greater at 25° C versus 4° C. Changes in P_{CO_2} and pH are accompanied by decreased glucose and increased lactate concentrations. Aerobic metabolism by white blood cells decreases P_{O_2}. These changes are minimized by cooling the blood sample. Prolonged venous stasis during venipuncture increases P_{CO_2} and decreases pH. Excessive heparin (> 10% of the sample volume) decreases pH, P_{CO_2}, and $[HCO_3^-]$, whereas citrate, oxalate, or EDTA may decrease pH. Blood gas analyzers calculate HCO_3^- from pH and P_{CO_2}, and T_{CO_2} is measured on autoanalyzers but calculated on many blood gas analyzers. The HCO_3^- value should be compared with the T_{CO_2} to verify accuracy of the HCO_3^- value. Normally, T_{CO_2} is approximately 1 to 2 mEq/L

higher than HCO_3^- (i.e., $T_{CO_2} = HCO_3^- + 0.03 \times P_{CO_2}$).

Drugs That May Alter Blood Gas Results ● Acetazolamide, salicylate (causing metabolic acidosis), NH_4Cl, and $CaCl_2$ may cause acidosis. Antacids, sodium bicarbonate, potassium citrate or gluconate, salicylate (causing respiratory alkalosis), and loop diuretics may cause alkalosis.

Analysis of Blood Gas Results ● If the pH is outside of the normal range, an acid-base disturbance is present. If the pH is within the normal range, an acid-base disturbance may or may not be present. If the pH is low and plasma HCO_3^- concentration decreased, *metabolic acidosis* is present. If the pH is low and P_{CO_2} increased, *respiratory acidosis* is present. If the pH is high and plasma HCO_3^- increased, *metabolic alkalosis* is present. If the pH is high and P_{CO_2} decreased, *respiratory alkalosis* is present.

Next, calculate the expected compensatory response in the opposing component of the system (e.g., respiratory alkalosis is compensation for metabolic acidosis, metabolic alkalosis is compensation for respiratory acidosis, and so on) using the guidelines in Table 6–8. (These guidelines were established with dogs and should not be used for cats.) If a patient's compensatory response falls within the expected range, a *simple* acid-base disturbance is probable. If the compensatory response falls outside of the expected range, a *mixed* disorder is present.

After classifying the type of disturbance and whether it is simple or mixed, one should determine whether the diagnosed acid-base disturbance is compatible with the patient's history and clinical findings. The interpretation of the blood gas must be questioned if the acid-base disturbance is not congruent with the patient's

Table 6–8 RENAL AND RESPIRATORY COMPENSATIONS FOR PRIMARY ACID-BASE DISORDERS IN DOGS

Disorder	Primary Change	Compensatory Response
Metabolic acidosis	↓ $[HCO_3^-]$	0.7 mm Hg decrement in P_{CO_2} for each 1 mEq/L decrement in $[HCO_3^-]$
Metabolic alkalosis	↑ $[HCO_3^-]$	0.7 mm Hg increment in P_{CO_2} for each 1 mEq/L increment in $[HCO_3^-]$
Acute respiratory acidosis	↑ P_{CO_2}	1.5 mEq/L increment in $[HCO_3^-]$ for each 10 mm Hg increment in P_{CO_2}
Chronic respiratory acidosis	↑ P_{CO_2}	3.5 mEq/L increment in $[HCO_3^-]$ for each 10 mm Hg increment in P_{CO_2}
Acute respiratory alkalosis	↓ P_{CO_2}	2.5 mEq/L decrement in $[HCO_3^-]$ for each 10 mm Hg decrement in P_{CO_2}
Chronic respiratory alkalosis	↓ P_{CO_2}	5.5 mEq/L decrement in $[HCO_3^-]$ for each 10 mm Hg decrement in P_{CO_2}

(From DiBartola SP: Fluid Therapy in Small Animal Practice. Philadelphia, WB Saunders, 1992, p 207.)

history, clinical findings, and other laboratory data.

Metabolic Acidosis (Table 6–9) • Metabolic acidosis is characterized by decreased plasma HCO_3^-, decreased pH, and a compensatory decrease in PCO_2. Metabolic acidosis is caused by loss of HCO_3^--rich fluid, addition of acid, acid production by metabolism, or diminished renal excretion of acid. Loss of HCO_3^--rich fluid usually occurs via the alimentary tract (e.g., small bowel diarrhea fluid HCO_3^- exceeds that of plasma while its Cl^- concentration is lower) but also may occur via the kidneys (e.g., carbonic anhydrase inhibitors, type II RTA). Loss of HCO_3^--rich fluid causes hyperchloremic metabolic acidosis. Addition of acid to the body may be due to ethylene glycol or salicylate intoxication or to drugs (e.g., NH_4Cl, cationic amino acids). Metabolic production of acid refers to lactic acidosis or diabetic ketoacidosis. Renal failure, hypoadrenocorticism, and type I RTA are examples of impaired urinary excretion of acid. The most common causes of metabolic acidosis are small bowel diarrhea, renal failure, hypoadrenocorticism, diabetic ketoacidosis, and lactic acidosis due to poor perfusion. The role of the anion gap in differentiation of causes of metabolic acidosis is discussed later.

Respiratory Acidosis (Table 6–10) • Respiratory

Table 6–9 CAUSES OF METABOLIC ACIDOSIS

Increased anion gap (normochloremic)
  Ethylene glycol intoxication
  Salicylate intoxication
  Other rare intoxications (e.g., paraldehyde, methanol)
  Diabetic ketoacidosis*
  Uremic acidosis†
  Lactic acidosis
Normal anion gap (hyperchloremic)
  Diarrhea
  Renal tubular acidosis
  Carbonic anhydrase inhibitors (e.g., acetazolamide)
  Ammonium chloride
  Cationic amino acids (e.g., lysine, arginine, histidine)
  Posthypocapnic metabolic acidosis
  Dilutional acidosis (e.g., rapid administration of 0.9% saline)
  Hypoadrenocorticism‡

*Patients with diabetic ketoacidosis may have some component of hyperchloremic metabolic acidosis in conjunction with increased anion gap acidosis.
†The metabolic acidosis early in renal failure may be hyperchloremic and later convert to increased anion gap acidosis.
‡Patients with hypoadrenocorticism typically present with uncorrected hypochloremia due to impaired water excretion (dilutional effect) and absence of aldosterone. Factors that may mask hyperchloremia include lactic acidosis and chronic vomiting.
(From DiBartola SP: Fluid Therapy in Small Animal Practice. Philadelphia, WB Saunders, 1992, p 218.)

Table 6–10 CAUSES OF RESPIRATORY ACIDOSIS

Airway obstruction
  Aspiration (e.g., foreign body, vomitus)
Respiratory center depression
  Neurologic disease (e.g., brainstem, high cervical spinal cord lesion)
  Drugs (e.g., narcotics, sedatives, barbiturates, inhalation anesthetics)
Cardiopulmonary arrest
Neuromuscular defects
  Myasthenia gravis
  Tetanus
  Botulism
  Polyradiculoneuritis
  Polymyositis
  Tick paralysis
  Hypokalemic periodic paralysis in Burmese
  Hypokalemic myopathy in cats
  Drug-induced (succinylcholine, pancuronium, aminoglycosides with anesthetics, organophosphates)
Restrictive defects
  Diaphragmatic hernia
  Pneumothorax
  Pleural effusion
  Hemothorax
  Chest wall trauma
  Pulmonary fibrosis
  Pyothorax
Pulmonary disease
  Respiratory distress syndrome
  Pneumonia
  Severe pulmonary edema
  Diffuse metastatic disease
  Smoke inhalation
  Pulmonary thromboembolism
  Chronic obstructive pulmonary disease
  Pulmonary fibrosis
Inadequate mechanical ventilation

(From DiBartola SP: Fluid Therapy in Small Animal Practice. Philadelphia, WB Saunders, 1992, p 267.)

acidosis is due to decreased effective ventilation (increased PCO_2). It is synonymous with "primary hypercapnia" and is characterized by increased PCO_2, decreased pH, and a compensatory increase in $[HCO_3^-]$.

Hypoventilation due to airway obstruction, cardiopulmonary arrest, and neuromuscular diseases (e.g., myasthenia gravis, tetanus, botulism, polyradiculoneuritis, tick paralysis, hypokalemic polymyopathy), neuromuscular blocking drugs (e.g., succinylcholine, pancuronium, aminoglycosides combined with anesthetics), restrictive defects (e.g., diaphragmatic hernia, pneumothorax, pleural effusion, hemothorax, chest wall trauma, pulmonary fibrosis, pyothorax), pulmonary diseases (e.g., pneumonia, severe pulmonary edema, diffuse pulmonary metastases, smoke inhalation, pulmonary thromboembolism, chronic obstructive pulmonary disease), and inadequate mechanical ventilation cause respiratory acidosis.

Table 6–11 CAUSES OF METABOLIC ALKALOSIS

Vomiting of gastric contents
Diuretic therapy (e.g., loop diuretics, thiazides)
Posthypercapnia
Primary hyperaldosteronism (rare)
Hyperadrenocorticism
Oral administration of sodium bicarbonate or other organic
  anions (lactate, citrate, gluconate, acetate, others)

(From DiBartola SP: Fluid Therapy in Small Animal Practice. Philadelphia, WB Saunders, 1992, p 249.)

Metabolic Alkalosis (Table 6–11) ● Metabolic alkalosis is characterized by increased plasma HCO_3^-, increased pH, and a compensatory increased Pco_2. Metabolic alkalosis is caused by loss of chloride-rich fluid via the alimentary tract or kidneys or by chronic administration of alkali. Renal excretion of exogenously administered alkali is very effective, making it difficult to create metabolic alkalosis by increasing HCO_3^- intake, unless there is renal dysfunction. Most cases of metabolic alkalosis are due to vomiting of gastric contents or administration of diuretics.

Respiratory Alkalosis (Table 6–12) ● Respiratory alkalosis results from increased ventilation (decreased Pco_2). It is synonymous with "primary hypocapnia" and is characterized by decreased Pco_2, increased pH, and a compensatory decrease in HCO_3^-.

Causes of respiratory alkalosis include tachypnea due to hypoxemia (e.g., right-to-left shunting of blood, decreased inspired oxygen concentration, congestive heart failure, anemia, hypotension, pulmonary diseases causing ventilation/perfusion mismatch), pulmonary disease with or without hypoxemia (e.g., pneumonia, pulmonary thromboembolism, pulmonary edema, pulmonary fibrosis), direct stimulation of the medullary respiratory center (e.g., gram-negative sepsis, hepatic disease, salicylates, xanthines, central nervous system disease, and heat stroke), and excessive mechanical ventilation. Unexplained respiratory alkalosis may suggest gram-negative sepsis or pain. Pulmonary edema may cause respiratory alkalosis, but metabolic acidosis and respiratory acidosis can also occur. Respiratory alkalosis may occur during recovery from metabolic acidosis because hyperventilation persists for 24 to 48 hours after correction of the acidosis.

TOTAL CARBON DIOXIDE

When samples are handled anaerobically, the Tco_2 determination is synonymous with $[HCO_3^-]$.

Frequent Indications ● In any severe systemic disease process, Tco_2 determination helps the clinician determine the need for blood gas analysis. Examples of diseases in which Tco_2 determinations and blood gas analysis would be indicated include uremia, ethylene glycol or salicylate intoxication, and diabetic ketoacidosis.

Advantages ● The Harleco apparatus for estimating Tco_2 is simple, rapid, inexpensive, and accurate. In this test, the sample is acidified and the amount of CO_2 released is measured by displacement of the plunger in the syringe portion of the apparatus. On autoanalyzers, released CO_2 is determined by a colorimetric method.

Disadvantages ● Tco_2 determination does not allow differentiation of metabolic and respiratory acid-base disorders. High Tco_2 suggests either metabolic alkalosis or respiratory aci-

Table 6–12 CAUSES OF TACHYPNEA RESULTING IN RESPIRATORY ALKALOSIS

Hypoxemia (stimulation of peripheral chemoreceptors by
  decreased oxygen delivery)
  Right-to-left shunting
  Decreased P_iO_2 (e.g., residence at high altitude)
  Congestive heart failure
  Severe anemia
  Hypotension
  Pulmonary diseases causing ventilation/perfusion
    inequality
    Pneumonia
    Pulmonary embolism
    Pulmonary fibrosis
    Pulmonary edema
Pulmonary disease (stimulation of nociceptive receptors
  independent of hypoxemia)
  Pneumonia
  Pulmonary embolism
  Interstitial lung disease
  Pulmonary edema
Central nervous system–mediated hypocapnia (direct
  stimulation of medullary respiratory center)
  Liver disease
  Gram-negative sepsis
  Drugs
    Salicylate intoxication
    Xanthines (e.g., aminophylline)
  Recovery from metabolic acidosis
  Central neurologic disease
    Trauma
    Tumor
    Infection
    Inflammation (e.g., granulomatous
      meningoencephalitis)
    Cerebrovascular accident
  Heat stroke
Mechanical ventilation

(From DiBartola SP: Fluid Therapy in Small Animal Practice. Philadelphia, WB Saunders, 1992, p 269.)

dosis. Low T_{CO_2} represents either metabolic acidosis or respiratory alkalosis. Evaluation of the clinical setting is necessary to decide which is most likely. If there is doubt about which is present, blood gas analysis is required. Metabolic acidosis is the most common acid-base disturbance, and most decreased T_{CO_2} measurements suggest this disorder.

Analysis • T_{CO_2} is measured in serum or plasma by colorimetric methods (autoanalyzers) or by volume displacement (Harleco apparatus; requires 1.0-ml sample). Serum or plasma collected anaerobically and analyzed within 15 to 20 minutes of collection is preferred. Samples may be stored in a capped syringe on ice at 4° C for up to 2 hours before analysis.

Normal Values • Dogs and cats, 17 to 23 mEq/L.

Danger Values • < 12 mEq/L (usually warns of severe metabolic acidosis).

Artifacts • T_{CO_2} values lower than $[HCO_3^-]$ may be reported in severely hyperlipidemic samples because T_{CO_2} is measured in the total volume of plasma but HCO_3^- is only distributed within the aqueous phase. Falsely decreased T_{CO_2} occurs when heparin anticoagulant occupies >10% of the sample volume. Falsely increased values occur if the sample stands at room temperature for > 20 to 30 minutes. Bromide causes increased T_{CO_2} measurement when using Ektachem reagents.

Drugs That May Alter T_{CO_2} • Acetazolamide and NH_4Cl reduce T_{CO_2} by causing metabolic acidosis. Furosemide and sodium bicarbonate may produce metabolic alkalosis and increased T_{CO_2}.

Causes of Decreased T_{CO_2} • T_{CO_2} concentrations are decreased in metabolic acidosis (most common cause) and respiratory alkalosis. Although a decreased T_{CO_2} concentration in a hyperventilating animal usually is due to compensated metabolic acidosis, it may also be due to compensated acute or chronic respiratory alkalosis. Blood gas analysis may be necessary to determine which is occurring. A severely decreased T_{CO_2} concentration in a patient with a recognized cause of metabolic acidosis may reasonably be assumed to represent metabolic acidosis. T_{CO_2} < 12 mEq/L in a patient with undiagnosed systemic disease is an indication for blood gas analysis and calculation of the anion gap. If blood gas analysis is not available, the clinician must correlate T_{CO_2} concentration with the clinical setting and decide if bicarbonate therapy is indicated. Measurement of serum electrolyte concentrations is indicated to plan fluid therapy, because acid-base disturbances often are associated with electrolyte abnormalities.

Causes of Increased T_{CO_2} • Metabolic alkalosis and respiratory acidosis are causes of increased T_{CO_2}. Metabolic alkalosis is more common and is usually due to chronic gastric vomiting, overzealous diuretic administration, or administration of sodium bicarbonate or other alkalizing organic anions (e.g., potassium citrate). Serum sodium, potassium, and chloride concentrations should be measured, because metabolic alkalosis is often accompanied by hypochloremia, hypokalemia, and hyponatremia. If these changes are present, the clinician should correct them (i.e., administer 0.9% NaCl + KCl) and diagnose the underlying cause (e.g., pyloric obstruction).

ANION GAP

The sum of the concentrations of commonly measured cations exceeds the sum of the concentrations of commonly measured anions; the difference is the anion gap:

$$(Na^+ + K^+) - (Cl^- + HCO_3^-)$$

The serum concentration of potassium varies little; therefore, the anion gap is sometimes defined as

$$Na^+ - (Cl^- + HCO_3^-)$$

There is no actual gap, because there are unmeasured cations (UC) and unmeasured anions (UA) that preserve electroneutrality:

$$\text{Electroneutrality: } Na^+ + K^+ + UC = Cl^- + HCO_3^- + UA$$

Thus, the anion gap is the difference between unmeasured anions and unmeasured cations:

$$\text{Anion gap} = UA - UC = (Na^+ + K^+) - (Cl^- + HCO_3^-)$$

Indications • Anion gap is used to help differentiate the causes of metabolic acidosis. Metabolic acidosis with a high anion gap is assumed to have arisen from an acid that does not contain chloride as an anion. Examples include inorganic acids (e.g., phosphates, sulfates) and organic acids (e.g., lactate, keto acids, salicylate, metabolites of ethylene glycol). Metabolic acidosis characterized by a normal anion gap is due to an increase in plasma chloride concentration. The anion gap may also be useful in identifying mixed acid-base disturbances (e.g., metabolic alkalosis plus lactic acidosis caused by chronic vomiting producing hypotension and decreased tissue perfusion: The pH could be normal if gastric HCl loss was counterbalanced by lactic acid accumulation. Increased anion gap would suggest the complicating organic acidosis).

Advantages ● It is a simple calculation that does not require additional blood samples from most patients. This calculation is often automatically provided in the chemistry report. Used carefully, it helps differentiate the causes of metabolic acidosis.

Disadvantages ● It is affected by several factors and has interpretive limitations.

Analysis ● The anion gap is calculated as $(Na^+ + K^+) - (Cl^- + HCO_3^-)$ or $Na^+ - (Cl^- + HCO_3^-)$, depending on the preference of the clinician or laboratory in question. The anion gap and all of its component values are expressed in milliequivalents per liter (mEq/L).

Normal Values ● The normal anion gap calculated as $(Na^+ + K^+) - (Cl^- + HCO_3^-)$ is approximately 12 to 24 mEq/L in dogs and 13 to 27 mEq/L in cats.

Danger Values ● No values are considered dangerous, but greatly increased values suggest acute ethylene glycol intoxication and warrant a careful review of the patient's history.

Causes of Decreased Anion Gap ● Hypoalbuminemia is probably the most common cause of a decreased anion gap. A decreased anion gap may also be observed in IgG multiple myeloma. The magnitude of increase in the unmeasured cations (e.g., calcium, magnesium) that would be necessary to change the anion gap would probably be fatal. Laboratory errors resulting in overestimation of TCO_2 or chloride or underestimation of sodium may result in an artifactually decreased anion gap. A decreased anion gap is seldom of clinical significance.

Causes of Normochloremic (Increased Anion Gap) Acidosis ● The most common causes of an increased anion gap in dogs and cats are laboratory error (i.e., a serum sample not analyzed until the next day), ethylene glycol intoxication, diabetic ketoacidosis, uremic acidosis, and lactic acidosis.

Causes of Hyperchloremic (Normal Anion Gap) Acidosis ● Severe, acute small bowel diarrhea causing HCO_3^- loss in excess of Cl^- produces a hyperchloremic (normal anion gap) acidosis. Carbonic anhydrase inhibitors (e.g., acetazolamide) inhibit proximal renal tubular reabsorption of HCO_3^- and produce a self-limiting hyperchloremic metabolic acidosis. Acidosis due to administration of NH_4Cl decreases HCO_3^- because H^+ ions are released during ureagenesis. There is a reciprocal increase in serum chloride and no change in the anion gap. Infusion of cationic amino acids (e.g., lysine HCl, arginine HCl) during total parenteral nutrition may cause hyperchloremic metabolic acidosis because H^+ ions are released as the ammonia from these amino acids is converted to urea. During compensation for chronic respiratory alkalosis, renal acid excretion decreases, with consequent reduction in plasma HCO_3^- and increase in Cl^-. When the stimulus for hyperventilation is removed and PCO_2 increases, pH decreases because it requires 1 to 3 days for the kidneys to increase acid excretion and increase plasma HCO_3^-. This transient phenomenon is called *posthypocapnic metabolic acidosis* and is associated with hyperchloremia. Dilutional acidosis occurs when extracellular volume is expanded using an alkali-free chloride-containing solution (e.g., 0.9% NaCl). The high Cl^- concentration of 0.9% NaCl (i.e., 154 mEq/L) and the highly resorbable nature of the chloride ion in the renal tubules contribute to decreased plasma HCO_3^- concentration and hyperchloremia in this situation. RTA is characterized by hyperchloremic metabolic acidosis due to either decreased HCO_3^- reabsorption (type II RTA) or defective acid excretion (type I RTA).

Other Causes of Increased Anion Gap ● Severe dehydration may increase serum albumin concentration and, consequently, the anion gap. Alkalemia may increase the anion gap slightly by increasing the electronegative charge of plasma proteins. Excessive exposure of serum to air also may increase the anion gap (a common error in samples not run until the next day).

General References

DiBartola SP: Fluid Therapy in Small Animal Practice. Philadelphia, WB Saunders, 1992.

Rose BD: Clinical Physiology of Acid-Base and Electrolyte Disorders. 3rd ed. New York, McGraw-Hill, 1989, 853 pp.

Schaer M (ed): Fluid and electrolyte disorders. Vet Clin North Am Small Anim Pract 1989; 19:203–385.

Specific References

Adams LG, Polzin DJ, Osborne CA, et al: Comparison of fractional excretion and 24-hour urinary excretion of sodium and potassium in clinically normal cats and cats with induced chronic renal failure. Am J Vet Res 1991;52:718–722.

Adrogue HJ, Madias NE: Changes in plasma potassium concentration during acute acid-base disturbances. Am J Med 1981;71:456–467.

Atkins CE, Tyler R, Greenlee P: Clinical, biochemical, acid-base, and electrolyte abnormalities in cats after hypertonic sodium phosphate enema administration. Am J Vet Res 1985;46:980–988.

Burrows CF, Bovee KC: Metabolic changes due to experimentally induced rupture of the canine urinary bladder. Am J Vet Res 1974;35:1083.

Crawford MA, Kittleson MD, Fink GD: Hypernatremia and adipsia in a dog. JAVMA 1984;184:818–821.

Degen M: Pseudohyperkalemia in Akitas. JAVMA 1987;190:541–543.

de Morais HSA: Chloride ion in small animal practice: The forgotten ion. Vet Emerg Crit Care 1992;2:11–24.

de Morais HSA, Chew DJ: Use and interpretation of serum and urine electrolytes. Semin Vet Med Surg (Small Anim) 1992;7:262–274.

DiBartola SP, Buffington CA, Chew DJ, Sparks RA: Development of chronic renal failure in cats fed a commercial diet low in potassium. JAVMA 1993;202:744–750.

DiBartola SP, Chew DJ, Jacobs G: Quantitative urinalysis including 24-hour protein excretion in the dog. JAAHA 1980;16:538.

DiBartola SP, Johnson SE, Davenport DJ, et al: Clinicopathologic findings resembling hypoadrenocorticism in dogs with primary gastrointestinal disease. JAVMA 1985;187:60.

Dow SW, Fettman MJ, LeCouter RA, et al: Potassium depletion in cats: Renal and dietary influences. JAVMA 1987;191:1569–1575.

Gentry PA, Black WD: Evaluation of Harleco CO_2 apparatus: Comparison with the Van Slyke method. JAVMA 1975;167:156–157.

Grauer GF, Thrall MA, Henre BA, et al: Early clinicopathologic findings in dogs ingesting ethylene glycol. Am J Vet Res 1984;45:2299–2303.

Hoskins JD, Turnwald GH, Kearney MT, et al: Quantitative urinalysis in kittens from four to thirty weeks after birth. Am J Vet Res 1991;52:1295–1299.

Hutchison AS, Ralston SH, Dryburgh FJ, et al: Too much heparin: Possible source of error in blood gas analysis. Br Med J 1983;287:1131–1132.

Ilkiw JE, Rose RJ, Martin ICA: A comparison of simultaneously collected arterial, mixed venous, jugular venous, and cephalic venous blood samples in assessment of blood gas and acid-base status in the dog. J Vet Intern Med 1991;5:294–298.

Jezyk PF: Hyperkalemic periodic paralysis in a dog. JAAHA 1982;18:977–980.

Madiedo G, Sciacca R, Hause L: Air bubbles and temperature effect on blood gas analysis. J Clin Pathol 1980;33:864–867.

Mason KV: A hereditary disease in Burmese cats manifested as an episodic weakness with head nodding and neck ventroflexion. J Am Anim Hosp Assoc 1988;24:147–151.

Middleton DJ, Ilkiw JE, Watson ADJ: Arterial and venous blood gas tensions in clinically healthy cats. Am J Vet Res 1981;42:1609–1611.

Reimann KA, Knowlen GG, Tvedten HW: Factitious hyperkalemia in dogs with thrombocytosis. J Vet Intern Med 1989;3:47–52.

Russo EA, Lees GE, Hightower D: Evaluation of renal function in cats, using quantitative urinalysis. Am J Vet Res 1986;47:1308.

Tyler RD, Qualls CW, Heald RD, et al: Renal concentrating ability in dehydrated hyponatremic dogs. JAVMA 1987;191:1095.

Willard MD, Refsal K, Thacker E: Evaluation of plasma aldosterone concentrations before and after ACTH administration in clinically normal dogs and in dogs with various diseases. Am J Vet Res 1987;48:1713–1718.

Willard MD, Fossum TW, Torrance A, et al: Hyponatremia and hyperkalemia associated with idiopathic or experimentally induced chylothorax in four dogs. JAVMA 1991;199:353–358.

George E. Lees
Michael D. Willard
Robert A. Green

7 Urinary Disorders

DIFFERENTIATION OF POLYURIA-POLYDIPSIA, POLLAKIURIA, AND INCONTINENCE

These three abnormalities must be differentiated early in the diagnostic workup, preferably by the history. *Polyuria-polydipsia* (pu-pd) means increased urine production and increased water consumption. *Pollakiuria* means unduly frequent urination and implies that small amounts are voided each time. Clients commonly assume that increased frequency means increased volume. The diagnostician must ascertain whether the amount of urine voided with each micturition is large, small, or unknown. Animals with pu-pd and pollakiuria are conscious of their voiding and do not wake up in puddles of urine unless they are too weak or too pained to get up. Patients with urinary incontinence often wake up soaked in urine or may dribble urine unconsciously or uncontrollably as they walk or run.

Polyuria-Polydipsia

A precise history from the client and multiple, consistently low urine specific gravities (≤1.017) are acceptable evidence of pu-pd.

115

Measurement of water consumption over a 24-hour period may be necessary in some animals to verify polydipsia (normal ≤ 100 ml/kg/day). This is often more accurate when done at the client's home because some polyuric patients will not drink water as readily at a clinic. Quantitation of urine production is difficult unless a metabolism cage is available (normal ≤ 50 ml/kg/day). Moreover, patients with several common causes of pu-pd can concentrate their urine if they choose not to drink, making a normal finding questionable.

Polyuria-polydipsia has many possible causes (Table 7–1). History and physical examination are crucial first steps in evaluating patients with pu-pd (Fig. 7–1). Iatrogenic causes must be sought from the history. Diuretics, high-salt diets, and improper thyroid supplementation should be obvious. Aminoglycosides tend to produce high-output (nonoliguric) renal failure. Corticosteroids often cause pu-pd, even when administered rectally or topically (especially the newer, more potent drugs). Pyometra is usually suggested by history (i.e., recent estrus) or physical examination findings (i.e., enlarged uterus or vaginal discharge). If in doubt, a complete blood count (CBC) and abdominal radiographs are usually definitive (i.e., neutrophilic leukocytosis with left shift and enlarged uterus). Weight loss plus pu-pd in a cat suggests hyperthyroidism, renal failure, or diabetes mellitus (hyperthyroidism also occurs in dogs but is rare). A urinalysis should be evaluated for glucosuria; however, serum thyroxine determinations are indicated in elderly cats (i.e., ≥ 10 years) before more extensive testing is begun. Postoliguric diuresis is usually diagnosed from the history (e.g., a male cat that has had a urethral obstruction removed). Additional diagnostics are not necessary in such obvious cases; however, spontaneous relief of a urethral obstruction or ingestion of just enough ethylene glycol to produce a nonlethal, spontaneously resolving oliguric renal failure may be more difficult to discern. Finally, patients with obvious hyperadrenocorticism (e.g., potbelly or bilaterally symmetric alopecia) should have adrenal function testing performed next (see Chapter 8).

If the cause is not obvious, complete urinalysis is the next step (see Fig. 7–1). Glucosuria suggests but does not diagnose diabetes mellitus, a common cause of pu-pd. Urinary tract infections (UTIs) are often secondary in patients with pu-pd, especially when due to hyperadrenocorticism or diabetes mellitus; but UTI can cause pu-pd if there is sufficient renal involvement. Neutrophilic leukocytosis, azotemia, white blood cell (WBC) casts, lumbar pain, or hyposthenuria (specific gravity < 1.007) may occur. However, pyelonephritis can also be occult and difficult to diagnose (i.e., exclude other causes, see changes on excretory urogram or renal ultrasonography, and obtain response to antibiotic therapy).

Because clinicopathologic screening often reveals changes suggestive of the more common causes of pu-pd (e.g., renal failure, hyperadrenocorticism, hepatic insufficiency, hypercalcemia, and diabetes mellitus), evaluating a CBC and serum chemistry profile usually is the most appropriate next step (see Fig. 7–1). Modified water deprivation testing is used mainly to evaluate patients with persistent hyposthenuria (≤1.007) that is thought to be caused by diabetes insipidus or excessive water consumption (i.e., apparent psychogenic polydipsia). These conditions are uncommon, and water deprivation testing is unwise unless results of clinicopathologic screening tests have been evaluated first. Not only are the other conditions more common, but patients with such conditions might be harmed by iatrogenic dehydration.

Many patients with hyperadrenocorticism are obviously cushingoid at physical examination. Cutaneous abnormalities are seen in approximately one half of these patients, and there are no invariable CBC or serum chemistry profile changes. Increased levels of serum alkaline phosphatase (SAP) and serum cholesterol, eosinopenia, and lymphopenia are common. Hepatomegaly and abnormal hepatic function tests (e.g., bile acids) are typical, making adrenal function tests (see Chapter 8) or hepatic biopsy necessary to distinguish hyperadrenocorticism from primary hepatic disease in most patients.

Renal failure, hypercalcemic nephropathy, and hypoadrenocorticism can also resemble each other. The first two usually produce pu-pd, whereas the last causes it in 15% to 25% of patients. Each may have various degrees of azotemia, isosthenuric or near-isosthenuric urine (e.g., specific gravity 1.012–1.020), and hypercalcemia (10–15% of renal failure and 30–40% of hypoadrenal patients). Most hypoadrenal patients that have not received prior therapy will have moderately concentrated urine (specific gravity 1.020–1.030) and serum Na:K ≤ 27:1 with hyponatremia and/or hyperkalemia. However, an adrenocorticotropic hormone (ACTH) stimulation test is needed to confirm the diagnosis, since other disorders (including renal failure) may have identical electrolyte changes. For example, chronic blood loss due to any

Table 7–1 CAUSES OF POLYURIA-POLYDIPSIA (pu-pd) OR PERSISTENTLY HYPOSTHENURIC OR ISOSTHENURIC URINE IN DOGS AND CATS

Causes	Remarks
Drugs (e.g., diuretics, corticosteroids, salt in diet, aminoglycoside, or amphotericin B)	History is informative
Renal disease (e.g., chronic renal failure or postoliguric diuresis)	Should be isosthenuric (or persistently < 1.030 [dogs] or 1.035 [cats]) May be azotemic or nonazotemic For nonazotemic renal failure, creatinine clearance is useful
Upper urinary tract infection	May be hyposthenuric Not a common cause, since both kidneys must be affected WBC casts, lumbar pain, contrast radiography, and ultrasonographic findings are helpful when present
Fanconi's syndrome	Usually nonazotemic, hyperchloremic acidosis, glucosuric and aminoaciduric
Diabetes mellitus	Hyperglycemic Note: Cats with severe illness may have stress-induced hyperglycemia with glucose > 250 mg/dl
Central diabetes insipidus	Hyposthenuric (see Fig. 7–7) Rarely may see partial diabetes insipidus
Nephrogenic diabetes insipidus	Hyposthenuric May be congenital, idiopathic, or due to myeloma, pyelonephritis, hyperadrenocorticism, hypercalcemia, hypokalemia, or amyloidosis
Pyometra or prostatic abscess	Usually hyposthenuric and seen 2–8 weeks after estrus, often with proteinuria Neutrophilic leukocytosis with left shift ± vaginal discharge Abdominal radiographs often diagnostic
Hyperadrenocorticism	Isosthenuric, hyposthenuric, or concentrated Common cause of pu-pd in old dogs, rare in cats Often resembles hepatic insufficiency with increased SAP and abnormal hepatic function tests
Hypoadrenocorticism	pu-pd seen in approx 20% of patients May closely resemble renal failure and/or hypercalcemic nephropathy
Hypercalcemia	Isosthenuric or hyposthenuric, azotemic or nonazotemic May mimic hypoadrenocorticism
Hepatic insufficiency	Isosthenuric, or hyposthenuric, or concentrated May resemble hyperadrenocorticism Can have normal ALT and SAP
Hyperthyroidism	Can concentrate urine if dehydrated Primarily in older cats but may be iatrogenic due to supplementation
Hyponatremia	Due to loss of sodium from any cause May cause isosthenuria whenever < 120 mEq/L
Thyroiditis	Poorly documented May be due to transient hyperthyroidism
Hypokalemia	Must be persistent and severe to cause polyuria
Polycythemia vera	Rare
Apparent psychogenic polydipsia	See Figure 7–7
Hypoglycemia associated with nonpancreatic neoplasia	This is an uncertain association
Syndrome of inappropriate ADH secretion (SIADH)	This is an uncertain association; see Chapter 6
Pheochromocytoma	This is an uncertain association
Acromegaly	Rare

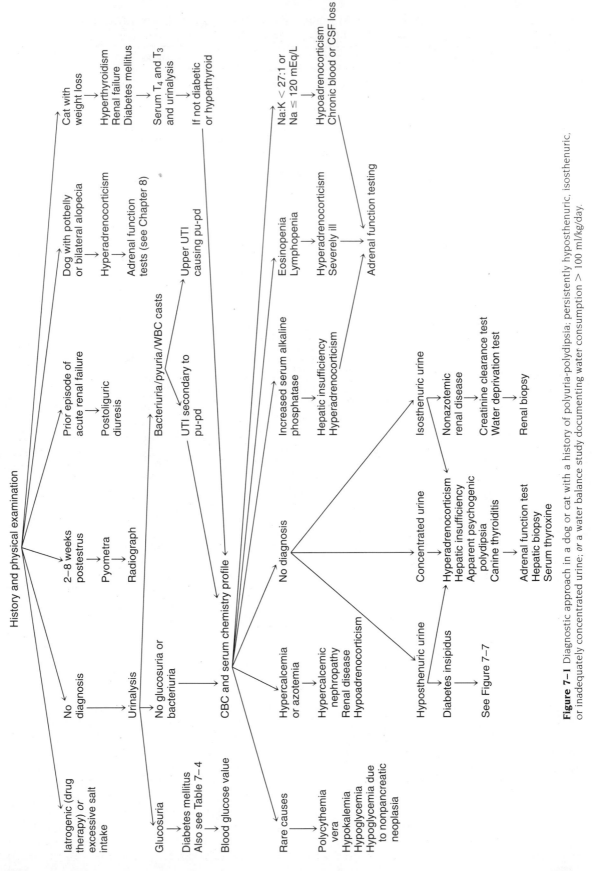

Figure 7–1 Diagnostic approach in a dog or cat with a history of polyuria-polydipsia: persistently hyposthenuric, isosthenuric, or inadequately concentrated urine; *or* a water balance study documenting water consumption > 100 ml/kg/day.

cause may produce severe hyponatremia (i.e., ≤ 120 mEq/L) resulting in isosthenuric urine despite dehydration. Most azotemic renal failure patients are isosthenuric and hyperphosphatemic; most patients with hypercalcemic nephropathy are hyposthenuric and hypophosphatemic before hypercalcemic renal failure occurs.

Rarely, polycythemia (packed cell volume [PCV] > 60%), severe persistent hypokalemia (potassium < 2.5 mEq/L), or a non–insulin-secreting tumor causing hypoglycemia may produce pu-pd.

More specialized testing is necessary if the diagnosis is still uncertain (see Fig. 7–1). Persistently isosthenuric urine (e.g., 1.008–1.012) suggests renal disease. Most patients with primary renal disease causing pu-pd are azotemic, but some are nonazotemic because of insufficient tubular function to concentrate urine despite adequate glomerular filtration to maintain blood urea nitrogen (BUN) and serum creatinine values in the normal range. These patients usually have normal radiographic renal silhouettes. A creatinine clearance test is a good noninvasive way to identify these patients. Water deprivation testing is also useful. However, elimination of other causes allows a reasonable tentative diagnosis. Note: Renal failure typically produces isosthenuria, but rare dogs in early failure may be hyposthenuric, and some cats may have urine specific gravity ≥ 1.030. Persistent hyposthenuria suggests diabetes insipidus, although hyperadrenocorticism, hepatic insufficiency, hyperthyroidism, and psychogenic polydipsia may have urine with any specific gravity. Adrenal, thyroid, or hepatic function testing and/or water deprivation is indicated.

Pollakiuria-Dysuria-Stranguria

Alteration in patterns of behavior associated with urination generally suggest disorders affecting the urinary bladder, urethra, or both (Fig. 7–2). Irritative or inflammatory (septic or nonseptic) lesions that do not impede urine flow typically cause animals to urinate more often (pollakiuria) and may cause apparent discomfort during urination (dysuria), but they usually do not cause voiding efforts to be excessively prolonged or forceful (stranguria). Urinary obstruction causes animals to make repeated voiding efforts that are either totally unproductive (i.e., with complete obstruction) or somewhat productive but unable to empty the bladder (i.e., with partial obstruction). Some animals with obstruction, however, are brought to veterinary attention for urinary incontinence instead of (or in addition to) stranguria and pollakiuria. Such paradoxical incontinence occurs when accumulated urine is forced past an obstruction that is located at or distal to effective sphincters.

Whenever it is a possibility, urinary obstruction must be promptly identified or reliably ruled out, because severe functional or structural damage may occur rapidly if obstruction is permitted to persist. The urinary bladder typically is enlarged, turgid, and inexpressible when completely obstructed. Partial obstruction may be more difficult to identify; however, careful observation of voiding integrated with assessment of postmicturition bladder volume (e.g., palpation, catheterization) usually is diagnostic. Mechanical obstructions, which may be intraluminal (e.g., uroliths, urethral plugs) or extraluminal (e.g., due to displacement caused by bladder entrapment in a perineal hernia), are most common, and in these cases, passing a urinary catheter can be both diagnostic and therapeutic. Functional obstruction is identified by finding that a urethral catheter can be passed without difficulty in a patient that cannot urinate. Neurologic examination usually detects deficits compatible with an upper motor neuron lesion or, rarely, a lower motor neuron lesion when the cause of functional obstruction is a neurogenic disorder of micturition. Nonneurogenic functional obstruction usually is caused by intramural lesions (e.g., neoplasia, stricture), which may be detected by palpation (e.g., digital rectal palpation of the pelvic urethra in dogs) or demonstrated by contrast radiography (i.e., urethrography, cystography).

Most dogs with pollakiuria-dysuria that are not obstructed have inflammation due to UTI. Bacteriuria, hematuria, and pyuria are the classic findings, but these are not invariable. If there is no evidence of UTI, then neoplasia, vaginitis, urethritis, and sterile cystic calculi must be considered. *Capillaria plica* ova are occasionally found. However, if there is any doubt, urine culture is the most definitive test for UTI (see Bacteriuria).

Cats with pollakiuria-dysuria may have UTI but more often have sterile cystitis, which is a diagnosis of exclusion. A urinalysis ± culture is indicated; otherwise, a treatable UTI may cause permanent changes while symptomatic therapy for sterile cystitis is being tried. Cats with sterile cystitis usually have hematuria with little or no pyuria. This condition is relatively frequent, and once UTI is eliminated, a therapeutic trial is reasonable. However, if the problem does not spontaneously resolve or cannot be controlled

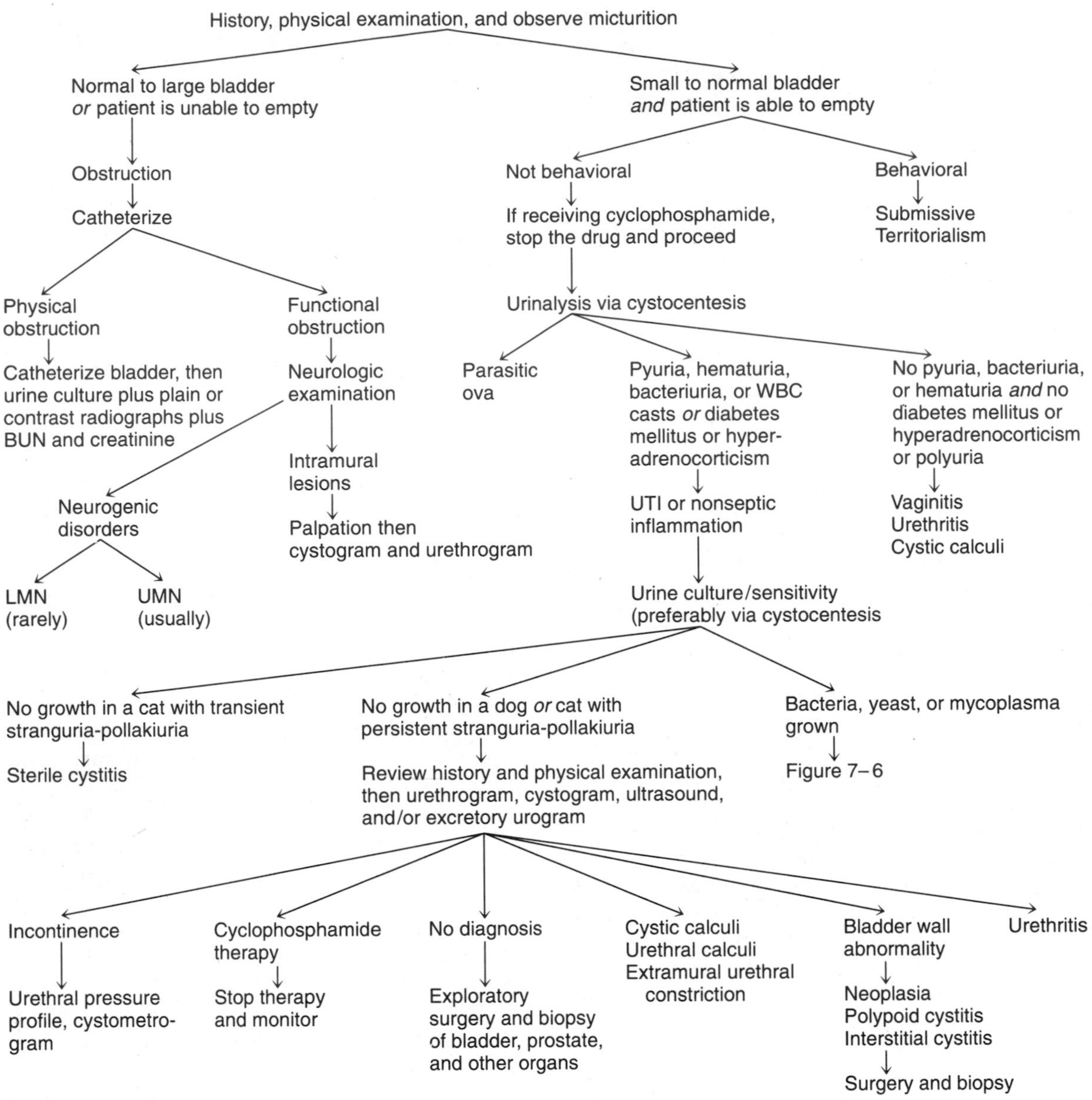

History, physical examination, and observe micturition

Normal to large bladder *or* patient is unable to empty

Small to normal bladder *and* patient is able to empty

Obstruction

Catheterize

Not behavioral

Behavioral

If receiving cyclophosphamide, stop the drug and proceed

Submissive
Territorialism

Physical obstruction

Functional obstruction

Catheterize bladder, then urine culture plus plain or contrast radiographs plus BUN and creatinine

Neurologic examination

Urinalysis via cystocentesis

Parasitic ova

Pyuria, hematuria, bacteriuria, or WBC casts *or* diabetes mellitus or hyper-adrenocorticism

No pyuria, bacteriuria, or hematuria *and* no diabetes mellitus or hyperadrenocorticism or polyuria

Intramural lesions

UTI or nonseptic inflammation

Vaginitis
Urethritis
Cystic calculi

Neurogenic disorders

Palpation then cystogram and urethrogram

LMN (rarely)   UMN (usually)

Urine culture/sensitivity (preferably via cystocentesis

No growth in a cat with transient stranguria-pollakiuria

No growth in a dog *or* cat with persistent stranguria-pollakiuria

Bacteria, yeast, or mycoplasma grown

Sterile cystitis

Review history and physical examination, then urethrogram, cystogram, ultrasound, and/or excretory urogram

Figure 7–6

Incontinence

Cyclophosphamide therapy

No diagnosis

Cystic calculi
Urethral calculi
Extramural urethral constriction

Bladder wall abnormality   Urethritis

Urethral pressure profile, cystometro-gram

Stop therapy and monitor

Exploratory surgery and biopsy of bladder, prostate, and other organs

Neoplasia
Polypoid cystitis
Interstitial cystitis

Surgery and biopsy

Figure 7–2 Diagnostic approach to nontraumatic pollakiuria-dysuria-stranguria in dogs and cats.

with symptomatic treatment, radiography ± ultrasonography of the urinary bladder is indicated.

Contrast radiographs are used to search for cystic or urethral calculi, urethritis, urethral constriction, and mass lesions. If an abnormality is found, surgery is indicated. If no abnormalities are found, one should review the history and physical examination. If incontinence is possible, a cystometrogram and urethral pressure profile may be considered. If incontinence does not appear to be present, exploratory surgery is indicated. However, UTI should be elim-

inated by culture first (see Fig. 7–2). Should surgery be performed, it is imperative that the bladder and prostate undergo biopsy regardless of how normal or how neoplastic they appear. Interstitial cystitis may not have any gross lesions, whereas polypoid cystitis may mimic malignancy.

URINALYSIS

Common Indications ● A screening test in any ill animal. Urinalysis should be performed in

Table 7–2 POTENTIAL CAUSES OF DISCOLORED URINE IN DOGS AND CATS

Urine Color	Causes	Urine Color	Causes
Deep yellow	Quinacrine	Red-purple	Porphyrins
Yellow-orange	Bilirubin		Phenolphthalein
	Fluorescein	Red-orange	Rifampin
	Concentrated urine		Phenazopyridine
	Sulfasalazine	Red	RBCs
Yellow-green	Bilirubin		Myoglobin
	Biliverdin		Dyes
Yellow-brown	Bilirubin		Porphyrins
	Biliverdin		Phenazopyridine
			Phenolsulfonphthalein
Brown-black	Methemoglobin		Beets
	Methocarbamol	Blue	Methylene blue
	Phenols	Blue-green	Urinary tract infection due to
Brown or rust-yellow	Nitrofurantoin		*Pseudomonas aeruginosa*
	Furazolidone		Indicanuria due to intestinal
	Metronidazole		bacterial overgrowth
	Sulfonamides	Dark green	Phenols
Red-brown	Methemoglobin	Milky	Pyuria
	Myoglobin		Lipiduria
	RBCs	Colorless	Dilute
	Hemoglobin		
	Dilantin		
	Dinitrophenol		
	Chronic lead or mercury intoxication		

every patient with any urinary tract disease or abnormality. Advantages: ability to perform this analysis in almost any clinic frequently provides clinically useful information in patients with various systemic diseases, as well as in patients with disorders of the urinary system.

Analysis • Uncontaminated urine should be obtained, preferably by cystocentesis. If cystocentesis cannot be performed, a clean-catch midstream voided sample from a male cat or a female, or a catheterized sample from a male dog (after discarding the first portion to lessen contamination) is the next best sample.

A standard volume of urine should be used for sedimentation (e.g., 10 ml). For greatest accuracy in detecting and differentiating casts and cellular components, urine sediment should be examined while the specimen is as fresh as possible.

If the urinalysis cannot be performed within 2 hours, the urine should be held at 4°C and brought back to room temperature just before analysis.

Analysis consists of (1) determining color and turbidity; (2) chemical analysis using multitest dipsticks or single chemical tests; and (3) microscopic analysis of the sediment. All three portions are important. The color and turbidity

should be determined first. Then 10 ml of urine should be centrifuged at 2000 rpm for 5 minutes. Standardization of volume, speed, and duration of centrifugation allows meaningful comparison of results from different samples. Dipstick analysis is performed on the supernatant or on well mixed urine, depending on the type of dipstick. Rapid, complete immersion of the test strip with immediate shaking off of excess urine plus holding the dipstick level to avoid runoff between pads is needed to avoid mixing reagents from different test pads. Preservatives (e.g., toluene) may alter some test results.

Color/Turbidity

Analysis • Visual inspection. Normal urine is clear to slightly turbid and amber-yellow. Dilute urine tends to be colorless, and concentrated urine is a darker yellow. Different colors and their significance are listed in Table 7–2. Review of the history for drug administration and careful examination of the urine sediment are indicated if urine discoloration is noted. Hematuria, hemoglobinuria, and bilirubinuria are the most common causes of discolored urine. Pyuria is a common cause of turbidity.

Specific Gravity

Analysis • Specific gravity is determined on the postcentrifugation supernatant with a refractometer. Calibration of the refractometer should be checked periodically by verifying that distilled water gives a reading of 1.000. Some dipsticks have a test pad that indicates specific gravity; however, these results often do not correlate well with results obtained by refractometer. Use of dipstick test pads to evaluate urine specific gravity in dogs and cats is not recommended.

Normal Values • Dogs, 1.015 to 1.040; cats, 1.015 to 1.050.

Danger Values • There are no danger values per se; but, values > 1.050 in dogs and > 1.060 in cats may reflect severe dehydration.

Artifacts • Falsely decreased: alkaline urine (dipstick). Falsely increased: dextran and radiographic contrast media (refractometer). Dipstick values may be increased by proteinuria (>100 mg/dl) and radiographic contrast agents used for excretory urograms, although there is controversy about whether the latter is always significant. Urine with a specific gravity >1.040 may not be affected by contrast agents, whereas urine with a specific gravity <1.040 will usually have the specific gravity increased for approximately 8 hours after intravenous injection. However, if the contrast medium is injected directly into the bladder, it will always increase the specific gravity.

Drug Therapy That May Alter Results • Low specific gravity may be caused by corticosteroids, selected diuretics, demeclocycline, colchicine, methoxyflurane, lithium, and fluid therapy. Increased specific gravity may be caused by radiographic contrast media. *It is important to obtain urine before treatment (especially fluid therapy) is begun.*

Causes of Altered Urine Specific Gravity • Urine that is ≤1.007 is hyposthenuric and implies that the kidneys are capable of diluting glomerular filtrate (especially if <1.004). Hyposthenuria suggests that renal failure is not present; however, some dogs with renal failure are able to excrete hyposthenuric urine. Persistent hyposthenuria suggests a lack of antidiuretic hormone (ADH) (excessive water consumption or central diabetes insipidus) or resistance to ADH

(nephrogenic diabetes insipidus). Resistance to ADH may be due to hyperadrenocorticism, hypercalcemia, hypokalemia, myeloma, amyloidosis, pyelonephritis, or drug therapy or may be congenital.

Urine that is 1.008 to 1.012 is isosthenuric, meaning that the kidneys have not altered the concentration of the glomerular filtrate. Urine that is 1.013 to 1.029 (dog) or 1.013 to 1.034 (cat) has been concentrated, but not enough to document adequacy of renal tubular function.

Urine that is ≥1.030 (dog) or ≥1.035 (cat) demonstrates urine concentrating ability indicating adequate renal function to maintain normal homeostasis. A patient could still have many of the diseases that cause pu-pd (e.g., hyperadrenocorticism, hepatic insufficiency, or hyperthyroidism), as well as renal glomerular disease. A single urine specific gravity >1.007 and <1.030 or 1.035 does not always imply renal tubular dysfunction or pu-pd unless the patient is clinically dehydrated, in which case such a specific gravity reflects deficient renal tubular function. Otherwise, repeated urine specific gravity measurements or failure to concentrate urine adequately during appropriate water deprivation testing may be needed to establish deficient renal tubular function. Persistently hyposthenuric, isosthenuric, or inadequately concentrated urine (<1.030 or <1.035 in dogs and cats, respectively) is an indication for further testing (see Fig. 7–1).

Urine pH

Analysis • Analysis is performed with a pH test pad on a urine dipstick.

Normal Values • Most normal dogs and cats have a urine pH of 5.5 to 7.0; however, some normal pets may have higher or lower values.

Danger Values • None.

Artifacts • Falsely increased: standing open at room temperature for a long time awaiting analysis. Certain urease-producing bacteria generate ammonia from urea, causing pH to increase when urine is allowed to stand at room temperature. Improper dipstick technique and prolonged waiting before reading the test strip may cause erroneous values.

Drug Therapy That May Alter Results • Decreased urine pH may be due to methionine, mandelate, ammonium phosphate, potassium

Table 7–3 CONVERSION OF SEMIQUANTITATIVE UNITS TO APPROXIMATE QUANTITATIVE UNITS (mg/dl) USING AMES DIPSTICKS

Semiquantitative Value	Protein Concentration (mg/dl)	Glucose Concentration (mg/dl)	Ketone Concentration (mg/dl)
Trace		100	5
1 + (small)	30	250	15
2 + (moderate)	100	500	40
3 + (large)	300	1000	80
4 +	>2000	>2000	160

phosphate, ammonium chloride, and ascorbic acid. Increased urine pH may be due to acetazolamide, bicarbonate, and perhaps amphotericin B.

Causes of Altered Urine pH • Urine pH does not reliably reflect body pH, especially in a hypochloremic vomiting patient that may have aciduria despite alkalosis. Ingestion of meats or acidic fruits, proximal renal tubular acidosis (RTA), Fanconi's syndrome, and metabolic alkalosis due to severe gastric vomiting tend to cause aciduria (pH ≤ 5.5). Ingestion of alkali (e.g., bicarbonate or citrate), UTI with urease-producing bacteria (e.g., *Staphylococcus aureus, Proteus* spp., and *Klebsiella* spp.), distal RTA, diets rich in vegetables, metabolic and respiratory alkalosis, and recent eating may cause an alkaline urine (e.g., pH > 7.0).

Persistently alkaline urine is an indication for complete urinalysis or urine culture and sensitivity testing. If no reason for alkaline urine is found on history, urinalysis, or urine culture, then distal renal RTA may be considered (rare). RTA is a rare syndrome that may be due to various drugs (i.e., acetazolamide, sulfanilamide, or old tetracycline) and diseases (i.e., systemic lupus erythematosus, hepatic cirrhosis, myeloma, nephrotic syndrome, heavy metal poisoning, and others) or may be idiopathic. Both distal and proximal RTA cause hyperchloremic metabolic acidosis with a normal anion gap and often produce hypokalemia (see Chapter 6). Diagnosis of distal RTA requires administering 0.1 g/kg ammonium chloride orally after an overnight fast. Urine pH is then measured at 1- to 2-hour intervals over the next 8 hours. Failure to achieve a urine pH <6.0 is diagnostic of distal RTA.

Proximal RTA causes urine with pH <6. Diagnosis requires infusion of 0.5 to 1.0 mEq/kg/hour sodium bicarbonate. With proximal RTA, a patient requires excessive amounts of bicarbonate to maintain a normal serum HCO_3. Diagnosis of RTA requires searching for a cause and symptomatically treating electrolyte and acid-base abnormalities.

Proteinuria

Analysis • Analysis is performed using a test pad on a urine dipstick, sulfosalicylic acid precipitation, spectrophotometric analysis, and protein electrophoresis. This section principally considers the first two. Quantitative spectrophotometric analysis is discussed under Urine Protein: Urine Creatinine Ratio. The test pad on the dipstick primarily detects albumin; the sulfosalicylic acid test also detects globulins.

Proteinuria must be interpreted in light of the urine specific gravity. Dilute or unconcentrated urine means there will be a greater daily volume of urine, and this greater volume requires that more protein (or other substance) be excreted into the urine before it reaches detectable concentrations. Therefore, a "small" reaction (e.g., 30 mg/dl) in urine from a patient with a specific gravity of 1.010 means that more protein is being lost into the urine each day than in an identical protein reaction in a patient with a 1.030 urine specific gravity. Therefore, patients with isosthenuria or hyposthenuria may have "trace" or "negative" protein reactions despite significant urinary protein loss. See Table 7–3 for conversion of semiquantitative values (i.e., trace, 1+, 2+, and so on) to approximate quantitative values (i.e., 100 mg/dl, 250 mg/dl, and so on).

Myelomas that produce free light chains (i.e., Bence Jones protein) do not cause a positive reaction with dipsticks but are positive on sulfosalicylic acid testing. Protein electrophoresis is indicated in these patients, in which case most of the urinary protein is a monoclonal spike in the β or γ regions. Rarely, immunoglobulinuria may occur.

Normal Values • In both dogs and cats, normal values are none in urine with specific gravity

Stop use of nephrotoxic drugs (see Table 7–8, especially those denoted ''important''). If proteinuria is clearly insignificant, stop. If not sure of significance, proceed.

Eliminate artifact due to alkaline urine, drugs, radiographic contrast agents, and contamination. Repeat urinalysis using cystocentesis-obtained urine.

If proteinuria persists and is not due to artifact or contamination, measure urine protein:creatinine ratio. If ratio < 1.0, do not proceed. If ratio > 1.0, obtain urinalysis, serum creatinine, BUN, and serum total protein and albumin.

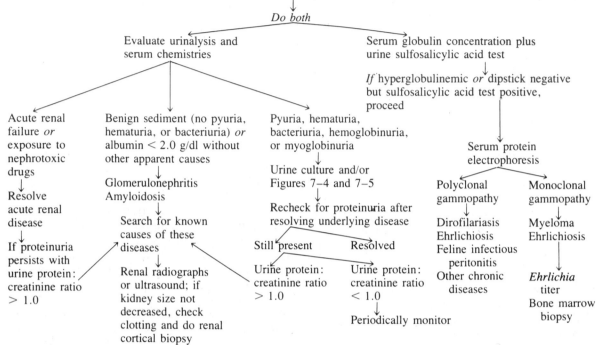

Figure 7–3 Diagnostic approach to proteinuria in dogs and cats.

≤ 1.020, ≤ 30 mg/dl in urine with specific gravity ≤ 1.035, and never more than 100 mg/dl. These values are approximations, and more precise tests may be needed (see 24-Hour Urine Protein Determination and Urine Protein: Urine Creatinine Ratio).

Danger Values • None.

Artifacts • Falsely decreased (sulfosalicylic acid): very alkaline urine. Falsely increased (dipstick): quaternary ammonium compounds, phenazopyridine, chlorhexidine, allowing the dipstick test pad to become wet during storage, allowing prolonged contact of the test pad with excessive amounts of urine during urinalysis, or highly alkaline urine (pH ≥ 9) due to acetazolamide, sodium bicarbonate, and some UTIs. Falsely increased (sulfosalicylic acid): radiographic contrast media, carbenicillin, penicillin G, cephalosporins, and sulfa drugs.

Drug Therapy That May Cause Proteinuria •

Certain penicillins (e.g., oxacillin), radiographic contrast agents, sulfonamides, amphotericin B, cephaloridine, aminoglycosides, and gold therapy may cause renal disease with subsequent proteinuria.

Causes of Proteinuria • Because small amounts may be normal, one must first decide if the proteinuria is potentially significant (Fig. 7–3). If it is clearly insignificant, one may ignore it unless the patient is receiving nephrotoxic drugs (e.g., aminoglycosides). These drugs should be stopped regardless of the amount of proteinuria, because mild proteinuria may be an early sign of nephrotoxicity and impending acute renal failure. Aminoglycoside and amphotericin B nephrotoxicities typically cause proteinuria or other changes in the urinalysis (e.g., glucosuria or cylindruria) before azotemia.

If the proteinuria may be significant, one should next consider artifacts and contamination. Repeating the urinalysis using a specimen obtained by cystocentesis eliminates contamination and allows one to determine if the protein-uria is transient or persistent. Transient protein-uria may be due to many causes (e.g., strenuous exercise, fever, or contamination) and is rarely significant. Persistent proteinuria should prompt both a search for potential nephrotoxins and determination of a urine protein:urine creatinine ratio to ascertain whether the proteinuria is significant. Hypertension, right-sided heart failure causing severe congestion, urinary tract inflammation, or urinary tract hemorrhage may cause proteinuria but usually produces insignificant losses of <30 mg/kg/day (i.e., urine protein:creatinine <1.0). However, some animals with UTI will have marked proteinuria (i.e., urine protein:creatinine >10.0).

If the proteinuria is significant, complete urinalysis and evaluation of serum albumin and globulin concentrations are indicated (see Fig. 7–3). Note: A normal serum albumin concentration does not necessarily mean that the proteinuria is insignificant.

Proteinuria associated with an inflammatory sediment (i.e., pyuria or hematuria) requires resolution of the inflammation and then rechecking for persistence of the proteinuria. The most common cause of inflammatory proteinuria is UTI. Urine culture should be performed if there is any possibility of infection.

Proteinuria associated with a benign sediment and normal serum globulins or a polyclonal gammopathy is usually due to renal glomerular disease: glomerulonephritis or amyloidosis. (Note: Feline amyloidosis usually affects the medulla and may not cause proteinuria.) Search should be made for known causes of glomerulonephropathy: heartworm disease (usually associated with polyclonal gammopathy), systemic lupus erythematosus, brucellosis, sarcoptic mange, feline leukemia virus (FeLV), feline infectious peritonitis (FIP), various neoplasias, ehrlichiosis (monoclonal-like or polyclonal gammopathy), pyometra, and other chronic inflammatory diseases (e.g., pancreatitis). Renal cortical biopsy is usually indicated to determine if glomerulonephritis or amyloidosis is present. Urine protein electrophoresis may be done to differentiate albuminuria from globulinuria, but this is usually not cost-effective.

Proteinuria detected by sulfosalicylic acid testing but not dipstick, or proteinuria associated with a monoclonal gammopathy may be due to Bence Jones proteins and necessitates a search for osteolytic lesions and lymphoproliferative disorders. Ehrlichiosis occasionally may mimic myeloma by producing glomerulonephritis and a monoclonal-like gammopathy as well as having plasmacytosis of the bone marrow. A titer may be diagnostic (see Chapter 15). If the patient does not have ehrlichiosis, urine protein electrophoresis is indicated. Albuminuria suggests glomerular disease; globulinuria suggests abnormal proteins. Both may coexist if abnormal globulins are causing glomerulonephritis.

24-Hour Urine Protein Determination

Occasional Indications • To determine the significance of proteinuria detected by urine dipstick; it can also be used to help monitor progression of glomerular disease, although the fractional albumin clearance is possibly more accurate. Advantages: better accuracy than dipstick procedures. Disadvantages: 24-hour urine collection required.

Analysis • Urine is collected for 24 hours. The total urine volume is determined, and the urine albumin concentration on a 1.5-ml aliquot of the pooled 24-hour sample is measured by spectrophotometric methods.

Urine vol (ml) × albumin conc (mg/ml) = 24-hour urine protein loss

Shorter time periods may be used, and the calculation adjusted; however, shorter collection times may render the test less accurate.

Normal Values • Dogs, < 250 to 500 mg/day or < 30 mg/kg/day; cats, < 100 mg/day.

Danger Values • Not determined.

Artifacts • See the section on total protein in Chapter 12.

Causes of Increased Urine Protein Loss • See the earlier discussion under Proteinuria.

Urine Protein:Urine Creatinine Ratio

Frequent Indications • To determine the approximate magnitude and therefore the significance of proteinuria; it can also monitor progression of glomerular disease, although fractional albumin clearance may be more accurate. Advantages: more accurate than dipstick procedures, needs only a spot urine sample, and shows close correlation with quantitative 24-hour determinations.

Analysis • Total protein and creatinine concentrations are measured in 3 ml of urine by spectrophotometric methods. Total protein is usually determined by Coomassie brilliant blue dye-binding or trichloroacetic acid–ponceau S methods. Measurements with the former tend to be higher than with the latter, but the latter can detect very small amounts of protein. The following ratio is calculated:

$$\frac{\text{Total protein (mg/dl)}}{\text{Creatinine (mg/dl)}}$$

Ratios of > 1.0 are abnormal and are typically associated with a protein loss of > 30 mg/kg/day. Using the urine protein:urine creatinine ratio, a dog's approximate daily urine protein loss (mg/kg/day) can be estimated using the following equations (where UP = urine protein and UC = urine creatinine):

$$\frac{\text{Coomassie brilliant blue method}}{\text{Daily loss} = (\text{UP/UC} \times 19.2) + 3.1}$$

$$\frac{\text{Trichloroacetic acid–ponceau S method}}{\text{Daily loss} = (\text{UP/UC} \times 28.7) + 2.8}$$

Normal Values • Dogs and cats < 0.6.

Danger Values • None.

Artifacts • See sections on total protein (Chapter 12) and Creatinine (this chapter).

Causes of Increased Urine Total Protein: Creatinine Ratio • See the earlier discussion under Proteinuria.

Fractional Albumin Clearance

Occasional Indications • To help monitor progression of renal glomerular disease.

Analysis: • Albumin and creatinine concentrations are measured in 0.5 ml of serum and 3 ml of urine and are used in the following formula:

$$\frac{\text{Urine albumin (mg/dl)} \times \text{serum creatinine (mg/dl)}}{\text{Urine creatinine (mg/dl)} \times \text{serum albumin (mg/dl)}}$$

The value obtained is used to compare losses in a given patient at different times. It is not used to compare different patients. Worsening glomerular disease may cause total urine protein losses to decrease (owing to decreased glomerular filtration rate [GFR]); however, the fractional albumin clearance should be increased, documenting worsening disease.

Glucosuria

Analysis • Test pad on urine dipstick or paper test strip (glucose oxidase method) or a test for reducing substances in urine (Clinitest). To avoid misinterpretations arising from artifacts, both tests should be performed.

Normal Values • Dog and cat urine should be negative for glucose by these tests (see Table 7–3).

Danger Values • None.

Artifacts • Falsely decreased: refrigerated urine, large amounts of ascorbic acid, tetracycline (due to ascorbic acid in formulation), salicylates, mercurial diuretics, or ketones (dipstick) plus low urine pH and increased urine salt concentrations (paper test strip). Falsely increased: hydrogen peroxide and hypochlorite or bleach (dipstick).

The Clinitest reaction is not specific for glucose. Falsely decreased: severe proteinuria. Falsely increased: galactose, pentose, lactose, fructose, formaldehyde (from mandelic acid), salicylates, chloramphenicol, penicillins, streptomycin, some cephalosporins, nalidixic acid, nitrofurans, uric acid, tetracyclines, radiographic contrast media, low specific gravity (slight), and large amounts of ascorbic acid, creatinine, and sulfonamides (Clinitest). Furthermore, very strong positive reactions may be read out low because the final color is less orange than that which occurred during the reaction ("pass-through" phenomenon).

Drug Therapy That May Cause Glucosuria • Drugs capable of causing hyperglycemia (see Chapter 8), intravenous infusion of dextrose-containing solutions, and selected nephrotoxins causing proximal renal tubular dysfunction (e.g., aminoglycoside nephrotoxicity typically produces glucosuria before azotemia).

Causes of Glucosuria • Glucosuria may be due to hyperglycemia, proximal renal tubular dysfunction, or urinary tract hemorrhage (Table 7–4). Glucosuria always is an indication for a

Table 7–4 CAUSES OF GLUCOSURIA IN DOGS AND CATS

Blood glucose concentration exceeding renal threshold	Diabetes mellitus Stress (especially in cats) Infusion of dextrose-containing fluids Hyperadrenocorticism (rarely causes glucose > 180 mg/dl) Pheochromocytoma (rare) Increased cardiac output plus mild hyperglycemia
Abnormal proximal renal tubular function	Early aminoglycoside toxicity Early amphotericin B toxicity Acute renal failure Fanconi's syndrome Primary renal glucosuria
Contamination	Urinary hemorrhage in a patient with hyperglycemia

blood glucose measurement except in cats that are stressed or animals that have severe cystic hemorrhage (e.g., blocked tomcats). The most common cause of persistent glucosuria due to hyperglycemia is diabetes mellitus, although stressed cats may have hyperglycemia for many days. If the blood glucose concentration is normal, then the urine should be reevaluated with both urine dipstick and the Clinitest. If glucosuria is still present, history should be reviewed and complete urinalysis, BUN, and serum creatinine concentrations determined to search for acute renal disease. Primary renal glucosuria is due to a defect in proximal renal tubular function. Occasionally, there are multiple tubular defects: Fanconi's syndrome (rare) occurs in some breeds (e.g., basenji), producing glucosuria despite normoglycemia, hyperchloremic metabolic acidosis, and hyperphosphaturia. Specific analysis also reveals aminoaciduria.

Ketonuria

Analysis • Test pad on urine dipstick (see Table 7–3), tablet (Acetest), or test tube procedure (Rothera's). These detect acetoacetate and acetone but not beta-hydroxybutyrate, which is principally responsible for acidosis. However, adding a few drops of 3% aqueous hydrogen peroxide to a 10-ml urine sample converts beta-hydroxybutyrate to acetoacetate.

Normal Values • Dog and cat urine should be negative for ketones.

Danger Values • Severity of ketoacidosis is not correlated with the degree of ketonuria; hence, there are no danger values. However, large amounts of urine ketones suggest possible ketoacidosis and warrant further evaluation of acid-base status (e.g., total carbon dioxide [Tco_2] determination or blood gas analysis).

Artifacts • Falsely increased: phenazopyridine, paraldehyde, phenolphthalein, BSP and phenolsulfonphthalein (PSP) dyes.

Drug Therapy That May Cause Ketonuria • Inositol, methionine, streptozotocin, mesna, and aspirin intoxication.

Causes of Ketonuria • Lipolysis is necessary to produce ketones. Starvation, fasting, and diabetic ketoacidosis are the most common causes. Only diabetic ketoacidosis also is associated with significant ketonemia. Ketonuria is an indication for blood glucose determination. Ketonuria does not need to be investigated in anorexic, nondiabetic patients. If a patient is ketonuric and hyperglycemic, diabetic ketoacidosis is diagnosed and serum sodium, potassium, phosphorus, and Tco_2 or blood gas determinations are indicated.

Bilirubinuria

Analysis • Test pad on urine dipstick (diazo method) and occasionally the oxidation method (Harrison's spot test). The tablet method is supposedly more sensitive than the dipstick.

Normal Values • Dogs (especially males) may normally have small amounts of bilirubinuria if the urine specific gravity is ≥ 1.020. Normal cats do not have bilirubinuria regardless of the urine specific gravity.

Danger Values • None.

Artifacts • Falsely decreased: prolonged exposure to ultraviolet-containing light (degrades bilirubin into biliverdin, which is not detected), ascorbic acid, chlorpromazine, nitrite (due to infection), and aspirin. Substantial hemoglobinuria also may cause falsely decreased readings by masking the bilirubin-induced color change on dipsticks. Falsely increased: large amounts of phenothiazines or phenazopyridine (the latter also causes falsely decreased readings because of urine discoloration, which may confuse the laboratory).

Drug Therapy That May Cause Bilirubinuria ● See Chapters 3 and 9 for causes of hemolytic anemia and icterus, respectively.

Causes of Bilirubinuria ● Bilirubin must be conjugated to be excreted into the urine. Excessive bilirubinuria may occur with some hepatic diseases. However, canine kidneys can also conjugate bilirubin formed from hemolysis, resulting in bilirubinuria. The most common causes of hyperbilirubinuria in dogs and cats are hepatic disease and posthepatic bile duct obstruction. However, hemolytic diseases must be considered, especially hemobartonellosis and immune-mediated hemolytic anemia.

Excessive bilirubinuria in a dog or any bilirubinuria in a cat is an indication for determination of total serum bilirubin concentrations, serum alkaline phosphatase and alanine transferase activities, and a hematocrit. If the hematocrit is more than 10% to 15% below the lower limit of normal, a CBC plus reticulocyte count is indicated. See Chapter 9 for the diagnostic approach to icterus.

Urobilinogen

Assay ● Test pad on urine dipstick.

Normal Values ● Normal dogs and cats have 0.1 to 1.0 Ehrlich unit. One cannot detect total absence of urobilinogen with this test.

Danger Values ● None.

Artifacts ● Falsely decreased: prolonged exposure to light and high nitrite concentrations. Falsely increased: acetazolamide, bilirubin, formaldehyde (from mandelic acid), phenazopyridine, sulfonamides, phenothiazines, procaine, and BSP dye.

Drug Therapy That May Alter Results ● Urobilinogen may be decreased by antibiotics that suppress intestinal bacterial flora and drugs that acidify the urine (e.g., ammonium chloride and ascorbic acid). Urobilinogen may be increased by drugs that alkalize the urine (bicarbonate and acetazolamide).

Causes of Altered Urobilinogen ● Decreased urobilinogen may be caused by complete biliary obstruction. Increased urobilinogen may be due to increased production of bilirubin (i.e., he-

molytic disease) and primary hepatic disease. Increased urobilinogen is a weak indication for determining the serum bilirubin, serum alkaline phosphatase, and alanine transferase activities plus a hematocrit. If the hemocrit is more than 10% to 15% below normal, a CBC and reticulocyte count are indicated.

Hemoglobinuria-Myoglobinuria

Analysis ● Test pad on most urine dipsticks detects hemoglobin, myoglobin, and, to a lesser extent, intact red blood cells (RBCs). The dipstick test usually detects hematuria as well as hemoglobinuria because some RBCs lyse, particularly when the urine is hypotonic or when uncentrifuged urine is used. However, if urine supernatant is used and there is no hemolysis, the dipstick test will be negative. The assay is sensitive, detecting 10 RBCs/μl or 0.03 mg/dl hemoglobin.

Normal Values ● Dogs and cats should not have hemoglobinuria.

Danger Values ● None.

Artifacts ● Falsely decreased: ascorbic acid, high urine specific gravity, and nitrites. Falsely increased: iodine, hypochlorite, and microbial or WBC peroxidases (also see Hematuria: Artifacts).

Causes of Hemoglobinuria ● Artifacts must be eliminated first. Next, hematuria with subsequent hemolysis should be sought, since it is the most common cause. If RBCs or RBC ghosts are found in the urine, hematuria is confirmed. Absence of RBCs or RBC ghosts in the sediment of urine that is not discolored is an indication for repeat urinalysis. If the hemoglobinuria does not recur, one may ignore the first result. If the hemoglobinuria persists or recurs or if the urine is grossly discolored, one should determine the hematocrit and check for hemoglobinemia (Fig. 7–4). If the plasma is pink or red despite proper venipuncture technique (hemoglobinemia), then hemoglobinuria is present. However, a patient may have had transient hemoglobinemia that has been totally cleared into the urine, resulting in clear plasma. Therefore, clear plasma does not rule out hemoglobinuria.

If there is no evidence of hemoglobinemia or recent hemolysis, then myoglobinuria must be considered. In confusing cases, one may test for myoglobinuria by requesting urine precipitation with 80% saturated ammonium sulfate. This is

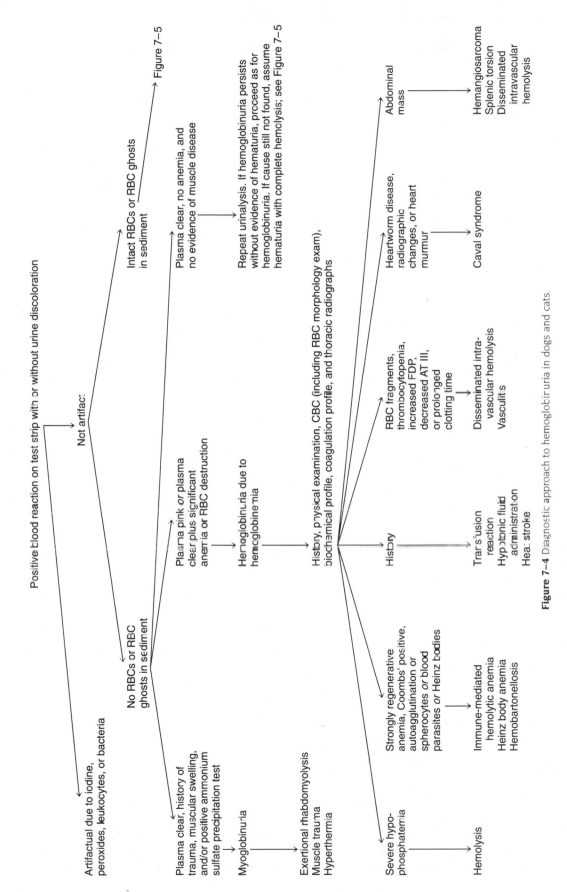

Figure 7-4 Diagnostic approach to hemoglobinuria in dogs and cats.

done by adding 2.8 g ammonium sulfate to 5 ml urine that remains reddish brown after centrifugation, mixing and recentrifuging the sample. If the supernatant becomes clear, it is hemoglobinuria; but if the supernatant remains dark, it is myoglobinuria. If there is no evidence of hematuria, hemoglobinemia, hemolysis, or muscle disease, one should recheck for artifacts. Persistent hemoglobinuria of unknown cause is an indication to look for occult urinary hemorrhage or muscular disease (e.g., creatine phosphokinase, electromyography, or muscle biopsy).

Hemoglobinuria due to hematuria is followed up as for hematuria (Fig. 7–5).

Hemoglobinuria due to hemoglobinemia mandates a search for hemolytic anemia (see Chapter 3). History, physical examination, and CBC are indicated.

Myoglobinuria requires a search for acute muscle trauma, hyperthermia, and myositis (see Chapter 14).

Hematuria

Analysis • Test pad on urine dipstick or, preferably, microscopic examination of urine sediment.

Normal Values • Urine obtained by cystocentesis should have 0 to 3 RBCs/high-power field (hpf), catheterized samples 0 to 5 RBCs/hpf, and midstream voided samples 0 to 7 RBCs/hpf by microscopic examination. In the first two methods, however, difficulty or trauma in obtaining the sample can result in gross or microscopic hematuria.

Danger Values • None.

Artifacts • Falsely decreased: hemolysis occurs rapidly in hyposthenuric or in very acidic or alkaline urine, in which it may be complete within 2 hours.

Causes of Hematuria • One must first rule out contamination with vaginal or preputial secretions as well as iatrogenic hemorrhage during sampling (see Fig. 7–5). Hematuria may result from UTI, nonseptic inflammation, coagulopathy, prostatic disease, trauma (exogenous, surgical, or calculi), neoplasia, cysts, leptospirosis, renal infarcts, urinary parasites, violent exercise, or glomerulonephritis (rare). In dogs, UTI is the most common cause of hematuria; therefore, a urine culture is indicated even if pyuria

and bacteriuria are absent. If there is a history of anticoagulant exposure, evidence of coagulopathy on history or physical examination, or hypovolemia or anemia due to hemorrhage, or if UTI has been precluded, coagulation screening tests are indicated. If these tests are unrevealing, positive-contrast radiography (or ultrasonography) is used to examine the kidneys, urethra, ureters, prostate, and urinary bladder. Exploratory surgery is indicated if bleeding remains occult after these tests and is severe or persistent. At surgery, urine from each ureter should be examined after intraoperative furosemide administration increases urine flow, allowing assessment of effluent from each ureter. If a lesion is not found, biopsies should be taken of both kidneys, the urinary bladder, and the prostate, regardless of their gross appearance.

In cats, nonseptic cystitis (e.g., feline urologic syndrome) is a common cause of hematuria. However, except for prostatic disease, the possibilities and indications for persistent or recurrent hematuria are the same as for dogs.

Nitrituria

Analysis • Test pad on urine dipstick.

Normal Values • Negative.

Danger Values • None.

Artifacts • Falsely decreased: frequent voiding and ascorbic acid. Falsely increased: phenazopyridine.

Causes of Nitrituria • UTIs with nitrate-reducing bacteria cause nitrituria if sufficient bacteria grow in the urine for at least 4 hours. This test does not seem to be as sensitive in dogs and cats as has been reported in persons. Nitrituria is an indication for urine sediment examination or urine culture.

Pyuria

Analysis • Test pad on dipstick or, preferably, microscopic examination of urine sediment. The dipstick test (for WBC esterase activity) has not been extensively tested in dogs and cats, although it appears to be a specific but insensitive screen for pyuria.

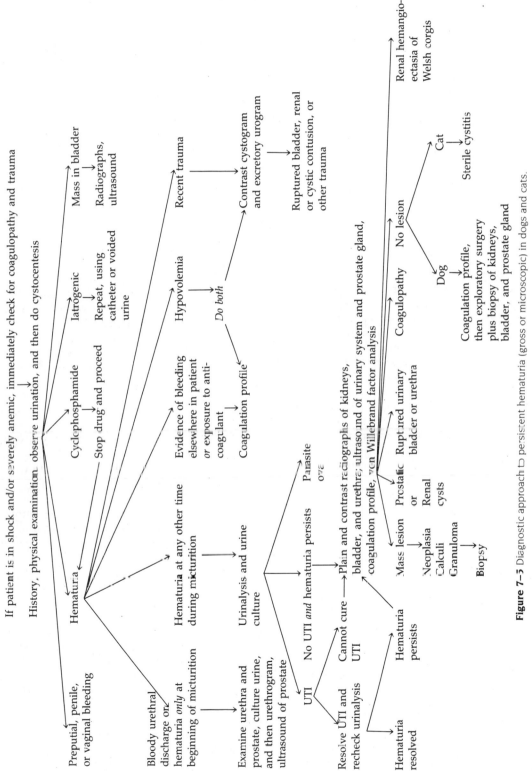

Figure 7-5 Diagnostic approach to persistent hematuria (gross or microscopic) in dogs and cats.

Normal Values • Urine obtained by cystocentesis should have 0 to 3 WBCs/hpf, catheterized samples 0 to 5 WBCs/hpf, and midstream voided samples 0 to 7 WBCs/hpf (except in male dogs) as determined by microscopic analysis.

Danger Values • None.

Artifacts • Falsely decreased: alkaline urine, dilute urine, or prolonged exposure to room temperature, causing WBC lysis (sediment examination). Falsely increased: oxidants such as nitrofurantoin, cephalosporins, and gentamicin (dipstick).

Causes of Pyuria • Pyuria occurs because of contamination with preputial or vaginal secretions, UTI, sterile cystitis, neoplasia, calculi, acute interstitial nephritis, glomerulonephritis (rare), fever, or exercise. A cystocentesis-obtained urine sample should be used to eliminate contamination and urethral inflammation. Fever and exercise should produce transient pyuria and are not indications for further testing. UTI is the most common cause of persistent pyuria; therefore, urine culture for bacteria, *Mycoplasma,* and yeast is the next step. (Note: Dilute urine or urine from patients with impaired WBC function such as hyperadrenocorticism or diabetes mellitus may not have pyuria despite a UTI.) If pyuria persists and bacteria, *Mycoplasma,* and yeast cannot be cultured, contrast radiographs of the urinary tract are indicated to eliminate neoplasia, granuloma, and calculi. If persistent, severe pyuria cannot be explained by these tests, exploratory surgery with renal, cystic, and prostatic biopsies and cultures should be considered.

Bacteriuria

Analysis • Microscopic examination of urine sediment or urine culture (see Chapter 15). Cystocentesis-obtained urine is preferred to avoid contamination. However, clean-catch midstream voided samples from females and midstream catheterized samples are usually acceptable.

Normal Values • Bacteriuria should not occur in urine obtained by cystocentesis. Contamination is frequent in urine obtained by catheter or free catch; therefore, quantitated urine culture may be needed to determine significance.

Danger Values • None.

Artifacts • Falsely decreased: recent antibiotic therapy (even if it was ineffective in resolving a UTI), diuresis, or contamination of urine with oxidants (e.g., bleach). Falsely increased: urine remaining at room temperature for more than 2 hours and contaminated centrifuge tubes or stain containers. Brownian motion of amorphous debris may be confused with bacteriuria in unstained wet mount preparations.

Causes of Bacteriuria • Mucus, degenerate WBCs, or bacteriuria without pyuria/hematuria suggests contamination if catheterized or voided urine is used. If there is any doubt, repeat urinalysis with cystocentesis-obtained urine is indicated. Once artifacts and contamination are eliminated, persistent bacteriuria diagnoses UTI (Fig. 7–6). Bacteriuria, pyuria, and hematuria in properly obtained urine are the classic findings in UTI; however, not all UTIs have detectable pyuria, hematuria, or bacteriuria. Dilute urine may have such a low concentration of cells that they are not found during examination of the sediment. Greater than 10^4 rods/ml or 10^5 cocci/ml must be present before they can readily be seen in the microscopic examination of the urine sediment. Patients with hyperadrenocorticism (endogenous or iatrogenic) or diabetes mellitus may not have any evidence of UTI on the urinalysis. Therefore, it is reasonable to culture urine from all patients with these conditions. Yeast infections typically have relatively few organisms per milliliter and therefore are easy to overlook on the urinalysis. Finally, *Mycoplasma* infections cannot be detected without appropriate culture because the organisms cannot be identified on urinalysis.

Urine culture and sensitivity testing, although useful, is not critical for proper treatment of most uncomplicated episodes of UTI in patients that have not been treated before. Bacterial morphology (e.g., gram positive or negative; rod or cocci) is usually sufficient for selecting appropriate therapy in these patients. If upper UTI is strongly suspected (e.g., fever, lumbar pain, leukocytosis, azotemia, or WBC casts), urine culture is indicated to help resolve the process quickly before permanent renal damage occurs. Medications are often stopped too early, and medications to be given three to four times per day are often given less frequently by clients. However, if a UTI has recurred (i.e., relapse or reinfection) after proper treatment, one cannot reliably predict antibiotic sensitivity based on morphology; therefore, a urine culture is mandated. Additionally, recurrent UTIs not attributable to bacterial resistance or lack of client compliance are indications for plain and positive-

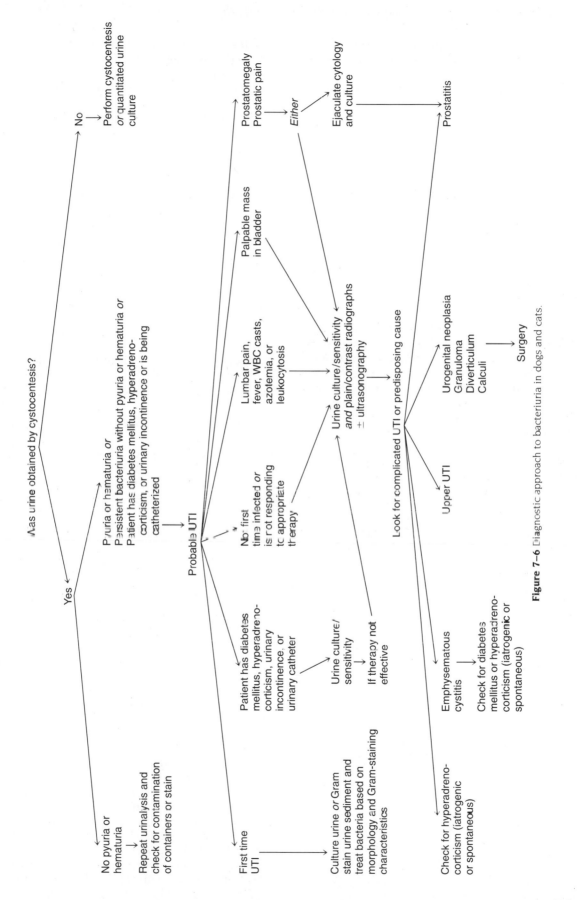

Figure 7-6 Diagnostic approach to bacteriuria in dogs and cats.

contrast radiographs, ultrasonography, and/or ejaculate cytology. Careful search must be made for underlying causes such as repeated or indwelling urinary catheterization, neoplasia, obstruction, renal infections, prostatitis, calculi, granulomas, diverticuli, incontinence, polyuria, urine retention, diabetes mellitus, hyperadrenocorticism, or other causes (Table 7–5). Exploratory surgery with biopsy and culture occasionally is necessary to detect diverticuli, interstitial cystitis, granulomas, and upper UTI.

Other Cells

Analysis • Microscopic examination of urine sediment. A few large and small round cells may be seen in the urine sediment of normal animals.

Causes of Other Cells • Neoplastic cells may be found in the urine of patients with malignancies (e.g., transitional cell carcinoma) of the bladder or urethra. If neoplastic cells are being sought in the urine, a large volume of fresh urine should be immediately centrifuged, the sediment smeared on a slide and allowed to dry, and the slide stained with new methylene blue or Wright-Giemsa stains. Collecting exfoliated cells in 0.9% saline solution using a bladder wash or catheter biopsy procedure, however, is the preferred method to obtain a specimen suitable for cytologic evaluation. Swelling and early degeneration of cells exposed to urine are common, and these changes may mimic malignancy (i.e., large or atypical nucleus and nucleolus). High concentrations of radiographic contrast agents produce similar changes. Rarely, funguria occurs in blastomycosis and disseminated aspergillosis.

Cylindruria

Analysis • Microscopic examination of urine sediment.

Normal Values • 0 to 2 hyaline casts/hpf or 0 to 1 granular casts/hpf.

Danger Values • None.

Artifacts • Casts rapidly disintegrate if the urine is stored too long (e.g., >2 hours) or subjected to vigorous mixing or handling.

Causes of Cylindruria • Casts support a diagnosis of renal disease but may be present in various primary or secondary conditions and do not automatically indicate a need for renal biopsy.

Hyaline casts may be found during diuresis, after dehydration, or in patients with proteinuria. These are the least significant casts.

WBC casts signify renal inflammation and are usually due to upper UTI, although nonseptic nephritis can rarely produce them. Few patients with upper UTI have them. These casts are an indication for urine culture.

RBC casts signify hemorrhage into renal tubules or severe glomerular inflammation allowing RBCs to enter the tubules (e.g., glomerulonephritis, vasculitis, and renal infarction). If persistent, these casts are a reasonable indication for excretory urogram, renal ultrasonography, or coagulation profile. If these tests are not informative and the casts persist, renal biopsy is indicated.

Renal tubular cell casts usually signify severe renal tubular disease such as heavy metal ingestion, tubular hypoxia, or acute oliguric renal failure of any cause.

Granular casts are composed of degenerating cells, proteins, and other substances. Various renal diseases may produce these, and large numbers can be seen when rehydrating a severely dehydrated patient.

Waxy casts represent older, degenerate granular casts and occur in various renal diseases.

Table 7–5 CAUSES OF RECURRENT OR RELAPSING URINARY TRACT INFECTIONS AND METHODS OF DIAGNOSIS

Lack of owner's compliance in drug administration	History (check for leftover medications)
Upper urinary tract infection	Excretory urogram showing dilated pelvis, culture urine from renal pelvis, renal biopsy, WBC casts, ultrasonography
Calculi	Plain and/or positive contrast radiographs, ultrasonography
Prostatitis	Ejaculate cytology and culture, prostatic aspirate, prostatic biopsy, ultrasonography
Neoplasm	Cytology of urine sediment, positive-contrast radiographs, biopsy, ultrasonography
Diverticulum	Positive-contrast radiographs, exploratory surgery
Granuloma	Positive-contrast radiographs, exploratory surgery
Urinary incontinence or urine retention due to any cause	History, physical examination
Decreased resistance to infection	Hyperadrenocorticism, diabetes mellitus (see Chapter 8)
Urinary catheterization	History, physical examination

Table 7–6 CRYSTALS THAT MAY BE FOUND IN CANINE AND FELINE URINE

Name	Description	Significance
Struvite (magnesium ammonium phosphate)	Colorless prisms with 3–6 sides (coffin lid)	Common in neutral to alkaline urine, usually does not signal UTI; may be associated with calculi
Calcium oxalate (monohydrate)	Dumbbells or small spindles	May be normal, due to ethylene glycol intoxication, or associated with calculi
Calcium oxalate (dihydrate)	Colorless envelopes or small stars	May be normal, due to ethylene glycol intoxication, or associated with calculi
Calcium phosphate	Prisms (long) or amorphous	May be normal or associated with calculi
Calcium carbonate	Yellow to colorless spherules or dumbbells	Rare in dogs and cats
Ammonium urate	Yellow-brown "thorn apples"	Normal in dalmatians; also associated with hepatic insufficiency; may be associated with calculi
Uric acid	Prisms or rosettes or oval with pointed ends	Common in dalmatians but may be found in other normal pets; may be associated with calculi
Bilirubin	Golden-yellow to brown needles or granules	May be present in normal dogs with concentrated urine or due to bilirubinuria
Cystine	Colorless, flat hexagonal plates	Due to cystinuria; may be associated with calculi
Cholesterol	Colorless, flat plates with notched cones	May be found in normal dogs and cats
Hippuric acid	Prisms (4–6 sides) with rounded corners	Uncertain; have been confused with calcium oxalate monohydrate crystals
Leucine	Yellow-brown laminated spheroids	May be associated with hepatic disease (?)
Tyrosine	Yellow or colorless needles in sheaves or rosettes	May be associated with hepatic disease (?)
Sulfonamide	Clear to brown eccentrically bound needles in sheaves	Associated with sulfonamide administration

(From Osborn CA: Canine urolithiasis. I. Vet Clin North Am, January 1986.)

Fatty casts are found in various renal diseases, especially in cats.

Crystalluria

Analysis ● Microscopic examination of urine sediment. Crystal habit (i.e., the characteristic shapes of mineral crystals) is used as an index of crystal composition; however, microscopic identification of urine crystals is imperfect because their appearance is altered by numerous factors. Definitive identification of crystal composition requires special analyses.

Artifacts ● Finding crystalluria proves that the urine specimen is oversaturated with crystallogenic substances; however, numerous variables operate *in vivo* and *in vitro* to influence crystalluria. The significance of crystalluria is easily misjudged if these factors are not considered. *In vivo* variables include urine concentration, urine pH, solubility of crystalloids, and excretion of medications or diagnostic agents. *In vitro* variables include temperature, evaporation, pH, and technique of specimen preparation. Solubility of crystals is so pH dependent that changing urine pH may cause some crystals to appear and others to disappear.

Causes of Crystalluria ● When knowledge of *in vivo* urine crystal type is potentially important, several fresh specimens should be examined. The number, size, and structure of crystals should be evaluated, as well as their tendency to aggregate (Table 7–6).

Detection of certain urine crystals sometimes aids discovery of a portosystemic shunt (i.e., ammonium urate crystals) or ethylene glycol ingestion (i.e., calcium oxalate crystals). Searching for crystalluria, however, is not a reliable way to diagnose these conditions.

The condition that most often causes concern about crystalluria is urolithiasis. Evaluation of urine crystals may aid in detection of conditions that predispose to urolith formation, help in estimating the mineral composition of uroliths, and assist evaluation of effectiveness of therapy intended to dissolve uroliths or prevent their formation. However, microscopic evaluation of crystalluria should not be used as the sole criterion for assessment of stone composition when uroliths are present. Additionally, animals that have crystalluria do not necessarily form uroliths, and finding crystalluria is not always an indication that treatment is needed.

MODIFIED WATER DEPRIVATION TESTING

Occasional Indications • Selected patients with pu-pd, especially when central diabetes insipidus or nephrogenic diabetes insipidus of unknown cause or apparent psychogenic polydipsia is considered. Advantages: specificity for central and congenital nephrogenic diabetes insipidus when the more common causes of pu-pd are eliminated. Disadvantages: the inability of the test to differentiate between many of the common causes of pu-pd and the need for close monitoring to avoid morbidity or mortality.

Analysis • This test is performed only in nonazotemic patients after using appropriate methods (i.e., history, physical examination, and laboratory testing, as needed) to rule out diuretic drug administration, dehydration, pyometra, glucosuria, hypercalcemia, hyperadrenocorticism (endogenous or iatrogenic), adrenal insufficiency, hepatic insufficiency, hyperthyroidism (in elderly cats), and hypokalemia (see the previous discussion of pu-pd).

A modified water deprivation test is conducted by gradually restricting a patient's water intake for several days (e.g., to 120 ml/kg/day beginning 72 hours before, then 90 ml/kg/day 48 hours before, and then 60–80 ml/kg/day 24 hours before), then evaluating the patient's response to complete water deprivation. While the patient is deprived of water, body weight and urine concentration (and preferably the urine and serum osmolality) are monitored every 2 hours (and up to every 30 minutes in severely polyuric patients). At each monitoring, the bladder is emptied of urine so that the most recent urine is not diluted with previously made urine. This is done until either

1. Adequate renal concentrating ability is documented by a urine specific gravity ≥1.030 in a dog or ≥1.035 in a cat or, preferably, a urine osmolality is achieved that is at least three times greater than a simultaneous serum sample; *or*

2. Serum osmolality ≥315 mOsm/kg (probably the best indication that maximum ADH release is occurring), the patient loses ≥5% of its body weight (not as accurate as serum osmolality in determining that ADH should be released), serum sodium ≥165 mEq/L, urine concentration plateaus for 2 to 4 hours, or azotemia (danger sign) occurs. If any of these occur and the urine is not adequately concentrated, 2 to 5 units of aqueous ADH are administered intramuscularly and additional urine samples are analyzed 30, 60, 90 and 120 minutes later.

Normal Values • Dogs, urine specific gravity ≥1.030 or urine:plasma osmolality of >3:1 (typically >5:1); cats, urine specific gravity ≥1.035, osmolality data assumed to be similar to dogs.

Danger Values • **Warning:** Failure to closely monitor patients may result in life-threatening hypernatremic dehydration, especially in small patients or those with severe pu-pd due to hyposthenuric disorders (e.g., diabetes insipidus). Also, unlimited access to water after administration of ADH can lead to water intoxication and central nervous system signs in patients that respond to the ADH.

Artifacts • Patients that are water loaded may lose 5% or more of their body weight without increasing their serum osmolality enough to stimulate pituitary ADH release. Urine specific gravity may be falsely increased by contamination, suggesting concentration.

Causes of Inability to Adequately Concentrate Urine • The water deprivation test is most useful in differentiating central diabetes insipidus and apparent psychogenic polydipsia from nephrogenic diabetes insipidus that is not due to hyperadrenocorticism, myeloma, hypercalcemia, pyelonephritis, pyometra, or hypokalemia. For the other more common causes of pu-pd, a CBC, serum chemistry profile, urinalysis, or selected endocrine analysis is easier, quicker, and more definitive. It is noteworthy that patients with hepatic insufficiency, hyperadrenocorticism, hypokalemia, polycythemia, hyperthyroidism, and hypercalcemia may be able to concentrate their urine, to varying degrees depending on whether renal medullary washout or renal tubular damage has occurred. To differentiate central and nephrogenic diabetes insipidus from psychogenic polydipsia, see Figure 7–7.

HYPERTONIC SALINE TESTING (HICKEY-HARE TEST)

Rare Indications • Differentiation of nephrogenic diabetes insipidus from central diabetes

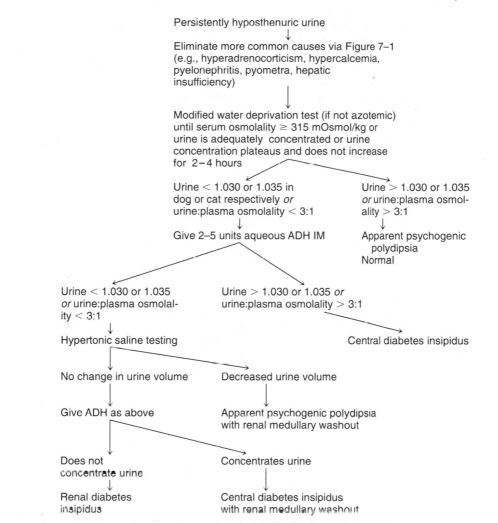

Persistently hyposthenuric urine
↓
Eliminate more common causes via Figure 7–1 (e.g., hyperadrenocorticism, hypercalcemia, pyelonephritis, pyometra, hepatic insufficiency)
↓
Modified water deprivation test (if not azotemic) until serum osmolality ≥ 315 mOsmol/kg or urine is adequately concentrated or urine concentration plateaus and does not increase for 2–4 hours

Urine < 1.030 or 1.035 in dog or cat respectively *or* urine:plasma osmolality < 3:1

Urine > 1.030 or 1.035 *or* urine:plasma osmolality > 3:1
↓
Apparent psychogenic polydipsia
Normal

Give 2–5 units aqueous ADH IM

Urine < 1.030 or 1.035 *or* urine:plasma osmolality < 3:1
↓
Hypertonic saline testing

Urine > 1.030 or 1.035 *or* urine:plasma osmolality > 3:1
↓
Central diabetes insipidus

No change in urine volume
↓
Give ADH as above

Decreased urine volume
↓
Apparent psychogenic polydipsia with renal medullary washout

Does not concentrate urine
↓
Renal diabetes insipidus

Concentrates urine
↓
Central diabetes insipidus with renal medullary washout

Figure 7–7 Use of water deprivation and hypertonic saline infusion tests for differentiation of renal and central diabetes insipidus ± renal medullary washout from apparent psychogenic polydipsia ± renal medullary washout.

insipidus complicated with renal medullary washout from apparent psychogenic polydipsia complicated with renal medullary washout. Advantages: the ability to detect renal medullary washout. Disadvantages: the cumbersome nature of the test. Note: Modified water deprivation testing (i.e., instead of abrupt water deprivation testing) has become the preferred method of overcoming medullary washout (instead of hypertonic saline infusion) when evaluating patients with pu-pd.

Analysis ● Water, 20 ml/kg, is given via stomach tube; a 2.5% saline solution is then infused at 0.25 ml/kg/minute for 45 minutes. Urine volume is measured over three 15-minute periods during the infusion and for one 45-minute period after the infusion.

Normal Values ● The volume of urine produced

by a patient with psychogenic polydipsia plus renal medullary washout should decrease because the pituitary is stimulated to release ADH and the renal medullary gradient is reestablished by the hypertonic saline infusion.

Danger Values ● None.

Causes of Inability to Decrease Urine Flow ● See Figure 7–7.

ANURIA-OLIGURIA

Anuria and oliguria necessitate aggressive diagnostic efforts, since the prognosis can be guarded to poor unless appropriate therapy is quickly begun. The clinician's immediate diagnostic aims are to simultaneously determine the presence of life-threatening secondary changes and the cause of the oliguria (Fig. 7–8). One must first determine from the history and physical examination if there is urinary obstruction or rupture, severe dehydration, or any likelihood of exposure to nephrotoxins. Obstruction and rupture can be ruled out by checking for abdominal fluid and passing a urethral catheter. If abdominal fluid is detected, its creatinine concentration should be compared with that of the serum (see Chapter 10). Urine for urinalysis should be obtained at this time or as soon as possible. Simultaneously, the clinician should check for hyperkalemia (chemistry analysis or electrocardiogram [ECG], although the ECG is not as sensitive or specific) and severe acidosis (blood gas is preferred, but TCO_2 is useful) as well as obtain blood for CBC and chemistry profile (to include at least serum sodium, potassium, calcium, osmolality, anion gap, glucose, total protein, albumin, BUN, and creatinine). Severe dehydration, hyperkalemia, and severe acidosis should be treated as soon as they are identified.

If UTI is present, one must consider bilateral pyelonephritis as the cause of the oliguria (rare), although secondary UTI (especially if the bladder has been repeatedly catheterized) is more likely.

Ethylene glycol intoxication must be considered in any dog or cat with acute oliguric renal failure, regardless of "lack of exposure." Calcium oxalate crystalluria is often present within the first 24 hours of ingestion. However, calcium oxalate monohydrate and dihydrate crystals are dissimilar, and monohydrate crystals may be mistaken for hippuric acid crystals. In early intoxications, patients have severe metabolic acidosis, have occasional central nervous system signs (i.e., seizures), and are often hypocalcemic. Hyperosmolality and increased osmolal and anion gaps (see Chapter 6) suggest ethylene glycol intoxication. If ethylene glycol is even a remote possibility, urine for toxicologic analysis should be saved. Anuria-oliguria and uremia are often not seen for 2 to 4 days after ingestion. By that time, calcium oxalate crystalluria and hypocalcemia may have resolved. Hyperkalemia is not invariable. Ultrasonography may detect renal hyperechogenicity due to deposition of calcium oxalate crystals. Renal biopsy may be needed to confirm the diagnosis.

Hypoadrenocorticism may mimic renal oliguria and hypercalcemic nephropathy. The hyponatremia, hyperkalemia, and decreased Na:K ratio seen in hypoadrenocorticism can occur in acute renal failure, and some hypoadrenal patients have near-isosthenuric urine. Therefore, if serum electrolyte concentrations suggest hypoadrenocorticism, one may begin appropriate fluid and hormonal replacement, but the diagnosis must be confirmed by an ACTH-stimulation test. Most patients with hypoadrenocorticism produce urine in response to intravenous fluids, which makes management easier while awaiting ACTH-stimulation test results.

Renal ischemia due to any cause (including dehydration and hypoadrenocorticism) may produce oliguria. Fortunately, most dogs and cats produce urine once they are properly rehydrated. However, in patients with severe, prolonged ischemia, it can be difficult to distinguish whether significant renal parenchymal destruction has occurred. If the clinician is unsure about the cause of the oliguria and the urine production remains inadequate despite appropriate fluid therapy, analysis of urine creatinine and fractional urine sodium excretion (see Chapter 6) may help determine if renal tubular necrosis has occurred and whether a renal biopsy may be warranted.

If oliguria persists despite appropriate intravenous fluid administration and the cause is still uncertain, the clinician must consider bilateral ureteral obstruction (rare), usually due to neoplasia. Abdominal ultrasonography is useful in quickly ruling out this possibility. If ultrasonography is not available, a positive-contrast cystogram may be done if the clinician's index of suspicion is high (e.g., palpable abnormality in the region of the trigone or a history of chronic hematuria-stranguria before the oliguric renal failure). Excretory urograms should be done only with extreme caution (if at all) in these patients, since they often worsen renal failure.

Hypercalcemia usually causes pu-pd. However, in severe or long-standing cases there may be enough renal calcification to cause oliguria. Also uncommon, hyperosmolar diabetes mellitus may cause acute oliguric renal failure in some patients. The blood glucose level in these patients is often >1000 mg/dl.

Patients that have anuric-oliguric renal failure of known or unknown cause and that do not have small kidneys and do not respond well to initial therapy or require prolonged, expensive therapy should have a clotting screen and a renal biopsy for diagnosis and prognostication. This is usually performed with a Vim-Silverman or Tru-Cut needle using a laparoscopy, ultrasonography or keyhole technique.

AZOTEMIA-UREMIA

Azotemia (increased BUN or serum creatinine level) and uremia (azotemia plus clinical

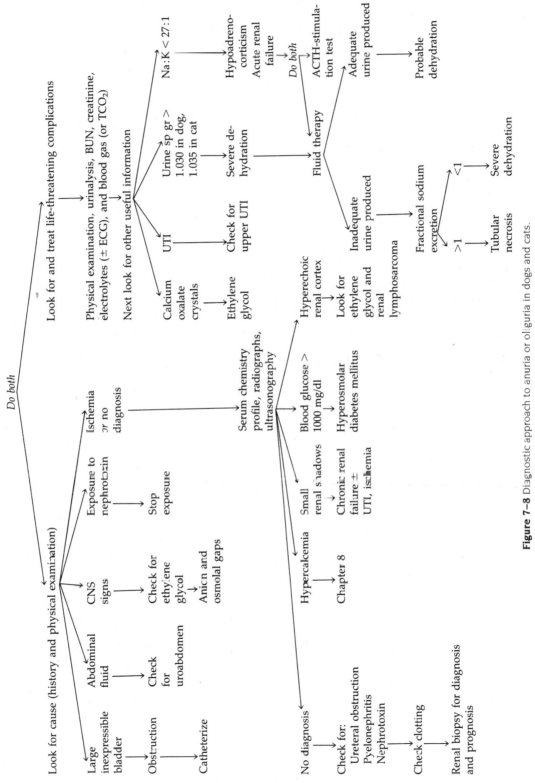

Figure 7–8 Diagnostic approach to anuria or oliguria in dogs and cats.

signs of renal failure such as lethargy, depression, reduced appetite, vomiting, weight loss) are due to decreased glomerular filtration. The clinician must remember three things. First, a mild increase in BUN or serum creatinine concentrations often signifies a substantial decrease in glomerular filtration. Second, extrarenal factors can affect these values (especially BUN). Third, there can be significant renal disease without azotemia. A complete urinalysis may document renal disease (i.e., proteinuria, glucosuria, casts, isosthenuria, pyuria, hematuria, or calcium oxalate crystals) before azotemia is detected. For example, aminoglycoside and amphotericin B nephrotoxicities typically cause isosthenuria, proteinuria, glycosuria, or cylindruria before causing azotemia. Therefore, patients treated with these drugs should be periodically evaluated with both urinalysis and serum creatinine.

Serum creatinine is preferable to BUN as an index of GFR because fewer extrarenal factors affect it. A simultaneous urinalysis should be determined to allow accurate evaluation of serum creatinine, BUN, or serum phosphorus concentrations. The first step in evaluating azotemia is to decide whether it is prerenal, renal,

or postrenal (see Table 7–7 and the later discussion under BUN). Renal azotemia is an indication for careful evaluation of history, physical examination, urinalysis, and serum chemistry profile (Fig. 7–9).

BLOOD UREA NITROGEN

Common Indications • As a screen for renal disease in any ill patient, especially those with vomiting, weight loss, chronic nonregenerative anemia, pu-pd, anuria-oliguria, chronic UTI, or dehydration. Measurement of BUN (preferably with serum creatinine) is indicated in every patient with renal disease. Advantages: ease and availability. Disadvantages: numerous extrarenal factors affect concentration.

Analysis • Measured in 0.5 ml of serum, plasma (heparin or EDTA), and urine by spectrophotometric, "dry reagent" reflectance meter, and ammonia-sensitive electrode methods as well as one drop of fresh whole blood on a dipstick. The different methods give comparable results except for the dipstick, which is a crude estimate.

Normal Values • Dogs, 6 to 24 mg/dl; cats, 5 to 30 mg/dl.

Danger Values • Although there is some correlation between BUN and the severity of renal disease, there are many exceptions. Further, the rapidity with which BUN increases may alter the severity of associated clinical signs.

Artifacts • Falsely decreased: high concentrations of sodium fluoride and sodium citrate (ammonia-sensitive electrodes) and chloramphenicol (Berthelot's method). Severe lipemia prevents accurate spectrophotometric analysis. Falsely increased: chloramphenicol (Nessler's method).

Drug Therapy That May Alter Results • Decreased BUN may be due to growth hormone or drugs that cause marked pu-pd. Increased BUN may be due to corticosteroids, arginine, and nephrotoxic drugs (Table 7–8).

Causes of Decreased BUN • BUN is decreased by inhibiting production (e.g., hepatic insufficiency or dietary protein restriction) or by increasing excretion (e.g., pu-pd, overhydration, or late pregnancy). The most common causes of severely decreased BUN (e.g., <5 mg/dl) are

Table 7–7 DISTINGUISHING CHARACTERISTICS OF PRERENAL, RENAL, AND POSTRENAL AZOTEMIA IN DOGS AND CATS

Prerenal azotemia	Urine specific gravity > 1.030 (dogs) or > 1.035 (cats) (Note, see below: Renal azotemia)
	BUN may increase before creatinine
	Warning: Significant proteinuria with a benign sediment may be due to primary glomerular disease, in which case a concentrated urine specific gravity does not rule out primary renal disease
Renal azotemia	Urine specific gravity 1.008–1.030 (dogs) or 1.008–1.035 (cats); however, cats in early renal failure occasionally have specific gravity > 1.035, whereas dogs in early renal failure may have specific gravity < 1.008
	Patient may be polyuric, oliguric, or anuric
Postrenal azotemia	Animal cannot urinate owing to urethral or ureteral obstruction *or* some urine is emptying into the abdomen because of a ruptured urinary tract
	Urine specific gravity may be any value

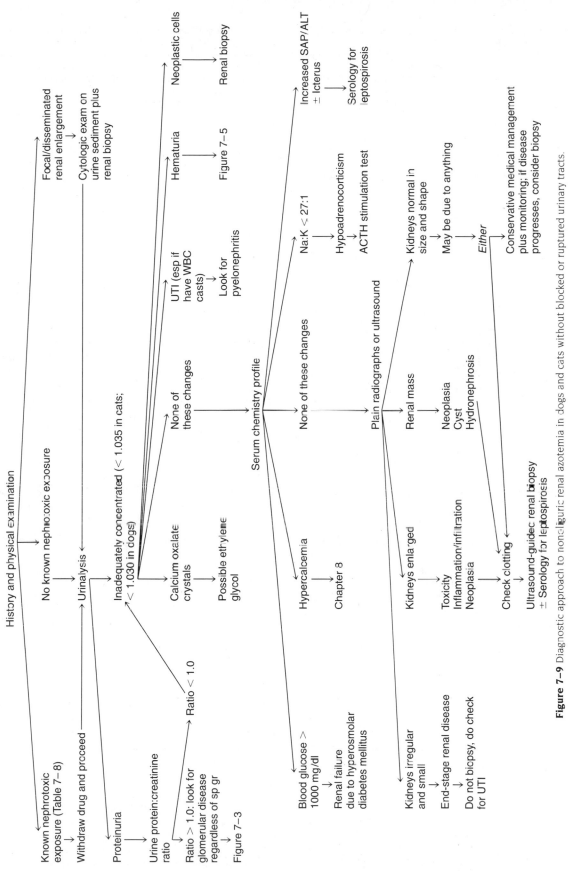

Figure 7–9 Diagnostic approach to nonoliguric renal azotemia in dogs and cats without blocked or ruptured urinary tracts.

Table 7–8 SELECTED POTENTIALLY NEPHROTOXIC DRUGS*

Aminoglycoside antibiotics such as neomycin, kanamycin, gentamicin, amikacin, and tobramycin (**important**)
Amphotericin B (**important**)
Arsenic
Cephalothin (uncommon)
Cisplatin (**important**)
Cyclophosphamide (nephrotoxicity is uncommon; sterile cystitis is more common)
Dextran (low molecular weight)
Ethylene glycol (**important**)
Furosemide (uncommon)
Lead
Mercury
Nonsteroidal anti-inflammatory drugs like aspirin, ibuprofen (**important** when there is preexisting renal disease)
Polymyxin B (**important**)
Radiographic contrast media (**important** when there is preexisting azotemia or oliguria)
Sulfonamides (uncommon if more soluble sulfonamides are used)
Tetracyclines (uncommon)
Thallium
Thiazides (uncommon)
Vancomycin (uncommon)
Zinc

*Not all of these drugs reliably produce nephrotoxicity. Those drugs recognized as the most dangerous are denoted **important**.

Table 7–9 CAUSES OF INCONGRUITIES BETWEEN BUN AND SERUM CREATININE CONCENTRATIONS

Increased BUN Plus Normal to Low Serum Creatinine	Increased Serum Creatinine Plus Normal to Low BUN
Early prerenal azotemia	
Falsely Increased BUN	**Falsely Decreased BUN**
High-protein diet	Hepatic insufficiency (important)
GI hemorrhage	Polyuria-polydipsia
Tetracycline or corticosteroid administration	Low-protein diet
Fever	
Severe muscle trauma (?)	
Falsely Decreased Creatinine	**Falsely Increased Creatinine**
Decreased muscle mass (severe cachexia needed to cause significant changes)	Myositis/muscle trauma (unlikely)
	Cooked meat diet (mild, transient changes)

chronic hepatic insufficiency (e.g., congenital portosystemic shunts or hepatic cirrhosis) and severe pu-pd due to hyperadrenocorticism or diabetes insipidus. A persistently decreased BUN is an indication for hepatic function tests (e.g., serum bile acids; see Chapter 9).

Causes of Increased BUN • An increased BUN requires concurrent pretreatment urinalysis for proper interpretation. A serum creatinine concentration should also be requested. If the serum creatinine concentration is normal, other factors must be considered (Table 7–9). BUN may be elevated 10 to 50 mg/dl by a recent high-protein (e.g., canned meat) meal. Other prerenal causes include increased synthesis due to extra protein intake (including hemorrhage into the gastrointestinal tract) or by catabolism of body tissues (e.g., due to fever, massive muscle trauma, corticosteroid or tetracycline therapy). These usually cause minor changes unless there is underlying occult renal disease. Finally, because of the highly diffusible nature of BUN, early prerenal azotemia due to decreased renal perfusion may increase BUN before it increases serum creatinine.

If both BUN and creatinine are increased, then decreased glomerular filtration is established. However, this decreased filtration may be due to prerenal causes (e.g., inadequate

renal perfusion due to shock, dehydration, or poor cardiac output), renal causes (e.g., renal parenchymal disease due to glomerular disease, tubular dysfunction, necrosis, or parenchymal scarring), or postrenal causes (e.g., urinary outflow tract disease due to urethral or ureteral obstruction or cystic or ureteral rupture; see Table 7–7).

Prerenal azotemia is typically associated with urine specific gravities of >1.030 in dogs and 1.035 in cats and similar increases in urine osmolality. However, cats with early renal disease may have azotemia and urine specific gravities of >1.035. It is important to obtain pretreatment urine for analysis. If a patient is receiving fluid therapy or drugs that alter renal concentrating ability (e.g., diuretics or corticosteroids) or has another disease inhibiting renal tubular function (e.g., hypercalcemia), the urine specific gravity may be inappropriately decreased, making it appear that renal azotemia is present when in fact prerenal disease is occurring. Occasionally, a clue may be the finding of hyposthenuric urine (i.e., specific gravity <1.007 and especially <1.004), which means that the renal tubules can function as seen by their ability to dilute the glomerular filtrate. However, some dogs with early renal failure may have hyposthenuric urine.

A special case involves azotemia and significant proteinuria in urine of any specific gravity. Glomerular lesions may impair glomerular filtration and cause azotemia despite adequately concentrated urine. Called *glomerulotubular imbalance*, the urine is concentrated because the glomerular lesions have not yet resulted in sufficient tubular injury to impair renal concentrating ability.

Isosthenuric or inadequately concentrated urine plus an increased BUN and serum creatinine concentration suggests primary renal disease. Many patients with renal azotemia have chronic renal disease of unknown cause. However, hypercalcemia, upper UTI, drug nephrotoxicity (e.g., aminoglycoside or amphotericin B), and hyperosmolar diabetes mellitus are causes of renal azotemia that, although potentially life threatening, may be resolved with early diagnosis and appropriate therapy. Hypoadrenocorticism may produce identical urine specific gravity, BUN, and serum creatinine values that are not due to morphologic renal lesions but are reversible with proper therapy. Therefore, after a complete urinalysis is performed, renal azotemia is an indication for carefully reviewing the history and physical examination plus determining at least a PCV, serum sodium, potassium, calcium, total protein, albumin, glucose, and TCO_2 values (see Fig. 7–9). Although of poor sensitivity, plain radiographs of the kidneys may reveal focal or diffuse enlargements, which are indications for renal biopsy. Small kidneys usually denote renal scarring and suggest that renal biopsy is unlikely to benefit the patient. Contrast radiographs (i.e., excretory urogram) are potentially dangerous in these patients and should be done only with extreme caution, if at all. Ultrasonography is more likely to reveal such abnormalities and is safer.

BUN in Abdominal Fluids • BUN is not as useful as creatinine in determining if an abdominal effusion contains urine, because BUN readily diffuses across the peritoneal membrane. Therefore, abdominal fluid could have a high urea nitrogen content because of urine leakage into it or because of urea nitrogen diffusing from the blood into abdominal fluid that is not contaminated with urine.

CREATININE

Common Indications • Same as for BUN; also, for determining whether increases in BUN are due to renal or nonrenal causes. Advantages: not altered by as many nonrenal factors as BUN.

Analysis • Measured in 0.5 ml of serum or plasma (heparin) by spectrophotometric or dry reagent reflectance meter methods. These give comparable results. More accurate techniques (e.g., mass fragmentography) are not readily available.

Normal Values • Dogs, 0.4 to 1.5 mg/dl; cats, 0.5 to 2.1 mg/dl.

Danger Values • Same as for BUN.

Artifacts • Falsely decreased: bilirubin concentrations >10 mg/dl. Falsely increased: bilirubin concentrations >10 mg/dl, hemoglobin, lipemia, ascorbic acid, and various "noncreatinine chromogens" (e.g., BSP, PSP, penicillins, cephalosporins, barbiturates, acetoacetate, fructose, and glucose). Note: Dry reagent methods are not affected by hyperbilirubinemia.

Drugs That May Alter Results • Nephrotoxic drugs (see Table 7–8) may increase the creatinine concentration.

Causes of Decreased Serum Creatinine • Significant loss of muscle (see Table 7–9) or pregnancy (which increases cardiac output and subsequently the GFR). A decreased or normal serum creatinine value despite increased BUN or serum phosphorus concentrations is an indication to check for severe muscle wasting or falsely increased BUN.

Causes of Increased Serum Creatinine • See Figure 7–9 and Table 7–9. Feeding cooked meat may increase serum creatinine by <1 mg/dl. Acute myositis and severe muscle trauma may also increase creatinine, but their significance is uncertain. Decreased glomerular filtration is the major cause of increased serum creatinine concentrations. Just as for BUN, the decreased filtration may be prerenal, renal, or postrenal. The urine specific gravity is essential for differentiating renal and prerenal causes, as described for BUN. Early or mild prerenal azotemia is often marked by increased BUN but a normal serum creatinine value, whereas more severe prerenal azotemia may be characterized by increased serum creatinine and phosphorus concentrations. Serum creatinine is more useful than BUN for serial monitoring of azotemic patients because of fewer nonrenal influences. An increased serum creatinine concentration is an indication for urinalysis and a BUN or phosphorus concentration. An increased serum creatinine concentration and BUN plus isosthenuric or inadequately concentrated urine is an indication for determining at least serum sodium, potassium, calcium, total protein, albumin, glucose, and TCO_2 values and possibly for plain radiographs or ultrasonography of the kidneys.

Creatinine Concentration in Abdominal Fluid • Because creatinine does not diffuse across membranes as readily as BUN, abdominal fluid creatinine concentrations are used to diagnose uroabdomen. Finding an abdominal fluid creatinine concentration substantially in excess of serum creatinine suggests uroabdomen and is an indication for an excretory urogram or urethrogram-cystogram.

URINE CREATININE

Frequent Indications • In calculations of clearance or fractional excretion and as an aid in differentiating oliguria due to renal tubular necrosis from that due to severe prerenal azotemia. Androgens and thiazides may decrease urine creatinine concentrations. Ascorbic acid, nitrofurans, and PSP may artifactually increase measured urine creatinine concentrations. Corticosteroids and nitrofurans may increase urine creatinine concentration.

Analysis • Measured in 3 ml of urine by spectrophotometric methods.

Causes of Altered Urine Creatinine • Severe prerenal azotemia in dogs and cats can *theoretically* cause an increased urine:plasma creatinine ratio (i.e., >20:1), whereas oliguric-anuric renal failure due to renal tubular necrosis can *theoretically* cause a smaller ratio (i.e., <20:1 and possibly <5:1).

URINE FRACTIONAL EXCRETION

Occasional Indications • To assess renal clearance of various substances (i.e., sodium, potassium, calcium, phosphorus, albumin). See respective sections for discussions of the uses of each.

Analysis • Use the following formula, in which all values are determined on simultaneous blood and urine samples.

$$\frac{\text{Urine substance}}{\text{Plasma substance}} \times \frac{\text{Plasma creatinine}}{\text{Urine creatinine}} \times 100$$

CREATININE CLEARANCE

Occasional Indications • Suspected nonazotemic renal disease or serial monitoring of patients with renal disease. In dogs and cats, creatinine clearance provides an estimate of GFR that is sufficiently accurate for any clinical purpose.

Analysis • For the *endogenous* clearance, a 24-hour urine collection plus a serum sample taken approximately midway through the urine collection is required. The total volume of urine produced in 24 hours is measured, and creatinine concentrations are determined on the serum and a 3-ml aliquot of the pooled urine. The clearance is calculated:

$$\text{Clearance} = \frac{\text{urine volume (ml)} \times \text{urine creatinine (mg/dl)}}{\text{time (min)} \times \text{serum creatinine (mg/dl)} \times \text{wt (kg)}}$$

which gives a value in ml/min/kg. Shorter collection periods may be used (e.g., 2 hours or 12 hours) but may be less accurate.

For the *exogenous* clearance, a creatinine solution (50 mg/dl) is administered subcutaneously at 100 mg/kg, with a maximum of 10 ml in any site. A stomach tube is passed, and water equal to 3% of the body weight is administered. The bladder is carefully emptied and rinsed with saline twice at 58 to 60 minutes after the subcutaneous injection. At 60 minutes after injection, a 20-minute urine collection is begun and a serum sample is obtained at the beginning and at the end of the urine collection. The volume of urine plus the serum and pooled urine creatinine concentrations are determined. The same formula is used as described for endogenous creatinine clearance, except that the serum creatinine concentration used in the calculation is the mean of the two measured serum values. It is best if several collections are performed and an average clearance is determined.

Normal Values • *Endogenous test:* dogs, 2.4 to 5.0 ml/min/kg; cats, 1.9 to 5.0 ml/min/kg. *Exogenous test:* dogs, 3.5 to 5.0 ml/min/kg; cats, 2.5 to 4.0 ml/min/kg.

Danger Values • Not established.

Artifacts • Anything that affects the measurement of creatinine may affect this test (see the earlier section on Artifacts under Creatinine). Failure to collect all urine produced during the time period may cause significant error.

Drug Therapy and Other Factors That May Alter Results • Decreased creatinine clearance may be due to thiazide diuretics, trimethoprim, cimetidine, procainamide, or nephrotoxic drugs (see Table 7–8). Increased creatinine clearance may be due to furosemide, methylprednisolone, and exercise during the test.

Causes of Decreased Creatinine Clearance • Renal disease is the major cause of decreased creatinine clearance, although decreased cardiac output may also be responsible. Decreased creatinine clearance in a patient that does not have small or scarred kidneys may be an indication for renal biopsy or serial monitoring of the creatinine clearance as well as measurement of blood pressure.

Causes of Increased Creatinine Clearance • Not significant.

PHOSPHORUS

Phosphorus levels may increase in patients with decreased GFR, similar to BUN and serum creatinine concentrations. Additionally, in patients with chronic renal failure, control of hyperphosphatemia is important to help combat renal secondary hyperparathyroidism. Evaluation of serum phosphorus is discussed in Chapter 8.

CALCULI

Urinary calculi may cause anuria-oliguria, urinary incontinence, stranguria-pollakiuria, discolored urine, or azotemia-uremia. Calculi should be considered in any patient with urinary obstruction, recurrent UTI, hematuria, or cystic mass. Stones are diagnosed by physical examination (i.e., palpation or urinary catheterization), plain or contrast radiographs (some calculi are radiolucent), or ultrasonography. Anytime a calculus is removed or spontaneously passed, it should be analyzed. Additionally, the urine of patients with urolithiasis should be cultured. Whereas many canine uroliths are struvite and form secondary to UTI, other types of stones may also cause a secondary UTI. Therefore, diagnosing UTI and urolithiasis does not allow presumption that an infection has caused a struvite calculus. Accurate determination of the crystalloid composition of calculi is essential if appropriate preventive measures are to be used.

Calculi Analysis

Common Indications • All urinary calculi should be analyzed for mineral content. Advantages: determine the type and cause of the calculi. Disadvantages: need to send calculi to laboratories equipped for proper analysis.

Analysis • Calculi are most commonly analyzed by optic crystallography, x-ray diffraction, and chemical analysis (e.g., the spot test). Less commonly used methods include scanning electron microscopy, electron microprobe, and infrared spectroscopy. Crystallography and diffraction seem to give accurate results, but chemical analysis is not dependable.

Artifacts • Chemical or qualitative analysis (e.g., the spot test) is fraught with inaccuracies. Calcium, silica, and oxalate are often falsely reported as absent; uric acid and calcium may be falsely reported as present.

Causes of Calculi • This subject is too extensive for discussion here. Interested readers are referred to recent reviews (Osborne et al., 1989a,c).

OTHER RENAL FUNCTION TESTS

The PSP and the sodium sulfanilate excretion tests have largely been replaced by creatinine clearance. Inulin clearance is used experimentally but rarely in clinical situations.

Bibliography

Barsanti JA, Johnson CA: Genitourinary infections. *In* Green CE (ed): Infectious Diseases of the Dog and Cat. Philadelphia, WB Saunders, 1990, pp 157–183.

Feldman EC, Nelson RW: Polyuria and polydipsia. *In* Feldman EC, Nelson RW (eds): Canine and Feline Endocrinology and Reproduction. Philadelphia, WB Saunders, 1987, pp 1–28.

Finco DR, Barsanti JA: Clinical evaluation of renal function: A critical appraisal of procedures and interpretations. *In* Kirk RW (ed): Current Veterinary Therapy X. Philadelphia, WB Saunders, 1989, pp 1123–1126.

Finco DR, Barsanti JA, Brown SA: Solute fractional excretion rates. *In* Kirk RW, Bonagura JD (eds): Current Veterinary Therapy XI. Philadelphia, WB Saunders, 1992, pp 818–820.

Hamilton GC: Use of the clinical laboratory in emergency medicine. I. Emerg Med Clin North Am 1986;4:1–210.

Lage AL: Diagnostic approach to canine and feline hematuria. *In* Kirk RW (ed): Current Veterinary Therapy X. Philadelphia, WB Saunders, 1989, pp 1117–1123.

Lulich JP, Osborne CA: Interpretation of urine protein-creatinine ratios in dogs with glomerular and nonglomerular disorders. Comp Cont Ed Pract Vet 1990; 12:59–72.

Osborne CA, Kruger JM, Johnston GR, Polzin DJ: Feline lower urinary tract disorders. *In* Ettinger SJ (ed): Textbook of Veterinary Internal Medicine. 3rd ed. Philadelphia, WB Saunders, 1989a, pp 2057–2082.

Osborne CA, O'Brien TD, Davenport MP, Clinton CW: Crystalluria: Causes, detection, and interpretation. *In* Kirk RW (ed): Current Veterinary Therapy X. Philadelphia, WB Saunders, 1989b, pp 1127–1133.

Osborne CA, Polzin DJ, Johnston GR, O'Brien TD: Canine urolithiasis. *In* Ettinger SJ (ed): Textbook of Veterinary Internal Medicine. 3rd ed. Philadelphia, WB Saunders, 1989c, pp 2083–2107.

Polzin DJ: Spectrum of clinical and laboratory abnormalities in uremia. *In* Kirk RW (ed): Current Veterinary Therapy X. Philadelphia, WB Saunders, 1989, pp 1133–1138.

Tietz NW: Clinical Guide to Laboratory Tests. 2nd ed. Philadelphia, WB Saunders, 1990.

White JV: Diagnostic approach to proteinuria. *In* Kirk RW (ed): Current Veterinary Therapy X. Philadelphia, WB Saunders, 1989, pp 1139–1142.

Willard MD: Urinary disorders. *In* Willard MD, Tvedten H, Turnwald GH (eds): Small Animal Clinical Diagnosis by Laboratory Methods. Philadelphia, WB Saunders, 1989, pp 121–153.

Richard W. Nelson
Grant H. Turnwald
Michael D. Willard

8 Endocrine, Metabolic, and Lipid Disorders

- ○ Calcium
- ○ Phosphorus
- ○ Magnesium
- ○ Parathyroid Hormone
- ○ Glucose
- ○ Insulin
- ○ Insulin Secretagogue Testing
- ○ Hyperlipidemia
- ○ Cholesterol
- ○ Triglycerides
- ○ Lipoprotein Electrophoresis
- ○ Thyroxine (T_4)
- ○ 3,5,3'-Triiodothyronine (T_3)
- ○ Free Thyroxine (fT_4)/Free 3,5,3'-Triiodothyronine (fT_3)

- ○ Thyroid Hormone Antibodies
- ○ T_3 Suppression Test
- ○ TSH-Stimulation Test
- ○ Endogenous Pituitary Adrenocorticotrophin (ACTH)
- ○ Plasma Cortisol
- ○ ACTH-Stimulation Test
- ○ Low-Dose Dexamethasone Suppression Test
- ○ Combined ACTH-Stimulation Test/Dexamethasone Suppression Test
- ○ High-Dose Dexamethasone Suppression Test
- ○ Urine Corticosteroid:Creatinine Ratio
- ○ Plasma Aldosterone

CALCIUM

Common Indications • Lethargy, anorexia, vomiting, constipation, weakness, polydipsia and polyuria (signs of hypercalcemia) or facial pruritus, restlessness, muscle tremors, fasciculations, cramping of rear legs, tetany or seizures (signs of hypocalcemia). Other indications include azotemia, diffuse bone disease, and selected electrocardiographic (ECG) abnormalities (i.e., prolonged QT interval with a normal QRS complex or unexplained premature ventricular contractions).

Analysis • Measured in 0.5 ml of serum, heparinized plasma, and urine by spectrophotometric methods. Most automated and in-house serum chemistry analyzers measure total serum cal-

cium concentration, which consists of biologically active, ionized calcium (50%), protein-bound calcium (40%), and calcium complexes (10%). Because of extensive protein binding, total serum calcium concentrations are decreased by hypoalbuminemia. In *dogs*, serum calcium should be corrected for hypoalbuminemia by use of either of these formulas (Meuten et al., 1982):

Corrected calcium (mg/dl) = measured calcium (mg/dl) − albumin (g/dl) + 3.5

Corrected calcium (mg/dl) = measured calcium (mg/dl) − [0.4 × serum protein (g/dl)] + 3.3

Similar adjustments for plasma protein concentration do not hold for cats (Flanders et al., 1989), but the trend is the same. The biologically active, ionized fraction of calcium can be determined directly. Special sample handling, use of specialized instrumentation, and adjustments for sample pH must be done to ensure accuracy in measuring serum ionized calcium concentration.

Normal Values ● Normal values for total and ionized serum calcium are as follows: Adult dogs: total Ca, 9.0 to 11.0 mg/dl; ionized Ca, 1.12 to 1.42 mmol/L. Adult cats: total Ca, 8.5 to 10.5 mg/dl; ionized Ca, 0.77 to 1.27 mmol/L. Note: An estimate of total Ca = ionized Ca × 8. In order to convert mg/dl to μmol/L, multiply mg/dl × 17.1.

Immature ● Young dogs (i.e., < 12 months), especially of the large and giant breeds, can have total serum calcium values as much as 1 mg/dl higher than adult dogs.

Danger Values ● Total serum Ca < 7.0 mg/dl (tetany). Note: This value depends on the blood pH. The lower the blood pH (i.e., the more acidemic), the lower the calcium can be without causing clinical signs and vice versa. Total serum Ca > 16 mg/dl (acute renal failure, cardiac toxicity).

Artifacts ● Falsely decreased: laboratory error, oxalate or EDTA anticoagulants, hyperbilirubinemia (spectrophotometric methods), and hypomagnesemia. Falsely increased: laboratory error, dehydration (mild increase), postprandial, lipemia, and hemolysis.

Drug therapy that may alter serum calcium: Hypocalcemia may be caused by mithramycin, EDTA, glucagon, anticonvulsants, citrate, fluoride, glucocorticoids, phosphate-containing enemas, and intravenous phosphate administration (i.e., potassium phosphate).

Hypercalcemia may be caused by vitamin D, cholecalciferol rodenticides, estrogen, progesterone, testosterone, anabolic steroids, parenteral calcium administration, and excess oral phosphate binders.

Causes of Hypercalcemia ● In dogs, nonparathyroid malignancy (i.e., hypercalcemia of malignancy), most notably lymphosarcoma, is the most common cause of hypercalcemia (Table 8–1). Other hemolymphatic malignant tumors (i.e., lymphocytic leukemia, multiple myeloma, myeloproliferative diseases), anal sac apocrine gland carcinoma, and soft tissue tumors metastasizing to bone (e.g., mammary gland adeno-

Table 8–1 CAUSES OF HYPERCALCEMIA IN DOGS AND CATS

*Malignancy**
  Hemolymphatic tumors
    Lymphoma/lymphocytic leukemia
    Multiple myeloma
  Myeloproliferative disease
  Solid tissue tumors, with or without bone metastasis
    Apocrine gland adenocarcinoma
    Mammary gland adenocarcinoma
    Prostatic adenocarcinoma
    Squamous cell carcinoma
    Thyroid gland adenocarcinoma
Endocrine disorders
  Primary hyperparathyroidism
  Hypoadrenocorticism
Toxicity
  Hypervitaminosis D
  Cholecalciferol rodenticides
  Hypervitaminosis A
  Plant ingestion (e.g., jasmine in cats)
Renal failure
Infection (rare)
  Neonatal sepsis
  Osteomyelitis
  Hypertrophic osteodystrophy
Granulomatous disease (rare)
  Fungal (e.g., blastomycosis)
Hematologic
  Hemoconcentration
  Hyperproteinemia
Factitious
  Lipemia
  Postprandial
  Young animal (< 6–12 months)
*Laboratory error**

*Common cause.

carcinoma) may also cause hypercalcemia. Less frequent causes include primary hyperparathyroidism, chronic renal failure, hypoadrenocorticism, and hypervitaminosis D (i.e., cholecalciferol rodenticide toxicity). Hypercalcemia is rare in cats and is usually caused by hypercalcemia of malignancy, especially lymphosarcoma, squamous cell carcinoma, or primary hyperparathyroidism.

Hypercalcemia should be confirmed, preferably by repeating the determination from a nonlipemic blood sample obtained from a fasted dog or cat, before initiating diagnostics to identify the cause. The history, physical findings (including a thorough rectal examination), and routine clinical pathology (i.e., complete blood count [CBC], serum biochemistry panel, urinalysis) often provide clues to the diagnosis (Fig. 8–1) and help eliminate artifacts and iatrogenic causes. Special attention should be paid to the serum phosphorus, urea nitrogen, and creatinine concentrations. The direction of the change in calcium is more consistent in various diseases than the change in phosphorus. Phos-

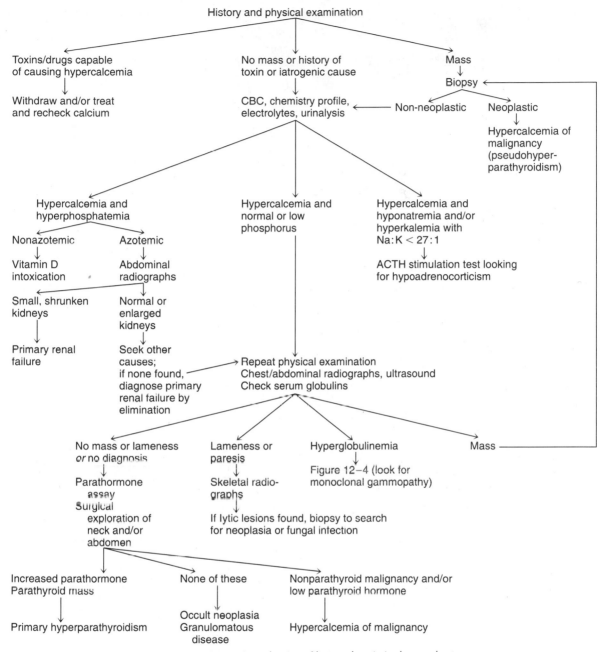

Figure 8–1 Diagnostic evaluation of hypercalcemia in dogs and cats.

phorus is more likely not to fit the predicted pattern. If the serum phosphorus concentration is normal or low, primary hyperparathyroidism or hypercalcemia of malignancy should be suspected first (Fig. 8–2). If the serum phosphorus concentration is increased and renal function is normal, hypervitaminosis D (including cholecalciferol rodenticides) or bone osteolysis from multiple myeloma should be considered. When hyperphosphatemia and hypercalcemia coexist with azotemia, one must differentiate primary renal failure from renal failure secondary to chronic hypercalcemia and metastatic mineralization of the renal tubules. When azotemia and hyperphosphatemia are present, all other potential causes of hypercalcemia must be ruled out before hypercalcemia induced by chronic renal failure can be diagnosed. Primary renal failure may be supported by finding other clinicopathologic abnormalities, including a nonregenerative anemia, isosthenuria, proteinuria, or small irregular kidneys.

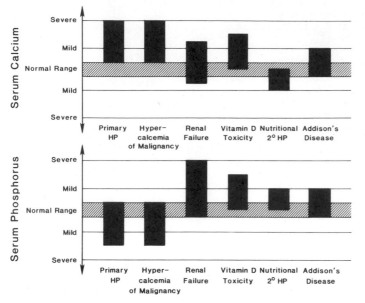

Figure 8–2 The range of serum calcium and phosphorus concentrations for the more common causes of hypercalcemia and for hyperparathyroidism in dogs. (HP, hyperparathyroidism; 2° HP, secondary hyperparathyroidism.) (From Feldman EC, Nelson RW: Canine and Feline Endocrinology and Reproduction. Philadelphia, WB Saunders, 1987, p 334. Reprinted with permission.)

Hypercalcemia of malignancy and primary hyperparathyroidism are the primary differentials if the history, physical findings, and clinical pathology do not establish the diagnosis. Radiographs of the thorax and abdomen and abdominal ultrasonography should be evaluated for soft tissue masses, organomegaly, lymphadenopathy, or abnormalities in organ echogenicity. If a mass is identified, histologic evaluation of a biopsy sample, obtained percutaneously or via exploratory surgery, should be performed to establish the diagnosis. Discrete lytic lesions in the vertebrae or long bones are suggestive of multiple myeloma. Hyperproteinemia, proteinuria (Bence Jones proteins, which may not show up on a dipstick), and plasma cell infiltration in the bone marrow suggest multiple myeloma. A bone core biopsy or bone marrow aspirate of a lytic lesion may be necessary to establish a definitive diagnosis of neoplasia or osseous fungal infection (e.g., blastomycosis).

Cytologic evaluation of peripheral lymph node and bone marrow aspirates should be done to rule out lymphoma. Involvement of the peripheral lymph nodes by lymphoma can be present without causing their enlargement. Ideally, a modestly to moderately enlarged lymph node should be evaluated because very large ones are often necrotic. Mesenteric and submandibular lymph nodes are often reactive. Normal lymph node and bone marrow aspirates, however, do not rule out lymphoma, especially involving other organs (e.g., liver and spleen). It may be necessary to excise and submit an entire lymph node to diagnose a well-differentiated lymphosarcoma.

Measurement of serum parathyroid hormone (PTH) concentration can be done if prior diagnostics have failed to identify the cause of hypercalcemia. High-normal to increased serum PTH concentration in a nonazotemic dog or cat is supportive of primary hyperparathyroidism (Fig. 8–3; Torrance and Nachreiner, 1989). Azotemia causes secondary renal hyperparathyroidism and increased serum PTH concentrations, making interpretation of increased serum PTH concentrations difficult in azotemic, hypercalcemic dogs and cats. If results of the serum PTH concentration are equivocal, ultrasonographic evaluation of the thyroid-parathyroid region of the neck, surgical exploration of the neck, and serum calcium determination after administration of L-asparaginase are additional diagnostic procedures to consider. A marked reduction in serum calcium should occur within 48 hours of L-asparaginase administration if hypercalcemia is due to lymphoma.

Causes of Hypocalcemia ● The most common cause of hypocalcemia is hypoalbuminemia, which is not a true hypocalcemic disease and is not associated with signs of hypocalcemia (Table 8–2). Causes and evaluation of hypoalbuminemia are discussed in Chapter 12. Profound, life-threatening hypocalcemia is usually caused by puerperal tetany, primary hypoparathyroidism, or thyroidectomy in cats with hyperthyroidism. Puerperal tetany may cause severe clinical signs despite modest hypocalcemia (i.e., 7 mg/dl) because concurrent alkalemia (due to panting) decreases ionized calcium concentration, resulting in clinical signs at higher than

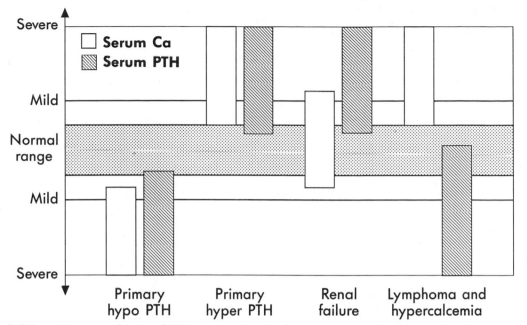

Figure 8–3 Range in serum calcium and PTH concentrations for the more common disorders causing alterations in serum calcium or parathyroid gland function. (PTH, parathyroid hormone; hypo PTH, hypoparathyroidism; hyper PTH, hyperparathyroidism.) (From Nelson RW, Couto CG: Essentials of Small Animal Internal Medicine. St. Louis, Mosby-Year Book, 1992, p 539 Reprinted with permission.)

expected total serum calcium concentration. Mild, usually asymptomatic, hypocalcemia may occur with acute and chronic renal failure, ethylene glycol toxicity, acute pancreatitis, and malabsorption syndromes.

Hypocalcemia should be confirmed by repeating the determination, and total serum calcium concentration adjusted for low serum total protein or albumin concentration in dogs be-

Table 8–2 CAUSES OF HYPOCALCEMIA IN DOGS AND CATS

Hypoproteinemia/Hypoalbuminemia*†
Endocrine disorders
  Primary hypoparathyroidism
  Puerperal tetany (eclampsia)*
  Nutritional secondary hyperparathyroidism†
  Renal secondary hyperparathyroidism*†
  Hyperthyroidism†
Toxicity
  Ethylene glycol*
Drugs
  See text
Acute pancreatitis†
Intestinal malabsorption syndromes†
Hypomagnesemia†
Iatrogenic
  Thyroidectomy (bilateral)*
  Thyroid surgery
Laboratory error

*Common cause of hypocalcemia.
†Rarely causes clinical *signs* of hypocalcemia.

fore initiating diagnostics to identify the cause. The history, physical findings, and routine clinical pathology (i.e., CBC, serum biochemical panel, urinalysis) usually provide the necessary clues to establish the diagnosis (Fig. 8–4) and eliminate artifacts and iatrogenic causes. Primary hypoparathyroidism is the most likely diagnosis in nonazotemic, nonlactating dogs or cats with clinical signs of hypocalcemia. Documenting a low baseline serum PTH concentration confirms this diagnosis (see Fig 8–3; Torrance and Nachreiner, 1989). Alternatively, response to vitamin D and calcium therapy can be used to establish a tentative diagnosis of hypoparathyroidism.

PHOSPHORUS

Common Indications ● Patients with any of the indications mentioned for calcium, plus unexplained hemolysis, seizures, or increased serum alkaline phosphatase (SAP).

Analysis ● Measured in 0.5 ml of serum, heparinized plasma, and urine as inorganic phosphorus by spectrophotometric methods.

Normal Values ● Adult dogs, 3.0 to 6.0 mg/dl; adult cats, 3.0 to 6.0 mg/dl. Immature young

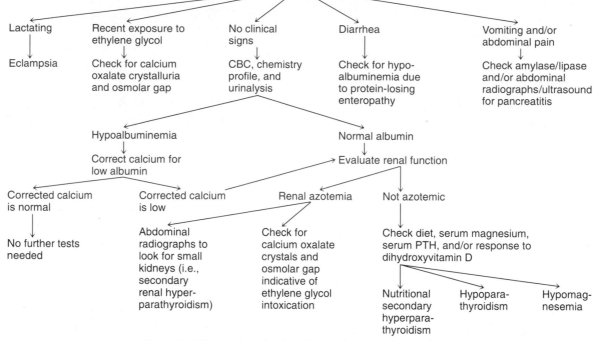

Figure 8–4 Diagnostic evaluation of hypocalcemia in dogs and cats.

dogs (i.e., < 12 months), especially of the large and giant breeds, and young cats (< 6 months) have higher serum phosphorus concentrations (dogs, 4–9 mg/dl; cats, 4–8 mg/dl) than adults. The serum phosphorus concentration should decrease to adult values by 12 months of age.

To convert mg/dl to mmol/L, multiply mg/dl × 0.323.

Danger Values ● < 1.5 mg/dl (hemolysis, neurologic signs).

Artifacts ● Falsely increased: hemolysis, postprandial (mild change), detergents, and sample handling error. Citrate, oxalate, and EDTA interfere with the measurement of phosphorus.

Drug Treatments That May Alter Phosphorus Values ● Hypophosphatemia may be caused by anabolic steroids, anesthetic agents, anticonvulsants, bicarbonate, diuretics, insulin, mithramycin, and salicylates. Hyperphosphatemia may be caused by phosphate-containing enemas in cats or obstipated small dogs, intravenous potassium phosphate supplementation, anabolic steroids, furosemide, hydrochlorothiazide, and minocycline. Tetracyclines have a variable effect on phosphorus.

Causes of Hyperphosphatemia ● Hyperphospha-

temia can result from increased intestinal phosphate absorption, decreased phosphate excretion in the urine, or a shift in phosphate from the intracellular to the extracellular compartment. Translocation of phosphate occurs between the intracellular and extracellular compartments, similar to what occurs with potassium. In dogs and cats, the most common causes of hyperphosphatemia are renal failure, vitamin D toxicosis (i.e., cholecalciferol rodenticide toxicosis), and hypoparathyroidism (Table 8–3). The history, physical examination, and routine clinical pathology (i.e., CBC, serum biochemical panel, urinalysis) usually enable the clinician to identify the cause. If a patient is azotemic, additional tests may be necessary to distinguish between prerenal, renal, and postrenal azotemia (see Chapter 7). Evaluation for primary hypoparathyroidism was discussed earlier under Causes of Hypocalcemia. Measurement of serum thyroxine concentration should be done in hyperphosphatemic, nonazotemic cats with signs of hyperthyroidism (i.e., weight loss, polyphagia, and restlessness). Survey skeletal radiographs may identify osseous neoplasia.

Causes of Hypophosphatemia ● Hypophosphatemia results from decreased phosphate absorption in the intestinal tract, increased urinary phosphate excretion, or a shift from the extra-

Table 8–3 CAUSES OF ALTERED SERUM PHOSPHORUS IN DOGS AND CATS

Hyperphosphatemia
  Young animal*
  Renal failure*
  Prerenal and postrenal azotemia*
  Endocrine
    Primary hypoparathyroidism
    Nutritional secondary hyperparathyroidism
    Hyperthyroidism (cats)
    Acromegaly
  Hypervitaminosis D
    Excess supplementation
    Cholecalciferol rodenticides
  Osteolytic bone lesions
  Rhabdomyolysis
    Trauma
    Necrosis
  Intravenous phosphorus supplementation (especially
    potassium phosphate)
  Laboratory error
Hypophosphatemia
  Endocrine
    Hypercalcemia of malignancy*
    Primary hyperparathyroidism*
    Diabetic ketoacidosis*
    Hyperinsulinism
  Respiratory/metabolic alkalosis
  Renal tubular defects
  Hypovitaminosis D
  Puerperal tetany (eclampsia)
  Hypomagnesemia
  Iatrogenic*
    Insulin therapy
    Bicarbonate therapy
    Diuretic therapy

*Common cause.

cellular to the intracellular compartment. Hypophosphatemia is commonly associated with hypercalcemia of malignancy (i.e., lymphoma) and primary hyperparathyroidism before renal failure develops, as well as the first 24 hours of therapy for diabetic ketoacidosis, especially if a patient is treated aggressively with insulin and bicarbonate (see Table 8–3). Translocation of phosphate between the intracellular and extracellular compartment is similar to potassium. Factors that promote a shift of potassium into the intracellular compartment (e.g., alkalosis, insulin, glucose infusion) also promote a similar shift in phosphate.

When hypophosphatemia is evaluated, artifacts and iatrogenic causes should be ruled out first. Mild hypophosphatemia (i.e., > 2.0 mg/dl) without hypercalcemia is often ignored unless a dog or cat is ketoacidotic (see Causes of Hyperglycemia). If concurrent hypercalcemia is present, diagnostic evaluation for hypercalcemia of malignancy and primary hyperparathyroidism should be done (see Causes of Hypercalcemia).

MAGNESIUM

Rare Indications • Unexplained hypocalcemia (hypomagnesemia may inhibit the actions of PTH and promote calcium uptake into bone), hypokalemia that is resistant to parenteral supplementation (hypomagnesemia may cause potassium-losing nephropathy), and unexplained myopathies, especially in patients receiving cisplatin and other nephrotoxic drugs. Also indicated in unexplained neuromyopathies (hypermagnesemia).

Analysis • Measured in 0.5 ml of serum or urine by spectrophotometric methods.

Normal Values • Dogs, 1.0 to 2.2 mg/dl; cats, 1.8 to 2.5 mg/dl. Note: 12 mg magnesium = 1 mEq magnesium; therefore, to convert from mg/dl to mEq/L, divide by 1.2. To convert mg/dl to mmol/L, multiply mg/dl × 0.411.

Danger Values • Unsure, but > 4 to 6 mEq/L causes toxicity and > 12 mEq/L causes respiratory arrest in people (magnesium salts have been used as an anesthetic). Values < 1 mEq/L cause weakness or convulsions in people.

Artifacts • Falsely decreased: hyperbilirubinemia, EDTA, sodium fluoride-oxalate, sodium citrate, and intravenous calcium gluconate. Falsely increased: hemolysis or use of metal containers for serum.

Drug Therapy That May Alter Serum Magnesium • Hypomagnesemia may be caused by excessive renal loss due to cisplatin, aminoglycosides, amphotericin B, and diuretics (furosemide and thiazides), as well as aggressive insulin therapy in diabetic ketoacidotic patients. Hypermagnesemia may be caused by magnesium-containing drugs (especially oral antacids), chronic aspirin therapy, lithium, and progesterones.

Causes of Hypomagnesemia • The primary cause is excessive renal loss, especially with certain drug therapies as described earlier. Hypoparathyroidism and inadequate supplementation during total parenteral nutrition may also cause hypomagnesemia. Serum calcium concentration and renal function should be evaluated and current drug therapy reviewed when hypomagnesemia is identified.

Causes of Hypermagnesemia • Hypermagnesemia occurs with hypoadrenocorticism and administration of magnesium-containing drugs to patients in renal failure. Adrenocortical and renal function should be evaluated and current drug therapy reviewed when hypermagnesemia is identified.

PARATHYROID HORMONE

Occasional Indications ● To document primary hyperparathyroidism and hypoparathyroidism in dogs and cats with hypercalcemia and hypocalcemia, respectively. Advantages: establishes a diagnosis of primary parathyroid disease without surgical intervention. Disadvantages: limited availability of validated PTH assays for dogs and cats, samples must be frozen during transit, and azotemia makes interpretation more difficult.

Analysis ● Measured in 0.5 ml of serum by radioimmunoassay (RIA). The sample should be centrifuged as soon as possible after clotting, frozen, and shipped frozen to the laboratory. Different PTH assays measure different parts of the PTH molecule and may give different results in the same patient. See Appendix I for availability of the test.

Normal Values ● Dogs, 2 to 13 pmol/L; cats, 2 to 13 pmol/L. Normal values may differ depending on the laboratory used.

Danger Values ● None.

Artifacts ● Prolonged storage or transport at temperatures above freezing may result in erroneous results.

Drug Treatment That May Alter PTH Concentrations ● Any drug therapy that affects serum calcium concentration can affect serum PTH concentration (see Calcium, Drug Therapy That May Alter Serum Calcium). Drugs that decrease serum calcium levels may increase serum PTH concentration, and vice versa.

Causes of Increased Serum PTH Concentration ● Disorders that cause increased serum PTH concentration include primary hyperparathyroidism, secondary renal hyperparathyroidism, secondary nutritional hyperparathyroidism, and nonparathyroid causes of hypocalcemia (see Calcium, Causes of Hypocalcemia). A high-normal or increased serum PTH concentration in a hypercalcemic dog or cat with normal renal

function is strongly suggestive of primary hyperparathyroidism (see Fig. 8–3; Torrance and Nachreiner, 1989; Kallet et al., 1991). Dogs and cats with non–parathyroid-induced hypercalcemia have low to low-normal serum PTH concentrations (i.e., < 5 pmol/L). Increased serum PTH concentrations can be found in dogs and cats with renal failure as a result of concurrent secondary renal hyperparathyroidism. Serum calcium concentration in these dogs and cats is usually in the normal range, although hypercalcemia may develop with chronic end-stage renal failure. Serum calcium is within the low-normal range in dogs and cats with secondary nutritional hyperparathyroidism.

Causes of Decreased Serum PTH Concentration ● Nondetectable serum PTH concentration in a hypocalcemic dog or cat is strongly suggestive of primary hypoparathyroidism. Dogs and cats with non–parathyroid-induced hypocalcemia should have normal or increased serum PTH concentrations. Nonparathyroid disorders that cause hypercalcemia (see Calcium, Causes of Hypercalcemia) also have low-normal to undetectable serum PTH concentrations. Notable exceptions to finding low PTH in a patient with hypercalcemia are primary hyperparathyroidism and hypercalcemia of chronic renal failure.

GLUCOSE

Common Indications ● Polyuria, polydipsia, weakness, coma, behavioral change or seizures (partial or complete). It should also be determined in patients with known hepatic or adrenal insufficiency, severe sepsis, pancreatic neoplasia, and glucosuria, as well as in patients receiving insulin or total parenteral nutrition. Advantages: availability of test. Disadvantages: insensitivity of single determination to detect disorders causing clinically significant hypoglycemia in some patients, and the need to rapidly separate serum from red blood cells (RBCs) to prevent artifacts when standard laboratory methods are used instead of reagent strips.

Analysis ● Measured in 1 drop of whole blood or 0.5 ml of serum or plasma (lithium heparin, sodium fluoride, or EDTA). There are two main ways to measure blood glucose: reagent strips (with or without a reflectance meter) and standard laboratory methods. The latter usually entail spectrophotometric analysis using either O-toluidine or enzymes (hexokinase or glucose oxidase). Newer reagent strips use whole blood and are quick, simple, inexpensive, and readily available. The correlation between results obtained with reagent strips and reflectance meter versus standard laboratory methods is quite variable. Differences between these methodologies are more pronounced at higher glucose concentrations (i.e., > 300 mg/dl). Blood glucose concentrations measured by reflectance meters are usually lower than corresponding results with standard laboratory methods.

Normal Values • Dogs, 65 to 120 mg/dl; cats, 65 to 120 mg/dl. To convert from mg/dl to mmol/L, multiply mg/dl × 0.055.

Danger Values • < 40 mg/dl (coma or seizures) or > 1000 mg/dl (hyperosmotic diabetes with impending coma, acute oliguric renal failure, or hyperkalemia).

Artifacts • With standard laboratory methods, hemolysis, icterus, or lipemia may interfere with results. Serum or plasma must be separated from RBCs and white blood cells (WBCs) within 30 minutes after collection to minimize consumption of glucose by cells. At 22° C, glucose concentration decreases approximately 10% every 30 to 60 minutes, and this may occur more rapidly if large concentrations of metabolically active cells (e.g., leukocytosis, leukemia) are present. Ascorbic acid, acetaminophen, and aspirin may decrease values when the glucose oxidase method is used. Azotemia can cause overestimation of blood glucose when using enzymatic methods.

When reagent strips are used, extremely increased or decreased packed cell volume (PCV) may alter the measured value. Reagent strips are less accurate at high glucose concentrations (i.e., > 300 mg/dl). Inadequate coverage of the reagent pad with blood may cause falsely low values. Expired reagent strips, meters that have not been properly calibrated, excessive washing or drying of the reagent strip, and inaccurate timing may also cause erroneous results.

Drug Therapy That May Alter Blood Glucose • Hypoglycemia may be caused by insulin, antihistamines, beta-blockers (i.e., propranolol), sulfonylureas (e.g., chlorpropamide), ethanol, and, in diabetics, salicylates and anabolic steroids. Hyperglycemia (especially in prediabetic patients) may be caused by asparaginase, beta-adrenergic drugs, corticosteroids, diazoxide, furosemide, acetazolamide, thiazides, salicylates, phenothiazines, nitrofurantoin, heparin, glucagon, thyroxine, progestagens, and estrogens.

Megestrol acetate may cause transient or persistent hyperglycemia in cats.

Causes of Hypoglycemia • Hypoglycemia typically results from excessive glucose utilization by normal (e.g., with hyperinsulinism) or neoplastic cells, impaired hepatic gluconeogenesis and glycogenolysis (e.g., portal shunt), a deficiency in diabetogenic hormones (e.g., hypocortisolism), inadequate dietary intake of glucose and other substrates required for hepatic gluconeogenesis (e.g., starvation), or a combination of these mechanisms (e.g., sepsis; Table 8–4). Iatrogenic hypoglycemia is a common problem with overzealous insulin administration in diabetic dogs and cats.

Table 8–4 CAUSES OF ALTERED BLOOD GLUCOSE IN DOGS AND CATS

Hypoglycemia
  Beta-cell tumor (insulinoma)
  Extrapancreatic neoplasia
    Hepatocellular carcinoma
    Leiomyosarcoma
    Hemangiosarcoma
  Hepatic insufficiency*
    Portacaval shunts
    Cirrhosis
  Sepsis*
  Hypoadrenocorticism
  Hypopituitarism
  Idiopathic hypoglycemia*
    Neonatal hypoglycemia
    Juvenile hypoglycemia (especially toy breeds)
    Hunting dog hypoglycemia
  Renal failure
  Exocrine pancreatic neoplasia
  Hepatic enzyme deficiencies
    Von Gierke's disease (type I glycogen storage disease)
    Cori's disease (type III glycogen storage disease)
  Prolonged starvation
  Prolonged sample storage/laboratory error*
  Iatrogenic*
    Insulin therapy
    Sulfonylurea therapy
    Ethanol
Hyperglycemia
  Diabetes mellitus*
  "Stress" (cat)*
  Postprandial (soft moist foods)
  Hyperadrenocorticism*
  Acromegaly (cat)
  Diestrus (bitch)
  Pheochromocytoma (dog)
  Glucagonoma (diabetic dermatopathy; dog)
  Pancreatitis
  Exocrine pancreatic neoplasia
  Renal insufficiency
  Drug therapy*
    Glucocorticoids
    Progestagens
    Megestrol acetate
    Thiazide diuretics

*Common cause.

Hypoglycemia should always be confirmed before beginning diagnostics to identify the cause. Careful evaluation of the history, physical findings, and routine clinical pathology (i.e., CBC, serum biochemical panel, urinalysis) usually provides clues to the underlying cause (Fig. 8–5) and helps to eliminate artifacts and iatrogenic causes. Hypoglycemia in a puppy or kitten is usually caused by idiopathic hypoglycemia, starvation, hepatic insufficiency (i.e., portal shunt), or sepsis. In a young adult dog or cat, hypoglycemia is usually caused by hepatic insufficiency, hypoadrenocorticism, or sepsis. In an older dog or cat, hepatic insufficiency, beta-cell neoplasia, extrapancreatic neoplasia, hypoadrenocorticism, and sepsis are the most common causes of hypoglycemia.

Hypoglycemia tends to be mild (i.e., > 45 mg/dl) and is often an incidental finding in dogs and cats with hypoadrenocorticism and hepatic insufficiency. Additional alterations in clinical pathology (e.g., hyponatremia/hyperkalemia, increased alanine transferase [ALT] activity, hypoproteinemia) are usually present. An adrenocorticotropic hormone (ACTH)-stimulation test or hepatic function test (see Chapter

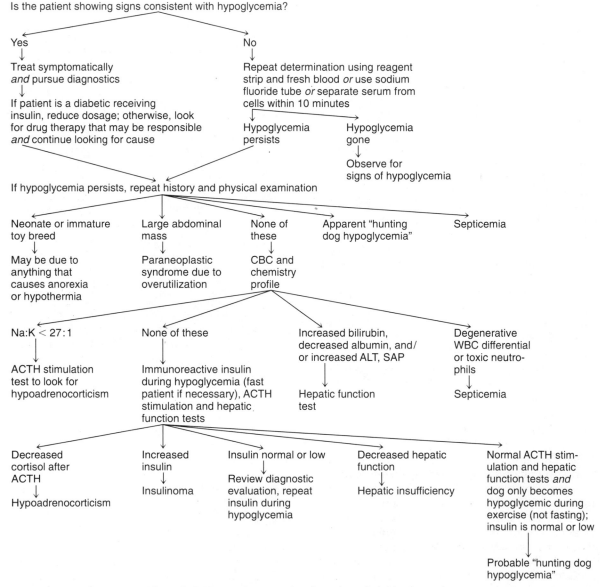

Figure 8–5 Diagnostic approach to hypoglycemia in the dog and cat.

9) may be required to confirm the diagnosis. Severe hypoglycemia (< 35 mg/dl) may develop in neonates and juvenile kittens and puppies (especially toy breeds) and with sepsis, beta-cell neoplasia, and extrapancreatic neoplasia, most notably hepatic adenocarcinoma. Sepsis is readily identified by physical findings and abnormalities on a CBC, including a neutrophilic leukocytosis (typically > 30,000/µl) or leukopenia (< 1,000–2,000/µl), a shift toward immaturity, and signs of toxicity. Extrapancreatic neoplasia can usually be identified on physical examination by palpating a large abdominal mass, abdominal or thoracic radiographs, and abdominal ultrasonography. Dogs with beta-cell neoplasia typically appear normal on physical examination and other than hypoglycemia show a lack of abnormalities on other diagnostic tests. Measurement of baseline serum insulin concentration when the blood glucose is < 60 mg/dl is necessary to confirm a beta-cell tumor (see Insulin).

Causes of Hyperglycemia • Hyperglycemia results from an absolute or relative insulin deficiency, impairment of insulin action in peripheral tissues (i.e., decreased glucose utilization), increased hepatic gluconeogenesis and glycogenolysis, or a combination of these (see Table 8–4). Iatrogenic causes of hyperglycemia include intravenous infusion of dextrose-containing fluids and the administration of diabetogenic drugs (e.g., glucocorticoids, megestrol acetate). Infusion of fluids containing as little as 2.5% dextrose may cause hyperglycemia, depending on the infusion rate and the presence of concurrent disorders that interfere with carbohydrate tolerance. Severe hyperglycemia, typically without glucosuria, occurs commonly in "stressed" cats, presumably from epinephrine secretion. Many diseases also cause carbohydrate intolerance and mild hyperglycemia, primarily by interfering with insulin action in peripheral tissues.

Hyperglycemia between 130 and 180 mg/dl does not cause glucosuria or corresponding signs of polyuria and polydipsia. Hyperglycemia in this range is clinically silent and is often an unsuspected finding on clinical pathology. If a dog or cat with mild hyperglycemia (< 180 mg/dl) presents for polyuria and polydipsia, a disorder other than insulin-requiring diabetes mellitus should be sought. Mild hyperglycemia can occur up to 2 hours after meals in some dogs and cats following consumption of soft moist foods, in stressed cats, with administration of diabetogenic medications, in early diabetes mellitus, and with disorders causing insulin in-

effectiveness (see Table 8–4). A diagnostic evaluation for disorders causing insulin ineffectiveness is indicated if mild hyperglycemia (< 180 mg/dl) persists in a fasted, unstressed dog or cat in which diabetogenic medications have been discontinued.

Urine should always be checked for glucose whenever hyperglycemia is identified. Persistent hyperglycemia and glucosuria in dogs and cats with polyuria and polydipsia establishes the diagnosis of diabetes mellitus. The persistence of diabetes mellitus is dependent, in part, on the pathology in the pancreatic islets, functional status of the beta-cells, and reversibility of concurrent diabetogenic diseases. Diabetogenic drugs (see Drug Therapy That May Alter Blood Glucose) should be stopped or adjusted, concurrent stresses minimized, and the effects on the blood glucose reevaluated in dogs and cats with suspected diabetes mellitus. A suspicion of concurrent diabetogenic disorders is usually gained from the history, physical examination, evaluation of routine clinical pathology (CBC, serum biochemical panel, urinalysis), and ease of glycemic regulation with insulin therapy. Concurrent diabetogenic disorders should always be suspected when glycemic control is difficult to attain with insulin therapy. The most common disorders interfering with glycemic regulation in dogs are hyperadrenocorticism, diestrus, and concurrent infection; in cats, hyperadrenocorticism, acromegaly, occult hyperthyroidism, and infection (Fig. 8–6). Additional diagnostic tests (e.g., ACTH-stimulation test, serum thyroxine concentration) may be necessary to identify these disorders. Problems with insulin therapy itself (e.g., poor absorption, Somogyi phenomenon, insulin-binding antibodies) should also be considered in poorly regulated diabetic dogs and cats. Assessment of insulin therapy in diabetic patients that are not responding to insulin as expected usually necessitates measuring the blood glucose concentration every 1 to 2 hours for 18 to 24 hours as the first diagnostic step in identifying problems with insulin therapy.

INSULIN

Occasional Indications • To confirm an insulin-secreting beta-cell tumor of the pancreas, to assess beta-cell function in dogs and cats with diabetes mellitus, and to increase the clinician's index of suspicion for circulating insulin-binding antibodies in dogs and cats with diabetes mellitus and insulin resistance. Advantages: insulin determination establishes preoperative diagnosis of beta-cell tumor that can be difficult

First, always ensure that faulty insulin and faulty administration technique are not responsible by buying a new bottle of insulin and observing the client mix, measure, and administer insulin. If a diluent is being used, one must ascertain that it is an acceptable diluent and not just unbuffered saline. If in doubt the veterinarian should treat the patient for 2 to 3 days to ensure that these factors are not responsible.

Gradually increase insulin dose up to 2.2–3.3 units/kg twice daily. If appropriate response by blood glucose is still not seen, check diet for too many calories or very high carbohydrate content (i.e., semimoist foods) and check for use of drugs that may antagonize insulin effects (e.g., steroids and others).

Next, measure blood glucose before insulin administration and around anticipated time of peak insulin effect to determine whether blood glucose does not decrease, decreases marginally, or decreases but only transiently. Note: Measuring blood glucose every 2 hours throughout the day (i.e., determining blood glucose curve from 7 AM to 9 PM) is preferable.

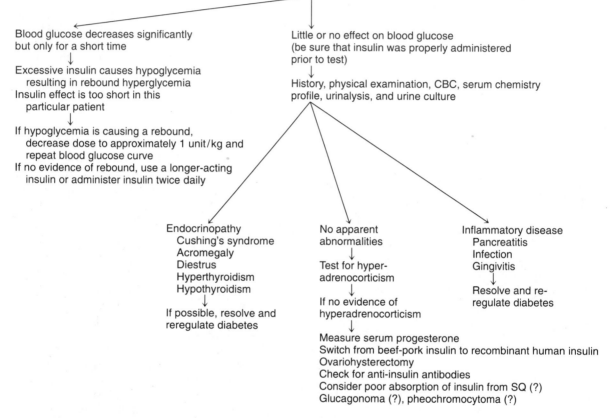

Figure 8–6 Diagnostic approach to persistent or inappropriate hyperglycemia in diabetics treated with insulin.

to find at surgery. Disadvantages: many variables can affect serum insulin concentration, interpretation must be done in conjunction with corresponding blood glucose concentration, and some RIAs for measuring insulin do not work in cats.

Analysis ● Measured in 0.5 ml of serum by RIA. Insulin concentrations measured in plasma tend to be higher than corresponding values in serum. Fasting samples are preferred to minimize the stimulatory effects of a meal on insulin secretion. Serum samples should be separated from cellular elements of blood and frozen before submission to the laboratory.

Normal Fasting Values ● Dogs, 5 to 20 μU/ml; cats, 5 to 20 μU/ml. To convert μU/ml to pmol/L, multiply μU/ml × 6.0.

Fasting serum insulin concentration > 20 μU/ml in an untreated diabetic dog or cat suggests type II diabetes or diabetes induced by concurrent insulin antagonistic disease.

Danger Values ● None, unless accompanied by hypoglycemia.

Artifacts and Effect of Drugs on Insulin ● Serum insulin concentration is increased for several hours after consumption of a meal. In addition, many of the drugs and disorders that affect blood glucose concentration also affect serum insulin concentration. Insulin derived from an insulin injection may be measured in blood samples obtained up to 24 hours after the insulin injection. Chronic exogenous insulin therapy in diabetic dogs and cats may cause insulin antibody formation, which can interfere with single antibody RIA systems, causing spuriously increased values (i.e., > 400 μU/ml).

Insulin and Hypoglycemia ● Confirmation of an insulin-secreting neoplasm requires documentation of inappropriate insulin secretion during hypoglycemia. If the blood glucose concentration is < 60 mg/dl and the serum insulin concentration is increased (i.e., > 20 μU/ml), the presence of an insulin-secreting neoplasm is likely. If the serum insulin is in the high-normal range (i.e., 10–20 μU/ml), the presence of an insulin-secreting tumor remains possible. Insulin values in the low-normal range (i.e., 5–10 μU/ml) may be found with other causes of hypoglycemia as well as insulin-secreting tumors. Careful assessment of the history, physical findings, clinical pathology, abdominal ultrasonography, and possibly repeated serum glucose and insulin values usually identify the cause of the hypoglycemia. A serum insulin concentration that is below the normal range (i.e., < 5 μU/ml) is consistent with insulinopenia and inconsistent with an insulin-secreting tumor.

Insulin and Hyperglycemia ● Serum insulin concentration should be increased (i.e., > 20 μU/ml) during periods of hyperglycemia in normal dogs and cats. Documenting serum insulin concentration > 20 μU/ml in dogs and cats with diabetes mellitus suggests residual beta-cell function and either type II (non–insulin-dependent diabetes mellitus [NIDDM]) or diabetes induced by concurrent insulin antagonistic disease. Most dogs and cats with type I (insulin-dependent diabetes mellitus [IDDM]) have serum insulin concentration < 10 μU/ml. Markedly increased serum insulin concentration (i.e., > 400 μU/ml) in blood obtained > 24 hours after the last insulin injection in a diabetic dog or cat would suggest insulin-binding antibodies if a single antibody RIA is used. Serum insulin concentration is typically < 50 μU/ml 24 hours after the previous insulin injection in diabetic dogs and cats without antibodies causing interference with the RIA.

INSULIN SECRETAGOGUE TESTING

Rare Indications ● To aid in differentiation of type I (IDDM) from type II (NIDDM) diabetes mellitus, to identify carbohydrate intolerance in dogs and cats with suspected preclinical diabetes mellitus, to identify an occult insulin-secreting tumor, and for the glucagon stimulation test, to identify hyperadrenocorticism and portosystemic shunts. The most common insulin secretagogue tests are the intravenous glucose tolerance test (IVGTT) and the intravenous glucagon stimulation test (IVGST). Advantages: none. Disadvantages: labor intensive and expensive tests that are often not effective in differentiating type I from type II diabetes mellitus. The tests are not recommended for the diagnosis of insulin-secreting tumor, hyperadrenocorticism, or portosystemic shunts.

Protocol ● The dog or cat should be fasted overnight. For the IVGTT, 0.5 g dextrose/kg of body weight (using 50% dextrose solution) is administered intravenously over 30 seconds, and blood samples are obtained before and 1, 5, 10, 15, 20, 30, 45, 60, 90, and 120 minutes after glucose administration. The IVGST is preferred if fasting hyperglycemia > 200 mg/dl is present. For the IVGST, 0.5 mg (cat) or 1.0 mg (dog) of glucagon per patient is given intravenously, and blood samples are obtained before and 1, 5, 10, 20, 30, 45, and 60 minutes after glucagon administration. For both tests, serum should be harvested from each blood sample and frozen until glucose and insulin can be assayed.

Interpretation ● Serum insulin concentration increases rapidly after intravenous administration of glucose or glucagon in normal dogs and cats, and is within 1 standard deviation (SD) of reference baseline mean serum insulin concentration by 60 minutes (Kaneko et al., 1977; Kirk et al., 1993). In diabetic dogs and cats, elevated fasting serum insulin concentration or any post-secretagogue insulin concentration > 1 SD above the reference mean (typically > 15 μU/ml) would suggest the existence of residual beta-cell function and the possibility of NIDDM. Identifying an increase in serum insulin concentration after intravenous administration of glucose or glucagon supports NIDDM, but failure to identify an increase in serum insulin concentration does not rule out NIDDM. The classification of a diabetic dog or cat as having IDDM or NIDDM ultimately depends on response to treatment.

For identification of carbohydrate intolerance, blood glucose concentration should return to normal by 60 minutes after intravenous glucose or glucagon administration. Persistent hyperglycemia (i.e., > 130 mg/dl) beyond this time would suggest carbohydrate intolerance and a possible prediabetic state. If desired, the glucose disappearance coefficient (K value) can be determined from the IVGTT using the following formula:

$$K = (0.693/t_{1/2}) \times 100$$

where $t_{1/2}$ is the half-time for glucose disappearance from serum (Kaneko et al., 1977). Linear regression analysis of a semilogarithmic plot of glucose concentration versus time is used to calculate the $t_{1/2}$, which is graphically estimated between 15 and 45 minutes after glucose injection. Normal dogs and cats typically have K values > 1.5 to 2.0%/min, whereas a K value < 1.0%/minute, is consistent with carbohydrate intolerance.

Artifacts ● Any of the drugs mentioned under Glucose, Drug Therapy That May Alter Blood Glucose, may alter the IVGTT and IVGST. Anesthetic agents may also produce glucose intolerance, a noteworthy fact in cats because of the difficulty in taking multiple blood samples in conscious cats unless an intravenous catheter is used.

Warning ● Glucagon administered to patients with pheochromocytoma may cause significant hypertension, and patients with insulin-secreting tumor may become severely hypoglycemic.

HYPERLIPIDEMIA

Increased concentrations of lipids, specifically cholesterol and triglycerides, and lipoproteins in the blood result in hyperlipidemia. Hyperlipidemia is often initially recognized by finding gross lipemia (i.e., milky plasma or serum) in a blood sample. Hyperlipidemia occasionally is suspected by finding opalescence of the anterior chamber of the eye (i.e., lipid-laden aqueous) or pinkish-white retinal vessels (i.e., lipemia retinalis) on physical examination.

Postprandial hyperlipidemia is normal; however, hyperlipidemia in a fasted (i.e., > 12 hours) dog or cat should be considered abnormal. Clear plasma or serum does not rule out hyperlipidemia, since hypercholesterolemia in the absence of hypertriglyceridemia does not cause lipemia. Lipemia is visible when serum triglyceride values are > 200 mg/dl. Lipemia implies hypertriglyceridemia and an increase in chylomicrons, very low-density lipoproteins (VLDLs), or both.

The chylomicron test can be used to evaluate for chylomicrons (exogenous hypertriglyceridemia) and VLDLs (endogenous hypertriglyceridemia) in lipemic serum. For this test, the lipemic serum sample should stand overnight in the refrigerator and then be assessed visually. Chylomicrons form a creamy layer at the top of the sample, whereas persistent lactescence of the serum is due to VLDLs.

Hyperlipidemia is also diagnosed after measurement of serum cholesterol and triglyceride concentrations. Hyperlipidemia should be suspected when serum cholesterol and triglyceride concentrations exceed 300 mg/dl and 150 mg/dl, respectively, in a fasted adult dog, and 200 mg/dl and 100 mg/dl, respectively, in a fasted adult cat.

Abnormal hyperlipidemic states may be idiopathic or secondary to an endocrine or metabolic disorder (Table 8–5). For most dogs and cats, hyperlipidemia is caused by an endocrine or metabolic disorder. The history, physical examination, routine clinical pathology (i.e., CBC, serum biochemical panel, urinalysis), lipase, and serum thyroxine concentration provide enough information to allow a tentative diagnosis to be established (Fig. 8–7). Tests of the pituitary-adrenocortical axis (e.g., ACTH-stimulation test) occasionally are necessary to identify hyperadrenocorticism.

A tentative diagnosis of idiopathic hyperlipidemia is made after ruling out secondary causes of persistent hyperlipidemia. These are ostensibly due to various enzymatic abnormalities in the lipid metabolism pathways. Although it can occur in any breed, miniature schnauzers seem to be predisposed. Idiopathic hyperlipidemias can be further characterized by determining al-

Table 8–5 CAUSES OF HYPERLIPIDEMIA IN DOGS AND CATS

Postprandial hyperlipidemia*
Secondary hyperlipidemia*
  Hypothyroidism
  Diabetes mellitus
  Hyperadrenocorticism
  Pancreatitis
  Cholestasis
  Hepatic insufficiency
  Nephrotic syndrome
Primary hyperlipidemia
  Idiopathic hyperlipoproteinemia (miniature schnauzers)*
  Idiopathic hyperchylomicronemia (cat)
  Lipoprotein lipase deficiency (cat)
  Idiopathic hypercholesterolemia
Drug-induced hyperlipidemia
  Glucocorticoids
  Megestrol acetate (cat)

*Common cause.

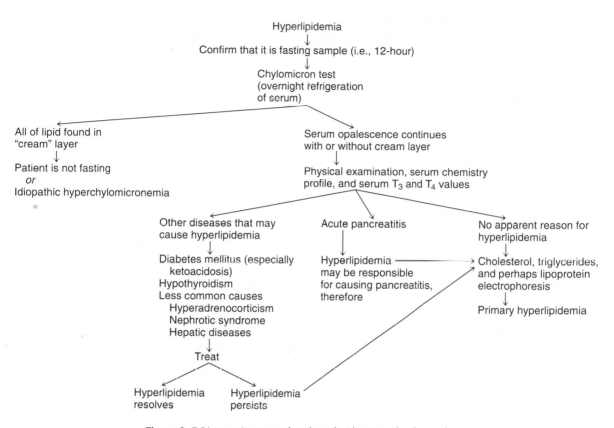

Figure 8–7 Diagnostic approach to hyperlipidemia in the dog and cat.

terations in serum lipoprotein concentrations by lipoprotein electrophoresis or lipoprotein ultracentrifugation. An idea of lipoprotein alterations can also be gained by measuring serum cholesterol and triglyceride concentrations and performing the chylomicron test.

CHOLESTEROL

Occasional Indications ● Hyperlipidemia in dogs and cats and as a screening test for hypothyroidism and hyperadrenocorticism. Hypercholesterolemia by itself does not cause lipemia.

Analysis ● Measured in 0.5 ml of serum or heparinized plasma by spectrophotometric, chromatographic, automated direct, and enzymatic methods. Automated direct techniques may slightly overestimate serum cholesterol concentration.

Normal Values ● Dogs, 125 to 300 mg/dl; cats, 50 to 200 mg/dl. To convert mg/dl to mmol/L, multiply mg/dl × 0.026.

Danger Values ● None.

Artifacts ● Falsely increased: icterus (spectrophotometric techniques), fluoride, and oxalate anticoagulants (enzymatic techniques). Lipemia may cause inaccurate measurement.

Drug Therapy That May Alter Serum Cholesterol ● Hypocholesterolemia may be caused by L-asparaginase, azathioprine, colchicine, cholestyramine, and oral aminoglycosides. Hypercholesterolemia may be caused by corticosteroids, methimazole, phenytoin, prochlorperazine, thiazides, and phenothiazines.

Causes of Hypocholesterolemia ● Rarely a problem, hypocholesterolemia primarily occurs with protein-losing enteropathy, hepatopathy (most notably portacaval shunt and cirrhosis), selected malignancies, and severe malnutrition.

Causes of Hypercholesterolemia ● Hypercholesterolemia may be caused by diet or spontaneous disease (see Table 8–5). Feeding a very high-fat diet or sampling blood shortly after eating may rarely cause minor elevations in serum cholesterol concentration. The diagnostic approach for persistent hypercholesterolemia in a fasted dog or cat is as outlined for hyperlipidemia (see Fig. 8–7). The primary differentials are diabetes mellitus, hypothyroidism, hyperadrenocorticism, and protein-losing nephropathies.

TRIGLYCERIDES

Occasional Indications • Hyperlipidemia or hypercholesterolemia. Lipemia implies hypertriglyceridemia.

Analysis • Measured in 0.5 ml of serum or EDTA plasma by spectrophotometric or enzymatic methods. Triglyceride values tend to be slightly less in plasma than in serum. Enzymatic methods may give slightly greater values than spectrophotometric methods.

Normal Values • Dogs, 10 to 150 mg/dl; cats, 5 to 100 mg/dl.

Danger Values • > 1000 mg/dl (neurologic signs, seizures).

Artifacts • Lipemia may cause inaccurate measurement.

Drug Therapy That May Alter Serum Triglycerides • Hypotriglyceridemia may be caused by ascorbic acid, L-asparaginase, and heparin. Different anabolic steroids have different effects. Hypertriglyceridemia may be caused by estrogens and cholestyramine (?).

Causes of Hypotriglyceridemia • Not clearly associated with any disease; it may rarely be seen in hyperthyroidism (?) and some malabsorptive protein-losing enteropathies (?).

Causes of Hypertriglyceridemia • Blood obtained from a nonfasted patient is the most common cause. Hypertriglyceridemia may be secondary to other disorders or be a primary idiopathic hyperlipidemic disorder (see Table 8–5). The diagnostic approach for persistent hypertriglyceridemia in a fasted dog or cat is as outlined for hyperlipidemia (see Fig. 8–7). The primary differentials are diabetes mellitus, hypothyroidism, acute pancreatitis, and dyslipoproteinemias. It is not known whether acute pancreatitis causes hypertriglyceridemia or vice versa.

LIPOPROTEIN ELECTROPHORESIS

Rare Indications • Unexplained persistent, fasting hyperlipidemia. Disadvantages: the need for specialized equipment and the lack of diagnostic specificity in most cases. Because of differences in dogs and cats versus people, a combination of laboratory methods may be necessary to specifically evaluate a given lipoprotein class and prevent erroneous interpretations of results.

Analysis • Performed on 0.5 ml of serum or EDTA plasma.

Normal Values • Dogs, see Zerbe (1986); cats, see Bauer (1992).

Danger Values • None.

Artifacts • Grossly lipemic serum or plasma should not be allowed to separate and have the "cream layer" (i.e., chylomicrons) discarded before testing.

Drug Treatment That May Alter Results • See Cholesterol and Triglycerides.

Causes of Altered Patterns • Although lipoprotein electrophoresis allows the diagnostician to determine if chylomicrons, VLDLs, low-density lipoproteins (LDLs), or high-density lipoproteins (HDLs) are responsible for the hyperlipidemia, it does not allow identification of a specific disease in most cases. This is not an accurate test for pancreatitis.

THYROXINE (T₄)

Common Indications • To diagnose hypothyroidism and hyperthyroidism and to monitor sodium levothyroxine therapy for hypothyroidism and methimazole therapy for hyperthyroidism. Clinical signs suggestive of hypothyroidism include endocrine alopecia, seborrhea, pyoderma, lethargy, obesity, exercise intolerance, weakness, neurologic signs (facial nerve paralysis, head tilt, ataxia, seizures), infertility, and failure to grow (i.e., cretinism). Clinical signs suggestive of hyperthyroidism include polyphagia, weight loss, hyperactivity, polyuria-polydipsia, and a palpable cervical mass. Advantages: readily available test, the hormone is stable during handling and shipping. Disadvantages: myriad variables can affect serum T_4 concentration, resulting in misinterpretation of results.

Analysis • Measured in 0.5 ml of serum by RIA. T_4 concentration in serum is stable for at least 8

Table 8–6 DRUGS (BESIDES THYROID HORMONE SUPPLEMENTS) THAT MAY ALTER SERUM T_4 AND/OR T_3 CONCENTRATIONS IN DOGS AND CATS

Decrease T_4 and T_3	Decrease T_4 Only	Decrease T_3 Only	Increase T_4 and T_3	Increase T_4 Only	Increase T_3 Only
Androgens	Phenothiazines	Radiocontrast agents	Estrogens	Fatty acids	Thiazides
Salicylates			Narcotic analgesics	Radiocontrast agents	
Heparin			5-Fluorouracil	Prostaglandins	
Diazepam			Halothane	Insulin	
Sulfonylureas					
Methimazole					
Propylthiouracil					
Phenylbutazone					
Phenytoin					
Carbamazepine					
Phenobarbital					
Primidone					
Glucocorticoids					
Iodide					
Nitroprusside					

(From Ferguson DC: Thyroid function tests in the dog. Recent concepts. Vet Clin North Am 1984; 14:793.)

days at room temperature, and hemolysis or freezing and thawing of serum does not affect T_4 concentrations. Despite stability, serum samples should be frozen and sent to the laboratory on cool packs. The laboratory must use a validated RIA for cats and dogs. When evaluating sodium levothyroxine therapy, serum should be obtained before and 4 to 6 hours after sodium levothyroxine administration. A single serum sample can be obtained at any time when evaluating methimazole therapy.

Normal Values • Dogs, 0.8 to 3.6 µg/dl; cats, 1.0 to 4.0 µg/dl. To convert µg/dl to nmol/L, multiply µg/dl × 12.87. Note: Different laboratories have different normal ranges.
Interpretation for hypothyroidism in dogs:

> 2.0 µg/dl:	hypothyroidism very unlikely
1.5 to 2.0 µg/dl:	hypothyroidism unlikely
1.0 to 1.5 µg/dl:	unknown
0.5 to 1.0 µg/dl:	hypothyroidism possible
< 0.5 µg/dl:	hypothyroidism very likely

Interpretation for hyperthyroidism in cats:

> 4.0 µg/dl:	hyperthyroidism very likely
3.0 to 4.0 µg/dl:	hyperthyroidism possible
2.5 to 3.0 µg/dl:	unknown
< 2.0 µg/dl:	hyperthyroidism very unlikely

Note: The clinician must also consider clinical signs, physical findings, clinical pathology changes, and index of suspicion when interpreting serum T_4 results.

Danger Values • None.

Variables That Affect Serum T_4 Concentration • Variables that affect serum T_4 concentration can be divided into physiologic, pharmacologic, and systemic illness. Serum T_4 concentration is higher in young dogs (< 1 year of age) and decreases with advancing age (Reimers et al., 1990). Small breeds have higher T_4 concentrations than large or giant breeds. Certain breeds (i.e., German shepherd, cocker spaniel, boxer, beagle, Labrador retriever, Alaskan malamute, Siberian husky, and perhaps greyhounds) have lower serum T_4 values than other breeds. Estrus, pregnancy, and obesity increase serum T_4 concentration, whereas hypoproteinemia may decrease serum T_4 concentration. Antithyroid hormone antibodies may develop in dogs with lymphocytic thyroiditis and cause spuriously increased or decreased serum T_4 values (Thacker et al., 1992). The effect of antithyroid hormone antibodies on the serum T_4 value depends on the type of assay being used by the laboratory. Drugs that may alter serum T_4 concentration are listed in Table 8–6. The most clinically relevant is concurrent glucocorticoid administration. Many nonthyroidal illnesses are associated with decreased serum T_4 concentration (Table 8–7). This phenomenon is called the *euthyroid sick syndrome.* The severity of illness has a direct corre-

Table 8–7 MAJOR CAUSES OF THE EUTHYROID SICK SYNDROME

Acute diseases
    Bacterial bronchopneumonia
    Distemper
    Autoimmune hemolytic anemia
    Systemic lupus erythematosus
    Intervertebral disk disease
    Polyradiculoneuritis
    Acute renal failure
Chronic diseases
    Generalized demodicosis
    Generalized bacterial furunculosis
    Lymphoma
    Chronic renal failure
    Diabetes mellitus
    Congestive heart failure
    Blastomycosis
    Hepatic insufficiency
    Obesity
    Gastrointestinal disturbances
    Megaesophagus

(Modified from Feldman EC, Nelson RW: Hypothyroidism. In Feldman EC, Nelson RW (eds): Canine and Feline Endocrinology and Reproduction. Philadelphia, WB Saunders, 1987, pp 55–90; Muller GH, Kirk RW, Scott DW: Cutaneous endocrinology. In Muller GH, Kirk RW, Scott DW (eds): Small Animal Dermatology. 3rd ed. Philadelphia, WB Saunders, 1983, pp 492–560.)

lation with the severity of suppression of serum T_4 concentration. The euthyroid sick syndrome is thought to be a protective mechanism during periods of negative energy balance.

Causes of Decreased Serum T_4 Concentration ● The primary disorder causing decreased serum T_4 concentration is hypothyroidism, which must be differentiated from all the earlier listed variables that can also suppress serum T_4 concentration (Table 8–8). In dogs, primary hypothyroidism may be due to lymphocytic thyroiditis, idiopathic atrophy, or neoplastic destruction of the thyroid gland. Secondary hypothyroidism results from a deficiency of TSH and may be

Table 8–8 CAUSES OF ALTERED SERUM T_3 AND T_4 VALUES IN DOGS AND CATS

Decreased serum thyroid hormone values
    Hypothyroidism (primary and secondary)
    Nonthyroidal illness (euthyroid sick syndrome) (see Table 8–7)
    Drugs (see Table 8–6)
    Iatrogenic
        Postthyroidectomy (bilateral)
Increased serum thyroid hormone values
    Hyperthyroidism
    Drugs (see Table 8–6)
    Thyroid hormone autoantibodies
    Iatrogenic
        Excess thyroid hormone supplementation

caused by pituitary malformation, destruction, or suppression. Hypothyroidism in cats is usually iatrogenic, resulting from bilateral thyroidectomy or overuse of methimazole for the treatment of hyperthyroidism. Congenital hypothyroidism is rare in dogs and cats and, when present, results in cretinism.

The diagnosis of hypothyroidism must take into account the history, physical findings, clinical pathology, serum T_4 concentration, and the clinician's index of suspicion for the disease (Fig. 8–8). Fasting lipemia, hypercholesterolemia, and less commonly mild normocytic-normochromic anemia (PCV = 30–35%) are the most common abnormalities identified on routine clinical pathology. Increases in ALT and SAP are less common. Proteinuria may be found in dogs with lymphocytic thyroiditis. Mild hypercalcemia may be noted in congenital hypothyroidism, and skeletal survey radiographs may identify decreased length of bones and incomplete ossification of epiphyseal centers. Additional diagnostic tests, including performance of a TSH-stimulation test or clinical response to trial therapy with sodium levothyroxine, may be required to establish a definitive diagnosis.

When monitoring dogs receiving sodium levothyroxine supplementation for hypothyroidism, blood for serum T_4 measurement should be obtained immediately before and 4 to 6 hours after oral T_4 administration. With appropriate supplementation, all serum T_4 concentrations should be in the upper half of normal or mildly increased (i.e., 2.5–6.0 μg/dl). Serum T_4 concentration < 2.5 μg/dl, especially < 1.5 μg/dl, suggests inadequate thyroid hormone supplementation, especially if clinical signs of hypothyroidism persist.

Causes of Increased Serum T_4 Concentrations ● The primary disorder causing increased serum T_4 concentration is hyperthyroidism (see Table 8–8). In cats, spontaneous hyperthyroidism is usually caused by functional thyroid adenoma(s). Functional thyroid tumors are uncommon in dogs but, when present, may be adenoma or carcinoma. Oversupplementation of sodium levothyroxine to dogs with hypothyroidism and spurious increase due to antithyroid hormone antibody interference with single antibody RIAs for serum T_4 measurement must also be considered. Oversupplementation is diagnosed by history. Antithyroid hormone antibodies should be suspected in dogs with clinical signs of hypothyroidism but increased serum T_4 concentration.

The history and physical examination are the basis for suspecting hyperthyroidism. CBC,

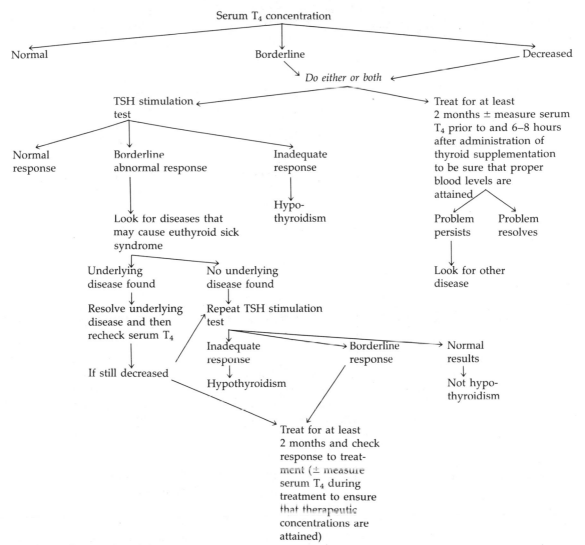

Figure 8–8 Evaluation of an adult patient with suspected hypothyroidism. History or clinical signs (dermatologic or reproductive disease, lethargy, or obesity) are suggestive of hypothyroidism.

serum biochemistry panel, urinalysis, ECG, thoracic radiographs, and echocardiogram may have suggestive changes but are not specific. Nearly 50% of cats with hyperthyroidism have an increased PCV and macrocytosis, and most have increased SAP and ALT. Less consistent findings include azotemia, hyperglycemia, hyperphosphatemia, and hypocalcemia. A wide variety of ECG changes may occur with hyperthyroidism, including sinus tachycardia, tall R-wave amplitude in lead II, intraventricular conduction defects, atrial and ventricular premature contractions, and atrial fibrillation. Hyperthyroidism may cause hyperdynamic function of the heart, hypertrophic cardiomyopathy, and, less frequently, dilatative cardiomyopathy. Cardiomegaly and radiographic signs of heart failure may be seen on thoracic radiographs.

Measurement of baseline serum T_4 concentration is reliable in establishing the diagnosis of hyperthyroidism in most cats and dogs (Fig. 8–9). Serum T_4 concentration may be normal in some cats with hyperthyroidism as a result of random fluctuation and the suppressive effects of concurrent illness. When nondiagnostic results are obtained and hyperthyroidism is suspected, the T_3-suppression test (discussed later) should be performed to clarify the status of the pituitary-thyroid axis.

3,5,3'-TRIIODOTHYRONINE (T_3)

Occasional Indications ● The indications for measurement of serum T_3 concentration are the same as for serum T_4. Although measurement

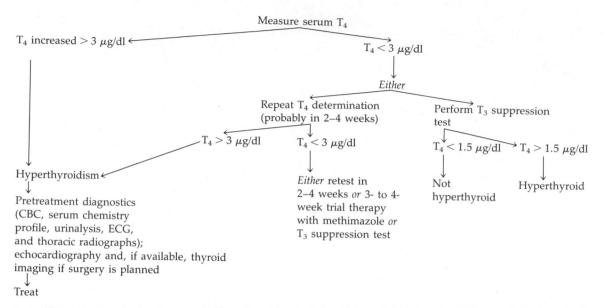

Figure 8–9 Evaluation of cats with suspected hyperthyroidism based on history, clinical signs (weight loss, polyphagia, polyuria-polydipsia, hyperactivity, cervical mass) or laboratory findings (increased serum alkaline phosphatase, increased serum phosphorus).

of baseline serum T_3 concentration is beneficial in identifying hyperthyroidism in cats, measurement of baseline serum T_3 is of minimal value in assessing thyroid gland function in dogs (Nelson et al., 1991). The poor reliability of serum T_3 concentration for identifying hypothyroidism may be due, in part, to a predominance of T_4 secretion by the normal thyroid gland, the primary intracellular location of T_3, and the increased thyroidal secretion of T_3 with progressive loss of thyroid gland function. Advantages: readily available test, hormone is stable during handling. Disadvantages: questionable diagnostic usefulness, myriad of variables that can affect serum T_3 concentration.

Analysis • Same as for serum T_4.

Normal Values • Dogs, 0.5 to 1.8 ng/ml; cats, 0.4 to 1.6 ng/ml. To convert ng/ml to nmol/L, multiply ng/ml × .536. Note: Different laboratories have different normal ranges.

Danger Values • None.

Variables That Affect Serum T_3 Concentration • Same as for serum T_4 concentration. The incidence of anti-T_3 antibodies is greater than anti-T_4 antibodies in dogs with lymphocytic thyroiditis.

Causes of Decreased Serum T_3 Concentration • Same as for serum T_4 concentration.

Causes of Increased Serum T_3 Concentrations • Same as for serum T_4 concentration. Spurious increase due to antithyroid hormone antibody interference with single antibody RIAs is more common with T_3 than T_4.

FREE THYROXINE (fT$_4$)/FREE 3,5,3'-TRIIODOTHYRONINE (fT$_3$)

Rare Indication • Suspected hypothyroidism. Theoretically, measurement of the non–protein-bound fraction of serum T_4 and T_3 may minimize some of the physiologic mechanisms involved with the euthyroid sick syndrome (e.g., altered plasma protein binding affinity) and improve the diagnostic accuracy of assessing thyroid gland function. Unfortunately, measurement of baseline serum fT$_4$ concentration by RIA in canine sera provides minimal additional information about thyroid gland function to that gained with measurement of serum T_4 concentration (Nelson et al., 1991). Results obtained with many of these RIAs underestimate serum fT$_4$ concentration when compared with equilibrium dialysis (Montgomery et al., 1991). In addition, serum fT$_4$ concentration as determined by RIA is affected by concurrent illness and drug therapy, often in a manner similar to serum T_4 concentration. A modified equilibrium dialysis technique* that has become avail-

---

*Nichols Institute, San Juan Capistrano, CA 92675.

able may be more amenable to commercial use than standard equilibrium dialysis methods and may offer a more accurate assessment of free thyroid hormone concentrations than currently available RIAs. Studies assessing the value of serum fT_3 have not been reported in dogs or cats. Advantages: none. Disadvantages: questionable diagnostic usefulness, myriad of variables that can affect serum concentration.

THYROID HORMONE ANTIBODIES

Occasional Indications • To explain unusual serum T_4 or T_3 values in dogs with suspected hypothyroidism and to identify lymphocytic thyroiditis. Circulating thyroid hormone antibodies may interfere with RIA techniques used to measure serum T_4 and T_3 concentrations, causing spurious numbers that are not reliable (Young et al., 1985; Thacker et al., 1992). The type of interference depends on the separation system used in the RIA. Falsely low results are obtained with nonspecific separation methods (e.g., ammonium sulfate, activated charcoal), whereas falsely increased values occur with single antibody systems using antibody-coated tubes. Determination of accurate T_4 or T_3 concentration in these patients requires special extraction techniques or removal of the endogenous immunoglobulin before assay.

Measurement of circulating antibodies directed against T_3 and T_4 is offered by Michigan State University (see Appendix I). A positive thyroid hormone antibody titer in a dog with appropriate clinical signs, clinical pathology, and low or high serum thyroid hormone concentration would support hypothyroidism caused by lymphocytic thyroiditis. Interpretation of a positive thyroid hormone antibody titer in an asymptomatic dog with no clinical pathology abnormalities and normal serum thyroid hormone concentrations needs further clarification. This may be an early marker for lymphocytic thyroiditis or may be a normal finding.

T_3 SUPPRESSION TEST

Occasional Indication • To confirm hyperthyroidism in cats with occult disease. The T_3 suppression test evaluates the responsiveness of pituitary TSH secretion to suppression by sodium liothyronine (synthetic T_3). Suppression of pituitary TSH secretion by the T_3 supplement decreases serum T_4 concentration in normal cats. In hyperthyroid cats, serum TSH is already suppressed and T_3 supplementation has no effect on the pituitary-thyroid axis. Serum T_4 concentration remains increased. Because T_3 cannot be converted to T_4, measurement of serum T_4 concentration provides an accurate assessment of the suppressibility of the pituitary-thyroid axis. Advantages: readily available, relatively inexpensive, and easy to interpret. Disadvantages: failure to ensure that a cat swallows T_3 supplement can result in unexpectedly high post-T_3 T_4 value and thereby cause a wrong diagnosis of hyperthyroidism.

Protocol • A baseline serum T_4 and T_3 concentration is obtained in the morning; then sodium liothyronine, 25 µg/cat, is administered per os three times a day for 2 days and then in the morning of the third day. Blood for measurement of serum T_4 and T_3 is obtained 2 to 4 hours after administration of the last dose of synthetic T_3.

Interpretation • In normal cats, the serum T_4 concentration following T_3 therapy is < 1.5 µg/dl and is typically < 50% of the serum T_4 concentration obtained before initiation of the test (Peterson et al., 1990). In cats with hyperthyroidism, there is minimal to no decline (usually < 35%) in serum T_4 concentration after T_3 supplementation compared with the pre-T_3 therapy serum T_4 concentration, despite an increase in serum T_3 concentration. Serum T_4 concentration typically remains > 1.5 µg/dl. If serum T_3 concentration fails to increase during the test, failure to give the T_3 supplement or failure of the cat to consume the supplement must be considered.

TSH-STIMULATION TEST

Occasional Indications • To confirm hypothyroidism in dogs. Advantages: easy to perform and usually accurate in differentiating hypothyroidism from other disorders decreasing serum thyroid hormone concentrations. Disadvantages: expense and availability of TSH.

Protocol • A blood sample is obtained immediately before and 6 hours after intravenous administration of 0.1 unit TSH per kg. Serum T_4 is measured in each blood sample. Serum T_3 concentration frequently does not increase after TSH administration, even in healthy dogs, and is not routinely measured. The remaining reconstituted TSH can be stored in the refrigerator for 3 weeks or frozen for 3 months without loss of biologic activity.

Interpretation ● Interpretation of the TSH-stimulation test should be based on absolute serum T_4 values. For the laboratory at the College of Veterinary Medicine, University of California at Davis, euthyroid dogs have a post-TSH serum T_4 concentration > 3.0 µg/dl and dogs with hypothyroidism have a post-TSH serum T_4 concentration below the normal baseline serum T_4 range (i.e., < 1.5 µg/dl; Fig. 8–10; Nelson et al., 1991). Post-TSH serum T_4 concentrations between 1.5 and 3.0 µg/dl are nondiagnostic and may be found in the early stages of hypothyroidism or may represent suppression of thyroid gland function due to concurrent illness or drug therapy in an otherwise euthyroid dog. Similarly, low baseline serum T_4 concentration and normal post-TSH serum T_4 concentration are also difficult to interpret. Assessment of history, physical findings, clinical pathology, and in some cases response to trial therapy may be required to ultimately determine the status of thyroid gland function. Pre- and post-TSH serum T_4 concentrations above baseline in conjunction with a lack of response of the thyroid gland to TSH (see Fig. 8–10) are occasionally noted in dogs with hypothyroidism and may reflect the presence of circulating thyroid hormone antibodies.

ENDOGENOUS PITUITARY ADRENOCORTICOTROPHIN (ACTH)

Occasional Indications ● To differentiate pituitary-dependent from adrenal-dependent hyperadrenocorticism in dogs with documented spontaneous hyperadrenocorticism and to differentiate primary versus secondary hypoadrenocorticism in dogs. Similar indications exist for cats; however, baseline ACTH concentration can be < 20 pg/ml (the lower limit of normal) in normal cats and cats with hyperadrenocorticism caused by adrenocortical tumor (Smith and Feldman, 1987). Measurement of baseline endogenous ACTH concentration is not indicated for the diagnosis of hyperadrenocorticism because of episodic secretion and overlapping values between normal and pituitary-dependent hyperadrenocorticism (PDH). Advantages: the most reliable test to differentiate PDH from adrenocortical tumor. Disadvantages: ACTH is a labile hormone, requiring *meticulous* care in specimen handling (discussed later). Plasma samples must remain frozen until assayed. Assay has limited availability and is expensive.

Protocol ● A blood sample should be drawn between 8 and 9 AM after a dog has been hospitalized overnight. Blood should be collected in a cold, heparinized plastic syringe and immediately transferred to cold plastic tubes and placed on ice until centrifuged. Alternatively, blood can be placed in special EDTA tubes obtained from the laboratory. These are precooled and, once filled with blood, placed on ice. Blood should be centrifuged immediately, and the plasma frozen in plastic tubes. This entire procedure should take < 10 minutes. Samples must be shipped frozen and must stay frozen until assayed for ACTH. ACTH assays validated for use in dogs are currently limited by their availability and cost.

Analysis ● Measured in 0.5 ml of plasma by RIA. The assay must be validated by the laboratory for dogs.

Normal Values ● Dogs, 20 to 100 pg/ml. Interpretation in dogs with hyperadrenocorticism:

< 20 pg/ml:	adrenal-dependent hyperadrenocorticism
20 to 50 pg/ml:	nondiagnostic
> 50 pg/ml:	pituitary-dependent hyperadrenocorticism

Interpretation in dogs with hypoadrenocorticism:

< 20 pg/ml:	secondary hypoadrenocorticism
20 to 50 pg/ml:	nondiagnostic
> 50 pg/ml:	primary hypoadrenocorticism

Danger Values ● None.

Artifacts ● Falsely decreased: storing plasma above freezing, sample thawing during transport to laboratory, using glass containers during collection or storage.

Drug Therapy That May Alter ACTH Values ● Decreased: administration of glucocorticoids (e.g., dexamethasone). Increased: insulin.

Causes of Altered Plasma ACTH Concentration ● Alterations in baseline endogenous ACTH concentration result from primary disorders of the pituitary gland or disorders affecting blood cortisol concentration and the negative inhibitory effects of blood cortisol on ACTH secretion (Table 8–9). Pituitary disorders include PDH,

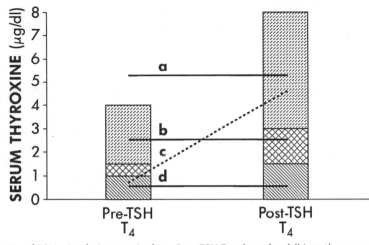

Figure 8-10 Interpretation of TSH stimulation test in dogs. Post-TSH T₄ values that fall into the normal range usually indicate normal thyroid gland function. Exceptions include high pre-TSH T₄ values with no increase in post-TSH T₄ (line a) and low pre-TSH T₄ values with normal response to TSH (line c). Primary hypothyroidism with anti-T₄ antibodies (lines a and b) and secondary hypothyroidism or the suppressive effects of concurrent disease (line c) should be considered. Low pre-TSH and post-TSH T₄ values (line d) and post-TSH T₄ values in the nondiagnostic range may be indicative of hypothyroidism or the suppressive effects of concurrent disease. ▨ s, Normal; ▧ s, nondiagnostic range; ▩ s, hypothyroid range. (From Nelson RW, Couto CG: Essentials of Small Animal Internal Medicine. St. Louis, Mosby-Year Book, 1992, p 549. Reprinted with permission.)

which is associated with increased ACTH secretion (Fig. 8-11), and secondary hypoadrenocorticism, which results from loss of function of the pituitary corticotroph cells and decreased ACTH secretion (Fig. 8-12). Functional adrenocortical tumors of the zona fasciculata have increased cortisol secretion, which inhibits pituitary ACTH secretion. Plasma ACTH concentration typically decreases to undetectable levels (see Fig. 8-11). A similar phenomenon occurs with excessive exogenous glucocorticoid administration (i.e., iatrogenic hyperadrenocorticism). Destruction of the zona fasciculata as occurs with primary hypoadrenocorticism results in decreased blood cortisol concentration, loss of feedback inhibition on pituitary ACTH secretion, and increased plasma ACTH concentrations (see Fig. 8-12). Preliminary evaluation of assays for endogenous ACTH in cats shows similar results (Peterson et al., 1989), although values in normal cats can be < 20 pg/ml. Similar

results can occur with adrenocortical tumor, bringing into question the usefulness of this assay for identifying adrenocortical tumors in cats.

PLASMA CORTISOL

Common Indications • To assess the pituitary-adrenocortical axis in dogs and cats with

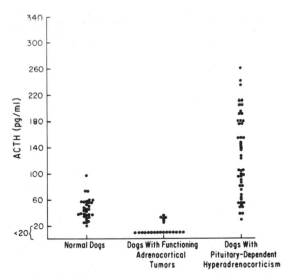

Figure 8-11 Endogenous plasma ACTH concentrations from clinically normal dogs, dogs with adrenal-dependent hyperadrenocorticism (adrenocortical carcinomas or adenomas), and dogs with pituitary-dependent hyperadrenocorticism. (From Feldman EC, Nelson RW: Canine and Feline Endocrinology and Reproduction. Philadelphia, WB Saunders, 1987, p 168. Reprinted with permission.)

Table 8-9 CAUSES OF ALTERED ENDOGENOUS PLASMA ACTH CONCENTRATION IN DOGS

Normal to increased
  Pituitary-dependent hyperadrenocorticism
  Primary hypoadrenocorticism
Normal to decreased
  Adrenal-dependent hyperadrenocorticism
  Iatrogenic hyperadrenocorticism
  Spontaneous secondary hypoadrenocorticism*
  Improper sample collection/storage

*Rare.

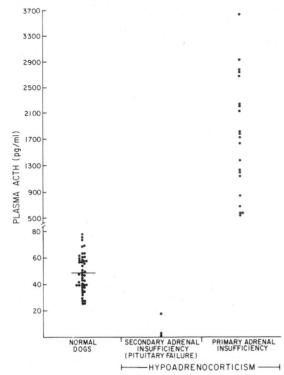

Figure 8-12 Endogenous plasma ACTH concentrations in normal dogs, dogs with secondary adrenal failure, and dogs with primary adrenal failure. (From Feldman EC, Peterson ME: Hypoadrenocorticism. Vet Clin North Am 1984;14:761. Reprinted with permission.)

suspected hyperadrenocorticism or hypoadrenocorticism. Findings suggestive of hyperadrenocorticism include polydipsia, polyuria, polyphagia, endocrine alopecia, calcinosis cutis, epidermal/dermal atrophy, conformational changes (e.g., potbellied appearance), anestrus, insulin-resistant diabetes mellitus, hepatomegaly, stress leukogram, increased SAP, hypercholesterolemia, persistent isosthenuria or hyposthenuria, and recurring urinary tract infection, especially in middle-aged to older patients. Findings suggestive of hypoadrenocorticism include lethargy, depression, anorexia, vomiting, weakness, weight loss, bradycardia, hypovolemia, hyponatremia, and hyperkalemia, especially in young to middle-aged dogs and cats. Advantages: the test is readily available, and the hormone is stable during handling. Disadvantages: baseline plasma cortisol concentration has absolutely *no* diagnostic significance; interpretation is only valid after manipulation of the pituitary-adrenocortical axis with ACTH or dexamethasone.

Analysis ● Measured in 0.5 ml of heparinized or EDTA plasma by RIA. RIAs measure free and protein bound cortisol. RIAs should be vali-

dated for dogs and cats. Plasma should be harvested and frozen soon after collection to minimize binding of cortisol to RBCs. If mailed, plasma samples should be shipped with cool packs. Repeated freezing and thawing or hemolysis of the sample does not alter cortisol concentrations. Fasting for up to 36 hours does not affect cortisol values, and no clinically detectable diurnal variation occurs in dogs or cats.

Normal Values ● Dogs, 1.0 to 5.0 μg/dl; cats, 0.5 to 5.5 μg/dl. To convert μg/dl to ng/ml, move the decimal point one place to the right. To convert μg/dl to nmol/L, multiply μg/dl × 27.59.

Danger Values ● None.

Artifacts Affecting Plasma Cortisol Concentration ● Environment, "stress," excitement, and chronic disease may increase baseline plasma cortisol concentrations. Exogenous glucocorticoid preparations that contain hydrocortisone, cortisone, prednisone, prednisolone, and possibly methylprednisone cross-react with many cortisol assays, causing spurious increase in measured cortisol values. Dexamethasone does not cross-react with cortisol assays. Plasma cortisol concentrations decrease by 21% after 2 days and 57% after 8 days at 22° C but do not decrease when stored at 4° C for 8 days.

Drug Therapy That May Alter Plasma Cortisol ● Estrogen administration may increase plasma cortisol. Chronic androgen or glucocorticoid administration and megestrol acetate can decrease plasma cortisol concentration.

Causes of Hypercortisolemia ● The most clinically relevant cause of hypercortisolemia is hyperadrenocorticism (Table 8–10). Additional causes include environmental factors that create stress or excitement, chronic illness (e.g., diabetes mellitus, renal insufficiency, congestive heart failure), and medications that contain glucocorticoid preparations that cross-react with the cortisol assay. For the latter to cause increased cortisol values, the medication must have been given within 12 to 24 hours of blood sampling and the steroid must still be present in the blood. Once the glucocorticoid in the preparation has been metabolized, plasma cortisol concentrations are decreased because of the negative inhibitory effects of the exogenous glucocorticoid on pituitary ACTH secretion. This phenomenon, termed *iatrogenic hyperadre-*

Table 8-10 CAUSES OF ALTERED RESTING PLASMA CORTISOL CONCENTRATION IN DOGS AND CATS

Increased
  Stress
    Environment
    Severe or chronic illness
  Drugs
    Cortisone, hydrocortisone, prednisone,
      and prednisolone (due to cross-
      reaction with cortisol assay)
    Anticonvulsants
  Hyperadrenocorticism
    Pituitary dependent
    Adrenal dependent
Decreased
  Improper storage
  Iatrogenic hyperadrenocorticism
  Hypoadrenocorticism
    Primary
    Secondary (i.e., pituitary insufficiency)
  Drugs
    Megestrol acetate

nocorticism, creates signs of hyperadrenocorticism, but the pituitary-adrenocortical axis is suppressed and resembles hypoadrenocorticism (Fig. 8–13; see Causes of Hypocortisolemia).

Hyperadrenocorticism occurs relatively frequently in dogs but rarely in cats. A tentative diagnosis of hyperadrenocorticism can be established based on results of the history, physical examination, and routine clinical pathology (i.e., CBC, serum biochemical panel, urinalysis; see description under Plasma Cortisol, Common Indications). In patients with hyperadrenocorticism, common abnormalities that may be identified on clinical pathology include a stress leukogram, increased SAP and ALT activities, hypercholesterolemia, mild hyperglycemia (120 –150 mg/dl), isosthenuria to hyposthenuria, proteinuria, and bacteriuria. In cats with hyperadrenocorticism, hyperglycemia and hypercholesterolemia are the most consistent findings on clinical pathology (Nelson et al., 1988). Additional abnormalities in dogs and cats may include increased serum amylase, lipase, and insulin concentrations and decreased baseline serum T_4 and T_3 concentrations. Some dogs with hyperadrenocorticism are misdiagnosed as having primary hepatic disease because of hepatomegaly, increased hepatic enzymes (especially SAP), increased serum bile acid concentrations, and vacuolar hepatopathy secondary to hyperadrenocorticism.

A definitive diagnosis of hyperadrenocorticism and differentiation between PDH and adrenocortical tumor require evaluation of plasma cortisol concentrations after manipulation of the pituitary-adrenocortical axis with ACTH or dex-

amethasone (Fig. 8–14). Baseline plasma cortisol concentration, by itself, has *no* diagnostic value. Tests to confirm hyperadrenocorticism include the ACTH-stimulation test, low-dose dexamethasone suppression test, and combination ACTH-stimulation/dexamethasone suppression test. Tests to differentiate between PDH and adrenocortical tumor include endogenous ACTH concentration, low-dose dexamethasone suppression test, high-dose dexamethasone suppression test, and abdominal ultrasonography. Diagnosis of iatrogenic hyperadrenocorticism is based on historical confirmation of glucocorticoid administration and results of the ACTH-stimulation test. Sections that follow have specific information on these tests.

Causes of Hypocortisolemia • The most clinically relevant cause of hypocortisolemia is primary hypoadrenocorticism (see Table 8–10), which results after destruction of the zona fasciculata (glucocorticoid-producing zone) plus the zona glomerulosa (mineralocorticoid-producing zone) of the adrenal cortex. Rarely, selective hypocortisolism occurs if only the zona fasciculata has been damaged. Additional causes include iatrogenic hyperadrenocorticism (see Causes of Hypercortisolemia), secondary hypoadrenocorticism (a deficiency of glucocorticoid secretion, which usually results from inadequate ACTH secretion secondary to pituitary disease),

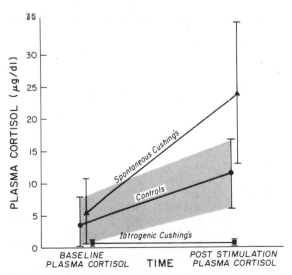

Figure 8–13 Mean plasma cortisol concentrations (± 2 SD) determined before and 1 hour after the administration of synthetic ACTH in control dogs, dogs with spontaneous hyperadrenocorticism, and dogs with iatrogenic hyperadrenocorticism. (From Feldman EC, Nelson RW: Canine and Feline Endocrinology and Reproduction. Philadelphia, WB Saunders, 1987, p 162. Reprinted with permission.)

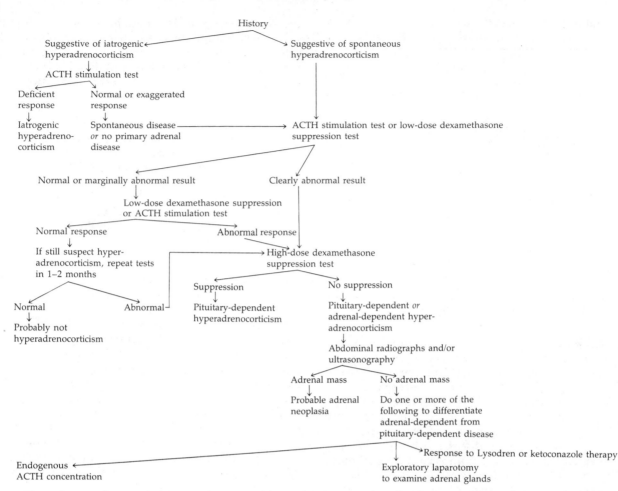

Figure 8–14 Evaluation of patients with suspected hyperadrenocorticism based on history (polyuria-polydipsia, polyphagia, anestrus, panting), physical examination (truncal alopecia, potbelly, calcinosis cutis, hepatomegaly), or laboratory findings (increased serum alkaline phosphatase, lymphopenia, eosinopenia, hypercholesterolemia, urinary tract infection).

megestrol acetate therapy, and artifact due to improper sample handling.

Primary hypoadrenocorticism typically occurs in young adult dogs and rarely in cats. A suspicion of hypoadrenocorticism can often be gained after careful evaluation of the history, physical examination, and routine clinical pathology (i.e., CBC, serum biochemical panel, urinalysis; see description under Plasma Cortisol, Common Indications). Abnormalities identified on clinical pathology may include a mild nonregenerative anemia, lack of a stress leukogram in a sick dog or cat, hyperkalemia, hyponatremia, hypochloremia, prerenal azotemia, hyperphosphatemia, mild hypercalcemia (12–14 mg/dl), mild hypoglycemia (45–60 mg/dl), or metabolic acidosis. Ideally, urine specific gravity is hypersthenuric (i.e., > 1.030), which allows differentiation of prerenal from renal azotemia. Unfortunately, urine specific gravity can be isosthenuric in primary hypoadrenocorticism because of renal sodium wasting and loss

of the renal medullary concentration gradient. Cardiac conduction disturbances may develop with severe hyperkalemia (i.e., > 7 mEq/L). These are readily identified on a lead II rhythm strip of an ECG and may include dampening of the P wave, prolongation of the PR interval and QRS complex, spiking of the T wave, or ventricular arrhythmias.

The hallmark abnormalities of hypoadrenocorticism are hyperkalemia, hyponatremia, and hypochloremia. The serum sodium:potassium ratio reflects changes in these electrolytes and has frequently been used to identify primary hypoadrenocorticism. The normal ratio varies between 27:1 and 40:1. Values are often well below 27:1 in primary hypoadrenocorticism. Normal serum electrolyte concentrations, however, do not rule out adrenal insufficiency. Serum electrolyte concentrations may be normal early in the course of disease, in selective hypocortisolism, in hypoadrenal patients that have recently received fluid therapy, and in

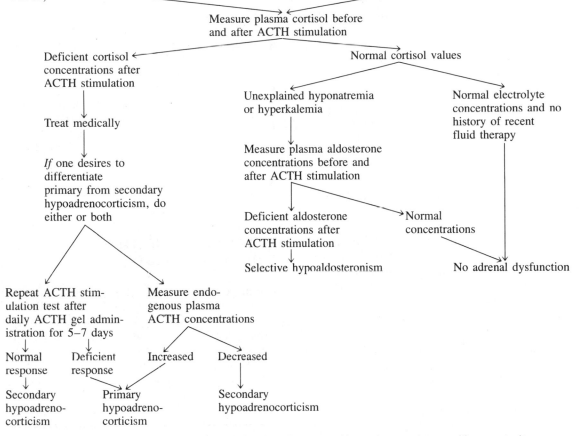

Hyponatremia and/or hyperkalemia (Na:K usually < 27:1)

History and/or physical examination suggestive of adrenoinsufficiency

Measure plasma cortisol before and after ACTH stimulation

Deficient cortisol concentrations after ACTH stimulation

Normal cortisol values

Unexplained hyponatremia or hyperkalemia

Normal electrolyte concentrations and no history of recent fluid therapy

Treat medically

Measure plasma aldosterone concentrations before and after ACTH stimulation

If one desires to differentiate primary from secondary hypoadrenocorticism, do either or both

Deficient aldosterone concentrations after ACTH stimulation

Normal concentrations

Selective hypoaldosteronism

No adrenal dysfunction

Repeat ACTH stimulation test after daily ACTH gel administration for 5–7 days

Measure endogenous plasma ACTH concentrations

Normal response

Deficient response

Increased

Decreased

Secondary hypoadrenocorticism

Primary hypoadrenocorticism

Secondary hypoadrenocorticism

Figure 8–15 Diagnostic evaluation of dogs and cats with suspected hypoadrenocorticism and hypocortisolism.

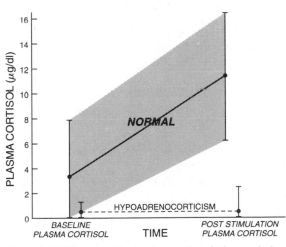

Figure 8–16 Plasma cortisol concentrations before and after exogenous ACTH stimulation in normal dogs and in dogs with hypoadrenocorticism. The ranges are means ± 2 SD. (From Feldman EC, Nelson RW: Canine and Feline Endocrinology and Reproduction. Philadelphia, WB Saunders, 1987, p 209. Reprinted with permission.)

secondary hypoadrenocorticism. In addition, other disorders, most notably affecting the kidneys, gastrointestinal system, and liver, can cause serum electrolyte alterations that mimic adrenal insufficiency. Refer to Chapter 6 for other causes of hyponatremia, hypochloremia, and hyperkalemia.

Confirmation of primary and secondary hypoadrenocorticism requires evaluation of an ACTH-stimulation test (Fig. 8–15). Dogs and cats with adrenal insufficiency have low or low-normal baseline plasma cortisol concentration and minimal to no increase in plasma cortisol after administration of ACTH (Fig. 8–16). The ACTH-stimulation test does not distinguish dogs and cats with primary versus secondary adrenal insufficiency. Concurrent electrolyte abnormalities would imply primary hypoadrenocorticism. Normal serum electrolyte concentrations do not differentiate early primary from secondary adrenal insufficiency. Differentiation requires measurement of baseline endogenous ACTH concentration (see Plasma Cortisol) or plasma aldosterone concentrations during the ACTH-stimulation test (see Fig. 8–15; see Aldosterone).

ACTH-STIMULATION TEST

Common Indications ● To confirm hypoadrenocorticism and iatrogenic hyperadrenocorticism, to screen for spontaneous hyperadrenocorticism, and to monitor mitotane (op'-DDD) therapy in dogs with PDH. The ACTH-stimulation test does not differentiate between PDH and adrenocortical tumor. Advantages: readily available, relatively inexpensive, and easy to interpret; 80% to 85% accuracy in identifying spontaneous hyperadrenocorticism. Disadvantages: may be affected (i.e., exaggerated) by chronic illness and stress, does not differentiate between primary and secondary hypoadrenocorticism. It is especially unreliable in diagnosing adrenal tumors.

Protocol ● The protocol for the ACTH-stimulation test differs between dogs and cats and with the type of ACTH used. When using ACTH gel, blood for cortisol assay is obtained before and 2 hours after (dogs) and before and 1 and 2 hours after (cats) intramuscular administration of 2.2 U ACTH gel/kg of body weight. When using synthetic ACTH, blood for cortisol assay is obtained before and 1 hour after intramuscular administration of 0.25 mg of synthetic ACTH per dog and before and 30 and 60 minutes after intramuscular administration of 0.125 mg synthetic ACTH per cat. The ACTH-stimulation test can be performed at any time of the day.

Artifacts and Drug Therapy That May Alter Results ● Anything that can alter plasma cortisol concentration can affect the results of the ACTH-stimulation test (see Plasma Cortisol, Artifacts That May Alter Plasma Cortisol Concentration). Anticonvulsant medications may spuriously increase results of the ACTH-stimulation test.

Interpretation in dogs:

Post-ACTH cortisol, < 5 µg/dl:	hypoadrenocorticism or iatrogenic hyperadrenocorticism
Post-ACTH cortisol, 6 to 18 µg/dl:	normal
Post-ACTH cortisol, 18 to 24 µg/dl:	suggestive of spontaneous hyperadrenocorticism
Post-ACTH cortisol, > 24 µg/dl:	strongly suggestive of spontaneous hyperadrenocorticism

Interpretation in cats:

post-ACTH cortisol, < 5 µg/dl:	hypoadrenocorticism or iatrogenic hyperadrenocorticism
Post-ACTH cortisol, 6 to 12 µg/dl:	normal
Post-ACTH cortisol, 13 to 16 µg/dl:	suggestive of spontaneous hyperadrenocorticism
Post-ACTH cortisol, > 16 µg/dl:	strongly suggestive of spontaneous hyperadrenocorticism

To convert µg/dl to ng/ml, see Plasma Cortisol, Analysis.

LOW-DOSE DEXAMETHASONE SUPPRESSION TEST

Common Indications ● To screen for spontaneous hyperadrenocorticism and to differentiate between PDH and adrenocortical tumor. This test does not identify iatrogenic hyperadrenocorticism, nor is it used to assess response to mitotane or ketoconazole therapy. Advantages: readily available, relatively inexpensive and easy to interpret; 95% to 98% accuracy in identifying spontaneous hyperadrenocorticism. Disadvantages: can be affected by acute stress, other procedures must be avoided until completion of the test, requires 8 hours to complete.

Protocol ● Ideally, this test should be started between 8 and 9 AM after a patient has been hospitalized overnight. In addition, the dog or cat should rest quietly in the cage except when walked outside or when blood samples are obtained for the test. In dogs, a plasma sample for cortisol analysis is obtained immediately before and 4 and 8 hours after intravenous administration of 0.01 mg dexamethasone per kg of body weight. The same dose of dexamethasone is used in cats; however, blood samples are obtained immediately before and 4, 6, and 8 hours after intravenous dexamethasone administration. Dexamethasone sodium phosphate or dexamethasone in polyethylene glycol can be used for this test.

Analysis and Artifacts ● See Plasma Cortisol.

Artifacts and Drug Therapy That May Alter Results ● Anything that can alter plasma cortisol concentration can affect the results of the low-dose dexamethasone suppression test (see Plasma Cortisol, Artifacts That May Alter Plasma Cortisol Concentration). Anticonvulsant medications may also spuriously increase results of this test.

Interpretation ● The 8-hour postdexamethasone plasma cortisol concentration is used to confirm hyperadrenocorticism (Fig. 8–17). Plasma cortisol values < 1.0 μg/dl 8 hours after dexamethasone administration are normal, between 1.0 and 1.5 μg/dl are nonconfirmatory, and > 1.5 μg/dl are consistent with spontaneous hyperadrenocorticism.

If the 8-hour postdexamethasone cortisol value supports hyperadrenocorticism, the 4-hour postdexamethasone plasma cortisol value may then be of value in distinguishing between PDH and adrenocortical tumor (Mack and Feldman, 1990). Low doses of dexamethasone may suppress pituitary ACTH secretion and plasma cortisol concentration in some dogs with PDH during the initial 2 to 6 hours of the test. Suppression does not occur in dogs with adrenocortical tumor, nor does it occur in 50% to 60% of dogs with PDH. Suppression, defined as either a 4-hour postdexamethasone cortisol concentration <1.0 μg/dl or a 4-hour postdexamethasone cortisol concentration < 50% of baseline cortisol concentration, would support PDH, but lack of suppression does not differentiate between PDH and adrenocortical tumor.

The low-dose dexamethasone suppression test

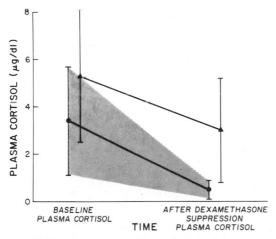

Figure 8–17 Mean plasma cortisol concentrations (± 2 SD) determined before and 8 hours after administration of a low dexamethasone dose (0.01 mg/kg) intravenously in control dogs (●) and in dogs with hyperadrenocorticism (▲). Note the slight overlap of values following dexamethasone. (From Feldman EC, Nelson RW: Canine and Feline Endocrinology and Reproduction. Philadelphia, WB Saunders, 1987, p 164. Reprinted with permission.)

is difficult to interpret in cats. An occasional normal cat escapes the suppressive effects of intravenous dexamethasone at 0.01 mg/kg, and falls outside the normal 8-hour postdexamethasone reference range (i.e., 8-hour postdexamethasone plasma cortisol > 1.5 μg/dl) (Smith and Feldman, 1987). Hyperadrenocorticism should be strongly suspected if the plasma cortisol concentration is > 1.5 μg/dl at 4, 6, and 8 hours after dexamethasone administration. The results are inconclusive if either the 4-hour (or 4- and 6-hour) cortisol value is < 1.5 μg/dl and the 6 and 8 (or 8-hour) cortisol value is > 1.5 μg/dl. The test should then be repeated using dexamethasone at 0.1 mg/kg (see High-Dose Dexamethasone Suppression Test). Because of the potential for escape in normal cats, the low-dose dexamethasone suppression test should never represent the sole evidence for hyperadrenocorticism in cats.

COMBINED ACTH-STIMULATION TEST/DEXAMETHASONE SUPPRESSION TEST

Rare Indications ● To screen for hyperadrenocorticism. This test does not reliably differentiate PDH from adrenocortical tumor and should not be used for this purpose. Advantages: readily available, relatively quick and easy to interpret; 75% to 85% accuracy in identifying spontaneous hyperadrenocorticism when the postdexamethasone and post-ACTH plasma cortisol concentrations are interpreted independently of each other. Disadvantages: more expensive and less reliable than ACTH-stimulation test or low-dose dexamethasone suppression test, may be affected by chronic illness and stress.

Protocol ● Ideally, this test should be started between 8 and 9 AM after a patient has been hospitalized overnight. In addition, the dog or cat should rest quietly in the cage except when blood samples are obtained for the test. A plasma sample for cortisol analysis is obtained immediately before and 2 hours after intravenous administration of 0.1 mg dexamethasone per kg. Immediately after the 2-hour blood sample is obtained, ACTH (either ACTH gel at 2.2 U/kg, 0.25 mg synthetic ACTH per dog, or 0.125 mg synthetic ACTH per cat) is administered intramuscularly and plasma samples for cortisol obtained 1 and 2 hours (ACTH gel) or 30 minutes and 1 hour (synthetic ACTH) after ACTH administration.

Analysis, Artifacts, and Drug Treatment That May Alter Values ● See Plasma Cortisol.

Interpretation ● In normal dogs, plasma cortisol concentration should be < 1.5 μg/dl, preferably < 1.0 μg/dl, 2 hours after dexamethasone administration and between 6 and 18 μg/dl after ACTH administration (Eiler et al., 1984). Plasma cortisol values > 1.5 μg/dl after dexamethasone administration or > 18 μg/dl after ACTH administration would suggest hyperadrenocorticism. Similar parameters are used for cats, except that post-ACTH cortisol concentrations > 15 μg/dl would suggest hyperadrenocorticism.

HIGH-DOSE DEXAMETHASONE SUPPRESSION TEST

Common Indications ● To distinguish PDH from adrenocortical tumor in dogs with confirmed spontaneous hyperadrenocorticism and to help confirm hyperadrenocorticism in cats with inconclusive low-dose dexamethasone suppression test results.

Protocol ● Ideally, this test should be started between 8 and 9 AM after a patient has been hospitalized overnight. In addition, the dog or cat should rest quietly in the cage except when walked outside or when blood samples are obtained for the test. In dogs, a plasma sample for cortisol analysis is obtained immediately before and 4 and 8 hours after intravenous administration of 0.1 mg dexamethasone per kg of body weight. The same dose of dexamethasone is used in cats; however, blood samples are obtained immediately before and 4, 6, and 8 hours after intravenous dexamethasone administration. Dexamethasone sodium phosphate or dexamethasone in polyethylene glycol can be used for this test.

Interpretation ● A higher dose of dexamethasone is used in this test in an attempt to suppress pituitary ACTH secretion in dogs with PDH. Suppression is defined as a 4- or 8-hour postdexamethasone plasma cortisol concentration that is < 50% of the predexamethasone plasma cortisol concentration. Suppression of plasma cortisol concentration is supportive of PDH (Fig. 8–18). Failure to induce suppression of the plasma cortisol concentration after administration of a high dose of dexamethasone is noted in 20% to 40% of dogs with PDH and virtually 100% of dogs with adrenocortical tumor. There-

fore, lack of suppression has provided no further information concerning etiology. Higher doses of dexamethasone could be administered in an attempt to suppress pituitary ACTH secretion in dogs with dexamethasone-resistant PDH (Fig. 8–19). However, higher doses of dexamethasone have not consistently yielded results that have been significantly easier to interpret. Alternatively, evaluation of abdominal radiographs, abdominal ultrasonography, and baseline plasma endogenous ACTH concentration may help differentiate PDH from adrenocortical tumor.

The high-dose dexamethasone suppression test is also used to diagnose hyperadrenocorticism in cats. In normal cats, the plasma cortisol concentrations should be < 1.5 μg/dl 4, 6, and 8 hours after dexamethasone administration. Similar results may be found in some cats with PDH. Hyperadrenocorticism should be suspected if the 8-hour, and ideally the 6-hour, plasma cortisol concentration is > 1.5 μg/dl. Any postdexamethasone plasma cortisol concentration < 50% of the precortisol value would support PDH once hyperadrenocorticism is confirmed.

URINE CORTICOSTEROID: CREATININE RATIO

Occasional Indication ● As a screening test for hyperadrenocorticism in dogs. The urine corticosteroid:creatinine ratio as determined from a random urine sample is significantly increased in dogs with spontaneous hyperadrenocorticism compared with healthy dogs (Stolp et al., 1983). Unfortunately, an increased urine corticosteroid:creatinine ratio is not specific for hyperadrenocorticism, because it is increased in dogs with nonadrenal illness and in dogs with clinical signs consistent with hyperadrenocorticism but with a normal pituitary-adrenocortical axis as evaluated by ACTH-stimulation and dexamethasone suppression tests (Feldman and Mack, 1992). Although a normal urine corticosteroid:creatinine ratio rules out spontaneous hyperadrenocorticism, an increased ratio is not diagnostic of hyperadrenocorticism.

Protocol ● Cortisol and creatinine concentrations are measured in urine. It is preferable to have the owner collect the urine at home with the dog in a "nonstressed" state. The urine corticosteroid:creatinine ratio is determined by dividing the urine cortisol concentration (in μmol/L) by the urine creatinine concentration (in μmol/L).

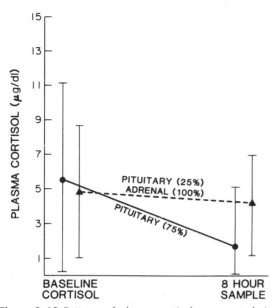

Figure 8–18 Patterns of plasma cortisol responses during high-dose (0.1 mg/kg) dexamethasone suppression testing in dogs with pituitary-dependent or adrenal-dependent hyperadrenocorticism. Note that suppression is diagnostic of pituitary dependency. Lack of suppression occurs in all adrenal tumor cases and in 25% of pituitary-dependent cases. (From Feldman EC, Nelson RW: Canine and Feline Endocrinology and Reproduction. Philadelphia, WB Saunders, 1987, p 169. Reprinted with permission.)

Interpretation • At the University of California at Davis Veterinary Endocrinology laboratory, the urine corticosteroid:creatinine ratio is $< 1.35 \times 10^{-5}$ in normal dogs, between 2 and 210×10^{-5} in dogs with spontaneous hyperadrenocorti-

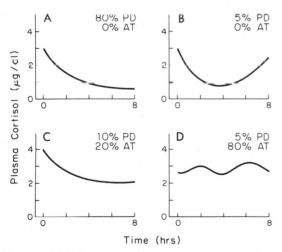

Figure 8–19 Patterns of plasma cortisol responses during megadose (1 mg/kg) dexamethasone suppression testing in dogs with hyperadrenocorticism. (PD, pituitary-dependent hyperadrenocorticism; AT, adrenal-dependent hyperadrenocorticism.) (From Peterson ME: Hyperadrenocorticism. Vet Clin North Am 1984;14:741. Reprinted with permission.)

cism, and between 0.8 and 15×10^{-5} in dogs with chronic illness and other disorders causing polyuria and polydipsia. Because of overlap in results between dogs with hyperadrenocorticism and dogs with other illnesses, the corticosteroid:creatinine ratio is best used as a screening test for hyperadrenocorticism, and test results must be interpreted cautiously.

PLASMA ALDOSTERONE

Rare Indications • To identify selective aldosterone deficiency in patients with hyponatremia, hyperkalemia, and normal plasma cortisol responsiveness to ACTH, to identify hyperaldosteronism (?), and to assess the hormonal function of an adrenal mass. Clinical findings with hyperaldosteronism include lethargy, weakness, hypokalemia, hypernatremia, hypertension, and adrenomegaly.

Analysis • Measured in 0.5 ml of EDTA plasma by RIA. Baseline plasma aldosterone concentration has little to no diagnostic value. Interpretation of plasma aldosterone is always done after stimulation of the zona glomerulosa with ACTH (see ACTH-Stimulation Test). Timing of blood sampling is the same as for plasma cortisol. For meaningful results, the aldosterone assay must be validated for use in dogs and cats, and normal values established. The assay is currently available for dogs (see Appendix I).

Artifacts • Storage at 22° C for $\geq$ 3 days or at 37° C for 1 day decreases the measured plasma aldosterone concentration.

Interpretation • Normal plasma aldosterone concentration in dogs: baseline, 5 to 345 pg/ml; 1 hour post-ACTH, 91 to 634 pg/ml; 2 hours post-ACTH, 71 to 758 pg/ml. To convert pg/ml to pmol/L, multiply pg/ml $\times$ 2.774.

After stimulation with ACTH, the plasma aldosterone value at 1 and 2 hours post-ACTH should be double baseline value, unless the baseline value is in the upper range of normal or above. Hypoaldosteronism is documented by finding a low baseline value and minimal to no increase in post-ACTH plasma aldosterone concentration (Golden and Lothrop, 1988). Markedly increased baseline and post-ACTH plasma aldosterone concentration would suggest primary hyperaldosteronism in a dog and cat with no other explanation for hypokalemia, hyperkaluria, hypernatremia, decreased natriuresis, and systemic hypertension. Identification of unilateral adrenomegaly with abdominal ultrasonography would further support the diagnosis.

References

Bauer JE: Diet-induced alterations of lipoprotein metabolism. JAVMA 1992;201:1691–1694.

Eiler H, Oliver JW, Legendre AM: Stages of hyperadrenocorticism: Response of hyperadrenocorticoid dogs to the combined dexamethasone suppression/ACTH stimulation test. JAVMA 1984;185:289–294.

Feldman EC, Mack RE: Urine cortisol:creatinine ratio as a screening test for hyperadrenocorticism in dogs. JAVMA 1992;200:1637–1641.

Feldman EC, Nelson RW: Hypothyroidism. In Feldman EC, Nelson RW (eds): Canine and Feline Endocrinology and Reproduction. Philadelphia, WB Saunders, 1987, pp 55–90.

Ferguson DC: Thyroid function tests in the dog. Recent concepts. Vet Clin North Am 1984;14:793.

Flanders JA, Scarlett JM, Blue JT, et al: Adjustment of total serum calcium concentration for binding to albumin and protein in cats: 291 cases (1986–1987). JAVMA 1989;194:1609–1611.

Golden DL, Lothrop CD: A retrospective study of aldosterone secretion in normal and adrenopathic dogs. J Vet Intern Med 1988;2:121–125.

Kallet AJ, Richter KP, Feldman EC, et al: Primary hyperparathyroidism in cats: Seven cases (1984–1989). JAVMA 1991;199:1767–1771.

Kaneko JJ, Mattheeuws D, Rottiers RP, et al: Glucose tolerance and insulin response in diabetes mellitus of dogs. J Small Anim Pract 1977;18:85–94.

Kirk CA, Feldman EC, Nelson RW: The diagnosis of naturally occurring Type I and Type II diabetes mellitus in the cat. Am J Vet Res 1993;54:463–467.

Mack RE, Feldman EC: Comparison of two low-dose dexamethasone suppression protocols as screening and discrimination tests in dogs with hyperadrenocorticism. JAVMA 1990;197:1603–1606.

Meuten DJ, Chew DJ, Capen CC, et al: Relationship of serum total calcium to albumin and total protein in dogs. JAVMA 1982;180:63–67.

Montgomery T, Nelson RW, Ferguson DC, et al: Comparison of five analog RIAs for free thyroxine in dogs (abstract). Proceedings, Annual Meeting, Veterinary College of Internal Medicine, New Orleans, May 1991.

Muller GH, Kirk RW, Scott DW: Cutaneous endocrinology. In Feldman EC, Nelson RW (eds): Small Animal Dermatology. 3rd ed. Philadelphia, WB Saunders, 1983, pp 492–560.

Nelson RW, Feldman EC, Smith MC: Hyperadrenocorticism in cats: Seven cases (1978–1987). JAVMA 1988;193:245–250.

Nelson RW, Ihle SL, Feldman EC, et al: Serum free thyroxine concentration in healthy dogs, dogs with hypothyroidism, and euthyroid dogs with concurrent illness. JAVMA 1991;198:1401–1407.

Peterson ME, Graves TK, Gamble DA: Triiodothyronine (T_3) suppression test. An aid in the diagnosis of mild hyperthyroidism in cats. J Vet Intern Med 1990;4:233–238.

Peterson ME, Greco DS, Orth DN: Primary hypoadrenocorticism in ten cats. J Vet Intern Med 1989;3:55–58.

Reimers TJ, Lawler DF, Sutaria PM, et al: Effects of age, sex, and body size on serum concentrations of thyroid and adrenocortical hormones in dogs. Am J Vet Res 1990;51:454–457.

Smith MC, Feldman EC: Plasma endogenous ACTH concentrations and plasma cortisol responses to synthetic ACTH and dexamethasone sodium phosphate in healthy cats. Am J Vet Res 1987;48:1719–1724.

Stolp R, Rijnberk A, Meijer JC, et al: Urinary corticoids in the diagnosis of canine hyperadrenocorticism. Res Vet Sci 1983;34:141–144.

Thacker EL, Refsal KR, Bull RW: Prevalence of autoantibodies to thyroglobulin, thyroxine, or triiodothyronine and relationship of autoantibodies and serum concentrations of iodothyronines in dogs. Am J Vet Res 1992;53:449–453.

Torrance AG, Nachreiner R: Intact parathyroid hormone assay and total calcium concentration in the diagnosis of disorders of calcium metabolism in dogs. J Vet Intern Med 1989;3:86–89.

Young DW, Sartin JL, Kemppainen RJ: Abnormal canine triiodothyronine-binding factor characterized as a possible triiodothyronine autoantibody. Am J Vet Res 1985;46:1346–1350.

Zerbe CA: Canine hyperlipidemias. In Kirk RW (ed): Current Veterinary Therapy IX. Philadelphia, WB Saunders, 1986, pp 1045–1053.

Michael D. Willard
David C. Twedt

9 Gastrointestinal, Pancreatic, and Hepatic Disorders

Gastrointestinal problems (e.g., vomiting, diarrhea, weight loss, anorexia, icterus, hepatomegaly, abnormal behavior associated with eating, and abdominal pain) typically necessitate laboratory testing. Dysphagia, regurgitation, ptyalism, halitosis, constipation, mucoid stools, hematochezia, and melena are best approached initially by other means (physical examination, radiology, endoscopy, or surgical biopsy).

DIFFERENTIATION OF EXPECTORATION, REGURGITATION, AND VOMITING

Whenever fluid, mucus, foam, food, or blood is expelled from the mouth, one must determine whether vomiting, regurgitation, gagging, or expectoration is occurring. The history is often sufficient to allow differentiation.

Expectoration

Expectoration is the coughing up of material from the lungs or major airways. The material typically is frothy mucus or red blood, but bile is absent. The characteristic sequence of coughing followed by oral expulsion must be determined from the history. Regurgitation and vomiting typically occur without simultaneous coughing, although regurgitation is often accompanied by tracheitis-aspiration pneumonia. Of the three, expectoration should be the easiest to identify.

Regurgitation

Regurgitation is due to oral, pharyngeal, or esophageal dysfunction and is typically characterized as a relatively passive expulsion of esophageal contents. Gagging is the expulsion of oral or pharyngeal material and may be associated with disorders of dysphagia (difficult swallowing) or with regurgitation. The relatively minor abdominal contractions associated with gagging can often be differentiated from the vigorous abdominal contractions that vomiting commonly produces. Regurgitation may occur seconds to hours after eating or drinking. If only saliva is regurgitated, eating may not have occurred for hours or even days before the act. Regurgitated food material may be in a tubular form conforming to the shape of the esophageal lumen, but this is rare. Most clients cannot reliably distinguish undigested from digested

food. Regurgitated material that has been in the esophagus for hours is macerated, is mixed with saliva and mucus, and may have a bad odor. Only blood that has been partially digested by gastric acid (e.g., "coffee grounds") can readily be distinguished from its undigested form.

It is sometimes difficult to differentiate vomiting from regurgitation, and a patient can have both processes occurring concurrently. Vomiting may cause secondary esophagitis with subsequent regurgitation, or a patient with longstanding esophageal disease may develop another concurrent disorder causing vomiting. It is important to clarify the chronologic order of occurrence of specific signs. Finally, some patients have signs suggestive of regurgitation but in fact are vomiting. To aid in differentiation, if time allows one may attempt to observe the act of expulsion. Watching the patient eat may be helpful because pharyngeal dysphagia becomes quite obvious and suggests oropharyngeal disease. Some patients with pharyngeal dysphagia have concurrent esophageal muscle weakness. If one cannot differentiate the two by history or physical examination, contrast radiographs of the pharynx and esophagus usually are definitive.

Regurgitation is usually best evaluated by history, physical examination, plain and contrast radiographs, or esophagoscopy (Fig. 9–1). Contrast radiographs should use barium instead of iodide contrast agents unless esophageal rupture is strongly suspected. The main purpose of a contrast esophagram is to distinguish esophageal weakness from esophageal obstruction, diverticulum, or fistula. Note: Some drugs (e.g., xylazine) commonly used for restraint cause esophageal paralysis, making the radiographs potentially misleading. Esophagoscopy is usually not a good way to diagnose esophageal muscle weakness, but it may be used to sample mass lesions, differentiate intramural from extramural obstruction, identify esophagitis that has been missed by radiographs, detect diverticuli, and remove foreign objects. Patients with acquired esophageal weakness should be evaluated for myopathies, neuropathies, and myasthenia gravis (generalized or localized to the esophagus). Occasionally hypoadrenocorticism, hyperkalemia, lead poisoning, *Spirocerca lupi*, and selected central nervous system (CNS) disorders (e.g., distemper or hydrocephalus) may be responsible. There are several causes of generalized or localized myopathies and neuropathies, such as trauma, dermatomyositis, thymoma, botulism, tick paralysis, hypothyroidism, hyperadrenocorticism, systemic lupus erythe-

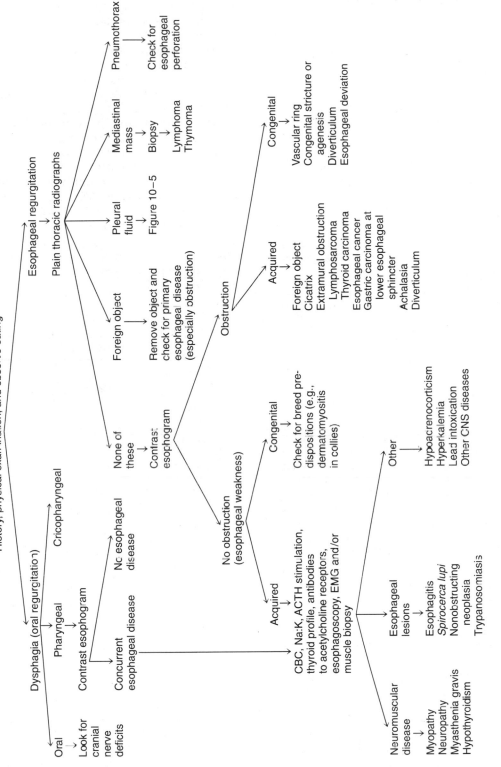

Figure 9–1 Diagnostic approach to chronic regurgitation in dogs and cats.

Table 9–1 MAJOR CAUSES OF ACUTE VOMITING IN
DOGS AND CATS

Motion sickness
Postoperative nausea
Acute gastritis-enteritis (various viral or
    bacterial agents or toxins)
    Parvoviral enteritis (dogs and cats)
    Hemorrhagic gastroenteritis
    Parasites
Gastrointestinal obstruction
    Obstructing foreign body
    Linear foreign body
    Intussusception
Dietary indiscretion
    Overeating
    Eating inappropriate or spoiled foods
Acute pancreatitis
Drug administration
    Adriamycin
    Chloramphenicol
    Cisplatin
    Cyclophosphamide
    Digitalis
    Erythromycin
    Narcotics
    Nitrofurantoin
    Tetracycline
    Theophylline
    Xylazine
Intoxications
    Ethylene glycol
    Herbicides
    Organophosphates
    Strychnine

matosus, nutritional factors, toxoplasmosis, and
trypanosomiasis. Dysautonomia has been recognized in both dogs and cats and is associated
with a generalized dysfunction of the autonomic
nervous system, which includes the regulation
of esophageal motility. Hypothyroidism and systemic lupus erythematosus in particular may exist without other obvious clinical signs. It is important to detect these underlying disorders lest
effective symptomatic therapy for the esophageal regurgitation allow progression of the underlying disease or death. It is also wise to evaluate patients with unexpected esophageal
foreign objects (e.g., a bolus of food) for partial
obstructions (i.e., a subclinical vascular ring
anomaly).

Vomiting

Vomiting is a reflex act originating in the
CNS. A number of conditions can stimulate
vomiting. One must consider both primary
gastrointestinal disease as well as nongastroin-
testinal disorders as causes. Examples of nongas-
trointestinal disorders include metabolic, in-

flammatory, and toxic conditions. Most patients
in clinical situations are in fact probably vomiting not from primary gastrointestinal problems
but rather from secondary conditions.

Vomiting is classically characterized by pro-
dromal salivation, licking of lips, or retching;
however, these signs are not consistent. Vomiting may occur any time after eating or drinking
(seconds to hours). A patient may vomit food,
water, fresh blood, or mucus that is indistinguishable from regurgitated material. Bile, partially digested blood, or expelled material with
a pH of 5 or less confirms that vomiting is occurring. Note: Vomited duodenal contents may
have a pH of 6 or more but might not be bile
colored. A urine dipstick with a pH indicator is
useful in making the determination.

Clinically, vomiting patients are best divided
into those with acute (<2 weeks) versus those
with chronic (>2 weeks) vomiting. The most
common categories of causes for each are listed
in Tables 9–1 and 9–2. Acute vomiting often

Table 9–2 MAJOR CAUSES OF CHRONIC VOMITING
IN DOGS AND CATS

Obstructive disease
    Foreign objects
    Intussusception
    Neoplasia
    Pyloric stenosis
    Gastric antral mucosal hyperplasia
    Inflammatory infiltrates
    Chronic partial gastric volvulus
    Idiopathic hypomotility of stomach and/or
        intestines (rare)
    Congenital structural abnormalities (rare)
Inflammatory disease
    Chronic gastritis
    Inflammatory bowel disease (small or large
        intestines)
    Gastrointestinal ulceration/erosion
    Peritonitis (sterile or septic)
    Pancreatitis
    Pharyngitis (due to upper respiratory virus in
        cats)
    Parasites
Other diseases that cause vomiting via the chemoreceptor
    trigger zone and/or vagal afferents
    Hepatic disease/insufficiency
    Hypoadrenocorticism
    Diabetic ketoacidosis
    Uremia
    Hypercalcemia
    Cholecystitis (rare)
Miscellaneous causes
    Feline heartworm disease
    Feline hyperthyroidism
    Central nervous system disease (e.g., limbic
        epilepsy, tumor, encephalitis, or increased
        intracranial pressure)
    Psychotic or behavioral changes
    Early congestive heart failure

spontaneously resolves if the patient is supported by fluid, electrolyte, and acid-base therapy, but one must determine if obstruction, shock, sepsis, or acute abdomen seems likely. A thorough history and physical examination are indicated first. Electrolyte and acid-base evaluations or radiographs should be considered next if the disease is severe. If vomiting persists, is progressive, or is attended by other clinical signs (e.g., polyuria-polydipsia, weight loss, icterus, painful abdomen, ascites, weakness, hematemesis), additional testing is indicated (Fig. 9–2).

Diet and Parasites

Diet and parasites commonly cause acute and chronic vomiting; hence, dietary change (to a bland or a hypoallergenic diet), fecal examination, and broad-spectrum anthelmintic therapy (such as febendazole) are reasonable initial choices in nonobstructed patients. Continued vomiting is an indication for laboratory tests or radiographs.

Obstruction

Gastric or intestinal obstruction does not require clinicopathologic testing for diagnosis. A complete blood count (CBC) may suggest sepsis, disseminated intravascular coagulation, or severe blood loss; renal function, electrolyte, and acid-base evaluations are recommended before anesthesia. One cannot reliably predict changes in these parameters even when the obstruction is known to be intestinal or gastric. Gastric vomiting infrequently causes a hypokalemic, hypochloremic metabolic alkalosis with aciduria. These changes generally occur secondary to either persistent and profuse vomiting, gastric outflow obstruction, or high duodenal obstruction. Most patients with gastric vomiting are not alkalotic. Insignificant acid-base changes or metabolic acidosis due to dehydration with resultant lactic acidosis is more common. Intestinal obstruction may cause acidosis owing to loss of pancreatic bicarbonate, although some patients have a normal blood pH or a metabolic alkalosis if the obstruction is high.

Abdominal palpation and radiography are the best initial diagnostic tests. In otherwise occult cases, contrast radiographs may be necessary. Barium is preferred over iodide compounds unless intestinal rupture is strongly suspected, in which case abdominal lavage (see Chapter 10) is indicated.

Extra-Alimentary Tract Disease

A serum chemistry profile should be obtained to help rule out acute pancreatitis (amylase and lipase are recommended, despite clear limitations), hepatic disease (alanine transferase [ALT], serum alkaline phosphatase [SAP], blood urea nitrogen [BUN], and albumin), hypoadrenocorticism (sodium and potassium), hypercalcemia (calcium and albumin), uremia (creatinine, BUN, and urinalysis), and diabetic ketoacidosis (glucose and urinalysis). Very young patients <12 to 14 weeks of age should have blood glucose monitored to avoid secondary hypoglycemia. More precise testing is occasionally required to diagnose these disorders (e.g., bile acids for hepatic insufficiency and adrenocorticotropic hormone (ACTH) stimulation test for hypocortisolemia). Other tests to consider are serum gastrin for gastrinoma, heartworm antigen enzyme-linked immunosorbent assay (ELISA) for feline heartworm disease, and serum thyroxine for feline hyperthyroidism.

Pancreatitis

Acute pancreatitis is relatively common in dogs but frequently unrecognized in cats. Predisposing causes in dogs include hyperlipidemia, fatty meals, or obesity. Pancreatitis can occur in any dog, but middle-aged obese female dogs, schnauzers, and Yorkshire terriers seem to be most commonly affected. Vomiting may or may not be associated with eating, abdominal pain, fasting hyperlipidemia, bloody diarrhea, and, rarely, diffuse subcutaneous fat necrosis. On radiographic examination, a mass or indistinctness (due to localized fluid) may be seen in the cranial right abdominal quadrant. Both serum amylase and lipase activities should be measured, but some affected dogs do not have an increase in either, in which case one must rely on other findings. Leukocytosis with or without a left shift (due to the sterile inflammation) and increased ALT and SAP concentrations (due to the proximity of the pancreas to the liver and obstruction of the biliary duct) are common. The latter may occasionally cause icterus. Mild to moderate hypocalcemia may occur. Abdominal ultrasonography may reveal abnormalities in the pancreatic region. If a pancreatic mass is discovered during surgery, it must be sampled because chronic pancreatitis is grossly indistinguishable from pancreatic neoplasia, and both may be associated with normal serum amylase and lipase values.

Feline pancreatitis is more difficult to diagnose. Vomiting may not be as prominent a sign as in dogs, and amylase and lipase values are more likely to be normal. Abdominal ultrasonography may be useful. A pancreatic biopsy

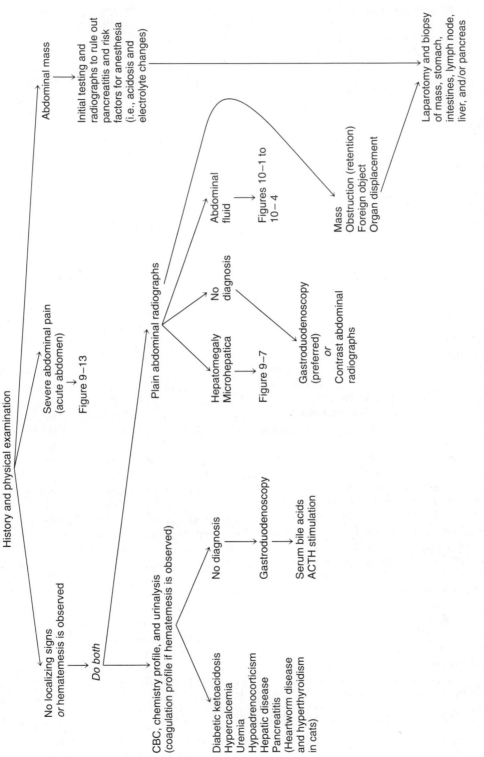

Figure 9-2 Diagnostic approach to chronic vomiting in a dog or cat that has been unresponsive to dietary change and anthelmintic therapy.

may be required for diagnosis. Feline pancreatitis may occasionally be due to toxoplasmosis (see Chapter 15) or to feline infectious peritonitis (FIP).

Gastritis, Enteritis, and Colitis

Chronic enteritis, colitis, or gastritis can cause various degrees of vomiting and may require mucosal biopsy for diagnosis. Plain and contrast abdominal radiographs may delineate infiltrative or inflammatory intestinal patterns. If gastritis or enteritis is suspected or if the other major causes of chronic vomiting have been ruled out, gastric and intestinal mucosal biopsies via endoscopy, biopsy capsule, or laparotomy are indicated. Inflammatory bowel disease is a significant cause of feline chronic vomiting. Duodenitis (without diarrhea) is also a significant cause in dogs; therefore, both gastric and intestinal biopsies should be performed. Finally, because 10% to 20% of patients with colitis vomit, it is useful to perform endoscopy routinely on both the upper and lower intestinal tracts in patients with chronic vomiting.

Hematemesis

Hematemesis is the vomiting of blood. It suggests gastric ulceration. The character of the vomitus may be either bright red blood or digested blood that resembles coffee grounds. Administration of nonsteroidal anti-inflammatory drugs (especially concurrently with corticosteroids) is a major reason for canine ulceration. Renal and hepatic failure, mast cell tumor, shock with poor mucosal perfusion, and coagulopathy must be considered. After these have been ruled out, endoscopy is indicated and allows diagnosis of ulceration (especially due to foreign object, inflammatory bowel disease, or neoplasia). Alternatively, one may treat symptomatically for ulceration; however, such treatment may allow progression of underlying disease.

Abdominal Inflammation

Septic or nonseptic peritonitis (or inflammation of any abdominal organ) may cause vomiting. Abdominocentesis or abdominal lavage (see Chapter 10) may be needed, especially if physical examination or abdominal radiographs suggest abdominal fluid. Occult cases may require exploratory surgery for diagnosis.

Gastrinoma

Gastrinoma (e.g., Zollinger-Ellison syndrome) is a gastrin-secreting tumor of the pancreatic islet cells; it causes a marked increase in gastric acid production and resultant duodenal ulceration. Gastrinoma is rare in dogs and cats but has been diagnosed more commonly since the advent of reliable serum gastrin assays. There are no other typical, unique clinicopathologic tests that suggest this disease. Any chronically vomiting middle-aged or older dog with weight loss or diarrhea is a reasonable suspect. Resting gastrin concentrations are typically increased. Duodenal ulceration and reflux esophagitis are commonly noted.

AMYLASE

Common Indications • Patients (especially obese) with vomiting, abdominal pain, nonseptic inflammatory abdominal exudate, icterus, or a prior history of pancreatitis. If pancreatitis is considered, it is recommended that both serum amylase and lipase values be determined. Disadvantages: poor sensitivity.

Analysis • Measured in 0.5 ml of serum, heparinized plasma, body fluid, and urine (?) by spectrophotometric methods using amyloclastic, saccharogenic, and chromogenic techniques. Turbidimetric, nephelometric, and "dry reagent" methods may also be used. Note: Different methods can give substantially different results in dogs. Some saccharogenic methods are affected by normal canine serum maltase concentrations and should not be used in dogs. Serum amylase activity is stable at room temperature for up to 7 days and at 4° C for as long as 1 month.

Normal Values • As with other enzymes, these vary between laboratories, depending on technique and units used.

Danger Values • None. The serum amylase activity does not correlate well with the severity of pancreatitis.

Artifacts • Falsely decreased: oxalate or citrate anticoagulants, lipemia, and increased serum pyruvate (Beckman's and Harleco's methods). Falsely increased: hemolysis.

Drug Therapy That May Cause Hyperamylasemia • Some drugs may occasionally cause pancreatitis (Table 9–3). Note that corticosteroids do not reliably cause an increase in serum amylase concentrations.

Table 9–3 DRUGS THAT MAY CAUSE ACUTE PANCREATITIS

Asparaginase
Azathioprine
Calcium
Estrogens
Furosemide
Glucocorticoids (especially dexamethasone)
Metronidazole
Salicylazosulfapyridine (Azulfidine)
Sulfonamides
Tetracycline
Thiazide diuretics

These drugs do not reliably cause pancreatitis, and the administration of one of these drugs plus signs of pancreatitis cannot be assumed to be cause and effect. However, a patient with acute pancreatitis or increased serum amylase or lipase determinations that is receiving one of these drugs should have the drug withdrawn, if possible, and the amylase and/or lipase rechecked later.

Causes of Hypoamylasemia ● Not significant. This finding does not support a diagnosis of pancreatic insufficiency.

Causes of Hyperamylasemia ● Decreased glomerular filtration (prerenal, renal, or postrenal azotemia) and pancreatitis are the two principal causes. Hyperamylasemia due to renal dysfunction usually is less than two to three times the upper limit of normal, whereas serum amylase values greater than this suggest pancreatic inflammation. However, patients with pancreatitis may have normal to markedly increased serum amylase values. Therefore, although a serum amylase value more than two to three times normal is suggestive, a normal value does not rule out pancreatitis.

Intestinal disease, ruptured intestines, and hepatic disease have been suspected of causing minor increases in serum amylase because of amylase present in these tissues. Serum amylase level appears to be an unreliable indicator of pancreatitis in cats.

Hyperamylasemia is an indication to search for pancreatitis by serum lipase, CBC, serum chemistry profile (including ALT and SAP), and abdominal radiographs/ultrasonography. In experimental pancreatitis in dogs, amylase concentrations increased rapidly and remained elevated for approximately 1 week. Once pancreatitis with hyperamylasemia has been diagnosed, following serum amylase values to monitor the progression of the disease is not useful.

Causes of Increased Urine Amylase ● This is not of proven value in dogs and cats and is not currently recommended.

Causes of Increased Fluid Amylase ● When ab-dominal fluid amylase is greater than serum amylase, a nonseptic exudate due to pancreatic disease is possible. Bowel rupture may also be possible.

LIPASE

Common Indications ● Same as for amylase. Serum lipase and amylase determinations should be done simultaneously to diagnose pancreatitis. Increased concentrations of amylase and lipase do not always parallel each other in cases of pancreatitis. Disadvantages: questionable sensitivity; some dogs with duodenal foreign objects or chronic gastritis have very increased serum lipase activities with no evidence of pancreatitis; 1 ml of serum is needed for some methods.

Analysis ● Measured in 1 ml of serum or body fluids using turbidimetric and titrimetric techniques. Methods using emulsified vegetable oils may be of greater clinical use than those using other substrates (e.g., stearate, palmitate, or laurate).

Normal Values ● As for other enzymes, these vary from laboratory to laboratory, depending on technique and units used.

Danger Values ● None. The severity of pancreatitis is not proportional to the increase in serum lipase activity.

Artifacts ● Falsely decreased: hemolysis and bilirubin (turbidimetric). Falsely increased: heavy metals and EDTA.

Drug Therapy That May Cause Hyperlipasemia ● Same as for amylase (see Table 9–3), plus heparin. Corticosteroids (dexamethasone) may increase serum lipase activity up to fivefold over baseline without histologic evidence of acute pancreatitis. However, many of these dogs still have lipase activities only slightly greater than the reference range.

Causes of Hypolipasemia ● Not significant. This finding does not support a diagnosis of pancreatic insufficiency.

Causes of Hyperlipasemia ● These are similar to the causes of hyperamylasemia (Fig. 9–3). Lipase may(?) be more specific for pancreatitis than is amylase, especially in cats. Renal dys-

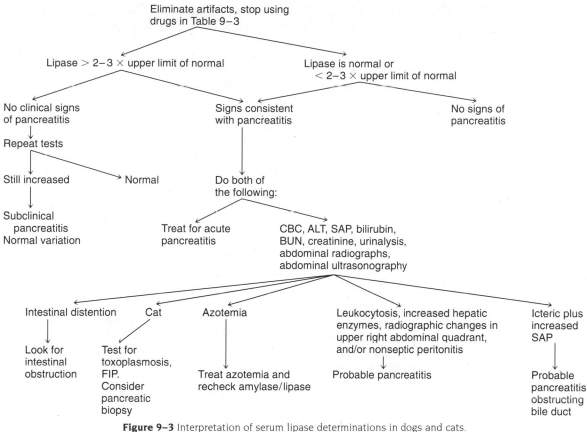

Figure 9–3 Interpretation of serum lipase determinations in dogs and cats.

function increases serum lipase, usually less than two to three times normal, although it may rarely be more than four times normal. Just as for amylase, not all patients with acute pancreatitis have increased serum lipase, and the increase in serum lipase activity is not proportional to the severity of the pancreatitis. Serum lipase and amylase determinations should be requested simultaneously to diagnose pancreatitis, and additional clinical and laboratory evaluation used to support the diagnosis. Serum trypsin-like immunoreactivity (TLI) and phospholipase A_2 have been investigated as tests for pancreatitis and show some promise.

GASTRIN

Occasional Indications ● Chronic vomiting, diarrhea, weight loss, suspected gastrinoma, or gastric bleeding of unknown cause. This test is usually not requested until more common diseases have been ruled out. Advantages: detects otherwise occult gastrinomas. Disadvantages: requires radioimmunoassay (RIA) method (long turnaround time).

Analysis ● Measured in 0.5 ml of serum by RIA. Serum should be frozen until assayed. See Appendix I for availability.

Normal Values ● Dogs, depends on laboratory (the assay must be validated for dogs); cats, not established.

Conversion of pg/ml to ng/L: multiply pg/ml × 1.0 = ng/L.

Danger Values ● None.

Artifacts ● Falsely decreased: hormone degradation due to storage for several days at temperatures above freezing.

Drug Therapy That May Increase Gastrin ● Antacids, including H_2 antagonist drugs, omeprazole, and others.

Causes of Hypogastrinemia ● Not significant.

Causes of Hypergastrinemia ● Atrophic gastritis (uncommon), antral G-cell hyperplasia (rare), short bowel syndrome, hyperparathyroidism, ulcers, gastric outlet obstruction, renal failure, and gastrinoma are the main causes. The last four are the most common. Hepatic insufficiency does not appear to directly increase serum gastrin concentrations. If gastrinoma is suspected in a patient that has a normal or equivocal serum gastrin concentration, secretin or calcium may be administered intravenously. A rise in the serum gastrin concentration after giving either of these drugs is indicative of gastrinoma.

ACUTE DIARRHEA

Patients with diarrhea are best classified into those with acute (<2 weeks) versus those with chronic (>2 weeks) diarrhea. Acute diarrhea (Table 9–4) is usually self-limiting, although some conditions may be severe, causing mortality, such as acute hemorrhagic gastroenteritis, parvoviral disease, parasites (e.g., hookworms), or intoxication. History should explore the possibility of recent dietary change or exposure to infectious agents. Diet, bacterial or viral agents, and parasites are the major identifiable causes of acute diarrhea in dogs and cats. Because intestinal parasites may contribute to any diarrheic state, multiple fecal examinations (direct and flotation) are warranted in all patients with diarrhea. Giardiasis may be particularly difficult to diagnose and may also require special techniques (see Fecal *Giardia* Detection).

Table 9–4 MAJOR CATEGORIES OF CAUSES OF ACUTE DIARRHEA IN DOGS AND CATS

Intestinal parasites
　Hookworms
　Roundworms
　Whipworms
　Coccidia
　Giardia (sometimes difficult to diagnose)
　Strongyloides
Dietary problems
　Poor quality food/food poisoning
　Sudden dietary change (especially young animals)
　Food intolerance
Acute viral or bacterial enteritis
　Feline panleukopenia
　Canine parvovirus
　Coronavirus
　Clostridium perfringens
　Campylobacteriosis
　Salmonellosis
Intussusception
Intoxication
　Garbage
　Food poisoning
　Heavy metal
　Organophosphate
Hemorrhagic gastroenteritis

Treatment with bland or hypoallergenic diets may be diagnostic as well as therapeutic. Depressed, weak, and dehydrated patients should have electrolyte and acid-base evaluations to aid in selecting fluid replacement therapy. All patients younger than 12 to 14 weeks should have blood glucose monitored to detect secondary hypoglycemia. Febrile or depressed patients should have CBC analysis to evaluate for sepsis or transmural inflammation. If canine parvovirus is suspected, it is rarely necessary to confirm the diagnosis, since therapy depends more on clinical signs (e.g., febrile and severely leukopenic patients require antibiotics, dehydrated patients require fluids and/or antidiarrheals) than on the diagnosis. To identify the cause of acute diarrhea that is not due to diet or parasites (e.g., in kennels, pet stores, shelters, and households where more than one member has diarrhea), fecal cultures for *Clostridium perfringens*, *Salmonella* spp., *Campylobacter jejuni*, *Yersinia enterocolitica*, and other pathogens plus viral identification methods (i.e., ELISA or electron microscopy) may be used.

With canine parvoviral diarrhea, not all patients are severely ill, have identifiable leukopenia, or have diarrhea or a fever. Leukopenia may persist as briefly as 24 to 36 hours and can easily be missed if a CBC is not performed during that period. Other diseases that cause severe sepsis (i.e., perforating linear foreign body with peritonitis or overwhelming salmonellosis) can cause leukopenia indistinguishable from that of canine parvoviral diarrhea. Routinely used vaccination schedules cannot guarantee protection against canine parvovirus. Finally, fecal shedding of viral particles decreases rapidly, and the virus may not be found by electron microscopy on feces. In-house ELISA tests for parvovirus can be performed on the feces and appear to be very accurate. The test should be strongly positive at the onset of clinical signs and remain positive for several days. A recent vaccination may give a faint reaction if any.

CHRONIC DIARRHEA

Chronic diarrhea should first be defined as either small intestinal or large intestinal, preferably by using the history and physical examination (Table 9–5). Occasionally the large and small intestines are involved concurrently. Patients with chronic diarrhea in which the clinical findings are determined not to be severe are often treated symptomatically before aggressive diagnostics are instituted. All patients should have at least three fecal examinations at 48-hour

Table 9–5 DIFFERENTIATION OF CHRONIC SMALL INTESTINAL FROM CHRONIC LARGE INTESTINAL DIARRHEA

	Small Intestinal Diarrhea	Large Intestinal Diarrhea
Weight loss	Common	Uncommon except with histoplasmosis, pythiosis, or cancer
Polyphagia	Common but not invariable	Uncommon
Vomiting	May occur	Occurs in 10–20% of patients
Volume of feces	May be larger than normal	May be smaller than normal
Frequency of defecation	Normal to slightly increased	Usually increased May have many small defecations per bowel movement
Slate-gray feces (steatorrhea)	Occasionally	No
Hematochezia	No	Common
Melena	Sometimes	No
Mucoid stools	Rare (unless ileum is diseased)	Common
Tenesmus/dyschezia	May occur	Common

intervals and should even be treated empirically for intestinal parasites (especially *Giardia* spp. and whipworms) before aggressive diagnostics are begun. Giardiasis may be particularly difficult to diagnose (see Fecal *Giardia* Detection).

Adverse reactions to food are also a cause of chronic diarrhea. Dietary food intolerances are a reaction to a particular substance in the diet, whereas true food allergies are immunologic reactions to a specific antigen. Food reactions are common, especially in cats. Dietary food trials are indicated in these cases. A failure of response to empirical therapy requires further diagnostic evaluation.

Large Intestinal Diarrhea

Once parasitism or dietary responsive disease is ruled out, additional simple diagnostic steps such as fecal cytology, rectal mucosal scrapings (not swabs) with cytologic examination, and fecal culture for *C. jejuni*, *Salmonella* spp., *C. perfringens* and/or *Y. enterocolitica* are appropriate. Large intestinal disease is usually an indication for colonoscopy plus biopsy, possibly the most cost-effective next step. Rigid colonoscopy of the descending colon is usually adequate for diagnosis. However, if available, flexible endoscopy allows evaluation and biopsy of the descending, transverse, and ascending colon, ileocolic valve, cecum, and ileum. If flexible endoscopy is unavailable, a barium enema may reveal lesions in this area and demonstrate the need for surgical biopsy.

Small Intestinal Diarrhea

Chronic and severe small intestinal diarrhea necessitates differentiation of maldigestion, bac-

terial overgrowth, protein-losing enteropathy, and non–protein-losing malabsorptive disease (Fig. 9–4). Weight loss and diarrhea are usually present.

Maldigestion

Maldigestion resulting from bile acid insufficiency due to biliary obstruction is possible but rare. Intestinal lactase deficiency is uncommon, but a lactose-free diet may be tried in selected patients (especially cats). Exocrine pancreatic insufficiency (EPI) is the most common cause of significant maldigestion in dogs but is rare in cats. Differentiation of EPI from malabsorptive disease is important, because this diagnosis is both overlooked in afflicted dogs and inappropriately made in patients without the malady. Clinical trials with pancreatic enzyme preparations are commonly used to diagnose EPI. Unfortunately, this method is not reliable, in part because of the different ways of supplementation. Powdered enzyme is superior to most tablet formulations, and some enzyme preparations are clearly superior to others. Even when appropriate therapy is administered, some dogs with EPI also require a low-fat diet, antacid therapy (rare), or treatment for concurrent intestinal bacterial overgrowth before proper enzyme replacement therapy is effective. Too often, failure of the initial enzyme trial replacement therapy may lead to unnecessary tests (i.e., exploratory laparotomy) because a definitive diagnosis of EPI was not established. There are no consistent hematologic or serum chemistry profile changes, and the serum amylase and lipase values are usually normal. Undigested fats are usually found in the feces; however, even this is not consistent. The fat absorption test is inexpensive but can have false results. The bentiro-

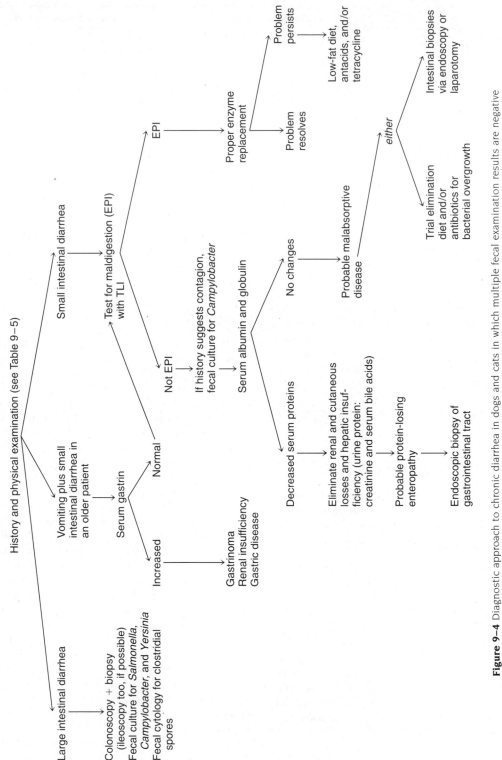

Figure 9–4 Diagnostic approach to chronic diarrhea in dogs and cats in which multiple fecal examination results are negative and empirical anthelmintic and antiprotozoal therapy and empirical dietary therapy do not resolve the diarrhea.

mide (BT-PABA) test appears to be accurate but is rarely performed. The TLI test is the most sensitive and specific test for EPI. This test has not been used extensively in cats; however, measurement of trypsin proteolytic activity appears to be an accurate means of diagnosing EPI in cats.

Malabsorption

Once maldigestion has been properly ruled out, malabsorption becomes the most likely diagnosis in an animal with diarrhea and weight loss. One must decide whether to perform diagnostic therapeutic trials or diagnostic tests. A definitive diagnosis ultimately necessitates intestinal biopsy in most patients. Tests such as fat absorption, D-xylose absorption, and upper gastrointestinal contrast radiographs are often used but are seldom essential. Patients that are critically ill should usually have intestinal biopsies (preferably via endoscopy). Patients that are not critically ill may be treated initially or may have testing initiated. However, because therapeutic trials may be chosen more rationally with the aid of some laboratory data, it is preferred at least to determine serum albumin and globulin concentrations before treatment.

Small Intestinal Bacterial Overgrowth

Intestinal bacterial overgrowth is probably a secondary occurrence. Bacterial overgrowth may prevent therapy aimed at the underlying problem from resolving clinical signs. There are no consistent CBC or serum chemistry profile changes in this syndrome. Altered D-xylose absorption and fat absorption are not reliable indicators of bacterial overgrowth. Fecal culture is not informative, and intestinal biopsy seldom helps. A barium contrast study may identify a segmental lesion or partial obstruction that may be responsible for a secondary bacterial overgrowth. Quantitated culture for aerobes and anaerobes in duodenal or proximal jejunal fluid is the most definitive test but is technically difficult. Serum vitamin B_{12} and folate concentrations are screening procedures for bacterial overgrowth once EPI has been ruled out. However, some patients with bacterial overgrowth have normal serum vitamin B_{12}/folate concentrations. Therefore, empirical antibiotic therapy may be chosen instead. Bacterial overgrowth usually responds to appropriate antibiotic therapy (e.g., tetracycline, tylosin, ampicillin, or metronidazole) unless there are irreversible mucosal changes or a primary underlying intestinal disease is present.

Non–Protein-Losing Disease

Many non–protein-losing malabsorptive diseases may be controlled by hypoallergenic diets (lamb and rice or rabbit and rice). At least 3 to 4 weeks should be allotted for such a dietary trial, during which time absolutely nothing else should be fed. If dietary, antibiotic, and repeated anthelmintic and antiprotozoal therapies are ineffective, small intestinal biopsy will probably be necessary. Laparotomy or endoscopy may be used. In most dogs and cats, the stomach, duodenum, ileum, and colon may be endoscopically sampled. Duodenal cytology is helpful in some disorders (e.g., eosinophilic enteritis, purulent enteritis, giardiasis, and lymphosarcoma). If laparotomy is performed, multiple representative full-thickness specimens (e.g., stomach, duodenum, jejunum, ileum, and mesenteric lymph node) are indicated because lesions can be sporadic. If endoscopy is performed, multiple specimens from each site are needed because of the small size of the samples.

Protein-Losing Enteropathy

Protein-losing enteropathies are often characterized by a decrease in serum concentrations of both serum albumin and globulin, which are lost through the gastrointestinal tract. Some patients (especially basenjis) may have only hypoalbuminemia. This can occur because the serum globulin concentration is greatly increased, and even though much of this fraction is lost into the intestines, the amount left in the blood is within the normal range.

Protein-losing enteropathy is a syndrome that may be due to various gastrointestinal diseases (eosinophilic, lymphocytic, plasmacytic, granulomatous or purulent enteritis, histoplasmosis, certain gastric diseases, and others). Intestinal lymphangiectasia is an example of severe protein-losing enteropathy and tends to produce some of the lowest serum protein levels (albumin levels possibly ≤ 1.0 g/dl) that occur in intestinal disease. Because of the loss of lymph into the intestines, peripheral lymphocyte counts may be decreased and hypocholesterolemia and steatorrhea are common. Fecal excretion of intravenously administered radiolabeled albumin or red blood cells is definitive for protein-losing enteropathy but impractical for most clinics. If renal protein loss and hepatic insufficiency have been eliminated, protein-losing enteropathy becomes the major differential. Intestinal biopsy is usually the definitive test. Full-thickness biopsy may risk dehiscence if the serum albumin level is <1.5 g/dl; however, serosal patch graft techniques will decrease the risk of dehiscence. Gastroduodenoscopy-ileoscopy plus biopsy is safe and often diagnostic. The intestinal lesion may occasionally be inaccessible via endoscopy. Dietary trial may be used in patients with protein-losing enteropathy. An ultra–low-fat diet with supplemented medium-chain triglycerides as an additional source of calories is recommended if lymphangiectasia is suspected.

Fecal Character

Mucoid feces should be approached as a large intestinal or a distal small intestinal problem. Fecal culture or cytology for *Clostridium* and colonoscopy plus biopsy are the most useful diagnostic tools after multiple fecal examinations have been performed. Hematochezia should also be considered as a large bowel problem. Melena signifies swallowed blood from any source, coagulopathy, or gastric–upper intestinal bleeding. Therefore, before performing an exploratory laparotomy, one should consider all the possible causes of oral bleeding (including coughing up blood from the respiratory tract as well as posterior nasal bleeding). Ingestion of bismuth subsalicylate (Pepto-Bismol) causes coal-black feces that resemble melenic stool. Use of dithiazanine (Dizan) causes the feces to become blue-green. Diet and changes in intestinal bacterial flora influence fecal color but do not generally signify disease.

FECAL ELISA FOR PARVOVIRUS

Occasional Indications • Dogs suspected of having parvoviral enteritis (especially those not displaying classic signs), acute neutropenia of unknown cause. Advantages: quick, available, and apparently has good sensitivity and specificity. Disadvantages: rare dogs with parvoviral enteritis have apparently false-negative reactions.

Analysis • Fresh feces, preferably taken from a dog that has begun to show signs recently, are used according to kit instructions (see Chapter 15, Enteric Viruses). The instructions must be followed, or false results might be obtained.

Normal Values • Dogs should not have parvoviral antigen in feces.

Interpretation • A positive result strongly suggests canine parvoviral enteritis. Not all dogs

affected with parvoviral enteritis have diarrhea and fever; some show only anorexia or vomiting or fever. Theoretically, if coproantibody binds all of the antigen in the feces, a false-negative result may occur (?). Shedding of viral particles decreases after the first week of disease, and a test performed too late in the disease might be negative (?).

FECAL ANALYSIS FOR CLOSTRIDIAL ENTEROTOXIN

Occasional Indications • Dogs with acute nosocomial diarrhea; dogs with chronic large bowel diarrhea of unknown cause; apparently contagious diarrhea. Advantages: quicker and easier than culture for *C. perfringens*, probably more definitive for *Clostridium* enterotoxemia than quantitated clostridial culture of feces. Disadvantages: uncertainty about positive and negative predictive values of test results and availability of the test.

Analysis • Fresh or frozen feces used according to the instructions on the test kit. Reversed passive latex agglutination and ELISA methodologies appear to be the most appropriate.

Interpretation • The presence of clostridial enterotoxin is taken as *prima facie* evidence of clostridial enteritis. Absence of toxin (as per the test) is assumed to preclude clostridial enteritis. However, production of enterotoxin may not be a consistent event (as indeed some of these diarrheas wax and wane); therefore, it might be useful to repeat the test in selected cases, especially when a patient is symptomatic.

It is believed that fecal spore counts probably correlate with clostridial toxin production. Therefore, examining fecal smears (see Fecal Microscopic Cytology) for this purpose seems to be an acceptable screening procedure.

FECAL CULTURE

Occasional Indications • Dogs and cats with persistent diarrhea (especially large bowel) of unknown origin, suspected contagious diarrhea, or a suspected infectious etiology (diarrhea with concurrent fever, leukocytosis, neutrophilic fecal cytology or bloody diarrhea). Common enteric pathogens include *C. perfringens*, *Salmonella* spp., *C. jejuni*, and *Y. enterocolitica*. Advantages: *Clostridium* enteritis may be a relatively frequent cause of chronic large bowel diarrhea in dogs.

Disadvantages: must specify which pathogen(s) to culture, must provide the laboratory with fresh feces or feces submitted in appropriate transport media, and requires a microbiology laboratory familiar with the specific enrichment/isolation techniques for each pathogen cultured for. Using culture swabs is not adequate for isolation of most enteric pathogens.

Analysis ● Fresh feces must be promptly submitted to the laboratory, and the laboratory must know the specific pathogen(s) sought. To submit old feces or feces that have not been collected or handled properly or to request a "general culture for pathogens" is generally a waste of time and money. Requires laboratories properly equipped to culture for the main enteric pathogens.

Culture for *C. perfringens* probably should use quantitative techniques. Even then, evidence of toxin production is probably more definitive for clostridial enteritis, as some strains do not produce toxin.

Interpretation ● Small numbers of any of the pathogens listed earlier may be found in a normal dog or cat, although *Y. enterocolitica* is particularly uncommon in the United States. Interpretation of the fecal culture must be done with consideration of the history, physical examination, laboratory data, and, in some cases, numbers of pathologic organisms (i.e., number of bacterial colony-forming units per gram of feces) found.

FECAL FAT

Common Indications ● To detect malabsorption or maldigestion in chronic small intestinal diarrhea or unexplained weight loss. *Semiqualitative analysis*: Advantages: minimal expense, availability, and reasonable accuracy as a screening test. Disadvantages: occasionally misleading results. *Quantitative analysis*: Advantages: very sensitive. Disadvantages: expense, difficulty in collecting and storing feces, and inability of test to differentiate between the causes of steatorrhea.

Analysis ● Semiqualitative analysis for undigested fats is performed by mixing a drop of fresh feces with a drop of Sudan III, heating the slide to a boil, and examining the smear microscopically. Analysis for digested fats is performed by mixing 1 drop of fresh feces, 1 drop of 36% acetic acid, and 1 drop of Sudan III. This is put on a microscope slide, heated to

boiling, and examined while still warm. In both cases, identifying orange droplets is a positive finding. When performing this test it is important that the patient has been eating a moderate to high fat diet. Diets low in fat content given to a malabsorptive dog may be negative for obvious fecal fat.

Quantitative analysis is performed by feeding a meat-based canned food at the rate of 50 g/kg/day for 3 days before the study. Then, all feces are collected for at least 24 and preferably for 72 hours while feeding this diet. Feces are refrigerated or preferably frozen while awaiting analysis. The entire collection of feces is submitted after carefully weighing it to the nearest gram. Gravimetric and titrimetric analyses may be used. This test is rarely performed.

Normal Values ● *Semiqualitative*: few or no undigested and digested fat globules per high power field (hpf). *Quantitative*: dogs, fat < 0.25 g/kg body weight/24 hours; cats, unknown.

Danger Values ● None.

Artifacts ● Falsely decreased (quantitative): not collecting all the feces. Falsely increased (quantitative): improper collection containers (e.g., wax paper, milk cartons, and other wax-coated objects) or administration of mineral oil. The semiqualitative analysis may have unexplained false-negative and false-positive reactions. Administration of barium sulfate, bismuth, Metamucil, mineral oil, or castor oil or feeding a low fat diet may also confuse semiqualitative analysis.

Drug Therapy That May Alter Measurement of Fat Excretion ● Decreased excretion may be due to medium-chain triglyceride oil supplements (titrimetric analysis). Increased quantitated fat excretion may be due to azathioprine, orally administered aminoglycosides, and cholestyramine.

Causes of Decreased Fecal Fat ● Do not exist.

Causes of Increased Fecal Fat ● Fat excretion of > 1.0 g/kg/24 hours or the finding of several orange globules/hpf, if repeatable on several examinations, is principally due to malabsorption or maldigestion. Quantitated fecal fat excretion is a sensitive, accurate indicator of these two conditions. Semiqualitative analysis is a reasonable screening test and helps distinguish maldigestion due to EPI (positive for undigested fats) from malabsorption (positive for digested fats). Despite occasional false-positive reactions, strongly positive results for undigested fecal fat in a dog with signs consistent with maldigestion are an indication for clinical enzyme replacement or more specific tests (e.g., TLI). Questionable results on the semiqualitative test should always be followed by more specific tests. Some dogs with EPI will not have fecal fat detectable with Sudan staining.

FECAL STARCH

Rare Indications • Chronic small bowel diarrhea or weight loss. Advantages: low cost and availability. Disadvantages: negative and positive results that do not correlate with malabsorption/maldigestion.

Analysis • Fecal smears are stained with 2% Lugol's iodine. Starch granules show up as dark blue-black granules when viewed microscopically.

Normal Values • Rare (0–5) granules/hpf although this may vary with the diet.

Danger Values • None.

Artifacts • Falsely increased: contamination of feces with food. Unexplained false-positive and false-negative results may also occur.

Drug Therapy That May Affect Fecal Starch • Some diets may have more fecal starch excretion than others.

Causes of No Amylorrhea • Normal finding.

Causes of Amylorrhea • EPI is most likely, but high-starch diets or conditions causing increased intestinal transit may cause amylorrhea. Amylorrhea is a weak indication of EPI unless supporting tests are positive. Amylorrhea in a patient with weight loss or diarrhea is an indication for serum TLI.

FECAL MUSCLE FIBERS

Rare Indications • Difficult-to-diagnose chronic small bowel diarrhea or unexplained weight loss. Advantages and disadvantages are the same as for fecal starch.

Analysis • A fresh fecal smear is stained with 2% Lugol's iodine, new methylene blue, or Wright's stain.

Normal Values • Dogs, muscle fibers should not be seen; cats, assumed to be similar to dogs.

Danger Values • None.

Artifacts • See the following section on effects of therapy.

Therapy That May Alter Fecal Muscle Fiber Determination • Some diets result in more fecal muscle fibers than others. Administration of barium sulfate, mineral oil, magnesium, or bismuth may make fiber identification difficult. A meat-free diet renders this test useless.

Causes of Creatorrhea • EPI is likely. However, more sensitive and specific tests are indicated to make this diagnosis.

FECAL PROTEOLYTIC ACTIVITY

Occasional Indications • To detect maldigestion in chronic small intestinal diarrhea or weight loss of unknown cause. Disadvantages: the unreliability of the readily available tests and the difficulty in performing the most reliable procedure, plus special specimen handling.

Analysis • Tests performed on *fresh* feces include film digestion, gelatin digestion, and biochemical analysis (para-tosyl-L-arginine methyl ester substrate) techniques. These do not give comparable results. Film digestion techniques are so undependable that the test is not recommended. Gelatin digestion is performed by mixing one part feces with nine parts of 5% sodium bicarbonate solution and adding 1 ml of this suspension to 2 ml of melted 7.5% gelatin. This tube is incubated 1 hour at 37° C and then allowed to cool. If it remains liquid, it signifies that trypsin is present, and vice versa. The biochemical test is performed on an aliquot of a mixed, 24-hour fecal collection, and the results are expressed as g trypsin per kg of body weight/day.

Performed on three sequential samples: Collect single fecal samples daily for 3 consecutive days in special containers and freeze before transport or rapidly deliver to the laboratory. Fecal proteolytic activity (FPA) assays fecal trypsin content by either azocasein hydrolysis or radial enzyme diffusion.

Normal Values • Dogs, gelatin is liquid, or trypsin, 4 to 6 g/kg/day; cats, azocasein hydrolysis is 20 to 207 azocasein units (ACU)/g feces. Radial enzyme diffusion is 5 to 16 mm gel clearing.

Danger Values • None.

Artifacts • The film digestion test is affected by so many factors that it should not be performed. The gelatin digestion test has fewer artifacts but is still of poor reliability. Artifacts in the biochemical test may be due to failure to collect all feces, failure to mix the sample properly before obtaining an aliquot, or improper storage of the feces (should be at 4° C or preferably frozen).

FPA as determined by azocasein hydrolysis or radial enzyme diffusion is a quantitative test and appears to have good reliability in cats with EPI. Fecal trypsin accounts for variable FPA and can be altered by pancreatic production as well as degradation of trypsin during passage through the intestinal tract. Accuracy increases when several fecal samples are evaluated.

Drug Therapy That May Alter Results • Dietary supplementation with pancreatic enzymes causes a positive reaction.

Causes of Decreased Fecal Trypsin • EPI is the major cause of true lack of trypsin.

FECAL MICROSCOPIC CYTOLOGY

Frequent Indications • Large or small intestinal diarrhea. Advantages: availability and ease of performing the test. Disadvantages: variable specificity for a particular etiologic factor.

Analysis • Thin, air-dried, fresh fecal smears are stained with new methylene blue or Wright's stain and examined using high power and oil immersion. Rectal and colonic mucosal scraping obtained with a curette is also a means of examining mucosal cells.

Normal Values • A mixed population of rod and cocci bacteria, few bacterial spores or yeast, occasional epithelial cells and amorphous debris.

Danger Values • None.

Artifacts • Old fecal sample (white blood cells [WBCs] do not remain identifiable in feces for long times, and the bacterial population changes and bacterial spores increase). Falsely increased: fecal debris may resemble degenerate WBCs.

Drug Therapy • Administration of barium and Metamucil may make interpretation difficult, and antibiotics change bacterial flora.

Causes of Abnormalities • Fecal WBCs (specifically neutrophils) are observed with bacterial (e.g., salmonellosis or campylobacterosis) and with inflammatory mucosal disease. Transmural colitides occasionally have increased fecal WBCs. Fecal WBCs are an indication for culture for specific bacterial pathogens or mucosal biopsy. Eosinophils may be observed with allergic or parasitic eosinophilic colitis. Increased numbers of yeast, fungal organisms, a uniform population of bacteria, or high numbers of bacterial spores (specifically *C. perfringens*) are abnormal and may help identify a cause.

FECAL OCCULT BLOOD

Rare Indications • To detect gastrointestinal bleeding that is not apparent grossly (melena or hematochezia). Disadvantages: see Artifacts.

Analysis • Fresh feces are smeared on a test pad. The patient must have been on a meat-free diet for at least 3 days before obtaining the feces. Sensitivity varies markedly between assays.

Normal Values • See Artifacts, next.

Artifacts • Falsely decreased: sampling unmixed feces (blood may not be distributed homogeneously throughout the feces). Falsely increased: Most diets contain meat or fecal peroxidases, which cause a positive reaction. Certain other foods may also cause positive reactions, depending on the assay (e.g., beets and tomatoes).

Causes of Fecal Occult Blood • Bleeding into the gastrointestinal tract at any level and due to any cause may result in fecal occult blood.

FAT ABSORPTION TEST

Occasional Indications • To detect and distinguish maldigestion from malabsorption in chronic small intestinal diarrhea or unex-

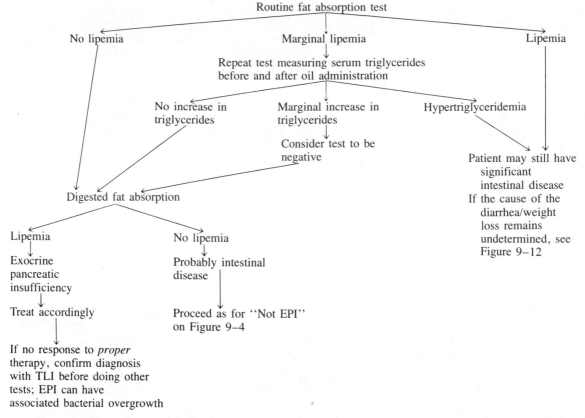

Figure 9–5 Diagnostic use of the fat absorption tests in dogs or cats with weight loss, chronic diarrhea, or both.

plained weight loss. Advantages: low cost and availability. Disadvantages: false-negative and false-positive results, difficulty in consistently ranking the degree of turbidity.

Analysis ● For the routine test: After a 12-hour fast and confirmation of nonlipemic plasma, corn oil, 3 ml/kg of body weight, is administered orally. If administration is with an oral syringe, do not allow the patient to aspirate the oil. Serum or plasma (any volume including microhematocrit tubes) is then examined at hourly intervals for up to 5 hours or at least at 2 and 4 hours after ingestion. Serum triglyceride concentrations or lipoprotein electrophoresis may be done on the plasma, or vitamin A (200,000 IU/dog) can be mixed with the oil to allow more quantitated measurement of absorption. However, these manipulations are seldom necessary. For the digested test, the same procedure is used except that the oil is mixed with 2 to 3 tsp of pancreatic enzyme powder. This may be done immediately after determining that the routine test is negative and the serum is still clear.

Normal Values ● Dogs and cats, marked lipemia

should be seen with either test within 5 hours (and usually within 2 hours).

Danger Values ● None. Do not allow the patient to aspirate the oil.

Artifacts ● Falsely decreased: vomiting after fat administration or delayed gastric emptying (due to the fat).

Drug Therapy That May Decrease or Delay Fat Absorption ● Oral aminoglycosides (rare) or drugs that delay gastric emptying.

Causes of Decreased Fat Absorption ● Classically, both maldigestion and malabsorption cause decreased routine fat absorption; malabsorption also causes decreased digested fat absorption (Fig. 9–5). If the results suggest maldigestion due to EPI, a therapeutic trial with appropriate pancreatic enzyme replacement or, preferentially, serum TLI may be done. If the fat absorption results suggest malabsorptive disease, a therapeutic dietary trial or additional tests may be performed (see Fig. 9–4). Tests may have false-negative and false-positive results. If the test results do not conform with those expected based on history, physical examination, and other laboratory tests or if the plasma becomes only slightly turbid, then additional testing should be considered. Malabsorptive diseases and protein-losing enteropathies severe enough to cause significant weight loss may allow enough functional intestinal mucosa to persist so that slight to moderate serum turbidity occurs.

Causes of Increased Fat Absorption • Normal finding (does not rule out intestinal disease).

BENTIROMIDE (BT-PABA)

Rare Indications • Difficult-to-diagnose chronic small bowel diarrhea or weight loss. Advantages: sensitivity and specificity for EPI, plus it may be combined with the D-xylose test. Disadvantages: multiple blood samples, expense, difficulty in getting the sample analyzed, and rare false-negative and false-positive results. Because of the accuracy and the increased availability of the TLI test, the bentiromide test is less commonly used.

Analysis • Measured in 1 ml heparinized plasma or urine using spectrophotometric methods. Bentiromide (also known as BT-PABA) is administered orally at the dose recommended by the laboratory performing the analysis. Samples are taken as recommended by the laboratory.

Normal Values • These vary with the laboratory and the technique.

Danger Values • None.

Artifacts • Unexplained false-positive and false-negative results may occur. Falsely decreased urine and falsely increased serum BT-PABA may be due to renal failure. Renal failure is an indication to use the TLI test instead of the BT-PABA test.

Drug Therapy That May Alter BT-PABA Measurements • Diuretics, sulfonamides, and chloramphenicol may interfere with measurement of urinary BT-PABA.

Causes of Decreased Plasma/Urine BT-PABA • EPI is the major reason plasma BT-PABA concentration does not increase over resting values after administration. However, vomiting or delayed gastric emptying may result in decreased or delayed plasma BT-PABA concentrations. Rare false-negative and false-positive results occur. Failure to find increased concentrations after BT-PABA administration is an indication for proper pancreatic enzyme replacement therapy. If proper therapy is inefficacious, confirmation of the diagnosis by TLI is indicated because malabsorptive disease rarely causes failure of BT-PABA absorption.

TRYPSIN-LIKE IMMUNOREACTIVITY

Common Indications • Difficult-to-diagnose chronic small bowel diarrhea or weight loss. Advantages: high sensitivity and specificity plus the need for only one serum sample that does not require special or cumbersome handling procedures, and most large veterinary diagnostic laboratories can perform this test. This test can sometimes detect loss of pancreatic acinar tissue at an earlier stage of disease than can gross examination or histopathology. Disadvantages: prolonged turnaround time for results.

Analysis • Performed on 1 ml serum using RIA. See Appendix I for availability.

Normal Values • Dogs, 5–35 µg/L (Fig. 9 6); cats, 28–115 µg/L.

Danger Values • None.

Artifacts • Theoretically, EPI due to an obstructed pancreatic duct instead of acinar cell atrophy would have a normal serum TLI.

Drug Therapy That May Alter TLI • Drugs causing acute pancreatitis (see Table 9–3) can increase serum TLI.

Causes of Decreased TLI • EPI is the major cause of serum TLI < 2.0 µg/L. A decreased serum TLI indicates treatment for EPI. The TLI should be considered the test of choice for EPI in dogs (Fig. 9–6).

Causes of Increased TLI • (Values > 35 µg/L in dogs, > 115 µg/L in cats.) Pancreatitis, renal failure, prerenal azotemia (may increase two times), and malnutrition.

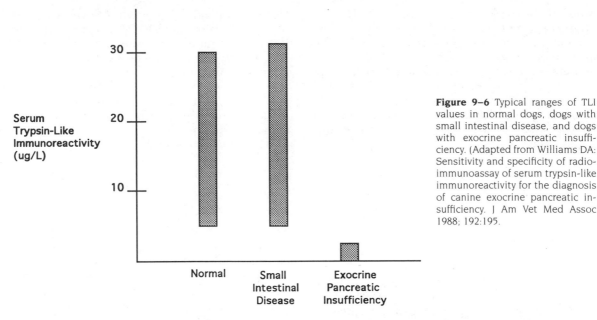

Figure 9–6 Typical ranges of TLI values in normal dogs, dogs with small intestinal disease, and dogs with exocrine pancreatic insufficiency. (Adapted from Williams DA: Sensitivity and specificity of radioimmunoassay of serum trypsin-like immunoreactivity for the diagnosis of canine exocrine pancreatic insufficiency. J Am Vet Med Assoc 1988; 192:195.

ORAL GLUCOSE ABSORPTION TEST

Rare Indications ● Difficult-to-diagnose chronic small bowel diarrhea or weight loss. Disadvantages: poor specificity and the need for multiple blood samples.

Analysis ● Glucose, 2 g/kg body weight, is given orally as a 12½% solution. Blood glucose is measured in serum or plasma obtained at 0, 15, 30, 60, 90, and 120 minutes after administration. Analysis is explained under Glucose in Chapter 8.

Normal Values ● Dogs, increases of at least 50 mg/dl by 30 minutes and return to normal at 120 minutes; cats, unknown.

Danger Values ● None.

Artifacts ● See Glucose in Chapter 8. Falsely decreased: vomiting or delayed gastric emptying.

Drug Therapy That May Alter Glucose Absorption Test ● See Glucose in Chapter 8.

Interpretation ● Because of the multiplicity of factors that affect this test, it is not recommended for evaluation of the gastrointestinal tract.

STARCH DIGESTION TEST

Rare Indications ● Same as for oral glucose absorption test. Disadvantages: same as for oral glucose absorption test.

Analysis ● Starch, 3 g/kg body weight, is administered orally. The starch must be mixed in a small amount of room temperature water; this solution is then added to water that has just finished boiling. This solution is then administered as soon as it is cool enough for the patient to tolerate. Blood samples are taken after 30, 60, 120, and 180 minutes and analyzed for glucose.

Values, Artifacts, Drug Effects, and Interpretation ● Same as for oral glucose absorption test, plus improper solution preparation may cause false-negative or false-positive results. Failure to increase blood glucose suggests EPI or malabsorptive disease. However, if there is no increase in the blood glucose concentration, an oral glucose absorption test must be done to differentiate maldigestion from malabsorption.

D-XYLOSE ABSORPTION TEST

Rare Indications ● Difficult-to-diagnose chronic small intestinal diarrhea, anorexia, or unexplained weight loss suspected to be from occult small intestinal disease. Advantages: relative specificity for primary and secondary intestinal diseases. Disadvantages: need for multiple blood samples, poor sensitivity for intestinal disease, inability to distinguish between different intestinal diseases, and rare test availability.

Analysis • Measured in 0.5 ml of serum, fluoride-treated blood, plasma (oxalate or heparin), or urine by colorimetric analysis. Drug is administered, and samples collected as per the laboratory.

Normal Values • Dogs, > 45 mg/dl at peak; cats, > 15 mg/dl at peak.

Danger Values • None.

Artifacts (for Blood Concentrations) • Lipemia or allowing the serum or plasma to remain with the cellular elements of the blood for protracted periods after sampling may alter test results. Falsely increased: renal failure.

Drugs That May Affect D-Xylose Absorption • Decreased D-xylose absorption may be due to atropine, salicylates, orally administered aminoglycosides, arsenicals, and digitalis.

Causes of Decreased D-Xylose Absorption • Delayed gastric emptying, decreased intestinal blood flow, third spaces (edema or ascites), intestinal bacterial overgrowth, and intestinal malabsorptive disease are the major causes of decreased D-xylose levels. However, D-xylose absorption may also be normal in any of these diseases. Decreased D-xylose absorption is an indication for serum vitamin B_{12} and folate determinations or other tests or antibiotic therapy to screen for intestinal bacterial overgrowth.

Causes of Increased D-Xylose Absorption • Renal failure may cause inappropriately increased serum D-xylose concentrations.

SERUM VITAMIN B₁₂/FOLATE

Occasional Indications • Chronic small bowel diarrhea or unexplained weight loss. Advantages: need only one serum sample. Disadvantages: few assays validated for dogs and uncertain sensitivity (some dogs with bacterial overgrowth and/or EPI have normal vitamin B_{12} and/or folate levels). This test should be used as an adjunct to other tests for maldigestion and malabsorption syndromes.

Analysis • Measured in 1 ml of serum by bioassay or RIA (RIA is recommended). "Charcoal boil" kits are most suitable for dogs. "No boil" methods are unreliable in dogs. Serum should be transported in a covered tube.

Normal Values • Depend on the laboratory. Normal ranges vary widely between laboratories. Assay must be validated by that particular laboratory for dogs.

Danger Values • None.

Artifacts • Falsely decreased vitamin B_{12}: degradation due to exposure of serum to sunlight.

Drug Therapy That May Alter Serum Vitamin B₁₂ Concentrations • Vitamin B_{12} may be decreased by H_2 blocker therapy, which allows intestinal bacterial overgrowth to occur. Vitamin B_{12} may be increased by vitamin B_{12} supplementation or antibacterial therapy that resolves bacterial overgrowth.

Causes of Decreased Serum Vitamin B₁₂ Concentrations • There are four major recognized reasons for decreased serum B_{12} concentrations: ileal disease or resection (rare), EPI, intestinal villus atrophy, and chronic intestinal bacterial overgrowth. The major differentiation to be made is among EPI, villus atrophy, and intestinal bacterial overgrowth; therefore, decreased serum B_{12} is an indication for serum TLI. Not all dogs with EPI, villus atrophy, or intestinal bacterial overgrowth have decreased serum vitamin B_{12}.

Causes of Increased Serum Vitamin B₁₂ Concentrations • Vitamin B_{12} supplementation.

Causes of Decreased Serum Folate • Severe mucosal disease of the proximal small intestine decreases serum folate. Not all patients with such disease have decreased folate levels.

Causes of Increased Serum Folate • Intestinal bacterial overgrowth and EPI are the major causes. Many patients with these diseases do not have increased folate levels.

HYDROGEN BREATH TEST

Occasional Indications • Chronic small bowel diarrhea or unexplained weight loss. Advantages: ease of the test and its lack of invasiveness.

Disadvantages: need for special equipment and unknown sensitivity and specificity. This is not a routine diagnostic test because it requires special hydrogen-analysis equipment.

Analysis • The concentration of hydrogen in expired air is measured after ingestion of food or oral administration of a carbohydrate such as D-xylose or lactulose.

Normal Values • Dogs, no increase in hydrogen after ingestion of food or xylose; cats, unknown.

Danger Values • None.

Artifacts • Abnormal intestinal motility may delay or hasten expiration of hydrogen owing to colonic bacterial fermentation of carbohydrates.

Drug Therapy That May Alter Hydrogen Breath Test • Decreased or delayed expiration of hydrogen may be due to antibiotics and drugs that delay intestinal transit.

Causes of Decreased Expired Hydrogen • Normal.

Causes of Increased Expired Hydrogen • Carbohydrate malabsorption and small intestinal bacterial overgrowth may result in increases in expired hydrogen. The only source of hydrogen is from certain bacterial fermentation of carbohydrates. The sensitivity and specificity of the hydrogen breath test for bacterial overgrowth in dogs are unknown. Not all animals with bacterial overgrowth have abnormal breath hydrogen.

FECAL SMEAR (WET MOUNT) FOR PARASITES

Common Indications • A screen for parasites and parasitic ova; any patient with diarrhea, melena, hematochezia, fecal mucus, weight loss, or vomiting. Advantages: availability, ease of performing the test, and low cost. Disadvantages: need for fresh feces and the frequency with which parasites and their ova or cysts are not detected.

Analysis • A thin smear is made of very fresh (< 5 minutes old) feces, usually mixed with a drop of saline solution and coverslipped to prevent dehydration. It should be examined immediately. If protozoa are seen and better cytologic

detail is desired, a drop of Lugol's iodine or Dobell and O'Connor's iodine (Kirkpatrick, 1987) may be placed at the corner of the coverslip. (Note: Iodine kills protozoa, thus stopping motility.)

Normal Values • Dogs and cats, no parasites or ova.

Artifacts • Cooling of the slide or dehydration inhibits the motility of some protozoa and bacteria.

Drug Therapy That May Alter Results • Orally administered compounds containing kaolin, pectin, barium sulfate, bismuth, and other intestinally active compounds (e.g., cathartics or enemas) may make it difficult to find and identify parasites, ova, and cysts.

Parasites, Bacteria, and Ova That May Be Identified • This test is most useful in identifying *Giardia* spp., *Pentatrichomonas* spp., *Entamoeba histolytica*, *Balantidium coli*, *Strongyloides stercoralis*, and *Aleurostrongylus abstrusus*. Any ova may be found, but this test may be useful for detecting *Spirocerca lupi* and *Trichuris vulpis* ova. With oil immersion, small motile bacterial spirochetes in conjunction with fecal WBCs suggest *Campylobacter* as a possible cause.

FECAL FLOTATION

Common Indications • As for fecal smear. Advantages: sensitivity, availability, and low cost.

Analysis • Feces are well mixed with either a saturated sugar solution or a zinc sulfate solution (Kirkpatrick, 1987). (Zinc sulfate solution is made by mixing 331 g $ZnSO_4 \cdot 7 H_2O$ in 1 L water. This is supposedly the best test for *Giardia* spp., because it does not distort the cysts.) Ova and cysts are allowed to rise to the surface and are retrieved with a coverslip. Samples for *Giardia* detection should be examined within 15 minutes to avoid distortion and lysis of cysts. Centrifugation of the sample increases the sensitivity of the procedure. Samples that will be sent to an outside laboratory for analysis may be refrigerated (not frozen) for 1 to 2 days or preserved by mixing 1 part feces with 3 parts sodium acetate–acetic acid–formalin. This is prepared by mixing 1.5 g sodium acetate + 2 ml glacial acetic acid + 4 ml 40% formaldehyde solution + 92.5 ml water (Kirkpatrick, 1987).

Normal Values • Dogs and cats, no ova or oocysts present.

Artifacts • Falsely decreased: diarrhea may decrease ova concentration within a sample.

Parasite Ova and Cysts That May Be Identified
• *Ancylostoma* spp., *Toxocara* spp., *Toxascaris leonina, T. vulpis, S. lupi, Physaloptera rara* (use dichromate solution), *Capillaria aerophilia, Capillaria plica, Onciola canis, Dioctophyma renale, Isospora* spp., *Giardia* spp., *Toxoplasma gondii, Cryptosporidia* sp., *Paragonimus kellicotti*, and some tapeworms.

FECAL SEDIMENTATION

Rare Indications • Same as for fecal smear and flotation, especially if flukes are being considered. If feces contain excessive fat, then formalin–ethyl acetate is probably better than a water sedimentation. Disadvantages: requires more time than direct fecal smear or fecal flotation.

Analysis • Feces are mixed with the sedimentation solution (e.g., water), usually strained once or twice to remove large debris, and allowed to settle for ½ to 2 hours. The sediment is then examined microscopically. When formalin–ethyl acetate is used, the strained feces are centrifuged, the pellet is resuspended in 9 ml of 5% formalin solution, 3 ml ethyl acetate is added, and the mixture is shaken vigorously. This is recentrifuged, the debris at the formalin–ethyl acetate interface is discarded, and the sediment is then examined (Kirkpatrick, 1987).

Normal Values • Dogs and cats, no ova.

Artifacts • Same as under Fecal Flotation.

Parasite Ova That May Be Identified • All the ova that may be found by fecal flotation, plus *Alaria canis* and *Nanophyetus salmincola*.

FECAL GIARDIA DETECTION

Occasional Indications • Chronic diarrhea, unexplained weight loss, intermittent bilious vomiting, or when *Giardia* is suspected clinically and routine zinc sulfate flotation tests are negative. Techniques include (1) duodenal aspiration and cytology and (2) fecal ELISA antigen

test. Advantages: Provides additional methods for detection of *Giardia*. Disadvantages: Duodenal aspirates require surgery or endoscopy. Fecal ELISA requires specialized laboratories. Neither test provides greater accuracy than multiple fecal flotation tests using zinc sulfate.

Analysis • Duodenal fluid aspirates require fresh direct wet mount observation of motile trophozoites. Fecal ELISA should have fresh fecal samples sent to referral laboratory for analysis.

Normal Values • No trophozoites or fecal antigen present.

Danger Values • None.

FECAL EXAMINATION FOR CRYPTOSPORIDIA

Rare Indications • Chronic diarrhea. Cats may(?) be more likely to have cryptosporidiosis than dogs, but the prevalence of this disorder is currently unknown. Disadvantages: oocysts are small and may be difficult to find.

Analysis • Fresh fecal samples should be sent to a referral laboratory experienced in finding cryptosporidia. Special fecal flotation techniques or direct fecal smears stained with an acid-fast stain are used.

Normal Values • Dog and cat feces should be negative for cryptosporidia.

HEPATIC ABNORMALITIES

Hepatic disease may be heralded by relatively specific signs (hepatomegaly, microhepatica, icterus, or hepatic encephalopathy associated with meals) or may be associated with very nonspecific signs (depression, weight loss, anorexia, vomiting, or ascites). The latter are common presenting complaints of many diseases, which is why serum biochemistry profiling is indicated in patients with signs of significant disease. It is important to note that no consistent signs or laboratory abnormalities are found in all patients with hepatic disease. When screening for hepatic disease, one should request at a minimum a CBC, serum ALT, SAP, albumin, BUN, and glucose, plus urinalysis and abdominal radiographs. Ultimately, hepatic function tests (bile acids, ammonia tolerance, others) ultra-

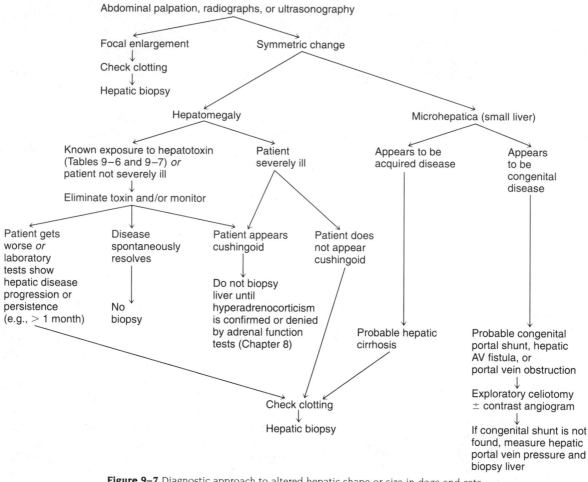

Figure 9–7 Diagnostic approach to altered hepatic shape or size in dogs and cats.

sonographic examination, hepatic biopsy, or contrast angiography will be necessary for definitive diagnosis in most cases. Abnormalities in liver-specific enzymes may result from primary hepatic disease but occur more frequently as the result of secondary hepatic involvement from a primary nonhepatic disease (e.g., glucocorticoid hepatopathy). After identifying abnormalities in ALT, aspartate transferase (AST), SAP, or gamma-glutamyl transpeptidase (GGT), one should investigate first for a primary nonhepatic disease because they are the most common cause of increased values. In such cases, the liver usually has reactive but reversible degenerative changes. Laboratory tests should be used to (1) identify the presence of hepatic disease and (2) determine if a biopsy or radiographic contrast procedure is indicated.

Microhepatica: Small Liver

A small liver suggests atrophy (due to portosystemic shunts, hepatic arteriovenous [AV] fis-

tulas), or fibrosis-cirrhosis (Fig. 9–7). Radiographically, hepatic atrophy tends to be characterized by sharp borders as opposed to the rounded or blunted hepatic margins typically associated with fibrosis and cirrhosis. However, some patients with hepatic fibrosis severe enough to cause portal hypertension also have sharp hepatic margins. Most patients with hepatic atrophy are relatively young (< 1–2 years) and have had signs of hepatic disease since or before weaning; most patients with cirrhosis are middle-aged or older and clearly have late onset of clinical signs. Acquired portosystemic shunts, hepatic vein obstruction, some hepatic AV fistulas, and rare congenital portosystemic shunts may cause clinical signs that are first detected in later life (4–10 years of age). Hepatic atrophy is accompanied by abnormalities in hepatic function tests (e.g., sulfobromophthalein [BSP], bile acids, ammonia, or ammonium chloride tolerance test) but may have normal or abnormal ALT, SAP, BUN, and serum albumin. Determining only one hepatic function test result to be normal or abnormal does not assure one that other hepatic function tests will have similar results. Pre- and postprandial serum bile acid concentrations seem to be the most sensitive function test. (Note: Bile acids are also increased by cholestatic diseases; therefore, they are not a "pure" test of hepatic function.) If hepatic disease is strongly suspected, one should not hesitate to perform multiple hepatic function tests. If hepatic atrophy is likely, abdominal ultrasonography, a radiographic contrast procedure (mesenteric venoportogram or splenic venoportogram), and a hepatic biopsy might be considered.

Small livers with clearly rounded or blunt hepatic margins are usually cirrhotic. Significant increases in serum ALT and SAP are usually present. Changes in serum albumin and BUN are more variable. If cirrhosis appears likely, a biopsy is indicated. Most cirrhotic livers can be identified grossly by their nodular or cobblestone appearance, although significant fibrosis can be present without major gross changes and severe nodular hyperplasia may appear as a cirrhotic liver. Evidence of acquired shunting seen grossly at laparoscopy or laparotomy is usually due to cirrhosis but can be secondary to congenital hepatic AV fistula, veno-occlusive disease, or portal vein obstruction. If the liver is not clearly cirrhotic or fibrotic, a mesenteric venoportogram may be indicated in patients with evidence of acquired shunting.

Hepatomegaly: Enlarged Liver

Focal or asymmetric hepatic enlargement generally necessitates further laboratory investigation, radiographic evaluation, and possibly biopsy. Neoplasia is a prominent but not invariable cause of hepatomegaly. The magnitude of the enlargement is not prognostic.

Generalized hepatomegaly necessitates careful clinicopathologic evaluation. Hepatomegaly may be due to primary or secondary hepatic disease. Diagnosis may be made with a history of exposure to certain toxins (Tables 9–6 and 9–7) or diagnosis of a systemic disease (e.g., hyperadrenocorticism) known to affect the liver. It is important to note that changes in ALT, SAP, hepatic function tests, and liver size, although suggestive of hepatic disease, are not diagnostic of specific entities. This is true even in breeds with specific predispositions (e.g., Doberman pinschers or Bedlington terriers). Changes in the SAP or serum ALT may be due to primary nonhepatic disease, which may be secondary to hyperadrenocorticism, inflamma-

tory bowel disease, diabetes mellitus, heart failure, or other causes. A definitive diagnosis usually requires hepatic biopsy. The clinician should seek to rule out nonhepatic causes of secondary hepatic dysfunction first. Hepatic bi-

Table 9–6 DRUGS THAT HAVE BEEN DOCUMENTED OR SUSPECTED TO CAUSE INCREASED ALT LEVELS DUE TO HEPATIC DISEASE

Acetaminophen **(important)**	Nitrofurantoin
L-Asparaginase	Oxacillin
Azathioprine	Oxybendazole
Barbiturates **(important)**	Phenobarbital **(important)**
	Phenylbutazone
Erythromycin estolate	Phenytoin
	Primidone **(important)**
Glucocorticoids in dogs only **(important)**	Propylthiouracil
	Quinidine
	Salicylate
Griseofulvin	Salicylazosulfapyridine
Halothane	Sulfonamides
Ibuprofen	Tetracycline
Ketoconazole	Thiacetarsamide **(important)**
Mebendazole	Trimethoprim-sulfamethoxazole
6-Mercaptopurine	
Methimazole	
Methotrexate	
Methoxyflurane	

These drugs do not reliably cause hepatic disease. A patient with an increased ALT that is receiving one of these drugs should probably have the medication stopped, if possible, and the ALT rechecked 2 to 4 weeks later. Those drugs that most reliably increase ALT are marked **(important)**. The other drugs are less consistent but may still cause severe hepatic disease.

Table 9–7 DRUGS THAT HAVE BEEN DOCUMENTED OR SUSPECTED TO CAUSE CHOLESTASIS OR HEPATIC ENZYME INDUCTION RESULTING IN INCREASED SAP LEVELS

Anabolic steroids	Nitrofurantoin
Androgens	Oxacillin
Asparaginase	Oxymetholone
Azathioprine	Phenobarbital **(important)**
Barbiturates **(important)**	Phenothiazines
Cephalosporins	Phenylbutazone
Cyclophosphamide	Phenytoin
Dapsone	Primidone **(important)**
Erythromycin estolate	Progesterone
Estrogens	Quinacrine
Glucocorticoids **(important in dogs only)**	Quinidine
	Salicylates
	Sulfur
Gold salts	Testosterone
Griseofulvin	Tetracyclines
Halothane	Thiabendazole
Ibuprofen	Trimethoprim-sulfamethoxazole
6-Mercaptopurine	Vitamin A
Methimazole	
Methotrexate	

Those drugs that most reliably increase SAP are marked **(important)**. The other drugs are less consistent.

opsy should be considered in patients with obviously significant hepatic disease, those that do not have hyperadrenocorticism, and those that have persistent (more than 1 month) changes in serum ALT or SAP consistent with chronic or progressive hepatic disease (see Fig. 9–7). It is not always possible to make these distinctions accurately; therefore, whenever hepatic biopsy is performed via laparotomy or laparoscopy, the rest of the abdomen should be explored and other organs sampled if there is any doubt of their involvement. Fine-needle aspirates with cytology are useful in detecting diffuse hepatic infiltrative disease and hepatic lipidosis (see Color Plate 3F).

Hepatic Encephalopathy

Abnormal behavior, sometimes associated with eating, may be due to hepatic encephalopathy, although hypoglycemia and epilepsy must also be considered. Whenever possible, glucose should be measured on blood obtained during an episode. Evaluation of hepatic function is indicated in patients with behavioral changes, transient blindness, seizures, coma, or vague CNS abnormalities. Congenital (portosystemic shunt) as well as severe acquired hepatic disease (cirrhosis) may cause encephalopathy. Routine biochemical profiling may be suggestive, but hepatic function testing is mandatory, since these diseases may not significantly change serum ALT, SAP, albumin, BUN, glucose, or bilirubin determinations. Resting plasma ammonia concentrations are meaningful only if they are increased. A patient in an episode of hepatic encephalopathy may have increased or normal resting plasma ammonia concentrations. Ammonia tolerance testing and pre- and postprandial serum bile acid concentrations appear to be the most sensitive and specific tests for hepatic dysfunction causing hepatic encephalopathy. A very rare congenital urea cycle enzyme deficiency may cause hepatic encephalopathy and hyperammonemia without affecting enzymes, bile acids, or BSP. Analysis of urea cycle enzymes in biopsy samples is necessary for diagnosis.

Icterus

Icterus is detected either during physical examination or when serum or plasma is inspected in the laboratory. Hyperbilirubinemia always denotes hepatobiliary or hematopoietic

disease (Fig. 9–8). Hepatic and hematopoietic diseases are not always associated with icterus, and disease in either system may be secondary to other disorders. The presence or absence of icterus is not diagnostic or prognostic. Sepsis, ruptured urinary bladder, and inflammatory bowel disease sometimes cause secondary hepatic dysfunction that may include icterus.

TOTAL SERUM BILIRUBIN

Occasional Indications ● Icterus (on either physical examination or inspection of nonhemolyzed serum or plasma), bilirubinuria (any amount in a cat or significant amounts in a dog), or suspected hepatic disease that is not apparent on other tests. It is questionable practice to request this test routinely because the sclera will have detectable icterus when the serum bilirubin is > 3 to 4 mg/dl, and the plasma will be icteric when the serum bilirubin is > 1.5 to 2 mg/dl. Note: Icterus is absent in many canine and feline hepatic diseases. Serum bilirubin is not a sensitive test for hepatic disease.

Measurement of direct (conjugated) and indirect (unconjugated) bilirubin fractions is not useful in determining the cause of increases in total bilirubin. Hemolytic, hepatic, and biliary tract diseases have unpredictable variation in the amount of each fraction. Other laboratory or diagnostic tests are required in order to identify the cause of the total bilirubin increase.

Analysis ● Measured in 0.5 ml of serum or heparinized plasma by spectrophotometric and dry reagent methods. The latter require dilutions if the bilirubin is > 7.5 mg/dl. Bilirubin is stable at 4° C for 7 days if not exposed to bright light. Measurement of urine bilirubin is discussed in Chapter 7.

Normal Values ● Dogs, < 1.0 mg/dl; cats, < 1.0 mg/dl.

Danger Values ● Dogs, > 40 mg/dl (kernicterus?); cats, unknown.

Artifacts ● Severe hemolysis may render spectrophotometric determinations inaccurate, and dry reagent methods may show increased results. Falsely decreased: fluorescent light and sunlight (lowered as much as 50% in 1 hour) and viscous serum (dry reagent). Falsely increased: lipemia and hemolysis (spectrophotometric).

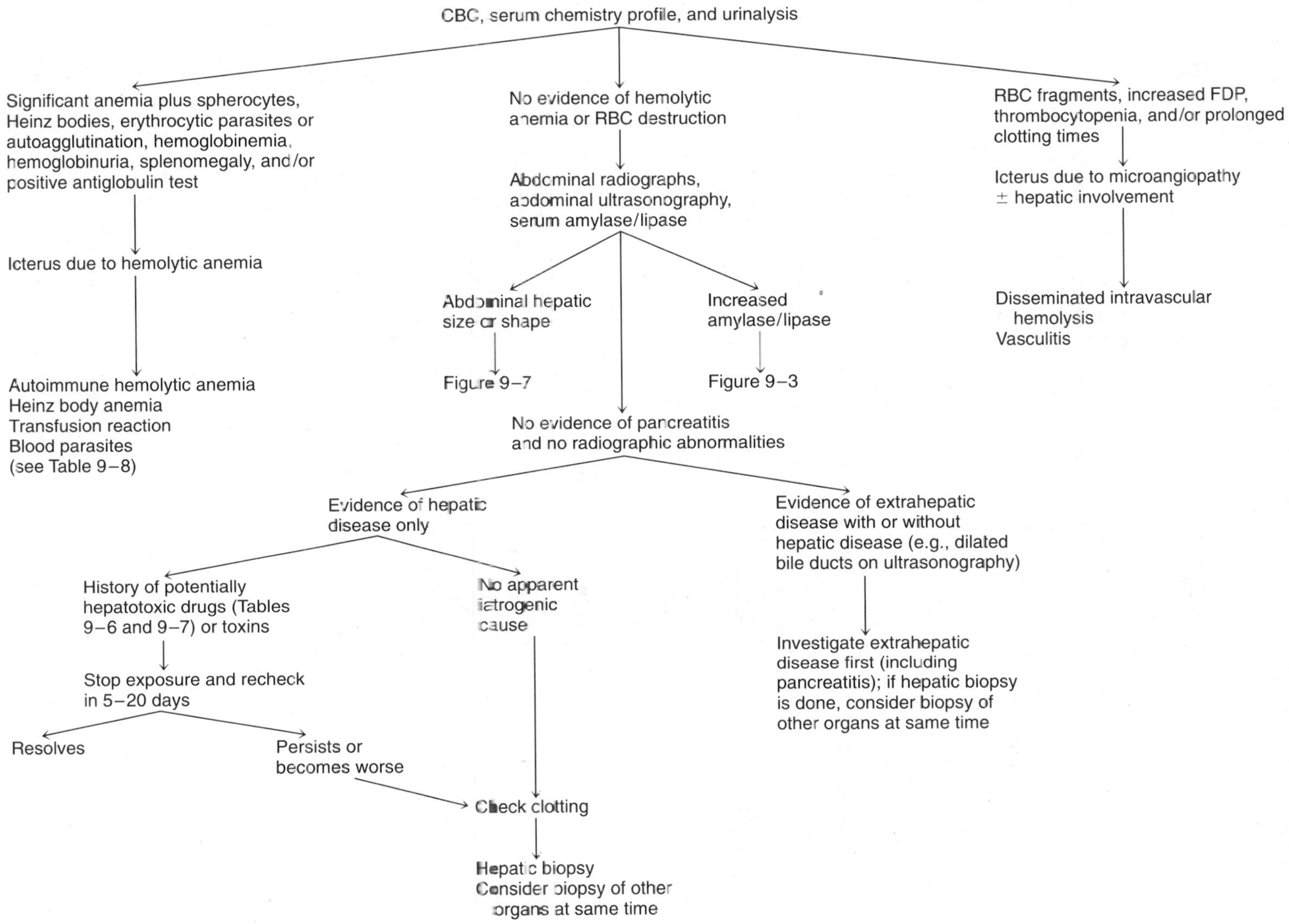

CBC, serum chemistry profile, and urinalysis

Significant anemia plus spherocytes, Heinz bodies, erythrocytic parasites or autoagglutination, hemoglobinemia, hemoglobinuria, splenomegaly, and/or positive antiglobulin test

Icterus due to hemolytic anemia

Autoimmune hemolytic anemia
Heinz body anemia
Transfusion reaction
Blood parasites
(see Table 9–8)

No evidence of hemolytic anemia or RBC destruction

RBC fragments, increased FDP, thrombocytopenia, and/or prolonged clotting times

Icterus due to microangiopathy ± hepatic involvement

Disseminated intravascular hemolysis
Vasculitis

Abdominal radiographs, abdominal ultrasonography, serum amylase/lipase

Increased amylase/lipase

Figure 9–3

Abdominal hepatic size or shape

Figure 9–7

No evidence of pancreatitis and no radiographic abnormalities

Evidence of extrahepatic disease with or without hepatic disease (e.g., dilated bile ducts on ultrasonography)

Investigate extrahepatic disease first (including pancreatitis); if hepatic biopsy is done, consider biopsy of other organs at same time

Evidence of hepatic disease only

No apparent iatrogenic cause

History of potentially hepatotoxic drugs (Tables 9–6 and 9–7) or toxins

Stop exposure and recheck in 5–20 days

Persists or becomes worse

Resolves

Check clotting

Hepatic biopsy
Consider biopsy of other organs at same time

Figure 9–8 Diagnostic approach to hyperbilirubinemia in dogs and cats.

Drug Therapy That May Alter Serum Bilirubin ● Decreased bilirubin may be due to drugs that displace bilirubin from albumin (rare but may be due to large doses of salicylates, sulfisoxazole, and penicillin) or that cause hepatic enzyme induction (e.g., phenobarbital). Increased bilirubin may be due to drugs causing hemolytic anemia (Table 9–8) or acute hepatic necrosis (see Table 9–6).

Causes of Hypobilirubinemia ● Do not exist.

Causes of Hyperbilirubinemia ● Hemolytic disease and hepatic disease (including extrahepatic obstruction) are the two main causes (see Fig. 9–8). A CBC should be determined in every icteric patient to rule out hemolytic disease. The red blood cell numbers must decrease rapidly and significantly to result in clinical icterus. Very regenerative anemias suggest that icterus is due to immune-mediated hemolytic anemia (IHA). Reticulocytosis, hemoglobinemia, hemoglobinuria, erythrocytic autoagglutination, spherocytosis, positive Coombs' test results, splenomegaly, or hepatomegaly is usually present. See Chapter 3 for further discussion of IHA and other regenerative anemias (e.g., Heinz body, zinc intoxication, *Haemobartonella*). Dividing the total serum bilirubin concentration into direct and indirect fractions (i.e., conjugated and unconjugated, respectively) is not useful in differentiating hemolytic from hepatic icterus and may even be misleading. Indirect bilirubin initially predominates in patients with hemolysis but is quickly replaced by direct bilirubin. Even when indirect bilirubin predominates, a patient

may have primary hepatic disease. Bilirubinuria theoretically should be absent in hemolytic disease but is often present in IHA because the canine kidneys can conjugate bilirubin. The clinician must not be misled by increases in ALT because severe, acute hemolytic anemia may have a simultaneously increased ALT, ostensibly due to acute hepatic hypoxia.

In some patients, severe hepatic disease (especially acute necrosis) may be accompanied by DIC and subsequent hemolytic anemia. These cases may be difficult to distinguish from IHA. However, anemia due to disseminated intravascular coagulation is usually not as regenerative as in IHA, and the presence of red blood cell fragments, thrombocytopenia, increased fibrin degradation products (FDP), decreased antithrombin III, prolonged clotting time, and abnormal hepatic function tests usually allows differentiation, as do vomiting, abdominal pain, and encephalopathy when present.

Dogs and cats often have relatively severe hepatic disease before icterus is observed. The magnitude of the total serum bilirubin is not prognostic or diagnostic, and the relative proportions of direct and indirect bilirubin are not helpful in distinguishing hepatic from extrahepatic disease. In both cases, the conjugated bilirubin may compose 95% + of the serum total bilirubin. Furthermore, secondary hepatic disease (reactive disease or so-called bystander phenomenon due to septicemia, toxemia, inflammation) may be marked by icterus similar to that seen in primary hepatic disease.

Most hepatic diseases may cause icterus in cats, but the most common causes are hepatic lipidosis, cholangitis-cholangiohepatitis, hepatic lymphosarcoma, and FIP. Icterus in cats is an indication for CBC and a serum biochemistry panel. Icterus in a cat that is not the result of hemolytic causes usually indicates a hepatic biopsy because most icteric cats have some sort of primary hepatic disease. Biopsy is necessary to differentiate cause(s) and institute specific treatment. Fine-needle aspirate is usually definitive for lipidosis.

Icterus in dogs is an indication for CBC and a serum biochemistry panel (to include at least ALT, SAP, BUN, albumin, amylase, and lipase). Common causes of nonhemolytic icterus in dogs include pancreatitis obstructing the bile duct, intrahepatic cholestasis, chronic hepatitis, hepatic lymphosarcoma, acute hepatic necrosis, and hepatic cirrhosis. Because many other diseases may also cause icterus, further testing (abdominal radiographs, hepatic ultrasonography, and hepatic function tests) is indicated to deter-

Table 9–8 SELECTED SUBSTANCES THAT HAVE BEEN DOCUMENTED OR SUSPECTED TO CAUSE HEMOLYTIC ANEMIA

Acetaminophen **(especially cats)**
Benzocaine **(especially cats)**
Cephalosporins
Dapsone
Methylene blue **(especially cats)**
Nitrofurantoin
Onions
Penicillins
Phenacetin **(especially cats)**
Phenazopyridine
Phenylbutazone
Propylthiouracil
Sulfonamides
Vitamin K_3
Zinc

These substances do not always cause anemia, but they have the potential and should be stopped, if possible, in patients with hemolytic anemia.

mine if primary hepatic disease exists. If there is primary hepatic disease, a hepatic biopsy is usually indicated. If pancreatitis is present, surgery is not indicated unless a chronic bile duct obstruction results and it becomes necessary to bypass the common bile duct with a cholecystoduodenostomy. If there is coexisting extrahepatic disease, it must also be investigated.

ALANINE TRANSFERASE

ALT was formerly known as serum glutamic-pyruvic transaminase (SGPT).

Common Indications • Systemic disease including weight loss, hepatomegaly, vomiting, diarrhea, icterus, ascites, depression, and anorexia; also, as a screening procedure for hepatic disease in any patient with undiagnosed illness. Most patients with known hepatic disease should have periodic ALT determinations to monitor the problem. Advantages: specificity for the liver. Disadvantages: lack of sensitivity (i.e., patients with significant hepatic disease such as cirrhosis or hepatic neoplasia may have normal ALT) and inability to distinguish between different hepatic diseases or when there is secondary nonhepatic disease involvement.

Analysis • Measured in 0.5 ml of serum (heparinized plasma in selected assays) by spectrophotometric and dry reagent methods. ALT is stable in separated serum for approximately 1 (at 22° C) to 7 (at 4° C) days.

Normal Values • Serum enzyme activity may vary markedly between laboratories, depending on the technique and the units used.

Danger Values • Despite correlation between ALT and active hepatic damage, there is no correlation between ALT and hepatic function; hence, there are no danger values.

Artifacts • Falsely increased: severe hemolysis and lipemia.

Drug Therapy That May Alter Serum ALT • Increased ALT may be due to any drug causing hepatocellular damage (i.e., drug-induced hepatopathy). The list of all drugs suspected to cause increased ALT is extensive and includes many that are safe in the majority of patients. A list of selected drugs documented to cause increased ALT in human beings, dogs, and cats is given in Table 9–6. Administration of one of these drugs does not automatically explain an increased ALT. Note: A patient could have an idiosyncratic reaction from almost any drug, resulting in an increased ALT.

Causes of Decreased ALT • Not significant.

Causes of Increased ALT • Increase in ALT is principally due to hepatocellular damage from any cause (Table 9–9). Red blood cells and striated muscle cells contain small amounts of ALT, and damage to these may cause relatively minor increases (i.e., less than two to three times normal) in serum ALT, as may exercise. Hepatocytes contain substantial amounts of ALT in the cytosol, and major increases in serum ALT (i.e., three or more times normal) indicate hepatocellular leakage of the enzyme but do not always signify primary or irreversible hepatic disease. Hepatic disease may have normal to significantly increased serum ALT activity. The magnitude of the increase in ALT does not correlate with the seriousness of the hepatic disease and is not a prognostic indicator unless a specific disease is being considered. The serum ALT half-life is approximately 1 to 2 days or less, and serum ALT is expected to decrease over 1 to 2 weeks once active hepatic damage ceases. It is thought ALT remains elevated during hepatic regeneration.

When identifying increased serum ALT, many factors must be considered (Fig. 9–9). If no other disease is present in the patient, the increased ALT indicates the need for periodic monitoring, since it may be the first detectable

Table 9–9 SELECTED CAUSES OF INCREASED SERUM ALT LEVELS

Dogs	Cats
Hepatic parenchymal disease	Hepatic parenchymal disease
Cholangitis	Cholangitis
Cholangiohepatitis	Cholangiohepatitis
Cirrhosis	Feline infectious peritonitis
Copper storage disease	
Hepatic malignancy	Hepatic lymphosarcoma
Chronic hepatitis	Cirrhosis
Hepatic toxin	Hepatic toxin
Trauma	Trauma
Other disorders	Other disorders
Anoxia due to anemia/ shock	Anoxia due to anemia/ shock
Iatrogenic (see Table 9–6)	Iatrogenic (see Table 9–6)

Almost any disease affecting the liver can cause increased ALT levels. The disorders listed above represent those that may be more likely to cause a significant increase. However, any of these diseases can exist with minor or no increase in ALT values.

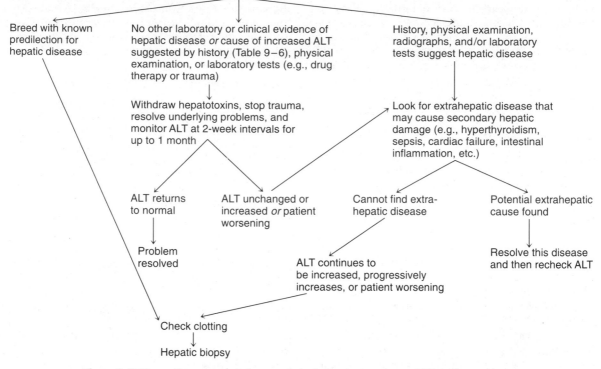

Figure 9–9 Diagnostic approach to increased alanine aminotransferase (ALT) in dogs and cats.

sign of significant hepatic disease. When other abnormalities consistent with hepatic disease are present, the approach is like that in any other patient with hepatic disease. Common causes of serum ALT more than three times normal include hepatic anoxia, poor hepatic perfusion, spontaneous and surgical trauma (e.g., hit by a car, or surgery), chronic hepatitis, cirrhosis, cholangitis-cholangiohepatitis, acute biliary obstruction, hepatic necrosis due to any cause, acute pancreatitis, hepatic neoplasia, sepsis, and certain drugs. Sepsis, especially septicemia and toxemia, may secondarily damage hepatocytes. Abdominal inflammation may do the same: The pancreas is in close proximity to the liver, and inflammation in the pancreas may cause mechanical damage to the liver. In Doberman pinschers, Bedlington terriers, and West Highland white terriers, an increased serum ALT suggests that copper storage disease may be present.

ASPARTATE TRANSFERASE

AST was formerly known as serum glutamic-oxaloacetic transaminase (SGOT).

Occasional Indications • Same as for ALT. Disadvantages: not as specific for the liver as ALT.

Analysis • Same as for ALT.

Artifacts • Falsely increased: hemolysis, lipemia, and ketoacidosis.

Drug Therapy That May Alter AST • Decreased AST may be due to metronidazole therapy and vitamin B_6 deficiency (rare). Increased AST may be due to hepatotoxic drugs (see Table 9–6).

Causes of Decreased AST • None.

Causes of Increased AST • Like ALT, AST is present in significant quantities in hepatocytes. Whereas ALT is present in the cytosol, AST is present in mitochondria. Increased serum ALT reflects cell membrane damage and leakage, whereas AST increases reflect more serious hepatic damage because mitochondria are not damaged as readily as the cell membrane is. AST is, however, present in significant quantities in many other tissues including muscle and red blood cells; therefore, increased AST is not as specific for hepatic injury as is increased ALT. Exercise and intramuscular injections may increase serum AST. The most common causes of increased AST include hepatic disease, muscle disease (inflammation or necrosis), or hemolysis (spontaneous or artifactual). Increased AST is an indication to check for ongoing hemolysis by measuring the hematocrit and observing the color of the plasma/serum on a centrifuged blood sample. If there is no hemolysis, the next step is to measure serum ALT to determine whether the increased AST is from the liver (significant increases in ALT and AST suggest that AST increases are of hepatic origin).

SERUM ALKALINE PHOSPHATASE

Common Indications • Systemic disease including weight loss, hepatomegaly, vomiting, diarrhea, ascites, icterus, depression, or anorexia; also as a screen for hepatic disease and hyperadrenocorticism. Advantages: useful in evaluating the liver for subtle cholestatic disease. Disadvantages: effects of corticosteroids, bone lesions, and osteoblastic activity from a bone source in young growing dogs.

Analysis • Measured in 0.5 ml of serum or heparinized plasma by spectrophotometric methods. Stability in heat (55° C) has been used to differentiate bone-origin (heat-sensitive) from hepatic-origin (heat-stable) SAP. However, it is difficult to obtain reproducible results with the heat-inactivation test. L-Phenylalanine inhibits steroid-induced SAP and can be used to help determine if increased SAP is due to corticosteroids. Alternatively, cellulose acetate electrophoresis may be used to separate the isoenzymes more definitively. The diagnostic usefulness of determining the per cent steroid fraction is questionable, since dogs with hepatic disease often have considerable steroid involvement.

Normal Values • May vary markedly from laboratory to laboratory. Immature dogs characteristically have SAP (bone origin) activities up to twice that of sexually mature dogs.

Danger Values • Due to lack of correlation with hepatic function, there are no danger values for SAP.

Artifacts • Falsely decreased: fluoride, oxalate, phosphate, arsenate, zinc, citrate, manganese, EDTA, beryllium, and sulfhydryl compounds. Falsely increased: bilirubin > 8 mg/dl, severe lipemia, storage, and hemolysis (slight).

Drug Therapy That May Increase SAP • Any drug that causes hepatic enzyme induction or cholestasis (see Table 9–7) may increase SAP. Glucocorticoids, primidone, and barbiturates typically increase SAP in dogs, but other drugs are less consistent. Although glucocorticoids can cause marked SAP increases in dogs, they do not in cats.

Causes of Decreased SAP • Hypothyroidism (not significant).

Causes of Increased SAP • Bone-origin SAP is commonly increased (SAP less than three times normal) in animals < 6 to 8 months old. Bone disease (e.g., osteosarcoma or osteomyelitis) seldom causes increased SAP (and then it is usually a minor increase).

Increased SAP is interpreted differently in dogs and cats (Table 9–10). Cats have less hepatocellular SAP, which is readily excreted by their kidneys. Therefore, any increase in feline

Table 9–10 CAUSES OF INCREASED SAP LEVELS

Dogs	Cats
Biliary tract abnormalities	Biliary tract abnormalities
Pancreatitis	Same as for dogs
Bile duct neoplasia	
Cholelithiasis	
Cholecystitis	
Ruptured gallbladder	
Hepatic parenchymal	Hepatic parenchymal
disease	disease
Cholangiohepatitis	Cholangiohepatitis
Chronic hepatitis	Hepatic lipidosis
Copper storage disease	Hepatic lymphosarcoma
Cirrhosis/fibrosis	Feline infectious
Hepatic neoplasia	peritonitis
Lymphosarcoma	
Hemangiosarcoma	
Hepatocellular	
carcinoma	
Metastatic carcinoma	
Toxic hepatitis	
Aflatoxin	
Other disorders	Other disorders
Diabetes mellitus	Diabetes mellitus
Hyperadrenocorticism	Hyperthyroidism
Chronic passive	
congestion due to	
right heart failure	
Diaphragmatic hernia	
Septicemia	
Ehrlichiosis	
Young dog with bone	
growth	
Osteomyelitis*	
Iatrogenic (see Table 9–7)	Iatrogenic (see Table 9–7)

Almost any disease affecting the liver can cause increased SAP levels. The disorders listed above represent those that may be more likely to cause a significant increase. However, any of these can exist with minor or no increase in SAP values.
*Rarely of importance.

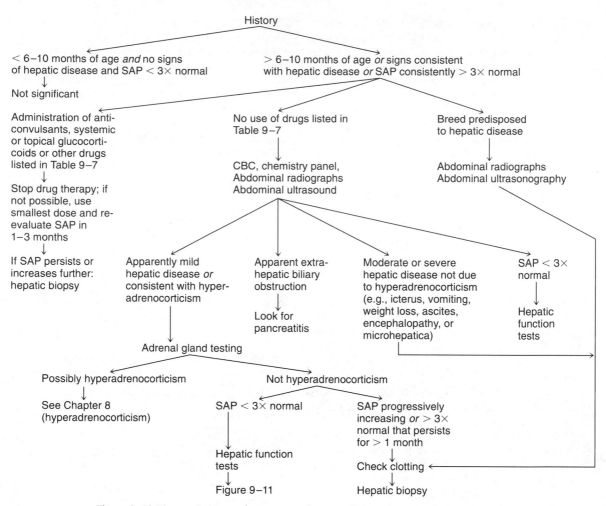

Figure 9–10 Diagnostic approach to increased serum alkaline phosphatase (SAP) in dogs.

SAP is considered significant, indicating further tests. Not all cats with hepatic disease have increased SAP, however. The major causes of increased SAP in cats are hepatic lipidosis, cholangitis-cholangiohepatitis, hyperthyroidism, and diabetes mellitus. SAP increases are generally more specific than GGT in cats with hepatic lipidosis. Hyperadrenocorticism (spontaneous and iatrogenic) is not expected to increase SAP in cats. Increased SAP in a cat is an indication for serum thyroid hormone determination, urinalysis, blood glucose and serum ALT measurement, and perhaps a hepatic function test (e.g., bile acid). If hepatic disease is the apparent cause of the increased SAP, one must determine if hepatic biopsy is indicated (see the later discussion under Bile Acids).

The major causes of SAP values more than three times normal in dogs are hepatic disease, hyperadrenocorticism, and therapy with glucocorticoids, anticonvulsants, or barbiturates. Hepatic disease with increased SAP usually has a cholestatic component; however, this does not imply icterus or gross obstruction of the biliary tract. Intrahepatic cholestasis due to diffuse or focal compression of bile canaliculi may occur in various hepatopathies, even those secondary to septicemia, toxemia, and chronic stress-induced vacuolar hepatopathy. Acute hepatocellular necrosis can transiently increase SAP (usually less than five times normal). Extrahepatic biliary obstruction and enzyme induction due to endogenous or exogenous glucocorticoids or drug administration may increase SAP more than 10 times normal. As with ALT, the magnitude of the increase in SAP does not correlate with the seriousness or prognosis of the hepatic disease.

In dogs, it is important first to rule out young age, drug therapy, and hyperadrenocorticism, lest an unnecessary hepatic biopsy be performed (Fig. 9–10). Hyperadrenocorticism can easily be confused with primary hepatic disease, since it typically causes hepatomegaly, polyuria-polydipsia, increased ALT, and possibly increased serum bile acids. Unless a patient has signs of hepatic failure, icterus, hepatoencephalopathy, hypoglycemia, weight loss, vomiting, hypoalbuminemia, ascites, or microhepatica, hyperadrenocorticism must be precluded by adrenal gland function testing. If a hepatic biopsy specimen is obtained from a patient with hyperadrenocorticism, vacuolar hepatopathy will be documented.

GAMMA-GLUTAMYL TRANSPEPTIDASE (GGT)

Occasional Indications ● Same as for SAP. SAP appears to be more sensitive for hepatobiliary disease in dogs, but GGT has slightly greater sensitivity in cats and perhaps greater specificity for hepatic disease except hepatic lipidosis. Therefore, it is more frequently indicated in cats than in dogs. GGT is less influenced than SAP by secondary hepatic disease conditions or enzyme-inducing drugs. The use of SAP and GGT together has a higher predictive value of hepatic disease.

Analysis ● Measured in 0.5 ml of serum, urine, and body fluids by spectrophotometric methods. GGT is stable in serum at 4° C for at least 3 days and at −20° C for up to 1 year.

Normal Values and Danger Values ● Same as for SAP.

Artifacts ● Lipemia may alter results.

Drug Therapy That May Affect GGT ● Same as for SAP, plus clofibrate may decrease GGT.

Causes of Decreased GGT ● Not significant.

Causes of Increased GGT ● Causes are similar to increased SAP, except bone lesions are not recognized to increase GGT. It is induced by glucocorticoid therapy and certain drugs, as is SAP. In cats, GGT may increase more than SAP. GGT does not tend to increase after acute hepatic necrosis, as does SAP. Increased GGT should be pursued as for increased SAP (see Fig. 9–10). Increased GGT may suggest pancreatitis causing obstruction of the bile duct, as for SAP.

Causes of Increased Urine GGT ● Increased 24-hour urinary excretion of GGT can be caused by various nephrotoxins (e.g., gentamicin).

LACTIC DEHYDROGENASE (LDH)

Rare Indications ● Disadvantages: lack of specificity.

Analysis ● Measured in 0.5 ml of serum, heparinized plasma, or cerebrospinal fluid (CSF) by spectrophotometric methods.

Normal Values and Danger Values ● Same as for ALT and SAP.

Artifacts ● Falsely decreased: oxalate, ascorbate, urea, and old test reagents. Falsely increased: hemolysis and severe lipemia.

Causes of Decreased LDH ● Not significant.

Causes of Increased LDH ● LDH is found in so many body tissues that serum LDH is of questionable diagnostic value. Inexplicable increases of small to great magnitude are not uncommon. Meals and exercise may increase LDH. If serum LDH is increased, more specific tests should be used (e.g., ALT, SAP, creatine kinase [CK]). Occasionally, serum LDH is significantly increased (more than three times normal) in some patients with malignancies who have no evidence of other organ dysfunction. Patients with hepatic disease (especially necrosis) often have significantly increased LDH. When LDH increase parallels SAP and ALT increases, it suggests the LDH source is the liver. In a patient that is otherwise normal, a significantly increased serum LDH can be ignored or one can repeat a serum chemistry profile within 3 to 4 weeks.

SULFOBROMOPHTHALEIN RETENTION

Rare Indications ● To evaluate hepatic function in patients with suspected hepatic disease and to monitor hepatic function in patients with known hepatic disease. There is no reason to measure BSP retention in icteric patients with hepatic disease because BSP and bilirubin compete for the same hepatic carrier proteins and hepatic icterus confirms hepatobiliary disease. Advantages: evaluates hepatic function. Disadvantages: many extrahepatic factors alter results, poor availability of BSP and laboratories performing the test.

Analysis • BSP dye, 5 mg/kg of lean body weight (in a 5% aqueous solution), is injected intravenously. Thirty minutes later, blood sufficient to provide 1.5 ml of serum or heparinized plasma is obtained. Spectrophotometric analysis is used.

Normal Values • Dogs, < 5% retention at 30 minutes; cats, < 3 to 5% retention at 30 minutes.

Danger Values • None recognized. **Warning**: Repeated administration of BSP may cause anaphylactoid reactions. If given perivascularly, inflammation may result (rarely significant).

Artifacts • Falsely decreased: improper dosing or improper sample collection. Falsely increased: improper dosing of BSP, hemolysis, lipemia, icterus, and certain drugs.

Drug Therapy That May Alter Percentage of BSP Retention • Decreased retention may be due to phenobarbital. Increased retention may be due to any drug causing severe hepatic disease (see Tables 9–6 and 9–7).

Causes of Decreased Percentage of BSP Retention • Hypoalbuminemia and enlarged third spaces (e.g., edema or ascites) increase drug distribution and thus result in a decreased measured serum concentration compared with what it would be if these conditions were not present.

Causes of Increased Percentage of BSP Retention • Either hepatic insufficiency or poor hepatic perfusion can increase BSP retention. Poor hepatic perfusion is usually caused by poor cardiac output (e.g., heart failure) or vascular anomalies such as portosystemic shunts, hepatic AV fistulas, or blocked portal veins. Hepatic disease (primary or secondary) may have any percentage of BSP dye retention (from normal to markedly increased), and one cannot reliably correlate the severity of clinical signs with the percentage of BSP retention.

INDOCYANINE GREEN (ICG)

Rare Indications • Same as for BSP. Advantages: may be somewhat more sensitive and specific than BSP, particularly in cats. Disadvantages: poor availability of test and relatively little clini-

cal experience with this test in dogs and cats, making it more difficult to interpret results.

Analysis • For the more commonly used retention study, 1 mg (dog) or 1.5 mg (cat) of ICG/kg of lean body weight (in a 0.5% solution made immediately before use) is injected intravenously. Thirty minutes later, sufficient blood to provide 1 ml of serum or heparinized plasma is obtained. A spectrophotometric analysis is used.

For clearance studies: ICG is injected as above, and blood samples are obtained at 0, 5, 10, and 15 minutes.

Normal Values • Dogs, < 20% to 25% retention or > 3 to 4 ml/min/kg clearance; cats, < 15% retention or > 4 to 12 ml/min/kg clearance.

Danger Values • None.

Artifacts • Falsely decreased: improper dosing or sampling error. Falsely increased: improper dosing, perivascular injection of the dye, lipemia, and serum bilirubin > 3 mg/dl.

Drug Therapy That May Alter ICG Retention • Same as for BSP.

Causes of Decreased ICG Retention • Same as for BSP.

Causes of Increased ICG Retention • Same as for BSP. However, there is less clinical experience with ICG in dogs and cats than there is with BSP. Therefore, there may be differences that are currently unrecognized.

BILE ACIDS

Frequent Indications • Suspected hepatic disease, chronic weight loss, abnormal CNS signs, icterus, hepatomegaly, and microhepatica; also to monitor hepatic function in patients with known hepatic diseases. Due to the ease of this test compared with BSP, ICG, and ammonia, it is used routinely as a screening test for hepatic dysfunction. Advantages: ease of use, few extrahepatic factors affect it. Disadvantages: does not reliably distinguish between different hepatobiliary diseases.

Analysis • Measured in 0.5 ml of serum by RIA, gas layer chromatography (GLC), and spectrophotometric methods. RIA is principally used to measure specific bile acids; spectrophotometric analysis usually measures total serum bile acids. GLC can measure either. It is important that the assay measure total bile acids or taurine conjugates, which are the predominant bile acid conjugates in dogs and cats. Assays that measure only choleglycine may be misleading.

Maximum information is obtained by determining a 12-hour fasting preprandial and 2-hour postprandial concentration. Dogs and cats should be fed canned food containing moderate fat content, causing the gallbladder to contract. Pre- and postprandial concentrations together improve the sensitivity of the test, making it more sensitive than other function tests (BSP, ICG, and ATT).

Normal Values ● Because of different techniques and assays (μmol/L or μg/ml), normal values must be established for each laboratory.

Danger Values ● None.

Artifacts ● Very increased serum dehydrogenase activities may require modification of the spectrophotometric technique. Severe lipemia (chylomicronemia) and hemolysis may falsely decrease bile acid measurements, and hypertriglyceridemia may falsely increase concentrations when spectrophotometric techniques are used, but they do not affect RIA. No further information is obtained in performing this test in icteric patients.

Drug Therapy and Other Factors That May Alter Serum Bile Acid Concentration ● Cholestyramine lowers serum concentrations by binding to bile acids in the intestinal lumen, preventing their reabsorption. Resection of the ileum (the principal site of bile acid reabsorption), severe ileal disease, or cholecystectomy may also cause serum bile acids to inaccurately reflect hepatic function. Prolonged anorexia (> 1 to 2 days) may cause fasting serum bile acid concentrations to be less than would be found if the patient were eating normally. Intestinal hypomotility may cause the 2-hour postprandial sample to be a less sensitive indicator of hepatic disease because of failure to deliver the bile acids to the ileum in a timely fashion. Hepatic insufficiency does not decrease serum bile acid concentrations.

Causes of Decreased Serum Bile Acid Concentration ● Not significant.

Causes of Increased Serum Bile Acid Concentration ● Serum bile acid concentrations are increased because of either hepatocellular disease, cholestatic disease, or portosystemic shunting. When both fasting and 2-hour postprandial serum bile acid levels are determined, the sensitivity of these tests becomes greater than other hepatic function tests. Because of the ease of performing the test and wide availability of the test, it has replaced other hepatic function tests used in clinical situations. Serum bile acids offer no additional information in icteric patients with hepatic or extrahepatic biliary tract disease. In nonicteric patients suspected of having hepatic disease, serum bile acids become a good screening test to support further diagnostic evaluations. Not all patients with hepatic disease have increased serum bile acid concentrations, and the relative increase in bile acids is not diagnostic for the type of disease or the prognosis. Reported fasting serum bile acids that are increased > 20 μmol/L or postprandial values of > 25 μmol/L suggest significant hepatic disease or portosystemic shunting and dictate further hepatic evaluation and possibly hepatic biopsy. Generally, pre- and postprandial bile acids are determined simultaneously; however, if only fasted values are determined and found to be normal, postprandial measurements are required. The magnitude of the rise or the per cent increase from pre- to postprandial values does not imply a specific diagnosis or prognosis. Most animals with chronic hepatitis, marked hepatic necrosis, cholestasis, and hepatic neoplasia have abnormal values. Bile acids are usually not markedly altered by secondary hepatic disease from a nonhepatic disorder or with glucocorticoid or anticonvulsant therapy. However, rarely they are markedly increased by such disorders.

Abnormal serum bile acids are possibly the most sensitive indicator of congenital portosystemic shunts. Almost all animals with congenital portal vascular anomalies have increased bile acids; some of the highest concentrations are observed in these cases.

AMMONIA AND AMMONIA TOLERANCE TESTING (ATT)

Rare Indications ● Same as for bile acids (i.e., where a sensitive function test is needed to prove hepatic disease in an animal in which easier tests do not allow diagnosis). Advantages: good sensitivity and specificity. Disadvantages: procedural requirements for submitting the samples, and the likelihood of vomiting or CNS signs with the ATT.

Analysis • Measured in 2.5 ml of blood, serum, plasma (heparinized is recommended), CSF, or urine by enzymatic, selective electrode, dry reagent, and resin absorption methods. There does not appear to be any advantage of arterial over venous blood. Blood must be drawn into an ice-chilled tube, which is stoppered tightly after filling, immediately put back on ice, and promptly taken to the laboratory. A control sample should be taken at the same time using the same technique. The test must be performed within 20 minutes, or the plasma must be frozen at $-20°$ C, which stabilizes the ammonia concentration for at least 2 days. If an ATT is to be performed, samples for ammonia determination should be taken before and 30 or 45 minutes after administration of NH_4Cl, 100 mg/kg of body weight. The NH_4Cl may be administered orally as a solution in 20 to 50 ml of water, as a 5% solution, as a dry powder in gelatin capsules, or rectally as a 5% solution. The use of orally administered gelatin capsules is the easiest and the least likely to result in expulsion (vomiting or defecation of the NH_4Cl).

Normal Values • *Resting ammonia*: dogs, 45 to 120 μg/dl; cats, 30 to 100 μg/dl. *ATT, ammonia at 30 minutes*: dogs, minimal change from normal values; cats, no change from normal values.

Danger Values • Dogs, > 1000 μg/dl (hepatic encephalopathy may be imminent, although there is poor correlation between clinical signs of encephalopathy and plasma ammonia concentrations); cats, unknown. **Warning**: Administration of NH_4Cl to patients with increased resting blood ammonia concentrations may cause encephalopathy. Do not perform ATT if a patient is showing obvious signs of encephalopathy. The lack of obvious clinical signs of encephalopathy does not predict blood ammonia levels to be in normal ranges.

Artifacts • Falsely increased: allowing the blood to stand, strenuous exercise, or the use of fluoride or oxalate anticoagulants. Lipemia and hemolysis may alter results.

Drug Therapy That May Alter Ammonia • Decreased serum ammonia may be due to intestinal antibiotics (e.g., aminoglycosides), lactulose, *Lactobacillus acidophilus* cultures, enemas, and diphenhydramine. Increased serum ammonia may be due to valproic acid, asparaginase, narcotics, diuretics causing hypokalemia or alkalosis, hyperalimentation, ammonium salts, and high-protein meals (including blood from spontaneous gastrointestinal bleeding).

Causes of Hypoammonemia • Not significant.

Causes of Hyperammonemia • Urea cycle disorders (rare), hepatic insufficiency, or portosystemic shunting (congenital or acquired). Resting blood ammonia concentrations are probably less sensitive than fasting serum bile acids in detecting hepatic dysfunction, whereas the ATT is possibly as sensitive as pre- and postprandial bile acids in detecting portosystemic shunting. A significantly increased fasting blood ammonia concentration renders an ATT unnecessary. Clinical signs are not well correlated with blood ammonia concentrations. An abnormal ATT result or resting ammonia value in a patient with hepatic disease is generally an indication for hepatic biopsy or a portogram (Fig. 9–11). Rarely, plasma ammonia may be increased as a result of urinary tract obstruction, especially if complicated by infection with urease-producing bacteria.

CHOLESTEROL (see Chapter 8)

WEIGHT LOSS OR ANOREXIA DUE TO UNKNOWN CAUSE

Weight loss may be due to many causes (Table 9–11). Concurrent problems with fewer potential causes (regurgitation, vomiting, diarrhea, icterus) should be considered first. If a patient had a reasonable appetite when it *first* began to lose weight, major differentials are intestinal disease, maldigestion, increased utilization of calories (e.g., hyperthyroidism, lactation), or increased loss of calories (e.g., diabetes mellitus). If no other identifiable problems other than weight loss or anorexia can be pursued, then a systematic search is indicated (Fig. 9–12). One should first preclude as many causes as possible with the history and physical examination (lack of food, calorie-deficient food, inability to eat, regurgitation, vomiting and diarrhea). Next, extensive clinicopathologic screening is indicated. Radiographs are considered an extension of the physical examination. If the abdomen can be palpated carefully, abdominal radiographs are seldom useful. However, thoracic radiographs may be very revealing even if a patient does not have coughing or abnormal lung sounds. If laboratory or radiographic abnormalities are not present or are unconvincing, one may repeat the tests at 1- to 3-week intervals, depending on the clinical condition of the patient, or immediately proceed to func-

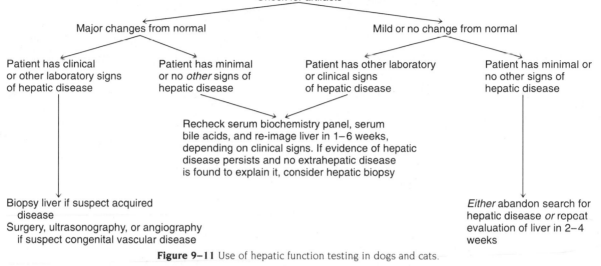

Figure 9–11 Use of hepatic function testing in dogs and cats.

tion tests and/or biopsies. Certain hepatic and adrenal gland diseases may require such tests. It is noteworthy that severe gastric or intestinal disease may cause anorexia or severe weight loss without vomiting or diarrhea. Gastroduodenoscopy-ileoscopy plus biopsy is reasonable in patients with severe weight loss of unknown cause. Some cases with gastric neoplasia may present only for anorexia and weight loss with no other gastrointestinal signs. Clinicians without access to endoscopic equipment may consider exploratory laparotomy. If surgery is done, gastric, duodenal, jejunal, ileal, mesenteric lymph node, hepatic, and splenic biopsies should be performed, regardless of a normal gross appearance of the organs.

Cancer cachexia can be particularly difficult to diagnose. It is a poorly defined, multifaceted syndrome that may involve loss of taste, malabsorption, increased metabolism with energy wasting, and other mechanisms. Almost any tumor can cause cancer cachexia. There are no consistent laboratory findings. Finding a neoplasia is required for the diagnosis. The causative cancer may be large or small, focal or diffuse. Lymphosarcomas and carcinomas are probably the most common causes.

Anorexia of unknown cause is similar to weight loss in being difficult to evaluate if there are no other identifiable abnormalities. The diagnostic approach is similar to that for chronic weight loss (Fig. 9–12 and Table 9–12). Anorexia can be divided into three categories: pseudoanorexia associated with inability to eat (oral, pharyngeal, or esophageal disease), primary anorexia (rare) associated with a primary CNS disorder, and secondary anorexia (the most common), which is the result of other systemic or metabolic disease.

If necessary, one may elect a therapeutic trial to treat for a suspected problem in a patient in whom a diagnosis cannot be made. However, it

Table 9–11 MAJOR CAUSES OF WEIGHT LOSS IN DOGS AND CATS

Calorie-deficient food or no food

Failure or refusal to eat
 Dysphagia
 Oral lesion
 Anorexia for any reason

Regurgitation
 Pharyngeal or esophageal disease

Vomiting (see Table 9–2)

Maldigestion
 Exocrine pancreatic insufficiency
 Bile salt deficiency?
 Lactase deficiency?

Intestinal malabsorption
 Does not always cause diarrhea

Malassimilation
 Hepatic failure
 Cardiac failure
 Diabetes mellitus
 Uremia
 Cancer cachexia syndrome
 Hypoadrenocorticism

Excessive use or loss of calories
 Hyperthyroidism
 Excessive demand for calories due to environment

Muscle wasting
 Myopathy
 Neuropathy

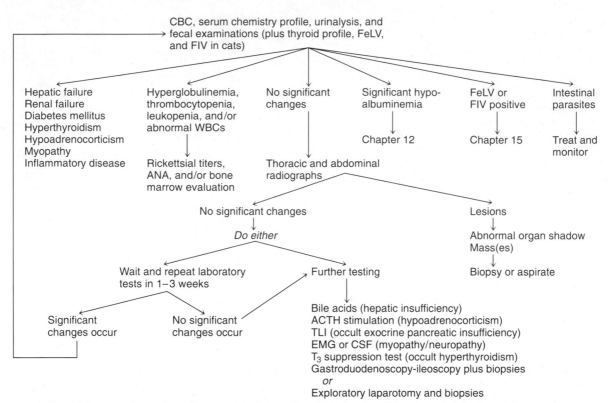

Figure 9–12 Diagnostic approach to chronic weight loss in dogs and cats when there are no other abnormalities on history or physical examination and the animal is not ingesting adequate calories (see Table 9–11).

Table 9–12 CATEGORIES OF DISEASES
THAT CAUSE ANOREXIA

Psychologic (especially cats)
Inability to smell food
Dysphagia (especially when it causes pain)
Inflammation
   Due to an etiologic agent
   Due to immune-mediated disease
   Due to neoplasia
   Due to necrosis
   Due to drugs
Alimentary and abdominal disease (especially that which
   causes nausea or abdominal pain)
Neoplasia
   Due to the neoplasia itself
   Due to secondary bacterial infection when the neoplasia
     impairs natural defense mechanisms
Toxins
   Exogenous (various ones)
   Endogenous (due to renal failure, hepatic failure, and
     other factors)
Endocrine disease
   Hypoadrenocorticism
   Hyperthyroidism
Central nervous system disease
   Primary
   Secondary

is vital that one design the therapy so that it is extremely likely to succeed if the presumptive disease is present. Then, if it fails, one may rule out that disease and go on to treat for something else. To do this, be sure that the dose is high enough and treatment is of sufficient duration. Avoid using polypharmacy, as one cannot determine which of the drugs was effective, an important concern if the animal improves but relapses when medications are withdrawn.

ABDOMINAL PAIN

History, physical examination, abdominal radiographs, and ultrasonography are the initial tools in diagnosing the cause of abdominal pain (Fig. 9–13). Extra-abdominal diseases such as spinal problems and patients predisposed to nonsurgical diseases (pancreatitis in diabetics) *must* be identified early. In patients with severe, progressive, acute abdomen (severe unrelenting pain or shock or stupor in a deteriorating pa-

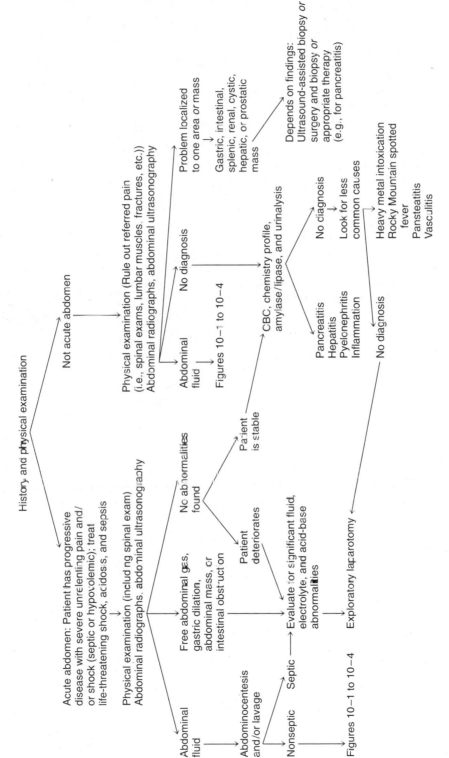

Figure 9–13 Diagnostic approach to abdominal pain in the dog and cat.

217

tient), surgery is usually indicated as soon as fluid, electrolyte, and acid-base status are determined and corrected. In these patients, extensive laboratory testing is unlikely to identify the more common causes of acute abdomen (intestinal obstruction, gastric dilation or volvulus, peritonitis, organ ischemia, tumor, sepsis, or bleeding) and usually only delays surgical resolution of the disease. Abdominal exploration offers a good chance for definitive diagnosis plus resolution of the disease process. Note: These maladies do not always present as surgical emergencies.

If a patient is not in severe pain and the disease is not progressing rapidly, one must differentiate between problems that ultimately necessitate surgery and those that usually do not (e.g., pancreatitis, hepatitis, upper urinary tract infection, prostatitis, pansteatitis, heavy metal intoxication, Rocky Mountain spotted fever, and others). Abdominal ultrasonography is useful to examine the liver, spleen, pancreas, kidneys, and prostate, as well as to detect peritoneal fluid. If abdominal fluid is present, abdominocentesis or abdominal lavage with cytologic analysis is indicated. If these procedures are not revealing and the problem continues, exploratory surgery may be necessary. Contrast radiographs are rarely useful, since thorough abdominal exploration should diagnose almost anything they will reveal; finding an abnormality on radiographs simply is an indication for surgery.

Bibliography

Grieve RB: Parasitic infections. Vet Clin North Am 1987; 17:1235–1518.

Hansten PD: Drug Interactions. 4th ed. Philadelphia, Lea and Febiger, 1983.

Jacobs DS, Kasten BL, Demott WR, Wolfson WL: Laboratory Test Handbook with DRG Index. St Louis, CV Mosby, 1984.

Johnson SE: Liver and biliary tract. *In* Anderson NV (ed): Veterinary Gastroenterology. 2nd ed. Philadelphia, Lea and Febiger, 1992, pp 504–569.

Kirkpatrick CE: Giardiasis. Vet Clin North Am 1987; 17:1377–1404.

Leib MS: Acute vomiting: A diagnostic approach and symptomatic management. *In* Kirk RW (ed): Current Veterinary Therapy XI. Philadelphia, WB Saunders, 1992, pp 583–587.

Sherding RG, Burrows CF: Diarrhea. *In* Anderson NV (ed): Veterinary Gastroenterology. 2nd ed. Philadelphia, Lea and Febiger, 1992, pp 399–477.

Speicher CE, Smith JW: Choosing Effective Laboratory Tests. Philadelphia, WB Saunders, 1983.

Strombeck DR, Guilford WG: Maldigestion, malabsorption, bacterial overgrowth, and protein-losing enteropathy. *In* Strombeck DR, Guilford WG (eds): Small Animal Gastroenterology. 2nd ed. Davis, CA, Stonegate Publishing, 1990, pp 296–317.

Tietz NW: Clinical Guide to Laboratory Tests. Philadelphia, WB Saunders, 1983.

Williams DA: Acute pancreatitis. *In* Kirk RW (ed): Current Veterinary Therapy XI. Philadelphia, WB Saunders, 1992, pp 631–639.

N. Bari Olivier
Michael D. Willard

10 Fluid Accumulation Disorders

All tissues require some degree of hydration for normal function. Optimum hydration is controlled by a balance between the rate at which fluid enters extravascular compartments and the rate of drainage. Either an increased influx of fluid, a decrease in drainage, or a combination can lead to excess fluid accumulation and various degrees of organ dysfunction. Increased influx can be caused by leakage from compromised blood or lymphatic vessels, alterations in microvascular Starling's forces (e.g., hypoalbuminemia or increased hydrostatic pressure), or increases in vascular permeability (e.g., inflammation). Less commonly, rupture of a normal fluid compartment such as the urinary bladder or gallbladder can lead to abnormal fluid accumulations. Impaired fluid drainage is usually caused by disorders of the lymphatic system.

The diagnostic approach to fluid accumulations is centered around localization and characterization of the fluid. Localization is often possible from physical examination findings such as visual evidence, palpation, ballottement of the abdomen, and auscultation or percussion of the thorax. Diagnostic images based on radiography and ultrasonography are also helpful in identifying excess fluid in body cavities and may reveal effusions not detected by physical examination. Exploratory centesis or lavage may be needed when fluid is suspected but cannot be confirmed using these other techniques. Centesis is ultimately required to sample the fluid for cytochemical characterization.

CHARACTERIZATION OF FLUIDS

Fluid Analysis • Routinely indicated in every effusion. The fluid should be sampled and analyzed for basic biochemical and cytologic characteristics. Whenever possible, paired 3-ml aliquots of the sample should be saved in an EDTA and clot tube for cytology and chemical analysis, respectively. Additional samples stored in refrigerated and sterile clot tubes provide a backup for most additional tests suggested by the results of the basic analysis. Basic analysis includes determination of specific gravity or total protein concentration, total and differential nucleated cell counts, and red blood cell (RBC) counts. If only a small volume is available (e.g., a joint aspirate), smears for cytologic examination are often the first priority. Nucleated cell counts and specific gravity are usually the next most important determinations.

Specific gravity and total protein concentrations

are routinely performed. The supernatant of the fluid (preferably without anticoagulant) is obtained after centrifugation is used.

Specific gravity is quick and easy to determine and serves as an estimate of total protein (solids) in a small drop of the fluid. Turbidity of a sample can artifactually change the specific gravity, as can sampling fluid contaminated by blood or chyle.

Total protein concentration is measured by spectrophotometric methods and is more accurate than specific gravity, but the latter is sufficient in most cases. Protein values may be falsely increased by contamination occurring at sampling or by hemolysis of RBCs during processing.

Total and differential nucleated cell counts are routinely performed. They are made from well-mixed anticoagulated noncentrifuged fluid. *Total cell counts* require a hemocytometer because there is often too much debris to use an automated cell counter. Falsely low cell counts can result from dilution if the sample volume is small compared with the volume of anticoagulant used. Other artifacts in the count can be caused by a poorly mixed sample, sampling contamination, prolonged setting, or storage. Prior or concurrent therapies (especially antibiotics, corticosteroids, or nonsteroidal anti-inflammatory drugs) may also affect cell counts by altering the disease process.

Differential cell counts are best performed on slides prepared from cytospin techniques that preserve morphologic detail. This is particularly true for many effusions that have relatively low total cell counts or high protein concentration. If cytospin technology is not available, either smears of sediment from centrifuged samples or sedimentation chambers on microscope slides (see Fig. 14–1) are useful. Smears of unconcentrated fluid are suitable and allow reasonable estimation of cell numbers when cell counts are > 1000 to 5000/μl. A search must be made for etiologic agents, especially those engulfed by white blood cells (WBCs). Wright-Giemsa is a good stain for WBCs and organisms; new methylene blue is best for evaluating nuclear detail of suspected neoplasms. Sepsis may be diagnosed by finding severely degenerative neutrophils and bacteria (especially engulfed by WBCs). Potential artifacts include microorganism-contaminated stains and postsampling degeneration of neutrophils (induced WBC degeneration mimicking sepsis) due to prolonged storage in EDTA or an effusion containing urine. Antibiotic therapy may cause a septic effusion caused by ongoing contamination to have so few bacteria that they cannot be found, plus prevent neutrophilic degeneration.

RBC counts or packed cell volumes (PCVs) are occasionally performed. Techniques similar to nucleated cell counts are used, as are microhematocrit tubes. The purpose is to quantitate the amount of blood in the sample. The major indication for this test is to compare the RBC content of the effusion with that of blood from a paired venipuncture when hemoabdomen or hemothorax is suspected (see the later discussion under Distinguishing Different Types of Effusions). Otherwise, it is not as useful as the specific gravity and total and differential nucleated cell counts. Values may be artifactually lowered by hemolysis if exposed to fluids with very high or low tonicity or by freezing and thawing, lipids, mechanical trauma, and some drugs. Prolonged standing or unmixed samples may give erroneous results.

CHEMISTRIES ON EFFUSIONS

Occasional Indications • See Table 10–1. Chemistry determinations (i.e., creatinine, bilirubin, and perhaps amylase) are best performed on the supernatant of a freshly collected sample of effusion. Analysis and artifacts for each test are explained in the specified chapters, as per Table 10–1. There are no "normal values"; the fluid value is compared with the blood or serum value to reach a conclusion.

Table 10–1 CLINICAL CHEMISTRY DETERMINATIONS INDICATED ON SELECTED EFFUSIONS

Determination	Indication(s)	Comments
Creatinine	Suspected uroabdomen	See Chapter 7; recommended for the diagnosis of uroabdomen
Bilirubin	Suspected ruptured biliary tract	See Chapter 9; usually suspected based on dark yellow-brown-green appearance of fluid
Amylase	Suspected pancreatic ascites	See Chapter 9; pancreatitis is not a common cause of ascites; intestinal leakage may (?) increase fluid amylase
Cholesterol/triglycerides	White or pink fluid (chylothorax or chyloabdomen)	See Chapter 8; chyle has more triglyceride but less cholesterol than serum; pseudochylous effusions are the opposite

ABDOMINAL LAVAGE

Occasional Indications • Patients with known or suspected abdominal fluid that cannot be recovered with abdominocentesis are candidates for abdominal lavage. The procedure is relatively easy and is associated with minimal risk and discomfort. Sterile, warmed physiologic saline solution (20 ml/kg) is rapidly administered into the peritoneal cavity via a catheter. The abdomen is then gently massaged for 1 to 2 minutes to expose the entire abdomen to the fluid. Lavage fluid is then aspirated and analyzed for the number and type of nucleated cells plus the presence of etiologic agents. Dogs normally have < 500 WBCs/μl. Normal values for cats have not yet been determined. Mild leukocytosis of the lavage fluid can be associated with recent trauma (i.e., surgery). Other forms of peritonitis may have WBC counts in the 1000 to 2000 WBCs/μl range. Bacteria should not be seen and, if present, indicate septic peritonitis.

DISTINGUISHING DIFFERENT TYPES OF EFFUSIONS

Most fluids can be categorized as either blood, chyle, pseudochyle, or a transudate, modified transudate, or exudate. There is some overlap between these categories, but the scheme helps focus the diagnostic approach.

Exudates and modified transudates may be confused with blood because they occasionally are red. Hemorrhage into a body cavity or space produces an effusion with a PCV and protein content similar to a paired blood sample taken by venipuncture. By comparison, the typical effusion containing RBCs secondary to inflammation or vascular congestion has a PCV $\leq$ 5% to 8%. Care must be taken to avoid hemorrhage resulting from traumatic sampling technique. Blood from traumatic sampling usually clots when exposed to an artificial surface, whereas most effusions do not. In the case of minor blood contamination of an effusion, small red clots may be seen floating in the effusion. Furthermore, cytologic examination of an effusion caused by recent or ongoing hemorrhage often reveals platelets. This is in contrast to other effusions that have chronic diapedesis of RBCs, which may also have erthyrophagocytosis (Color Plate 4C) or macrophages that contain hemosiderin.

Chyle is a turbid, white to pink fluid that is caused by leakage of lymphatics that drain the intestinal tract. It is characterized by a triglyceride concentration that exceeds that of serum and a cholesterol concentration less than that of serum. A simpler, qualitative test for high triglyceride content involves incubation of the fluid (pretreated with 1 to 2 drops of sodium hydroxide) with an equal volume of ether. Ether-soluble triglycerides rise to the top of the tube as a white band. Another method is to stain a fluid smear with oil red O or Sudan and look for fat droplets (i.e., chylomicrons) (Color Plate 4B). Nucleated cell counts can vary considerably and are usually dominated by lymphocytes, although neutrophils predominate in some chronic cases.

Pseudochylous effusion has been described. If it exists in animals, it is rare. Similar to true chylous effusion in gross appearance, it has high cholesterol and low triglyceride concentrations relative to serum, a pattern opposite that of chyle. The cause and pathogenesis of pseudochylous effusions have not been well documented.

Transudates are characterized by low cell counts (< 1000/μl), low protein content (< 2.5 g/dl), and a low specific gravity (< 1.017) (Table 10–2). Exudates have relatively high protein concentration (> 3.0 g/dl), high specific gravity (> 1.025), and relatively high WBC counts (> 5000/μl) dominated by neutrophils and mac-

MODIFIED TRANSUDATES, AND EXUDATES

	Transudate	Modified Transudate	Exudate
Specific gravity	<1.017	1.017–1.025	>1.025
Total protein (g/dl)	<2.5	2.5–5.0	>3.0
Nucleated cells (per μl)	<1000	500–10,000	>5000
Predominant cell types	Mononuclear	Lymphocytes	Neutrophils
	Mesothelial	Monocytes	Mononuclear
		Mesothelial	RBCs
		RBCs	
		Neutrophils	
Bacteria	Absent	Absent	Variable

rophages. Modified transudates compose an intermediate fluid type somewhere between the description of a transudate and an exudate. They have intermediate specific gravity, protein concentrations, and nucleated cell counts. Cell populations tend to be lymphocytic and monocytic with fewer neutrophils than exudates and variable numbers of RBCs.

HEMOABDOMEN/HEMOTHORAX

Causes of abdominal and thoracic hemorrhage include trauma, bleeding neoplasms, and coagulation disorders. Trauma is often suggested by a confirmatory history or evidence of superficial wounds or pain. Radiographs can be helpful, if time permits, in identifying occult trauma. If there is no evidence of trauma, a complete blood count (CBC) and coagulation profile are indicated to rule out coagulation disorders (Fig. 10–1). Neoplasms should be considered in older patients and those with a more chronic (weeks to months) history of illness. Ultrasonography is very cost-effective in screening the thorax and abdomen for neoplastic masses in the presence of fluid, although multiple radiographic views before and after centesis can also identify a focal source but are more cumbersome and take more time. If the cause of bleeding is not evident and does not respond to symptomatic therapy, exploratory surgery is indicated. This is more difficult for the thorax, which is hard to expose thoroughly by any single surgical approach. In the abdomen, the spleen, liver, and kidneys should be examined first; if these are normal, the entire intestinal tract, but especially the pancreas, ileum, and root of the mesentery, should be explored next.

CHYLOABDOMEN

Rarely found, chyloabdomen is principally associated with intestinal lymphangiectasia or a lymphoproliferative process involving the mesentery.

ABDOMINAL EFFUSIONS

An abdominal effusion is not an animal's major problem; it is a sign of another, underlying disease. Abdominal *transudates* are usually due to decreased plasma oncotic pressure. Measuring serum total protein and albumin concentrations is the first diagnostic step for transudates (Fig. 10–2). Transudates do not usually form until serum albumin falls to < 1.5 g/dl. Excessive albumin loss from protein-losing nephropathy or enteropathy or decreased synthesis resulting from hepatic insufficiency are the most likely causes. Rarely, exudative skin lesions may cause hypoalbuminemia, but this should be obvious at physical examination. Anorexia and emaciation by themselves are not adequate reasons for a serum albumin value < 2.0 g/dl. A urinalysis, urine total protein:creatinine ratio,

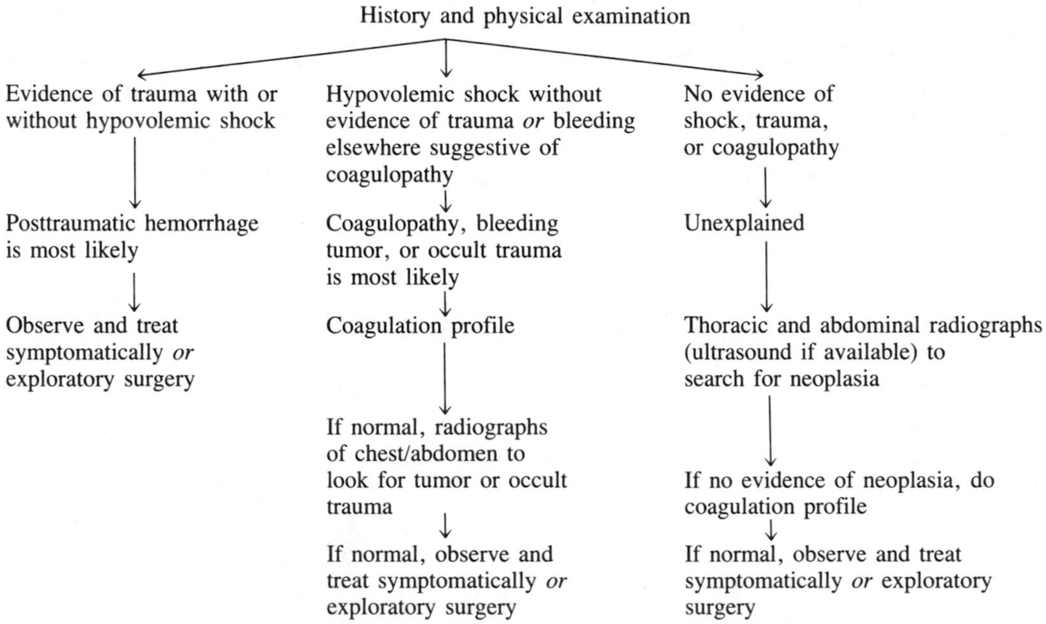

History and physical examination

Evidence of trauma with or without hypovolemic shock	Hypovolemic shock without evidence of trauma *or* bleeding elsewhere suggestive of coagulopathy	No evidence of shock, trauma, or coagulopathy
Posttraumatic hemorrhage is most likely	Coagulopathy, bleeding tumor, or occult trauma is most likely	Unexplained
Observe and treat symptomatically *or* exploratory surgery	Coagulation profile	Thoracic and abdominal radiographs (ultrasound if available) to search for neoplasia
	If normal, radiographs of chest/abdomen to look for tumor or occult trauma	If no evidence of neoplasia, do coagulation profile
	If normal, observe and treat symptomatically *or* exploratory surgery	If normal, observe and treat symptomatically *or* exploratory surgery

Figure 10–1 Diagnostic approach to hemoabdomen and hemothorax in the dog and cat.

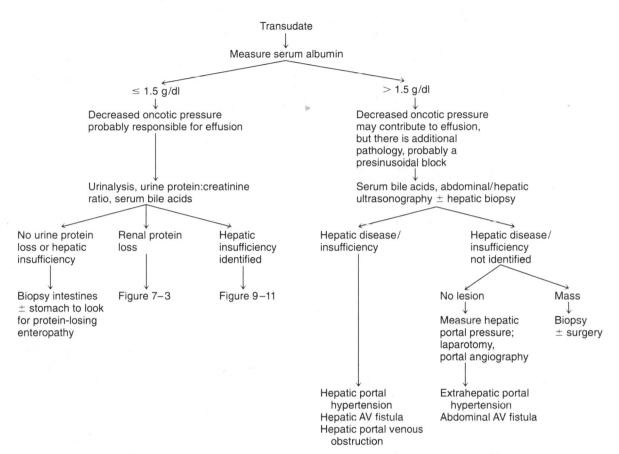

Figure 10–2 Diagnostic approach to abdominal transudates in dogs and cats.

and hepatic function test (e.g., bile acids) should be done. If all results are normal, gastrointestinal protein loss is probable and should be followed by biopsy of the stomach and intestine, even if there is no vomiting or diarrhea.

If serum albumin is > 1.5 g/dl, other factors such as portal hypertension are probably present. Portal hypertension causing a pure transudate in the presence of a normal or nearly normal serum albumin concentration suggests a presinusoidal obstruction of the portal vein, such as occurs in some types of hepatic fibrosis, a portal thrombosis, or a mass impinging on the portal vein. Congenital hepatic arteriovenous fistulas are a well-documented cause of finding a pure transudate in an animal with a serum albumin concentration ≥ 2.0 g/dl.

Modified transudates are principally secondary to increased venous (capillary) hydrostatic pressure due to cardiac failure or chronic hepatic failure. Compression of abdominal veins by neoplasms, other masses, or organ malposition can also result in venous hypertension and ascites. Neoplasia is rarely diagnosed by cytologic examination of the fluid, because reactive mesothelial cells often mimic malignancy. Nevertheless, Cytospin techniques should be used if available to allow evaluation of maximal numbers of cells.

The most cost-effective step in looking for right-sided heart failure causing an effusion is to examine the neck carefully for a jugular pulse. Many animals with right-sided congestive heart failure have this finding, although it is missing in a few (especially those with diseases like cor triatriatum dextrum). If one is unsure about whether a jugular pulse is present or whether there is enough of a jugular pulse to be concerned about, measurement of central venous pressure (CVP) is a quick and accurate method to test for right-sided heart failure. Values > 8 cm H_2O are suggestive, whereas values ≥ 14 cm are diagnostic of right heart failure (Fig. 10–3). However, CVP does not detect venous hypertension due to causes originating caudal to the heart (e.g., hepatic disease, venous thrombosis, neoplastic vascular compression).

If CVP is normal, hepatic function tests should be performed and abdominal ultrasono-

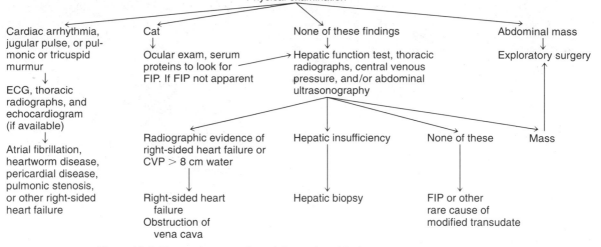

Figure 10–3 Diagnostic approach to abdominal modified transudates in dogs and cats.

graphic examinations conducted (if available) to assess liver size and architecture and caudal vena cava diameter and to scan for an abdominal mass. Abdominal radiography is generally less sensitive than ultrasonography in animals with abdominal fluid but can be helpful when performed after drainage of the abdomen. However, effusions can quickly re-form after drainage and reduce effective circulating blood volume. Repeated drainage decreases serum albumin. Patients need to be monitored carefully under these circumstances. If the diagnosis is still in question, an exploratory laparotomy may be indicated. If a tumor or granuloma is not found, hepatic, mesenteric lymph node, intestinal, and splenic biopsy samples plus portal pressure measurements should be obtained.

Exudates should be categorized as *septic exudates* or without evidence of sepsis (Fig. 10–4). Plant fibers in the abdominal fluid indicate alimentary tract rupture. Degenerate WBCs (Color Plate 4E) are suggestive but are not diagnostic of sepsis by themselves since there are many artifactual causes of WBC degeneration and some bacteria may not cause degenerative changes in WBCs, even cells that contain bacteria. Trauma (e.g., recent surgery) can cause mild and transient neutrophilic degeneration. Finding bacteria is highly suggestive of sepsis; intracellular bacteria are confirmatory in a fresh stain (Color Plate 4D). It is sometimes difficult to document that an effusion is septic, especially if there are low bacterial numbers due to prior antibiotic therapy. Even if the therapy was unable to resolve the infection or stabilize the patient, it may decrease bacterial counts to almost undetectable numbers and reduce the degree of neutrophil degeneration. *Actinomyces* and *No-*

cardia (Color Plate 4E) are sometimes difficult to find. Unless there is a specific reason to the contrary, all exudates should be cultured for aerobic and anaerobic bacteria (see Chapter 15). A spontaneous septic abdominal effusion indicates surgical exploration to search for alimentary tract rupture or leakage. Foreign bodies or abscesses may occasionally be found.

Some septic exudates can be attributed to contamination from previous surgery or repeated sampling or drainage of an initially sterile effusion. The history is usually suggestive in these cases. Cultures are mandatory, but surgical exploration may not be because many of these patients can be effectively treated medically.

When a *nonseptic abdominal exudate* is detected, one should first review the history for trauma, even that which occurred weeks before the effusion was noticed. Radiography can sometimes reveal minor fractures of the pelvis or associated bony structures if trauma is suspected but not confirmed by the history. Traumatic exudates are occasionally associated with uroabdomen and bilious ascites (both are relatively rare as spontaneous occurrences).

Uroabdomen classically is an exudate but may be a modified transudate in some animals. Simultaneous creatinine determinations on the fluid and serum diagnose uroabdomen. If uroabdomen is present, an excretory urogram is indicated before surgery to localize the site or sites of rupture.

Bilious ascites may be suspected because of its yellow to greenish-brown appearance. Bilirubin determinations on fluid and serum may confirm that excess bilirubin is present in the effusion. Bilious ascites is an indication for exploratory

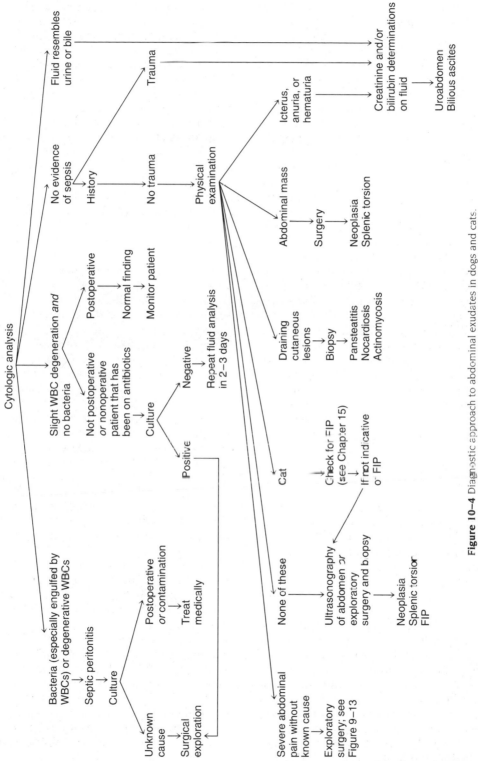

Figure 10—4 Diagnostic approach to abdominal exudates in dogs and cats.

225

surgery. Pancreatitis may rarely cause ascites. Supposedly, such an effusion should have high amylase concentration.

Feline infectious peritonitis (FIP) must be considered in any cat with a nonseptic exudate. High serum globulin concentrations ($\geq$ 4.5 g/dl), ocular lesions, high fluid protein values ($\geq$ 4.5 g/dl), plus an effusion with a wide range of nucleated cell counts but usually $\leq$ 15,000/μl, consisting of mixed inflammatory cells, are adequate for a presumptive diagnosis. FIP effusions occasionally are not definitive (e.g., principally have neutrophils but not mononuclear cells; or are a modified transudate). Antibody titers to FIP are currently dubious because cross-reactivity with other relatively nonpathogenic coronaviruses is considered common (see Chapter 15).

Once these causes are eliminated, neoplasia becomes a prominent concern. Diagnosis of malignancy by abdominal fluid cytology is desirable but difficult. Cell exfoliation from many neoplasms is too low to be detected in the fluid. False-positive cytology results are possible owing to reactive mesothelial cells, which commonly have cellular characteristics similar to malignancies, especially carcinomas. Again, abdominal ultrasonography or postdrainage radiography may illustrate a neoplastic mass. If not, abdominal exploration may be needed. Abdominal exploration has the advantage of also detecting other less common causes (e.g., *Mesocestoides* sp. infection, splenic torsion).

PLEURAL EFFUSIONS

Pleural effusions are approached in much the same manner as for abdominal effusions (Fig. 10–5). However, there are several differences. First, exploratory surgery does not readily allow exploration of the entire chest.

Mediastinal neoplasia is relatively common in cats and also occurs in dogs. In cats, such masses may be identified at physical examination by palpation of the cranial mediastinal area. Radiography is usually diagnostic of a mediastinal mass in dogs and cats. It is important to define the mass because thymomas (which may have a better prognosis) can mimic lymphosarcoma radiographically and also cause a lymphocytic (as opposed to a lymphoblastic) effusion. Diagnosis of lymphoma requires demonstration of *malignant* lymphoid cells. In cats, malignancy can often be diagnosed by fluid cytology. However, canine thoracic lymphosarcoma is harder to confirm by cytologic examination of the effusion and often requires percutaneous fine-needle aspirate cytology of the mediastinal mass.

Diaphragmatic hernias can cause modified transudates. A history of trauma is helpful, and radiographic displacement of the liver, intestines, or stomach into the thorax is definitive. Patients should not have their rear quarters elevated while the clinician is auscultating for gut sounds in the chest. In uncertain situations, contrast radiographs of the alimentary tract or contrast celiography are indicated.

Right-sided congestive heart failure usually causes ascites in dogs. Cats, in contrast, often develop pleural effusion secondary to either right- or left-sided congestive heart failure. A cardiac murmur or gallop rhythm is suggestive of feline cardiomyopathy, which can be confirmed echocardiographically.

Chyle causing a pleural effusion may be idiopathic or may be associated with feline heartworm disease, congestive heart failure, thoracic duct laceration, pleuritis, and neoplastic or granulomatous disease of the mediastinum. Some breeds (e.g., Afghan hounds) may have a congenital predisposition to chylous effusions. Ultrasonography of the thorax or postdrainage radiography is indicated. Contrast lymphangiography during a laparotomy can sometimes elucidate the site of leakage, but success seems to be quite variable.

Lung lobe torsions are uncommon but are suggested by a nonseptic exudate or pathologic hemorrhage and radiographic displacement of mainstem bronchi, especially the right middle lung lobe. Bronchoscopy is indicated and is diagnostic when it detects a twisted-off bronchus. Alternatively, the chest may be drained and reradiographed; however, pleural effusion is often associated with right middle lung lobe collapse that is not due to torsion.

Actinomycosis-nocardiosis is principally found in dogs, usually in the chest, although it may occur in the abdomen. Exudates due to pure actinomycosis may have minimal or no WBC degeneration. However, there is often a mixed population of organisms with a thick exudate of degenerate WBCs, which may or may not have typical, grossly visible "sulfur granules" (i.e., bacterial colonies). Finding beaded, branching filaments is adequate for presumptive diagnosis. These bacteria are best found on smears containing these sulfur granules. The effusion sometimes resembles hemothorax, and care must be taken to look for the organisms.

Pyothorax is principally found in cats and is diagnosed by finding obvious pus or seropurulent fluid with degenerate WBCs with or without

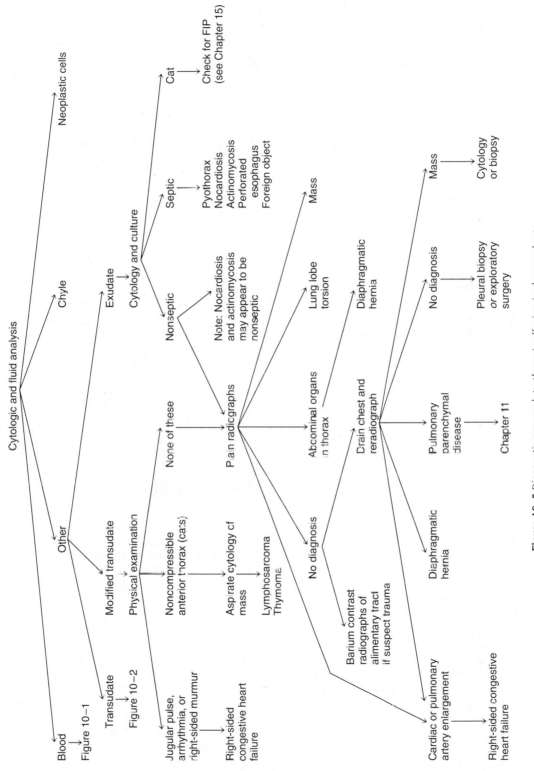

Figure 10-5 Diagnostic approach to thoracic effusion in dogs and cats.

multiple bacterial forms. The cause is seldom identified in cats. However, in both dogs and cats, esophageal perforation must also be considered, especially if a patient has been regurgitating. Exudate secondary to severe bacterial pneumonia occasionally occurs. This type of exudate may be sterile or septic, but it usually does not have grossly visible sulfur granules. Thoracic radiographs typically reveal pulmonary parenchymal involvement.

PERICARDIAL EFFUSIONS

Pericardiocentesis is performed by inserting a 20- to 23-gauge needle between the third to fifth intercostal spaces on the right side, at the level of the costochondral junction. Pericardial effusions should be analyzed as described for thoracic and abdominal effusions. Modified transudates due to right-sided heart failure or uremia, transudate due to hypoalbuminemia, exudate due to FIP, chylopericardium, or hemopericardium due to trauma, tumor, or coagulopathy is occasionally detected. Most pericardial effusions are port wine colored. Some are exudates (inflammatory), whereas others are more hemorrhagic. The major questions are, Is it septic or nonseptic? and Is it neoplastic? The first question is answered by cytologic examination and routine bacterial and mycotic culture. Coccidioidomycosis is a potential cause, and serologic testing is indicated in patients from endemic areas. Most nonseptic pericardial effusions are due to idiopathic pericarditis or neoplasia. Cytologic examination of malignant effusions rarely reveals neoplastic cells, although nonneoplastic reactive mesothelial cells often mimic neoplasia. Contrast radiography, ultrasonography, or exploratory surgery is usually needed to differentiate benign from malignant disease. The diagnosis in some cases requires exploratory surgery for pericardial biopsies.

SCROTAL EFFUSIONS

Scrotal effusion usually occurs when abdominal fluid enters the scrotum via the inguinal rings. However, severe orchitis or testicular torsion may be responsible. If effusion is localized to the scrotum, castration may be diagnostic and therapeutic.

JOINT EFFUSIONS

Joint fluid should be analyzed in patients with fever of unknown origin or excessive joint fluid.

In the former, swollen joints should be sampled if possible. If no joints are swollen, then at least two or three joints should be sampled, especially the carpi and tarsi. If enough fluid is obtained, culture, nucleated cell counts, differential cell counts, and mucin tests should be done (Fig. 10–6). If lesser amounts are obtained, smears should be made to determine relative cellularity and predominant cell type. The major questions are, Is there inflammation? and Is there sepsis? Inflammation is determined by finding > 3000 WBCs/μl^3 or $> 15\%$ of the cells as neutrophils. Sepsis is suggested by degenerative neutrophils in the fluid and is confirmed if bacteria are seen cytologically or cultured from the fluid. Concurrent antibiotic therapy may result in the neutrophils being nondegenerative despite persisting infection. Some agents (e.g., mycoplasma) may not be associated with highly degenerative neutrophils (see Chapter 15). In chronic low-grade infections, culture of synovial tissue obtained by biopsy seems to be more reliable than culture of the synovial fluid alone. If joint sepsis is found, one must determine if it is due to hematologic spread or mechanical invasion of the joint. Local extension of an infection to include a joint (from trauma or foreign body) does not necessitate additional diagnostics. Hematogenous spread suggested by multiple joint involvement or cardiac murmur suggests bacterial endocarditis and indicates echocardiography plus joint fluid cultures and blood cultures. Urine cultures are another good screening test for systemic infection.

Serologic testing for borreliosis (Lyme disease) may be helpful in patients with inflammatory arthritis of unknown cause. However, interpretation of titers for Lyme disease is difficult, at best. Correlation between serum titers and clinical signs is poor in experimentally infected dogs. Paired samples separated by 2 weeks or more may help confirm recent exposure and possibly active infection. The response to therapy may be the most compelling basis for a diagnosis.

Nonseptic inflammatory joint effusions can be categorized as either erosive or nonerosive based on the radiographic appearance of subchondral bone. Rheumatoid arthritis is often erosive. The nonerosive arthritides are more difficult to diagnose definitively, but systemic lupus erythematosus (Color Plate 4A) and rheumatoid-like arthritis due to various underlying causes are most likely. Antinuclear antibody, rheumatoid factor, lupus erythematosus (LE) cell preparations, and synovial biopsies may help determine the cause (see Chapter 12).

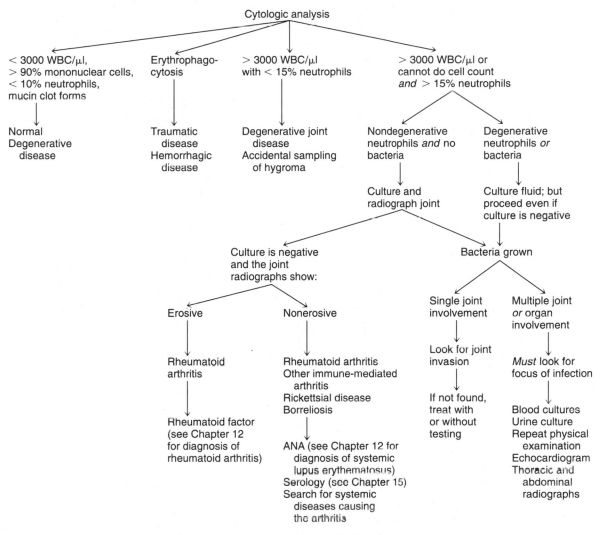

Figure 10–6 Diagnostic approach to joint fluid analysis in dogs and cats.

EDEMA

Like ascites, edema is always a sign of underlying disease. *Generalized edema* is often dependent and is principally found in the lower extremities. Overhydration, right-sided congestive heart failure, and decreased plasma oncotic pressure due to hypoalbuminemia are the most common causes. History, physical examination, serum albumin determination, thoracic radiographs, or CVP measurement usually allows diagnosis (Fig. 10–7). If these causes are ruled out, a skin biopsy to evaluate for vasculitis and analysis of edema fluid are indicated. Retinal examinations provide a unique opportunity to see small vessels that may be involved in systemic vascular disease.

Regional edema is usually due to either inflammation, vascular obstruction, or lymphatic flow obstruction (Fig. 10–8). Inflammation is suggested by redness, heat, and various degrees of pain in the affected region. Venous occlusion causes regional edema that is usually associated with cool extremities, peripheral cyanosis, or pallor. Careful palpation, ultrasonography, and radiography can be used to search for compressive granulomatous or neoplastic masses. Congenital or acquired arteriovenous fistulas are a rare cause of localized edema. They are often detected by a palpable fremitus or bruit but may require selective angiography for confirmation.

Lymphatic dysfunction is a common cause of regional edema and is considered after ruling out inflammatory or vascular causes. It can follow trauma, surgery, or regional infections. Extensive tests such as lymphangiograms are usually not indicated, although cytology of fine-needle aspirates from lymph nodes draining the area are routinely indicated. In equivocal cases, analysis of edema fluid (total protein, nucleated

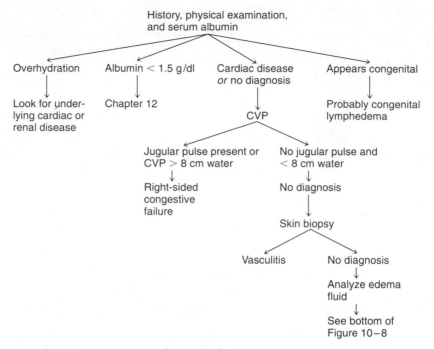

Figure 10–7 Diagnostic approach to generalized or dependent edema in dogs and cats.

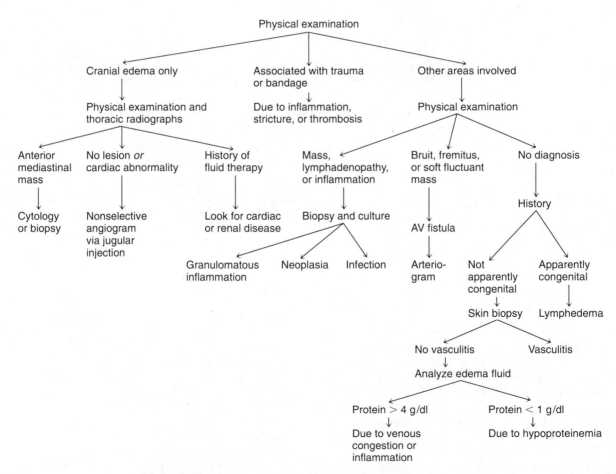

Figure 10–8 Diagnostic approach to regional or local edema in dogs and cats.

cell counts, and differential cell counts) may provide clues to the etiology.

Collection of Edema Fluid • A 22- to 25-gauge needle is gently introduced into the affected tissues. Fluid often drains spontaneously by gravity but can be assisted by *gentle* massage or aspiration. Hypoproteinemia causes edema fluid with a total protein < 1 g/dl, whereas venous congestion, lymphedema, or inflammation usually generates fluid with > 2.5 g/dl of protein. In the latter case, total and differential cell counts distinguish inflammatory (e.g., vasculitis) from noninflammatory causes.

CYSTS

When a cyst is found, the primary questions are, Is there malignancy?, Is there inflammation?, and Is there sepsis? These questions are answered by total and differential nucleated cell counts plus searching for etiologic agents. Intra-abdominal cysts can be carefully aspirated percutaneously using palpation or ultrasonography as a guide. Biochemical analysis of the fluid for amylase, bilirubin, and creatinine may identify the cyst as pancreatic, hepatobiliary, or renal, respectively. Fluid from perirectal cysts should always be examined for creatinine, to be sure the cyst is not a displaced bladder. Prostatic and paraprostatic cysts frequently do not have unique features allowing preoperative diagnosis but should be cultured and examined cytologically. Finding malignant cells in any cystic fluid is strong evidence of cancer. Failure to find such cells does not rule out cancer. If the diagnosis is uncertain, drainage of a cyst by aspiration may be curative. Recurrence signifies the need for resumption of tests, which may include surgical exploration for biopsy and histopathology.

Bibliography

Bauer T: Mediastinal, pleural, and extrapleural disease. *In* Ettinger SJ (ed): Textbook of Veterinary Internal Medicine. 3rd ed. Philadelphia, WB Saunders, 1989, pp 867–898.

Bolton GR, Ettinger SJ: Peripheral edema. *In* Ettinger SJ (ed): Textbook of Veterinary Internal Medicine. 3rd ed. Philadelphia, WB Saunders, 1989, pp 41–45.

Bunch SE: Abdominal effusion. *In* Ford RB (ed): Clinical Signs and Diagnosis in Small Animal Practice. New York, Churchill Livingstone, 1988, pp 521–540.

Ettinger SJ: Ascites, peritonitis, and other causes of abdominal enlargement. *In* Ettinger SJ (ed): Textbook of Veterinary Internal Medicine. 3rd ed. Philadelphia, WB Saunders, 1989, pp 131–138.

Pederson NC, Wind A, Morgan JP, Pool RR: Joint diseases of dogs and cats. *In* Ettinger SJ (ed): Textbook of Veterinary Internal Medicine. 3rd ed. Philadelphia, WB Saunders, 1989, pp 2329–2377.

Reed JR: Pericardial disease. *In* Fox PR (ed): Canine and Feline Cardiology. New York, Churchill Livingstone, 1988, pp 467–494.

Alice M. Wolf
Grant H. Turnwald

11 Respiratory Disorders

RESPIRATORY PROBLEMS

Abnormal Breathing Patterns

Respiratory distress (also called *dyspnea*) is an inappropriate degree of breathing effort based on the respiratory rate, rhythm, and character. Physical examination is the first step in diagnosis. Patients with obstructive respiratory diseases have a breathing pattern characterized by increased depth and rate. Obstructive lesions tend to accentuate the normal dynamic decrease of the airway diameter. Dynamic obstruction (e.g., laryngeal paralysis) cranial to the thoracic inlet (i.e., the upper airway) causes increased inspiratory effort. Dynamic obstruction (e.g., collapsing trachea) caudal to the thoracic inlet (i.e., lower airway) causes increased expiratory effort.

Fixed obstructions (e.g., tracheal tumor) may not exhibit such a difference. Nasal cavity obstruction only causes an obstructive breathing pattern if the animal cannot mouth breathe. Auscultation of wheezes also suggests airway obstruction, but wheezes are not always found when obstruction is present. Monophonic wheezes (of a single tone) may be noted with an elongated soft palate. Alternatively, wheezes can have multiple tones (polyphonic wheezes), as heard in asthmatic cats.

Patients with respiratory distress from extra-respiratory causes (e.g., severe anemia or severe metabolic acidosis) can have what may appear to be an obstructive breathing pattern with an increased intensity of normal lung sounds (i.e., bronchovesicular sounds) but do not have wheezes.

233

Diseases limiting the ability of the lungs to expand cause a restrictive breathing pattern characterized by an increased rate but a normal to decreased depth. Auscultation may reveal crackles, particularly during inspiration. Note that it may be difficult to auscultate pulmonary parenchymal abnormalities, especially in small patients with low tidal volumes. Thoracic radiographs from these patients can reveal a surprising amount of pulmonary parenchymal disease despite the apparent absence of abnormal respiratory sounds. The distinction between obstructive and restrictive breathing patterns may not always be clear; the pattern of breathing exhibited depends on the relative amount of pathologic change in affected tissues. For example, a dog with severe pulmonary edema may have obstructive disease (airway fluid) and restrictive disease (interstitial fluid).

Patients with disorders such as flail chest occasionally have paradoxical breathing movements, with a section of the chest wall collapsing during inspiration and expanding during expiration.

Common causes of abnormal breathing patterns in dogs and cats are listed in Table 11–1.

Most Useful Tests • After the cause of an abnormal breathing pattern has been localized by physical examination, tracheal and thoracic radiographs are usually the most useful next diagnostic step (Fig. 11–1). However, although a

collapsed trachea can be diagnosed by radiographs, it cannot be ruled out by radiographs, even if inspiratory and expiratory films are made. Transtracheal aspiration, bronchoalveolar lavage, or transthoracic fine-needle aspiration may follow if radiography suggests the need for cytologic analysis or culture of the lower airway, especially if coughing is present (Rebar et al., 1992). Direct examination of the pharynx and larynx is useful in upper airway obstruction. Endoscopy is useful in tracheal and bronchial disorders (particularly if a collapsed trachea or other obstructive disease is present) and mandatory in most pharyngeal and laryngeal abnormalities (see Fig. 11–1). If pleural effusion is present, fluid analysis is indicated (see Chapter 10). If dirofilariasis is suspected, a Knott's test, filter test, or *Dirofilaria* antigen test is indicated (see Chapter 15). Although they do not usually allow diagnosis, fecal flotation and Baermann's fecal analysis are inexpensive and noninvasive and, if positive, definitively diagnose pulmonary and tracheal parasites. Serologic testing for systemic mycoses (except histoplasmosis) may be useful in dogs if radiographic signs are compatible with such disease (see Chapter 15).

A complete blood count (CBC) is useful but rarely diagnostic unless severe pulmonary inflammatory disease (e.g., bronchopneumonia) is present. Allergic or parasitic disease in dogs may be reflected by eosinophilia, but this finding is inconsistent in cats (Moise et al., 1989). Serum chemistry profile and arterial blood gas analysis are less cost-effective in most of these patients unless the abnormal breathing pattern is nonrespiratory in origin (e.g., severe anemia or severe metabolic acidosis). Percutaneous fine-needle pulmonary aspiration biopsy is occasionally diagnostic in disseminated disease (e.g., blastomycosis, histoplasmosis) and can be useful if the organism cannot be demonstrated in more superficial structures (e.g., lymph node). Fine-needle aspiration can also be used to diagnose neoplasia, but there is some risk of morbidity and mortality.

PATTERNS IN DOGS AND CATS

Respiratory disorders
Nasal cavity/sinus disease; see Table 11–3
Trachea/lower airway disease
Pulmonary parenchymal disease; see Table 11–2
Mediastinal disease
Pleural cavity disorders
  Space-occupying masses
    Neoplasia
    Pleuroperitoneal hernia
    Pericardioperitoneal hernia
  Other space-occupying lesions
    Pleural effusion
    Pneumothorax
    Reduction in pleural cavity size by abdominal space-occupying masses
Body wall disorders
  Flail chest

Nonrespiratory disorders
Anemia
Cardiac disease
Pulmonary thromboembolism
Hemoglobin disorders
Hyperthermia
Metabolic acidosis
Seizures, including status epilepticus

Coughing, Including Hemoptysis

Common causes of coughing in dogs and cats are listed in Table 11–2. The history is used first to eliminate contagious infectious causes that tend to be self-limiting. Differentiation of a productive cough (as in bronchopneumonia) from a nonproductive cough (as in viral tracheobronchitis) and identification of abnormal breathing patterns (see Table 11–1 and Fig. 11–1) are also helpful. Tracheal and thoracic radiographs are

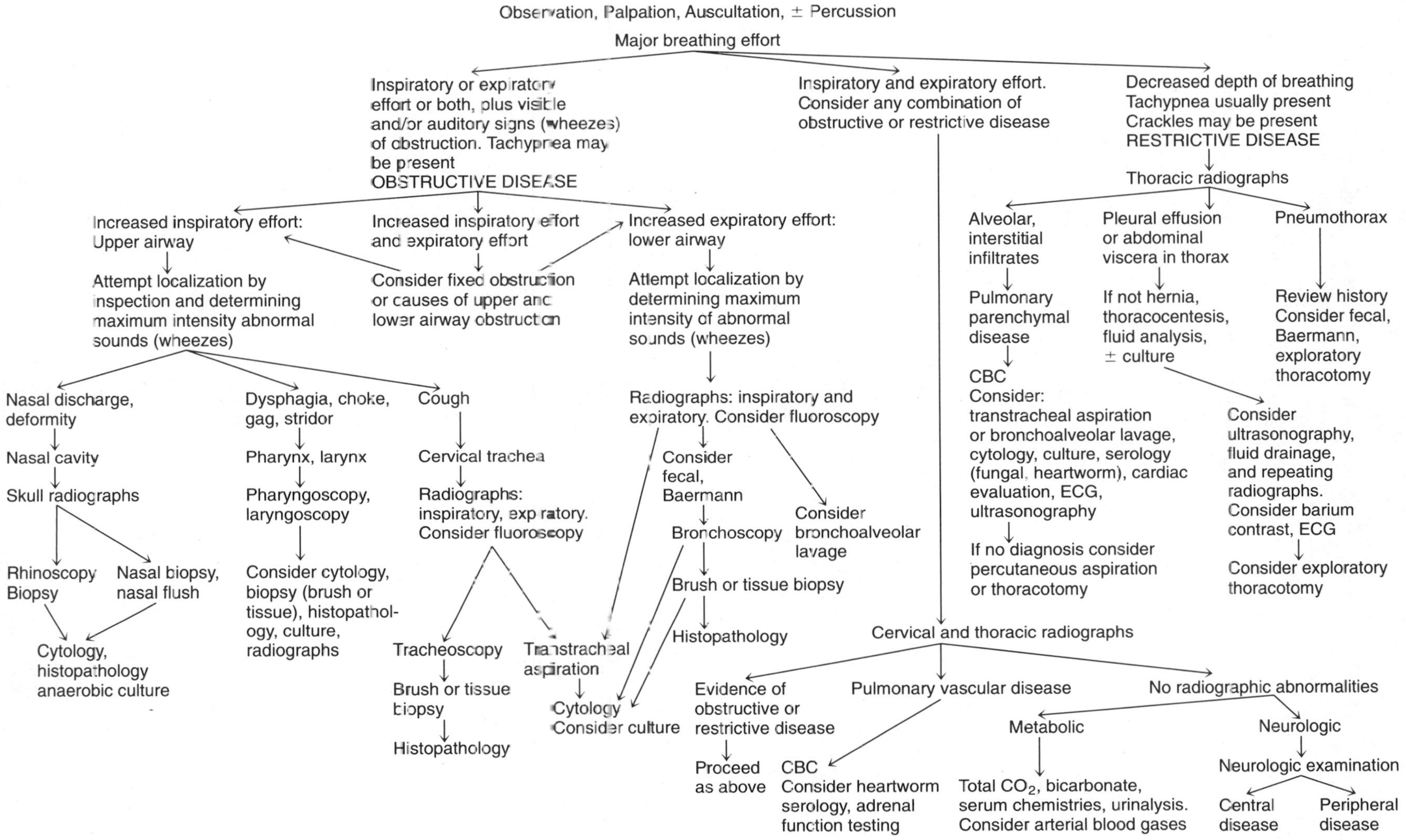

Observation, Palpation, Auscultation, ± Percussion

Major breathing effort

Inspiratory or expiratory effort or both, plus visible and/or auditory signs (wheezes) of obstruction. Tachypnea may be present
OBSTRUCTIVE DISEASE

Inspiratory and expiratory effort. Consider any combination of obstructive or restrictive disease

Decreased depth of breathing Tachypnea usually present Crackles may be present
RESTRICTIVE DISEASE

Thoracic radiographs

Pneumothorax → Review history Consider fecal, Baermann, exploratory thoracotomy

Pleural effusion or abdominal viscera in thorax → If not hernia, thoracocentesis, fluid analysis, ± culture → Consider ultrasonography, fluid drainage, and repeating radiographs. Consider barium contrast, ECG → Consider exploratory thoracotomy

Alveolar, interstitial infiltrates → Pulmonary parenchymal disease → CBC Consider: transtracheal aspiration or bronchoalveolar lavage, cytology, culture, serology (fungal, heartworm), cardiac evaluation, ECG, ultrasonography. If no diagnosis consider percutaneous aspiration or thoracotomy

Cervical and thoracic radiographs

No radiographic abnormalities

Pulmonary vascular disease → CBC Consider heartworm serology, adrenal function testing

Evidence of obstructive or restrictive disease → Proceed as above

Neurologic → Neurologic examination → Central disease / Peripheral disease

Metabolic → Total CO$_2$, bicarbonate, serum chemistries, urinalysis. Consider arterial blood gases

OBSTRUCTIVE DISEASE

Increased inspiratory effort: Upper airway

Increased inspiratory effort and expiratory effort → Consider fixed obstruction or causes of upper and lower airway obstruction

Increased expiratory effort: lower airway → Attempt localization by determining maximum intensity of abnormal sounds (wheezes) → Radiographs: inspiratory and expiratory. Consider fluoroscopy → Consider fecal, Baermann; Bronchoscopy → Consider bronchoalveolar lavage; Brush or tissue biopsy → Histopathology → Transtracheal aspiration → Cytology Consider culture

Increased inspiratory effort: Upper airway → Attempt localization by inspection and determining maximum intensity abnormal sounds (wheezes)

Nasal discharge, deformity → Nasal cavity → Skull radiographs → Rhinoscopy Biopsy → Nasal biopsy, nasal flush → Cytology, histopathology anaerobic culture

Dysphagia, choke, gag, stridor → Pharynx, larynx → Pharyngoscopy, laryngoscopy → Consider cytology, biopsy (brush or tissue), histopathology, culture, radiographs

Cough → Cervical trachea → Radiographs: inspiratory, expiratory. Consider fluoroscopy → Tracheoscopy → Brush or tissue biopsy → Histopathology; Transtracheal aspiration → Cytology Consider culture

Figure 11–1 Approach to respiratory distress and tachypnea in dogs and cats.

235

Table 11–2 CAUSES OF COUGHING IN DOGS AND CATS

Nasal cavity/sinus disease with postnasal drip
See Table 11–3

Pharynx/larynx
Trauma
Foreign body
Infection (bacterial or viral)
Neoplasia
Laryngeal paralysis (congenital or acquired)
Eversion of laryngeal saccules
Laryngeal collapse
Granulomatous laryngitis
Eosinophilic granuloma

Trachea/lower airway
Trauma
Foreign body
Allergy (allergic bronchitis/asthma)
Infection
Viral (see Table 11–3)
Bacterial (*Bordetella bronchiseptica*)
Parasitic (*Filaroides* spp., *Osleri osleri, Capillaria aerophilia*)
Anomalies (collapse, hypoplasia, primary ciliary dyskinesia, or segmental stenosis)
Neoplasia (osteochondral dysplasia [osteochondroma])
Degenerative disease (bronchiectasis)

Pulmonary parenchymal disease
Trauma
Allergy (pulmonary infiltrates with eosinophilia)
Infection
  Viral (see Table 11–3)
  Bacterial
  Fungal (*Blastomyces dermatitidis, Histoplasma capsulatum, Coccidioides immitis, Cryptococcus neoformans,* or *Aspergillus* spp.)
  Protozoal (*Toxoplasma gondii, Pneumocystis carinii*)
  Parasitic (*Filaroides hirthi, Filaroides milksi, Dirofilaria immitis, Angiostrongylus vasorum,* or *Paragonimus kellicotti*)
Degenerative disease (emphysema)
Neoplasia (primary or metastatic)
Noninfectious granulomatous disorders (eosinophilic pulmonary granulomatosis, pulmonary lymphomatoid granulomatosis)

Cardiovascular disease
Pulmonary edema
Left atrial enlargement causing bronchial compression
Thromboembolism (dirofilariasis, hyperadrenocorticism, protein-losing nephropathy, neoplasia, cardiac disease)

Mediastinal disease (causing airway compression)
Lymphosarcoma (especially cats)
Thymoma

usually the most useful next tests in patients with chronic cough, hemoptysis, or cardiovascular disease but are less useful in acute infectious tracheobronchial diseases (Fig. 11–2). Furthermore, radiographs can diagnose but cannot reliably rule out a collapsed trachea. Transtracheal aspiration or bronchoalveolar lavage (especially if combined with bronchoscopy) is often diagnostic in patients with chronic bronchial disease, allergic disease, parasitic infections, or bacterial infections. Bronchoscopy is

often needed for foreign body or obstructive disease. A CBC is frequently performed but is seldom of diagnostic value unless eosinophilia (suggestive of allergic or parasitic disease) is present. Fecal flotation and Baermann's fecal analysis are usually less revealing but are indicated because they are easy and cost-effective. Arterial blood gas analysis is rarely diagnostic or cost-effective in coughing patients without respiratory distress.

Nasal Discharge, Sneezing, and Epistaxis

Nasal discharge, sneezing, and epistaxis may be due to primary nasal cavity disease or may be secondary to distal airway disease. Epistaxis may be due to a local problem or a systemic problem (e.g., coagulopathy) (Dhupa and Littman, 1992). Common causes of these problems are listed in Table 11–3.

When epistaxis occurs, evaluation for a coagulopathy should be the initial diagnostic step (see Chapter 5). Radiographic examination of the nasal cavity is usually performed next (Fig. 11–3), but findings are seldom diagnostic in

Table 11–3 CAUSES OF NASAL DISCHARGE, SNEEZING, AND EPISTAXIS IN DOGS AND CATS

Structural anomalies
Cleft palate
Oronasal fistula
Cricopharyngeal achalasia
Megaesophagus

Allergic/immunologic
Allergic rhinitis
Lymphoplasmacytic rhinitis

Bleeding disorders
Factor deficiency (congenital and acquired)
Thrombocytopenia (infectious and immune-mediated)
Vessel wall (trauma and vasculitis)

Foreign bodies/trauma

Infections
Viral: Dogs: distemper, parainfluenza, or adenovirus type 2
        Cats: herpesvirus or calicivirus
Bacterial: including dental disease, chronic feline rhinosinusitis
Fungal: *Aspergillus* spp., *Penicillium* spp., *Cryptococcus neoformans,* or *Rhinosporidium seeberi*; other opportunistic fungi are rare (e.g., *Trichosporon*)
Rickettsial (*Ehrlichia canis, Ehrlichia ehrlichii,* Rocky Mountain spotted fever)
Parasitic (*Pneumonyssoides caninum, Linguatula serrata, Capillaria aerophila,* or *Cuterebra* spp.)
Other (*Chlamydia* spp.)

Neoplasia/polyps
Carcinomas, sarcomas, transmissible venereal tumor
Polyp (nasopharyngeal in cats)

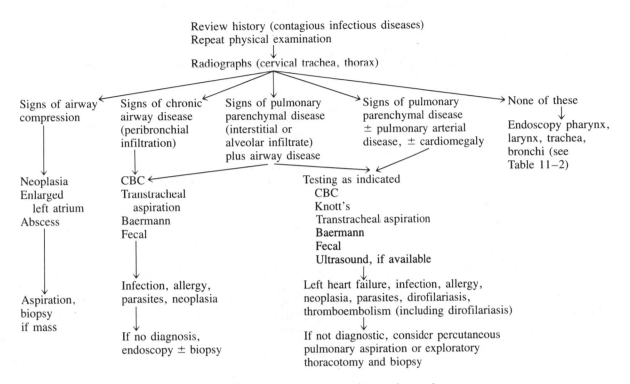

Figure 11-2 Diagnostic approach to coughing in dogs and cats.

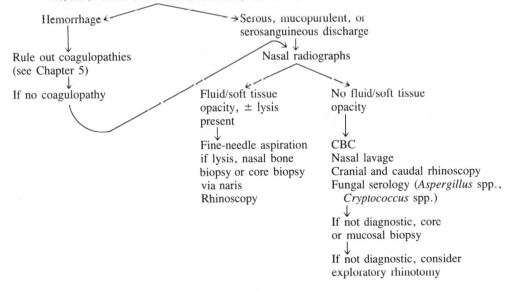

Figure 11-3 Diagnostic approach to nasal discharge/epistaxis in dogs and cats.

acute disease. If a mass lesion or bone lysis is identified, biopsy via the naris is indicated. Rhinoscopy to look for foreign objects is next and can be done while a patient is anesthetized for radiographs. Direct examination may reveal adult *Pneumonyssoides caninum*. Serologic testing for nasal aspergillosis is helpful but can be falsely negative and should not be relied on for a diagnosis (see Chapter 15). Direct examination of the nasal cavity can be performed with rigid instruments. The nasopharynx and posterior portion of the nasal cavity can be visualized with a dental mirror and penlight or more efficiently with a flexible fiberoptic endoscope. Endoscopy of the anterior portion of the nasal cavity in small dogs and cats is limited by the endoscope's diameter. Nasal lavage is rarely helpful in diagnosis. Bacterial culture is often done but is difficult to interpret because of the resident bacterial population of the nasal cavity (see Chapter 15). Fungal culture for aspergillosis can have both false-positive and false-negative results. Cultures for fungi are generally more reliable if performed on nasal biopsy specimens rather than from swabs of the nasal cavity. Nasal biopsy samples should be obtained with alligator-type clamshell instruments or by catheter core procedures (described later). If these procedures are not diagnostic and the condition persists, exploratory rhinotomy should be considered.

NASAL RADIOGRAPHY

Common Indications • Chronic nasal discharge, epistaxis, severe acute undiagnosed sneezing, facial deformity, nasal obstruction, or pawing at the face or nose (see Table 11–3). Advantages: noninvasive. Neoplasia and *Aspergillus* often cause bone lysis, a finding seldom present in other disorders. Disadvantages: General anesthesia is required, and excessive fluid (e.g., nasal hemorrhage or exudate) may obscure other soft tissue abnormalities.

Readers are referred to a radiology text for additional information. If available, computed tomography or magnetic resonance imaging can provide superior detail in the evaluation of the nasal cavity (Ogilvie et al., 1992; Codner et al., 1993).

RHINOSCOPY

Occasional Indications • As for nasal radiographs. Advantages: relatively noninvasive, may follow nasal radiographs during same anesthetic procedure, may provide definitive diagnosis. Disadvantages: Anesthesia is required, and if an otoscope cone is used, only the rostral nares can be visualized. Even with a fiberscope, arthroscope, or cystoscope overall visualization is limited, necessitating a careful, methodic examination that does not always result in a diagnosis. In small dogs, rhinoscopy is difficult unless an arthroscope is available. Care must be taken to avoid hemorrhage, which can obscure the field of view.

Procedure • Radiographs should be obtained before performing rhinoscopy. Under general anesthesia, anterior rhinoscopy may be performed with an otoscope, nasal speculum, fiberscope, arthroscope, or cystoscope (the last two are preferred). Posterior rhinoscopy is performed by retracting the soft palate with an ovariectomy hook and visualizing the area with a dental mirror, nasopharyngeal illuminator, or fiberscope (preferred). Tissue or brush biopsies can be obtained for cytologic analysis, histologic examination, or culture.

Analysis and Interpretation • Refer to the following sections, Nasal Lavage and Nasal Core Biopsy.

NASAL LAVAGE

Occasional Indications • As for nasal radiography. Advantages: less invasive than a core biopsy, and small possibility of complications. Disadvantage: seldom diagnostic.

Procedure • Under general anesthesia with endotracheal intubation, the nasopharynx is packed off with gauze sponges and the nasal cavity is vigorously lavaged with saline via a soft rubber tube.* The fluid is recovered in a dish placed at the nares. A foreign body may occasionally be dislodged and recovered from the naris or the gauze sponges in the nasopharynx.

Analysis • The recovered fluid is centrifuged, and the sediment is stained and examined. A Wright-Giemsa or Gram's stain is preferred when looking for organisms like *Cryptococcus* spp. If the lavaged material appears to be an exudate, it can be cultured for fungi. Bacterial culture is rarely useful. Direct examination of lavage fluid may reveal adult or larval *P. caninum*.

---

*Rob-Nel catheter, Sherwood Medical, St. Louis, MO 63103.

Interpretation • In allergic rhinitis, a predominance of eosinophils is seen (see Nasal Core Biopsy, next, for additional interpretation of nasal specimens).

NASAL CORE BIOPSY

Common Indications • As for nasal lavage. The decision to do a core biopsy is often based on nasal radiographic findings of a mass lesion or bone lysis. In the absence of these, the procedure is only occasionally diagnostic. Advantage: Tissue can be obtained for histopathologic evaluation. Disadvantages: The procedure is invasive, and although unlikely, penetration of the cribriform plate is possible if one is careless.

Procedure • If a dog's coagulation status is questionable, a platelet count, bleeding time, and activated clotting time should be performed (see Chapter 5). Nasal core biopsy is done under general anesthesia with endotracheal intubation. The nasopharynx is packed off as for nasal lavage. The biopsy instrument can be either a large-bore tube that covers one type of peripheral vein indwelling catheter* (medium or large dog) or an 8-gauge polypropylene urinary catheter† (small dog or cat) cut at 45° about 12 to 15 cm from the end that attaches to the syringe. If the large-bore tube is used, this is attached to the syringe by the cutoff hub of the needle supplied with the catheter (Fig. 11–4). The distance from the naris to the medial canthus of the eye is marked on the tube, because this approximates the distance to the cribriform

*Sovereign indwelling catheter, Monoject Division of Sherwood Medical, St. Louis, MO 63103.

†Polypropylene catheter, Monoject Division of Sherwood Medical, St. Louis, MO 63103.

plate. The tube is advanced into the affected tissue, suction is applied, and the tube containing a core of tissue is withdrawn. If a cutoff 8-gauge catheter is used, it is marked as for the tube and moved vigorously back and forth to dislodge tissue. Take special care to avoid penetration of the cribriform plate. A syringe containing saline (35 ml in a large dog, 10 ml in a cat or small dog) is attached, and the dislodged tissue is flushed out through the naris or into the nasopharynx. In addition, material can be obtained by aspiration.

Alternatively, bone curettes or alligator-type clamshell forceps may be used instead of a tube or catheter.

A portion of the biopsy specimen obtained from either method can be submitted for fungal culture (see Chapter 15). Impression smears can be made for cytologic examination, and the remainder of the tissue submitted for histopathologic examination. Mild bleeding from the naris after biopsy is expected but usually subsides within 30 minutes. Uncommonly, the bleeding is profuse for the first 10 to 15 minutes. In cases of profuse or prolonged nasal bleeding, the affected area can be packed with cotton-tipped swabs that have been dipped in dilute (1:10,000) epinephrine solution.

Caution! • It is imperative that the tube not be advanced beyond the level of the medial canthus because of potential cribriform plate perforation.

Interpretation of Impression Cytology

Infection • Because the nasal cavity in both health and disease contains a varied population of bacteria (see Chapter 15), identification of bacteria is rarely of diagnostic significance. *Aspergillus* spp. and *Penicillium* spp. can occasionally be recovered from the nasal cavity of normal animals

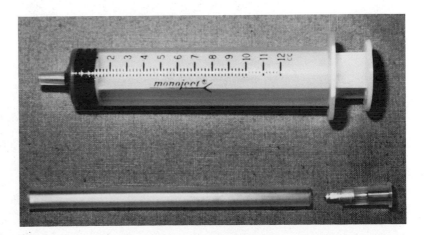

Figure 11–4 Plastic tube and needle hub used to obtain nasal biopsy specimen.

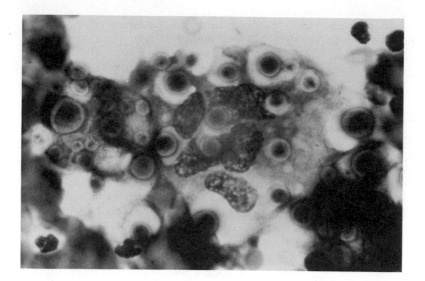

Figure 11–5 *Cryptococcus neoformans* from an impression smear from a nasal biopsy specimen. (Courtesy Dr S.D. Gaunt, Louisiana State University.)

as well as from some with other disorders (e.g., tumors); therefore, a diagnosis of aspergillosis or penicilliosis must be confirmed by histopathologic evaluation. However, finding *Cryptococcus* spp. in a cat with chronic nasal discharge is diagnostic (Fig. 11–5).

Neoplasia • The most common nasal tumors are adenocarcinomas and carcinomas (Fig. 11–6), although round cell tumors (i.e., transmissible venereal tumor, mast cell tumor, and lymphosarcoma) occasionally occur. Other malignant mesenchymal tissue tumors (e.g., fibrosarcoma) may occur in the nasal cavity but are less exfoliative and more difficult to diagnose cytologically (see Chapter 16 for cytologic evaluation of neoplastic cells).

Hemorrhage • In nasal hemorrhage, proportions of erythrocytes and leukocytes are approximately equivalent to whole blood.

NASAL MUCOSAL BIOPSY

Occasional Indications • Undiagnosed nasal discharge without radiographic evidence of masses or bone lysis. Two diseases that may be diagnosed by this method are lymphocytic-plasmacytic rhinitis and primary ciliary dyskinesia (immotile cilia syndrome), although the latter requires electron microscopy to be definitive.

Procedure • Specimens are obtained with alligator biopsy forceps (usually via an otoscope) or a bone curette, fixed in formalin or other

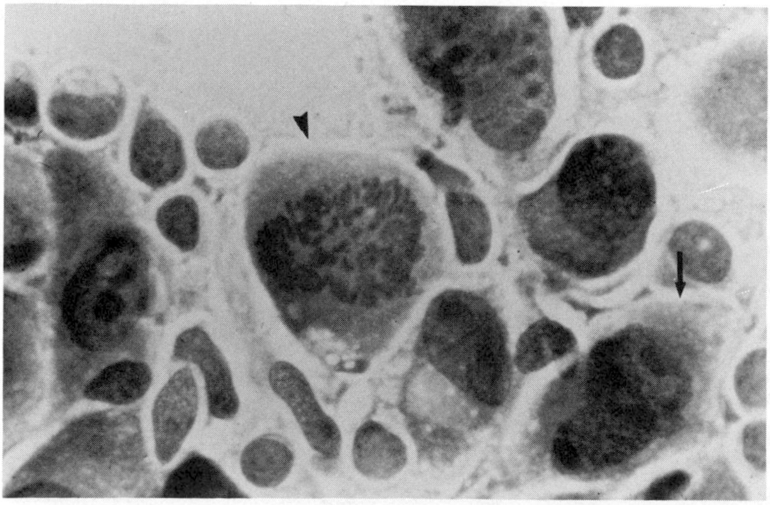

Figure 11–6 Carcinoma cell (arrow) from an impression smear of a nasal biopsy. Notice the mitotic figure (arrowhead). (Courtesy Dr C.L. Barton, Texas A&M University.)

appropriate fixative, and submitted for histo-pathologic examination.

NASAL FINE-NEEDLE ASPIRATION BIOPSY

Occasional Indications • Nasal bone destruction that permits a needle to be introduced into the nasal cavity without going through the naris. Advantages: Anesthesia is not required, and the procedure is minimally invasive. Disadvantage: Some tumors (mesenchymal) are poorly exfoliative.

Procedure • The area of bone lysis is identified by palpation or by nasal radiographs. A 23- or 25-gauge needle is inserted through the lytic area of bone, and aspiration is performed. Specimens are submitted for cytologic examination.

Interpretation • See Interpretation of Impression Cytology under Nasal Core Biopsy, earlier.

EXPLORATORY RHINOTOMY

Occasional Indications • Sneezing, nasal discharge, or epistaxis whose cause has not been established by one or more of the preceding procedures. Advantages: Allows excellent visualization, biopsy, and culture of the nasal cavity, plus it is useful in identifying nasal foreign bodies. Disadvantage: invasive.

Procedure • Readers are referred to a surgical text for a description of the procedure. Impression smears are made of specimens obtained, and the smears are submitted for cytologic examination. Tissue specimens are cultured for fungi and/or fixed in formalin and submitted for histopathologic evaluation.

SEROLOGY FOR NASAL FUNGAL DISORDERS

Occasional Indications • Chronic, undiagnosed nasal discharge that may be due to aspergillosis or cryptococcosis (and rarely other fungi) (see Chapter 15 for additional information on these tests).

COAGULATION TESTS FOR EPISTAXIS

Occasional Indications • Undiagnosed nasal cavity hemorrhage, especially before surgery or aggressive biopsy (see Chapter 5).

LARYNGEAL AND PHARYNGEAL EXAMINATION

Occasional Indications • Respiratory stertor, stridor, or gagging suggestive of upper airway obstructive disorder (e.g., nasopharyngeal polyp, laryngeal paralysis) or foreign body. Advantage: definitive treatment of the problem if polyp or foreign body. Disadvantage: requires anesthesia.

Procedure • The larynx should be examined under a light plane of anesthesia in order to evaluate movement of the laryngeal cartilages. The pharynx and nasopharynx are examined as described for posterior rhinoscopy.

TRACHEAL AND THORACIC RADIOGRAPHY

Common Indications • Chronic or severe cough or other bronchopulmonary disease (used early in evaluation). Advantages: noninvasive and often localizes problems. Disadvantage: rarely of value in acute inflammatory disorders (e.g., viral tracheobronchitis) or thromboembolism not due to dirofilariasis (LaRue and Murtaugh, 1990).

Procedure and Interpretation • Readers are referred to a radiology text for additional information. Evaluation of both right and left lateral views will improve chances of detecting pulmonary mass lesions (Biller and Myer, 1987; Steyn and Green, 1990).

TRANSTRACHEAL ASPIRATION

Common Indications • As for thoracic radiographs. Advantages: relatively noninvasive yet samples the tracheobronchial tree without anesthesia. Disadvantages: Complications can include subcutaneous emphysema originating at the site of needle penetration, esophageal perforation, hemorrhage, and catheter stylet trauma to the lower airway. Drowning is theoretically possible but unlikely because the injected fluid is rapidly absorbed. The procedure is contraindicated in patients with severe respiratory distress because restraint can worsen the distress, with potential mortality.

Procedure • Dogs often tolerate transtracheal aspiration (TTA) without sedation, but tranquilizers (e.g., acepromazine) can be used if necessary. However, sedation (e.g., 1–2 mg/kg ketamine intravenously) is routine for cats. The patient is restrained in sternal recumbency. After clipping and surgical preparation of the skin over the larynx, a bleb of lidocaine is injected over the cricothyroid membrane. A through-the-needle type of catheter* (20 gauge for cats and small dogs, 16 gauge for medium and large dogs) is inserted through the cricothyroid membrane and advanced to approximately the level of the mainstem bronchi. Alternatively, a sterile 3.5 French polypropylene urinary catheter can be inserted through a 14-gauge needle in large dogs. In anesthetized animals, the catheter can be inserted through a sterile endotracheal tube. This method is recommended for cats if anesthesia can be tolerated.

Depending on the animal's size, 0.5 to 1.0 ml/kg of sterile 0.9% saline is injected into the catheter. After the animal coughs, aspiration is performed. Chest coupage after fluid instillation may improve recovery of debris from the airways. Usually only a small amount of the injected material is recovered. If a low-pressure (i.e., < 5 mm Hg) suction pump is available, the yield is higher. Using the suction pump method, material can be aspirated into a suction trap†. Multiple aliquots of saline can be injected until a sample is obtained. Aliquots of the aspirate may be submitted for cytologic analysis and aerobic, anaerobic, or fungal culture. The decision to culture is best based on cytologic findings (see Interpretation, next).

Interpretation • Normal cats and dogs typically have occasional ciliated columnar or cuboidal

---

*Intracath, Deseret Medical Inc., Sandy, UT 84070.

†Dee Lee suction catheter, American Hospital Supply, McGaw Park, IL 60084.

epithelial cells, occasional undifferentiated macrophages with few or no vacuoles, rare neutrophils, and small amounts of mucus. Some normal epithelial cells may appear smudged or may lack cilia because of trauma during sample preparation. TTA aspirates from animals with bronchopulmonary disease may be classified as mucopurulent inflammation, nonpurulent inflammation, neoplastic, or hemorrhagic (see Chapter 16).

Mucopurulent Inflammation • This aspirate is a mixture of neutrophilic inflammation (see Chapter 16, Neutrophilic Inflammation) and abundant mucus, often plus a few macrophages (Fig. 11–7). A thorough search for bacteria (especially intracellular) should be made if degenerate neutrophils are seen (Fig. 11–8). Causes of nonseptic mucopurulent inflammation include fungal, viral, mycoplasmal, and protozoal infection as well as chronic bronchitis, tumors, foreign bodies, and aspiration (Padrid et al., 1991). In mucopurulent inflammation, the mucoid material may stain basophilic (blue) or become eosinophilic (pink) as the inflammation becomes more severe.

A portion of the TTA sample should be placed in a culture transport medium before cytologic evaluation. If the cytologic diagnosis is mucopurulent inflammation, this portion should be submitted for culture and sensitivity tests (see Chapter 15).

Nonpurulent Inflammation • This aspirate includes a higher percentage of macrophages (see Chapter 16, Granulomatous and Pyogranulomatous Inflammation) and eosinophils (see Chapter 16, Eosinophilic Inflammation) than

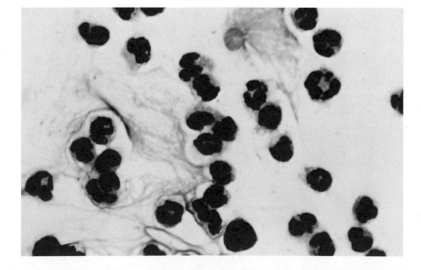

Figure 11–7 Mucopurulent inflammation from a transtracheal aspirate of a dog with chronic obstructive pulmonary disease associated with collapsed trachea. Notice large numbers of nondegenerate neutrophils and abundant mucus.

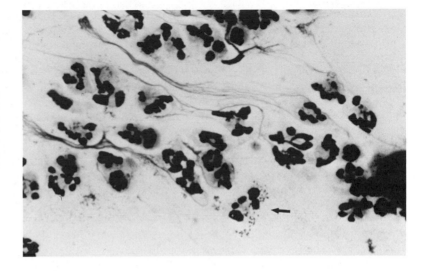

Figure 11–8 Septic inflammation in a transtracheal aspiration specimen from a dog with bacterial pneumonia. Notice the large number of degenerate neutrophils, some containing intracellular bacteria (arrow). (Courtesy Dr P.S. MacWilliams, University of Wisconsin.)

that found in mucopurulent exudates. Nonpurulent exudates may contain a predominance of eosinophils or macrophages or a mixture of eosinophils, macrophages, and neutrophils. Eosinophilic inflammation (Fig. 11–9) suggests hypersensitivity, due to either inhaled allergens, parasites, or eosinophilic pulmonary granulomatosis (Neer et al., 1986, Calvert et al., 1988). Parasitic causes include *Dirofilaria immitis, Aleurostrongylus abstrusus, Capillaria aerophilia, Osleri osleri, Filaroides* spp., *Paragonimus kellicotti*, or migrating parasites such as *Toxocara* spp. or *Ancylostoma* spp. Small numbers of mast cells are often found in eosinophilic inflammation. A predominance of differentiated macrophages (i.e., larger macrophages with abundant cytoplasm and numerous cytoplasmic vacuoles) suggests a subacute to chronic condition, such as granulomatous pneumonia due to fungi and lipid.

Fungal organisms are rarely recovered because of their localization in the interstitium rather than in the airways.

Other Cells That May Be Found in Transtracheal Aspirates • Reactive epithelial cells may be found in any inflammatory process, especially in cats. The cytoplasm of the cells is more basophilic (blue) than that in normal epithelial cells, and the nuclei have fine chromatin and visible nucleoli. The cells may be single or clustered.

Goblet cells may occasionally be seen in inflammatory disease. They contain granules of intracellular mucus and are often seen in conjunction with abundant extracellular mucus.

Neoplastic cells are occasionally seen in TTA samples from animals with primary lung tumors, particularly adenocarcinomas. Primary lung tumors are, however, much less common than are

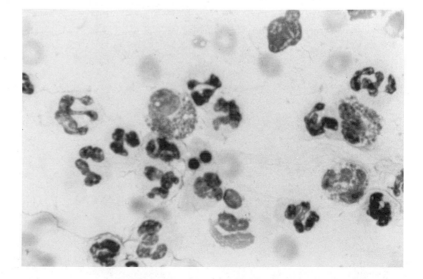

Figure 11–9 Eosinophilic inflammation in a transtracheal aspiration specimen from a cat with asthma. (Courtesy Dr K.A. Gossett, Louisiana State University.)

metastatic tumors. Cells from metastatic pulmonary tumors are unlikely to be seen in TTA specimens because of the interstitial location of the tumor.

Aspirated material from the oral cavity is suggested by squamous epithelial cells (which may be coated with bacteria) or certain large bacteria such as *Simonsiella* spp. (Fig. 11–10).

Lymphocytes may be seen in acute viral tracheobronchitis; lymphocytes plus plasma cells may be seen in chronic progressive septic bronchopneumonitis, sterile bronchopneumonitis, or pulmonary lymphoid granulomatosis (Berry et al., 1990).

Respiratory Parasites ● Ova of *C. aerophilia, P. kellicotti,* and *Filaroides hirthi* may occasionally be found, as may larvae of *Osleri osleri* (also known as *Filaroides osleri*), *Crenosoma vulpis, A. abstrusus, Toxocara canis, Toxocara cati,* and *Strongyloides stercoralis,* as well as microfilariae of *D. immitis.*

Anthracotic pigment appears as dense black granules within macrophages and is an incidental finding in dogs in industrial areas.

BRONCHOALVEOLAR LAVAGE

Common Indications ● Same as for transtracheal aspiration.

Procedure ● Patients should be selected carefully because bronchoalveolar lavage (BAL) is a more invasive technique, requires general anesthesia, and causes temporary respiratory compromise (Hawkins and DeNicola, 1989; Hawkins et al., 1990). Although not technically difficult, some practice is required to acquire confidence and skill in performing BAL. BAL can be per-

formed through an endotracheal tube; however, endoscopic BAL is recommended because of improved site selectivity for collection of specimens and enhanced retrieval of lavage fluid.

Animals undergoing BAL should receive atropine as a preanesthetic and be anesthetized with ketamine/acepromazine or ketamine/valium intravenously (cats) or other intravenous short-acting anesthetic agents (dogs). Additional anesthetic can be given intravenously if needed to maintain sufficient anesthesia to perform the procedure. An endotracheal tube (4-mm internal diameter for cats, appropriate size for dogs) is placed rostral to the carina, and the cuff is inflated. Oxygen (100% O_2) is administered for 10 minutes before lavage.

After preoxygenation, a patient is placed in lateral recumbency with the most affected side down, and a syringe adapter is attached to the endotracheal tube. Three aliquots (5 ml/kg) of warm, sterile 0.9% saline are gently infused into the lung and immediately retrieved with gentle suction. Elevating the hindquarters of the patient improves retrieval of BAL fluid. Each aliquot is kept in a separate syringe for analysis. O_2 (100%) is administered for 20 minutes after the BAL procedure.

If an endoscope is used, an endotracheal tube is not placed in cats or small dogs, but the endoscope is passed into the trachea and O_2 is delivered through the endoscopic biopsy channel or through an adaptor adjacent to the endoscope. In larger dogs, an endotracheal tube can be placed, the endoscope passed through it, and O_2/inhalant anesthesia administered around the endoscope with a T adapter. The distal end of the endoscope is "wedged" in a mainstem bronchus or airway of interest. Three aliquots (2 ml/kg) of warmed, sterile 0.9% sa-

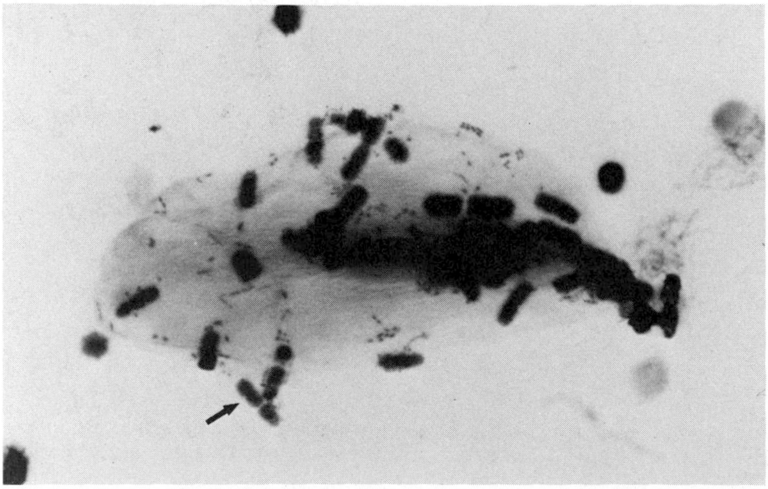

Figure 11–10 *Simonsiella* spp. (arrow) and a squamous epithelial cell in a transtracheal aspiration specimen from a dog. (Courtesy Dr D. Baker, Colorado State University.)

line are flushed through the endoscopic biopsy channel and immediately retrieved as previously described. Pre- and post-BAL oxygenation is also used with this procedure.

BAL specimens should be placed on ice immediately and transferred to the laboratory for analysis. BAL fluid often appears foamy because of pulmonary surfactant recovered by the BAL procedure. Cytologic specimens should be prepared immediately by Cytospin or centrifugation to concentrate cells present.

The cellular character of BAL preparations is vastly different from TTA specimens. The predominant cell type is the alveolar macrophage; however, large numbers of eosinophils (up to 30%) can apparently be present in BAL specimens from clinically normal cats (Padrid et al., 1991). Other cell types and infectious organisms (e.g., yeast, fungal hyphae, bacteria) may be present, depending on the pathologic process present in the patient, and interpretation is similar to that described for TTA (Hawkins and DeNicola, 1990).

Because of the inevitable oral contamination of the instruments used for BAL procedures, BAL specimens are not useful for accurate bacteriologic culture. Specimens for culture should be collected by TTA or with a guarded swab.

TRACHEOBRONCHOSCOPY

Occasional Indications • Tracheobronchoscopy is indicated in patients with persistent undiagnosed coughing, hemoptysis, or a suspected obstructive lesion or whenever direct visualization of the larger airways is required to look for obstruction or collapse or to sample one area of the tracheobronchial tree selectively. It is the procedure of choice to diagnose collapsed trachea if the diagnosis has not been established radiographically. Either a rigid or flexible bronchoscope can be used, but the latter is preferred. Advantages: direct visualization of major airways and ability to biopsy specific sites. This is the technique of choice to diagnose *O. osleri* infection. Cytologic specimens obtained by brush biopsy are usually superior to those obtained by TTA. As an extension of fiberoptic endoscopy, pulmonary biopsy can be performed via a transbronchial biopsy. Disadvantages: Requires general anesthesia; pulmonary biopsy has the potential risk of pneumomediastinum, pneumothorax, and pulmonary hemorrhage.

Procedure • The endoscope is either passed through an endotracheal tube (large dog) or passed directly into the trachea (small dog or cat). A thorough systematic examination is made of all accessible parts of the tracheobronchial tree.

Interpretation • In a collapsed trachea, a mainstem bronchus, or bronchi, the severity of the lesion is assessed. Other lesions are visualized and may be sampled by either brush or endoscopic forceps. Specimens obtained may be submitted for bacteriologic culture or for cytologic and histopathologic examination as appropriate.

FECAL EXAMINATION

Occasional Indications • Undiagnosed coughing or respiratory distress, particularly if an unexplained eosinophilia is present or if radiographic signs suggest pulmonary parasitism. Advantage: noninvasive. Disadvantage: Ova of some pulmonary parasites (e.g., *F. hirthi*) are not reliably recovered.

Procedure • Fecal flotation is performed using zinc sulfate solution (see Chapter 9).

Interpretation • Ova of *C. aerophilia* (Fig. 11–11), *F. hirthi*, *Eucoleus boehmi*, and *P. kellicotti* (Fig. 11–12) may be detected.

BAERMANN'S FUNNEL APPARATUS

Occasional Indications • Same as for fecal flotation for respiratory parasites. Advantage: nonin-

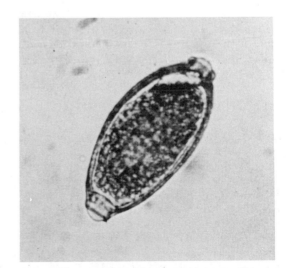

Figure 11–11 *Capillaria aerophilia* egg in a fecal specimen from a dog with chronic cough. (Courtesy Dr J.B. Malone, Louisiana State University.)

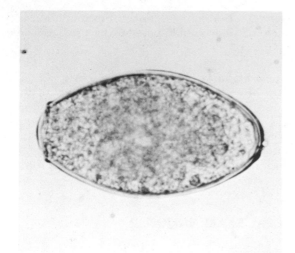

Figure 11-12 *Paragonimus kellicotti* egg in a fecal specimen from a cat with chronic cough. (Courtesy Dr J.B. Malone, Louisiana State University.)

vasive. Disadvantages: not as convenient as flotation; some parasites (e.g., *O. osleri*) shed larvae erratically.

Procedure • Fresh feces are placed on a cheesecloth in a strainer and then placed in the Baermann's apparatus (a funnel with a clamped rubber tube at the stem end). Water is added to the funnel to cover the feces, which are then broken up into small pieces. After a few hours, a small aliquot of water is drained through the rubber tube and examined microscopically for larvae.

Interpretation • Larvae of *Filaroides milksi, O. osleri, C. vulpis, A. abstrusus,* and *S. stercoralis* may be identified, but a negative test result does not rule out these parasites. The method of choice to diagnose *O. osleri* infection is bronchoscopy.

PULMONARY ASPIRATION BIOPSY

Occasional Indications • To investigate masses, procure material for culture, and evaluate diffuse parenchymal disease. Advantage: Samples pulmonary parenchyma without thoracotomy. Disadvantages: Possible complications include pneumothorax, pulmonary hemorrhage, hemoptysis, and (if the myocardium is inadvertently penetrated) cardiac arrhythmias, any of which may cause death.

Contraindications • Thrombocytopenia, bleeding disorders, severe uncontrolled coughing,

uncooperative patient, and pulmonary bullae or cysts.

Procedure • Coagulation status should be screened (see Chapter 5). For diffuse pulmonary disease, the recommended aspiration site is between the seventh and ninth intercostal spaces, two thirds of the distance from the costochondral junction to the vertebral bodies. A 25-gauge hypodermic or spinal needle* with the stylet removed and 12-ml syringe is used. After clipping and surgical preparation of the skin, the needle is attached to the syringe, inserted into the pulmonary parenchyma, and aspiration is performed. The procedure should be done quickly, the actual aspiration not taking more than a few seconds. Very little material is usually aspirated, and what is present typically remains in the needle hub. The needle should be removed from the syringe, air introduced into the syringe, the needle reattached, and the aspirated material quickly "blown" onto a clean glass slide. Another clean slide is used to prepare a horizontal "pull-apart" specimen for cytologic examination. Pulmonary aspiration should be performed early in the day so the patient can be monitored for respiratory distress caused by pneumothorax, pulmonary hemorrhage, or hemoptysis. Ultrasonography is generally not a useful tool for evaluating the pulmonary parenchyma. However, if a mass lesion is present, ultrasonographic or fluoroscopic guidance may be helpful in placement of the needle.

Larger lung tissue specimens for histopathologic examination can be obtained with a similar technique using a modified Menghini's aspiration biopsy needle† (Teske et al., 1991).

Interpretation • Fine-needle aspiration biopsy specimens are examined cytologically and classified as inflammatory, neoplastic, or hemorrhagic (see Chapter 16). Larger specimens are submitted for histopathologic examination.

Inflammatory • Neutrophils, monocytes, or eosinophils predominate. Abundant erythrocytes are commonly found. In fungal pneumonia, especially if caused by *Blastomyces* or *Histoplasma*, free or engulfed yeasts may be seen (Fig. 11-13). Increased numbers of eosinophils can occur in aspirates from animals with pulmonary infiltrates with eosinophilia, as well as other hypersensitivities and parasitism.

---

*Spinal needle, Becton-Dickinson, Rutherford, NJ 07070.
†Modified Menghini Biopsy needle, Becton-Dickinson, Rutherford, NJ 07070.

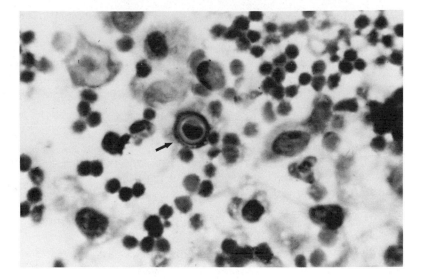

Figure 11–13 *Blastomyces dermatitidis* (arrow) in a fine-needle pulmonary aspiration specimen from a dog with weight loss and respiratory distress. (Courtesy Dr J.D. Hoskins, Louisiana State University.)

Neoplastic • Neoplastic cells may occasionally be seen in aspirates. Malignant epithelial cells tend to appear in clusters (e.g., rafts), and inflammatory cells may be present.

Hemorrhagic • Hemorrhage frequently occurs in pulmonary aspiration biopsy and is usually iatrogenic.

Parasites • Adult *F. hirthi* organisms are rarely recovered by pulmonary fine-needle aspiration.

SEROLOGY FOR PULMONARY DISEASES

In histoplasmosis, blastomycosis, cryptococcosis, and coccidioidomycosis, the finding of organisms is diagnostic. However, the pulmonary disease caused by these organisms is usually interstitial and TTA rarely demonstrates the organism. Positive serologic results, particularly for coccidioidomycosis and blastomycosis, may establish a tentative diagnosis when TTA, BAL, and pulmonary aspiration biopsy do not (check characteristics of individual tests in Chapter 15). Serologic testing for antibodies to *Toxoplasma gondii* is rarely indicated in patients with pulmonary disease.

THORACOTOMY

If the cause of severe pulmonary disease cannot be established by other procedures, exploratory thoracotomy and biopsy can provide tissue for histopathologic examination or culture.

ARTERIAL BLOOD GASES

Alveolar ventilation refers to the ability of inspired air to enter and leave alveoli. *Ventilatory failure* refers to inadequate airflow into and out of alveoli and results in an inability to maintain carbon dioxide (CO_2) homeostasis in the body. *Respiratory failure* refers to failure of ventilation, perfusion, or diffusion.

In normal animals, increased arterial CO_2 (hypercapnia) and decreased arterial O_2 (hypoxemia) are the main stimuli for respiration. Minor elevations in arterial CO_2 cause increased ventilation, whereas decreased arterial O_2 does not have a major effect on ventilation until the partial pressure of arterial O_2 (PaO_2) is < 55 mm Hg. Lesser degrees of hypoxemia increase ventilation, but the response is initially limited by the ensuing hypocapnia (Rose, 1984a).

Rare Indications • Airway or pulmonary parenchymal disease resulting in respiratory insufficiency, or ventilatory failure due to any cause. Advantages: Quantitates the degree of respiratory impairment, evaluates compensatory changes, and monitors response to treatment. Disadvantages: inability to determine focal versus disseminated respiratory disease, inability to diagnose or prognosticate, need for arterial puncture, necessity of prompt submission of the specimen, and expense.

Sample Procurement • The femoral artery is the usual site for arteriotomy. After the hair is clipped and the skin is swabbed with alcohol, the sample is obtained with a 25-gauge needle and heparinized syringe. The amount of heparin should be just enough to fill the needle and hub of the syringe; 1 ml of blood is preferred. Any air bubbles obtained during collection must be eliminated as quickly as possible, the needle point inserted into a rubber stopper (e.g., from a Vacutainer), and the specimen submitted in the same syringe in which it was collected. Analysis should be performed within 10 to 20 minutes of sampling but can be prolonged for up to 3 hours if the specimen is stored in an ice bath (0° C) (Ventriglia, 1986). Direct pressure is applied to the arteriotomy site for at least 5 minutes after sampling.

Analysis ● An arterial blood sample is necessary for evaluation of the respiratory system. Use of venous blood gas analysis for determination of acid-base status is discussed in Chapter 6; venous O_2 tension ($P\bar{v}O_2$) is discussed in the next section.

Normal Arterial Values ● See Table 11–4.

Danger Values ● PaO_2 < 60 mm Hg; $PaCO_2$ > 70 mm Hg. Note: The danger values depend on the duration of the problem: chronicity allows compensatory mechanisms, enabling tolerance of greater abnormalities.

Artifacts ● Improper sample storage before analysis or failing to remove air bubbles causes a decrease in PaO_2 (see Chapter 6, Blood Gas Analysis for Acid-Base Status [Venous Blood]).

Drug Treatment That May Alter Values ● Excessive heparin decreases both the pH and PaO_2, whereas citrate, oxalate, or EDTA decreases pH. Any drugs that alter control of the respiratory drive (e.g., anesthetic agents) may alter the PaO_2.

Partial Pressure of Oxygen

PaO_2 is measured to evaluate the degree of respiratory dysfunction, but it is only one factor affecting O_2 delivery to the tissues. Other pa-

Table 11–5 CAUSES OF HYPOXEMIA IN DOGS AND CATS

Respiratory disorders
Ventilation: perfusion mismatch
Airway or ventilation disorders
  Alveolar hypoventilation
  Decreased alveolar oxygen
  Drug-induced respiratory center depression
  Brainstem disorders causing hypoventilation
  Respiratory muscle disorders
  Thoracic cage disorders
  Airway obstruction disorders
  Pleural cavity disorders
  Inadequate mechanical ventilation
Impaired diffusion
  Pulmonary parenchymal disease
Vascular shunting
  Congenital heart disease with right-to-left shunting

Other disorders
Metabolic acidosis
Compensation for metabolic alkalosis
Increased metabolic rate
Hypothermia
High altitude (decreased alveolar oxygen)

rameters, such as cardiac output, blood pressure, regional blood flow, position of the hemoglobin dissociation curve, and hemoglobin concentration, are also important (Table 11–5).

Causes of Hypoxemia ● These include respiratory and nonrespiratory causes (see Table 11–5). Respiratory disease is the most common cause of hypoxemia and may be classified as ventilation/perfusion mismatching, alveolar hypoventilation, impaired diffusion, or vascular shunting (see Table 11–5). Characterization and evaluation of hypoxemia and accompanying PCO_2 and HCO_3^- changes are discussed later under Diagnostic Evaluation of Blood Gases.

Partial Pressure of Carbon Dioxide

$PaCO_2$ is controlled primarily by the rate at which CO_2 is eliminated from the lungs. Therefore, an increase or decrease in $PaCO_2$ is associated with a decrease or increase in ventilation, respectively (Table 11–6). Because increased $PaCO_2$ decreases pH, the condition is also known as *respiratory acidosis*. The reverse occurs with a decrease in $PaCO_2$ (respiratory alkalosis).

Causes of Hypercapnia (Hypercarbia) ● Hypercapnic patients breathing room air are also hypoxemic, because there is a concomitant decrease in O_2 uptake. Hypoxemia usually occurs much earlier than does hypercapnia because (1) CO_2 diffuses across the alveolar capillary 20

Table 11–4 NORMAL ARTERIAL BLOOD GAS VALUES

	Dogs	Cats
pH	7.36–7.44	7.36–7.44
PaO_2	85–95 mm Hg	100–110 mm Hg
$PaCO_2$	36–44 mm Hg	28–32 mm Hg
HCO_3^-	24–26 mEq/L	20–22 mEq/L

Table 11-6 CAUSES OF HYPOCAPNIA (RESPIRATORY ALKALOSIS) IN DOGS AND CATS

Hypoxemia (see Table 11-5)
Compensation for metabolic
  acidosis
Respiratory center stimulation
  Fear, anxiety, pain
  Brain disease
  Fever
  Heat stroke
  Hyperthyroidism
  Hepatic failure
  Gram-negative septicemia
Iatrogenic
  Mechanical ventilation

times more quickly than O_2 and (2) as patients attempt to increase ventilation in more functional lung, more CO_2 can be excreted but only a small amount of additional O_2 can be taken up, because O_2 saturation of hemoglobin in these areas approximates 100% (Rose, 1984a).

Alveolar hypoventilation is the major cause of hypercapnia, although other causes of hypoxemia may be responsible (see Table 11-5). Hypercapnia may be primary or secondary to metabolic alkalosis. Any disorder capable of producing hypoxemia is also capable of producing either hypercapnia or hypocapnia. The clinical significance of the $PaO_2/PaCO_2$ relationship is that in airway/pulmonary parenchymal disease with hypoxemia, there may be an initial hypocapnia. As the disease process worsens, there may be a normalization of $PaCO_2$ and eventual hypercapnia.

Causes of Hypocapnia (Hypocarbia) • Decreased $PaCO_2$ occurs when effective alveolar ventilation is increased beyond that needed to eliminate the metabolically produced CO_2. Major causes of hypocapnia are listed in Table 11-6.

Compensatory Responses to Alterations in Blood Gases • Decreased PaO_2 is associated with either increased or decreased $PaCO_2$. In humans, predictable changes in HCO_3^- are associated with alterations in $PaCO_2$ (Rose, 1984a,b), and similar changes may occur in dogs and cats (see Table 6-8).

Diagnostic Evaluation of Blood Gases

First, decide if the abnormality is significant. Minor elevations in PaO_2 are not an indication for additional evaluation other than characterization of the underlying disorder. In patients breathing an enriched O_2 mixture, a PaO_2 less than five times the inspired O_2 concentration requires additional diagnostics. Similarly, evaluation of extrarespiratory causes of hypocapnia depends on the underlying disorder.

If further evaluation of the blood gas analysis is indicated, one should first characterize the abnormality as a primary or secondary, compensated or uncompensated disorder, and then seek to determine the underlying cause (Table 11-7). A three-step process is recommended to characterize the abnormality. A brief overview of the three steps is given next. For additional information, readers are referred to Shapiro and colleagues (1982b).

Explanation of pH (Dogs)

pH normal	7.36 to 7.44
pH ↑	7.45 to 7.50
pH ↑ ↑	>7.50
pH ↓	7.30 to 7.35
pH ↓ ↓	<7.30

Explanation of HCO_3^- • No attempt is made to quantitate HCO_3^- changes.

Step 1: Evaluation of the Ventilatory Status • This is done by evaluation of $PaCO_2$. Ventilation is classified as acceptable (normal $PaCO_2$), hyperventilation (decreased $PaCO_2$), or hypoventilation (increased $PaCO_2$). From Table 11-7, the abnormality can be assessed as respiratory or metabolic in origin.

Step 2: Assessment of the Hypoxemic State • Decreased PaO_2 confirms arterial hypoxemia and suggests tissue hypoxia (see Table 11-5).

Step 3: Assessment of the Tissue Oxygen State • Normal tissue oxygenation requires perfusion by adequately oxygenated blood. Therefore, this step involves assessment of cardiac status, peripheral perfusion, and blood O_2 transport.

PARTIAL PRESSURE OF OXYGEN IN VENOUS BLOOD

Occasional Indications • In evaluating adequacy of O_2 delivery to tissues and monitoring cardiac output.

Analysis and Interpretation • If pulmonary edema is present, PaO_2 should be measured. If

Table 11-7 ASSESSMENT OF VENTILATION BASED ON BLOOD GAS ANALYSIS

Decreased Pa_{CO_2} *(hyperventilation)*			
pH ↓ – ↓↓	pH normal	pH ↑	pH ↑↑
HCO_3^- ↓↓	HCO_3^- ↓	HCO_3^- ↓	HCO_3^- normal
Partially compensated metabolic acidosis	Compensated metabolic acidosis	Chronic hyperventilation (partially compensated respiratory alkalosis)	Acute hyperventilation (uncompensated respiratory alkalosis)
Normal Pa_{CO_2}			
pH ↓ – ↓↓		pH ↑ – ↑↑	
HCO_3^- ↓		HCO_3^- ↑	
Uncompensated metabolic acidosis		Uncompensated metabolic alkalosis	
Increased Pa_{CO_2} *(hypoventilation)*			
pH ↓ – ↓↓	pH normal	pH ↑	
HCO_3^- normal	HCO_3^- ↑	HCO_3^- ↑	
Acute ventilatory failure (uncompensated respiratory acidosis)	Chronic ventilatory failure (compensated respiratory acidosis)	Partially compensated metabolic alkalosis	

Explanation of pH (dogs)

pH normal	7.36–7.44
pH ↑	7.45–7.50
pH ↑↑	>7.50
pH ↓	7.30–7.35
pH ↓↓	<7.30

Explanation of HCO_3^-: No attempt is made to quantitate HCO_3^- changes.

the Pa_{O_2} is > 65 mm Hg, the $P\bar{v}_{O_2}$ will reflect cardiac output (Kittleson, 1983). The sample should be taken from the jugular vein. Occlusion of the vein for longer than 5 to 10 seconds artifactually decreases $P\bar{v}_{O_2}$. Normal $P\bar{v}_{O_2}$ is > 40 mm Hg. Precautions for obtaining and storing the blood sample before analysis are the same as for arterial blood gases.

If the $P\bar{v}_{O_2}$ is < 30 mm Hg, O_2 delivery to the tissues is inadequate. Cardiac output, O_2 saturation, hemoglobin concentration, and peripheral arteriovenous shunts should be considered as causes of low $P\bar{v}_{O_2}$ and evaluated as described previously. In patients with cardiac disease, a $P\bar{v}_{O_2}$ cannot be correlated to a specific cardiac output, but increases or decreases in $P\bar{v}_{O_2}$ reflect improving or worsening cardiac output (respectively) relative to the initial value.

THORACOCENTESIS

Occasional Indications ● Pleural effusions or mass lesions of the pleural cavity or mediastinum. Advantage: relatively noninvasive. Disadvantages: potential for pneumothorax, hemothorax, or cardiac arrhythmias.

Procedure ● Skin over the right 5th to 11th intercostal spaces (or elsewhere if effusion is localized) is clipped and prepared surgically. The needle of a butterfly-type catheter is inserted in the seventh to eighth intercostal space at approximately the level of the costochondral junc-

tion, and fluid is aspirated into a syringe. A three-way stopcock can be attached to the syringe if the procedure is to be therapeutic as well as diagnostic. The method of analysis is described in Chapter 10. Masses may also be aspirated for cytologic evaluation, ideally with fluoroscopic or ultrasonographic guidance.

Interpretation ● See Chapter 10. Once the fluid has been analyzed, it may be useful to aspirate as much as possible of the remaining fluid and reradiograph the thorax to reveal structures (e.g., mediastinal masses) that were not previously evident.

THORACOTOMY

Rare Indications ● In patients with nocardiosis or actinomycosis to look for a foreign body (e.g., grass awn). It is also indicated in chronic or progressive undiagnosed pleural effusion to look for lesions and to obtain biopsy samples of affected tissue.

Bibliography

Barsanti JA, Prestwood AK: Parasitic diseases of the respiratory tract. *In* Kirk RW (ed): Current Veterinary Therapy VIII. Philadelphia, WB Saunders, 1983, pp 241–246.

Berry CR, Moore PF, Thomas WP, et al: Pulmonary lymphomatoid granulomatosis in seven dogs (1976–1987). J Vet Intern Med 1990; 4:157–166.

Biller DS, Myer CW: Case examples demonstrating the clinical utility of obtaining both right and left lateral thoracic radiographs in small animals. JAAHA 1987; 23:381–386.

Calvert CA, Mahaffey MB, Lappin MR, et al: Pulmonary and disseminated eosinophilic granulomatosis in dogs. JAAHA 1988; 24:311–320.

Chew DJ: Disorders in acid-base balance. *In* Fenner WR (ed): Quick Reference to Veterinary Medicine. Philadelphia, JB Lippincott, 1982, pp 419–431.

Codner EC, Lurus AG, Miller JB, et al: Comparison of computed tomography with radiography as a noninvasive diagnostic technique for chronic nasal disease in dogs. JAVMA 1993;202:1106–1110.

Dhupa N, Littman MP: Epistaxis. Comp Cont Ed Pract Vet 1992;14:1033–1042.

Duncan JR, Prasse K (eds): Cytology. *In* Veterinary Laboratory Medicine. 2nd ed. Ames, Iowa State University Press, 1987, pp 201–226.

Hawkins EC, DeNicola: Collection of bronchoalveolar lavage fluid in cats, using an endotracheal tube. Am J Vet Res 1989; 50:855–859.

Hawkins EC, DeNicola DB, Kuehn NF: Bronchoalveolar lavage in the evaluation of pulmonary disease in the dog and cat. J Vet Intern Med 1990; 4:267–274.

Hawkins EC, DeNicola: Cytologic diagnosis of tracheal wash specimens and bronchoalveolar lavage fluid in the diagnosis of mycotic infections in dogs. JAVMA 1990; 197:79–83.

Hirsch DC: Bacteriology of the lower respiratory tract. *In* Kirk RW (ed): Current Veterinary Therapy IX. Philadelphia, WB Saunders, 1986, pp 247–250.

Kittleson ME: Concepts and therapeutic strategies in the management of heart failure. *In* Kirk RW (ed): Current Veterinary Therapy VIII. Philadelphia, WB Saunders, 1983, pp 279–284.

Krotje JL: Cyanosis: Physiology and pathogenesis. Comp Cont Ed 1987; 9:271–278.

LaRue MJ, Murtaugh RJ: Pulmonary thromboembolism in dogs: 47 cases (1986–1987). JAVMA 1990;197:1368–1372.

Moise NS, Blue J: Bronchial washings in the cat: Procedure and cytologic evaluation. Comp Cont Ed 1983;8:621–630.

Moise NS, Weidenkeller D, Yeager AE, et al: Clinical, radiographic, and bronchial cytologic features of cats with bronchial disease: 65 cases (1980–1986). JAVMA 1989; 194:1467–1471.

Neer TM, Waldron DR, Miller RI: Eosinophilic pulmonary granulomatosis in two dogs and literature review. JAAHA 1986;22:593–599.

Ogilvie GK, LaRue SM: Canine and feline nasal and paranasal sinus tumors. Vet Clin North Am 1992;22:1133–1144.

Padrid PA, Feldman BF, Funk K, et al: Cytologic, microbiologic, and biochemical analysis of bronchoalveolar lavage fluid obtained from 24 healthy cats. Am J Vet Res 1991;52:1300–1307.

Rebar AH, Hawkins EC, DeNicola DB: Cytologic evaluation of the respiratory tract. Vet Clin North Am 1992;22:1065–1085.

Rose DB (ed): Respiratory acidosis. *In* Clinical Physiology of Acid Base and Electrolyte Disorders. 2nd ed. New York, McGraw-Hill, 1984a, pp 440–461.

Rose DB (ed): Respiratory alkalosis. *In* Clinical Physiology of Acid Base and Electrolyte Disorders. 2nd ed. New York, McGraw-Hill, 1984b, pp 462–470.

Roudebush P: Diagnostics for respiratory disease. *In* Kirk RW (ed): Current Therapy VIII. Philadelphia, WB Saunders, 1983, pp 222–230.

Shapiro BA, Harrison RA, Cane RD, Kozlowski-Templin R (eds): Clinical approach to interpretation of arterial blood gases. *In* Clinical Application of Blood Gases. 4th ed. Chicago, Year Book Medical Publishers, 1989, pp 77–98.

Steyn PF, Green RW: How patient positioning affects radiographic signs of canine lung disease. Vet Med 1990; 85:796–806.

Teske E, Stokhof AA, van den Ingh TSGAM, et al: Transthoracic needle aspiration biopsy of the lung in dogs with pulmonic diseases. JAAHA 1991;27:289–294.

Ventriglia WJ: Arterial blood gases. Emerg Med Clin North Am 1986;4:235–251.

Linda L. Werner
Grant H. Turnwald
Ota Barta

12 Immunologic and Plasma Protein Disorders

○ **Serum Total Protein and Albumin**
○ **Protein Electrophoresis**
   Electrophoresis
   Immunoelectrophoresis
○ **Serum Viscosity**
○ **Cryoprecipitation**
○ **Antinuclear Antibody**
○ **Lupus Erythematosus Test (LE Cell Test)**
○ **Antiglobulin (Coombs') Test**
○ **Tests for Immune-Mediated**
   Thrombocytopenia (IMT)

○ **Rheumatoid Factor Test**
○ **Direct Immunofluorescent Testing**
○ **Indirect Immunofluorescent Testing**
○ **Testing for Cellular Functions in Immunity**
   Evaluation of Phagocytes
   Enumeration of Proportions of T and B
    Lymphocytes
   Evaluation of Lymphocyte Functions *In*
    Vitro

A laboratory framework for the evaluation of patients with suspected immunologic disease as well as plasma/serum protein disorders is presented in this chapter.

SERUM TOTAL PROTEIN AND ALBUMIN

Common Indications • As an initial laboratory screening test in most ill patients but especially those with known or suspected anemia, edema, ascites, coagulopathies, diarrhea, weight loss, and hepatic or renal disease. Advantage: technically easy to perform. Disadvantage: Additional testing is required to establish a cause of altered protein concentrations.

Analysis • Total protein can be estimated in fluid, serum, or plasma (EDTA or heparinized) by a refractometer that measures total solids. It

can also be measured in 0.5 ml of serum, urine, or fluid by spectrophotometric methods.

Albumin is measured in 0.5 ml of serum or fluid by bromcresol green dye binding. Serum globulin concentration is calculated by subtracting the serum albumin from the serum total protein.

Normal Values • See Table 12–1. Note: Lower values are normal for perinates and very young animals. Values gradually increase with increasing age; the higher values are average normal

Table 12–1 NORMAL SERUM TOTAL PROTEIN AND ALBUMIN VALUES (g/dl)

	Dogs	Cats
Plasma total protein	6.0–7.8	6.0–7.5
Serum total protein	5.5–7.5	5.5–7.8
Serum albumin	2.5–4.0	2.5–4.0
Serum globulin	3.0–3.5	3.0–3.8

Table 12–2 CAUSES OF HYPERGLOBULINEMIA IN DOGS AND CATS

Polyclonal
  Infections
    Bacterial†
      Brucellosis
      Pyoderma
    Viral‡
      Feline infectious peritonitis
    Fungal†
      Systemic fungal infections (e.g., blastomycosis, histoplasmosis, coccidioidomycosis)
    Rickettsial‡
      Ehrlichiosis
    Parasitic†
      Dirofilariasis
      Demodicosis
      Scabies
  Immune-mediated disease
    Infections (immune complex)†
      Dirofilariasis
      Pyometra
    Systemic lupus erythematosus (SLE) including glomerulonephritis, immune-mediated hemolytic anemia (IHA) and thrombocytopenia (IMT), polyarthritis*
    IHA, IMT (not due to SLE)*
    Pemphigus complex, bullous pemphigoid*
    Rheumatoid arthritis*
  Neoplasia†

Monoclonal
  Infection‡
    Ehrlichiosis
    Feline infectious peritonitis (rare)
  Idiopathic*†
  Neoplasia†‡
    Multiple myeloma
    Macroglobulinemia
    Lymphosarcoma

*Mild (4–5 g/dl).
†Moderate (5–6 g/dl).
‡Severe (>6 g/dl).
Note: The effect of age should be considered when assessing globulin values (see Causes of Hypoglobulinemia).

The effects of hormonal changes on serum proteins are generally considered slight or minimal, even though physical changes such as alteration in body weight or muscle mass may be marked. Hyperproteinemia may be due to anabolic steroids, corticosteroids, progesterone, insulin, and thyroid hormones in human beings. Prolonged high-dose corticosteroid therapy can cause hyperproteinemia and hyperalbuminemia in normal dogs, but values return to normal within weeks after cessation of therapy (Moore et al., 1992). Hypoproteinemia may be due to estrogens, whereas hypoalbuminemia may be due to anticonvulsants, acetaminophen, estrogens, and various antineoplastic agents in human beings.

Causes of Alteration in Plasma/Serum Protein • Hyperproteinemia is caused by hyperalbuminemia (see following) or hyperglobulinemia (see Table 12–2 and Protein Electrophoresis). Decreased plasma protein is caused by hypoalbuminemia (Table 12–3) or hypoglobulinemia. Albumin and globulin must be evaluated separately, since alterations in each may have different causes.

Causes of Hyperalbuminemia • Dehydration and laboratory error can result in apparent hyperalbuminemia.

Causes of Hypoalbuminemia • These are best identified by concurrently evaluating serum globulin. If both the albumin and globulin values are decreased, hemorrhage, exudation from severe skin lesions, protein-losing enteropathy,

values for adult animals. Both albumin and globulin values tend to decline with advancing old age.

Danger Values • Albumin < 1.5 g/dl, depending on portal vein pressure: Increased portal vein pressures increase the possibility of hypoalbuminemia-induced effusion.

Artifacts • Falsely increased (refractometer): hyperlipemia, hyperbilirubinemia, hemolysis, severe hyperglycemia, azotemia, hypernatremia, and hyperchloremia. In spectrophotometric methods, hyperbilirubinemia also falsely increases total protein.

Drug Therapy That May Alter Protein Values •

Table 12–3 CAUSES OF HYPOALBUMINEMIA IN DOGS AND CATS

Decreased production
  Chronic hepatic insufficiency*
  Inadequate intake
  Maldigestion
  Malabsorption

Hypergammaglobulinemia

Sequestration
  Body cavity effusion
  Vasculopathy

Increased loss
  Renal: glomerular*
  Gastrointestinal: protein-losing enteropathy*
  Cutaneous
  Whole blood loss

Dilution

*Most common and important causes of serum albumin ≤2.0 g/dl. The other causes rarely if ever cause serum albumin ≤2.0 g/dl.

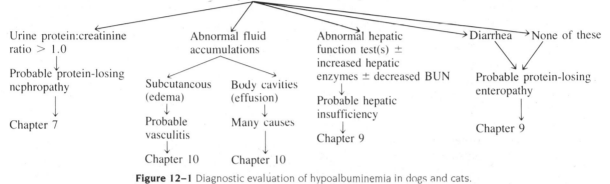

Physical examination
↓
If severely exudative lesion is found,
this may be the cause; however, proceed
with next tests in case additional disease
is present
↓
CBC, chemistry profile, urinalysis,
urine protein:creatinine ratio (Chapter 7),
and hepatic function tests (Chapter 9)

Urine protein:creatinine ratio > 1.0
↓
Probable protein-losing nephropathy
↓
Chapter 7

Abnormal fluid accumulations

Subcutaneous (edema)
↓
Probable vasculitis
↓
Chapter 10

Body cavities (effusion)
↓
Many causes
↓
Chapter 10

Abnormal hepatic function test(s) ± increased hepatic enzymes ± decreased BUN
↓
Probable hepatic insufficiency
↓
Chapter 9

Diarrhea

None of these
↓
Probable protein-losing enteropathy
↓
Chapter 9

Figure 12–1 Diagnostic evaluation of hypoalbuminemia in dogs and cats.

and dilution are the major considerations (see Table 12–3). Dilution usually causes mild decreases (albumin 2.0–2.4 g/dl); protein-losing enteropathy can cause a moderate (1.5–1.9 g/dl) to severe (< 1.5 g/dl) decrease. Although both serum albumin and globulin are usually decreased in protein-losing enteropathy, the globulin concentration may be normal to increased in some cases (e.g., lymphocytic plasmacytic enteritis in basenjis or other breeds; causes of protein-losing enteropathy in animals with chronic diseases associated with hyperglobulinemia as listed in Table 12–2).

Hypoalbuminemia plus normal to increased globulins suggests decreased albumin production, increased loss, or sequestration (see Tables 12–2 and 12–3). Decreased production is due to chronic hepatic insufficiency or hyperglobulinemia. The latter usually causes mild hypoalbuminemia, whereas chronic hepatic insufficiency can cause moderate to severe decreases. Inadequate protein intake (including poorly digestible protein), maldigestion, and malabsorption are rare causes of mildly decreased albumin production by themselves but are occasionally accompanied by conditions causing hepatic insufficiency or increased protein loss. Therefore, significant decreases in albumin should not be attributed solely to causes of deprived nutritional states without looking for additional contributing factors such as hepatic insufficiency or protein-losing disorders. In hyperglobulinemia, albumin synthesis may be decreased (i.e.,

"down regulation") irrespective of the cause of hyperglobulinemia.

Increased loss of albumin from the body occurs in glomerular disease (may be severe; see Chapter 7). Albuminuria due to glomerulopathy is occasionally associated with significant globulin loss. Sequestration may occur in pleural or peritoneal cavities or subcutaneous tissues as a consequence of hypoalbuminemia and loss of oncotic pressure. Alternatively, sequestration can be secondary to increased hydrostatic pressure, as noted in portal hypertension or in right-sided cardiac failure. Immune-mediated or infectious vasculopathies (e.g., endotoxemia/bacteremia, ehrlichiosis, or Rocky Mountain spotted fever) also allow loss from the vascular compartment. Hypoalbuminemia due to sequestration or vasculopathy is usually mild.

A diagnostic approach to hypoalbuminemic patients is outlined (Fig. 12–1). A urinalysis (preferably including urine protein:creatinine ratio, see Chapter 7) and measurement of postprandial serum bile acids (Chapter 9) are indicated. Severe cutaneous exudative lesions may be diagnosed by physical examination, but renal, hepatic, and alimentary disease should still be ruled out. Ascites and pleural effusion are indications for fluid analysis (see Chapter 10), with the expected result being a transudate. Significant proteinuria indicates a diagnostic workup for protein-losing nephropathy (see Chapter 7, Fig. 7–3). Hypoalbuminemia associated with hepatomegaly, microhepatica, neurologic signs, icterus, decreased blood urea nitrogen (BUN), increased alanine aminotransferase (ALT) or serum alkaline phosphatase (SAP), or abnormal hepatic function test results requires a diagnostic workup for hepatic insufficiency (see Chapter 9, Figs. 9–7 to 9–11). Note that ALT and SAP values are not always increased in patients with hepatic disease, even when it is severe. In younger animals, a portosystemic shunt is probable; acquired hepatic disease is more likely in adults and is an indication for hepatic biopsy. Hypoalbuminemia with or without diarrhea, normal liver function test results, and absence of proteinuria indicates diagnostic tests for protein-losing enteropathy (see Chapter 9). Intestinal biopsy may provide confirmation and an etiopathologic diagnosis. Endoscopic biopsies are safer for patients, but specimens may be obtained by exploratory laparotomy. When laparotomy is performed, hepatic biopsy should be done simultaneously. It is important to obtain biopsy specimens at several sites along the small intestine, even when there are no apparent gross lesions, because significant microscopic pathology may be localized or exist without visible evidence of a localizing lesion for biopsy.

Edematous subcutaneous fluid accumulations associated with hypoalbuminemia are usually transudates: Protein-losing nephropathy or enteropathy, chronic hepatic insufficiency, and immune-mediated or infectious vasculitis may be responsible. Refer to the later section in this chapter on immunofluorescent testing, Chapter 15 for evaluation of infectious disorders (especially rickettsial disorders), and Chapter 10 for edema.

Causes of Altered Globulins • See Protein Electrophoresis, next.

PROTEIN ELECTROPHORESIS

Occasional Indications • Protein electrophoresis should be done when hyperglobulinemia is not due to blood volume depletion, and when humoral immunodeficiencies are suspected. Although a specific diagnosis is seldom obtained from electrophoresis, patterns in the electrophoretic fractions can be valuable when interpreted with clinical signs and other laboratory tests. Electrophoresis is quantitative, whereas immunoelectrophoresis is qualitative, identifying specific proteins including immunoglobulins but not detecting slight increases or decreases. Immunoelectrophoresis is the method

of choice to detect urinary and serum Bence Jones protein, a monoclonal protein equivalent to immunoglobulin light chains that occasionally occurs in multiple myeloma and macroglobulinemia. Another indication for protein electrophoresis is the finding of a pale blue background on stained blood or bone marrow smears. This can represent the presence of increased plasma protein. Advantage: a useful screening test. Disadvantage: Specific diagnosis is seldom obtained.

Analysis • Measured in 0.5 ml of serum, which may be refrigerated or frozen.

Electrophoresis

The cellulose acetate technique is the method of choice. Interpretation of electrophoretograms is based on densitometric measurements of the intensity of staining of protein bands on the cellulose acetate strips. The serum separates into four fractions: albumin, alpha (α) globulins, beta (β) globulins, and gamma (γ) globulins. Canine and feline alpha and beta globulins are usually divided into two subfractions each: alpha-1, alpha-2, beta-1, and beta-2 (Table 12–4). Normal electrophoretograms from dogs and cats are illustrated in Figures 12–2 and 12–3.

A depression on an electrophoretogram at the spot of sample application should *not* be mistaken for a separation point between two subfractions of gamma globulin. The concentration of albumin is usually underestimated by electrophoresis in comparison with a chemical determination. Therefore, the A:G ratio is usually higher by chemical determination than by electrophoretic determination.

Immunoelectrophoresis

After electrophoresis in agar gel, polyclonal antiserum to specific proteins, including immunoglobulins, is added to a trough parallel with the separated serum proteins. The reagents are allowed to diffuse. To obtain quantitation of the individual immunoglobulins, radial immunodiffusion (RID), electroimmunodiffusion (rocket electrophoresis), or laser nephelometry is performed. These procedures, when available, can also be used to quantitate immunoglobulin subclasses.

Normal Values • Values vary among laboratories and the different techniques for quantitating

Table 12–4 NORMAL VALUES (MEAN ± 1 SD) FOR SERUM PROTEIN ELECTROPHORESIS IN DOGS AND CATS

Dogs	Mean	Limits	Mean	Limits	
	Breitschwerdt et al., 1987		Kaneko, 1980*		Rice, 1968
Total protein (g/dl)	6.84 ± 0.66	(6.0–7.6)	6.10 ± 0.52	(5.4–7.1)	6.71
Albumin†	3.20 ± 0.34	(2.72–3.67)	2.91 ± 0.11	(2.6–3.3)	3.43
α_1 globulin	0.33 ± 0.11	(0.25–0.60)	0.30 ± 0.03	(0.2–0.5)	α globulin 0.76
α_2 globulin	1.13 ± 0.25	(0.72–1.40)	0.62 ± 0.21	(0.3–1.1)	
β_1 globulin	0.74 ± 0.10	(0.63–0.89)	0.82 ± 0.23	(0.7–1.3)	β globulin 1.19
β_2 globulin	0.79 ± 0.14	(0.59–0.96)	0.89 ± 0.33	(0.6–1.4)	
γ globulin	0.64 ± 0.15	(0.49–0.83)			γ globulin 1.33
γ_1 globulin			0.80 ± 0.25	(0.5–1.3)	
γ_2 globulin			0.70 ± 0.14	(0.4–0.9)	
A:G ratio	0.89 ± 0.10	(0.79–1.02)	0.83 ± 0.16	(0.59–1.11)	1.04

Cats	Mean	Limits	Mean	Limits	
	Turnwald, Barta, 1989		Kaneko, 1980*		Rice, 1968
Total protein (g/dl)	7.66 ± 0.10	(7.3–7.8)	6.60 ± 0.70	(5.4–7.8)	6.79
Albumin†	3.41 ± 0.18	(2.82–4.18)	2.70 ± 0.17	(2.1–3.9)	3.33
α_1 globulin	0.47 ± 0.03	(0.30–0.64)	0.70 ± 0.02	(0.2–1.1)	α globulin 1.68
α_2 globulin	0.55 ± 0.04	(0.41–0.68)	0.70 ± 0.02	(0.4–0.9)	
β_1 globulin	0.91 ± 0.06	(0.77–1.25)	0.70 ± 0.03	(0.3–0.9)	β globulin 0.60
β_2 globulin	0.40 ± 0.02	(0.35–0.47)	0.70 ± 0.02	(0.6–1.0)	
γ globulin	1.92 ± 0.12	(1.39–2.22)			γ globulin 1.18
γ_1 globulin			1.60 ± 0.77	(0.30–2.50)	
γ_2 globulin			1.70 ± 0.36	(1.40–1.90)	
A:G ratio	0.80 ± 0.11	(0.63–1.15)	0.71 ± 0.20	(0.45–1.19)	0.96

*Note: The numbers do not add up to the total protein values and A:G ratios as given in the table.
†The concentration of albumin is usually underestimated by electrophoresis in comparison with a chemical determination. Therefore, the A:G ratio is usually higher by chemical determination than by electrophoretic determination.

individual immunoglobulins. Immunoglobulins migrate in the beta-2 and gamma regions of electrophoresis. Average concentrations of immunoglobulin classes in dogs and cats are listed in Table 12–5. Note that normal values for puppies differ substantially from those for adult dogs.

Artifacts • Electrophoretic bands with high-intensity staining (e.g., albumin) are underestimated, and bands of low-intensity staining are overestimated; consequently, the albumin to globulin (A:G) ratio determined by spectrophotometric methods is usually higher than that determined by electrophoresis.

Immunoglobulin G (IgG) migrates in the beta and gamma globulin regions; therefore, IgG concentrations determined by RID are usually higher than the gamma globulin fraction determined by electrophoresis. This discrepancy increases when IgG hyperproduction occurs (e.g., myelomas, canine ehrlichiosis, feline infectious peritonitis [FIP], and other chronic infections).

Causes of Altered Electrophoretic Patterns • Increases and decreases in protein fractions and associated disease conditions are summarized in

Table 12–6. Diagnostic evaluation of patients with abnormal electrophoretograms is discussed under Causes of Hyperglobulinemia, next.

Causes of Hyperglobulinemia • Polyclonal hyperglobulinemias, also referred to as *gammopathies*, have a broad-based peak in the beta and gamma regions and suggest chronic inflammatory disease (e.g., chronic bacterial, viral, fungal, or rickettsial disorders), parasitism (e.g., cutaneous parasites or dirofilariasis), neoplasia, or immune-mediated disease (see Table 12–2). In dogs, the most common causes are cutaneous parasitism, pyoderma, dirofilariasis, and ehrlichiosis, depending on geographic location (see Fig. 12–2 and Table 12–2). The increases are commonly in the beta and gamma regions. In cats, the most common cause of polyclonal gammopathy is FIP (see Fig. 12–3). The increases in globulins in cats are commonly in the gamma region. A concurrent decrease in albumin synthesis may occur in patients with hyperglobulinemia, perhaps to maintain oncotic pressure (Thomas and Brown, 1992) or viscosity; in hypoalbuminemic states, globulin may increase secondarily.

Monoclonal hyperglobulinemias have a narrow-based electrophoretic peak (''spike'') in the

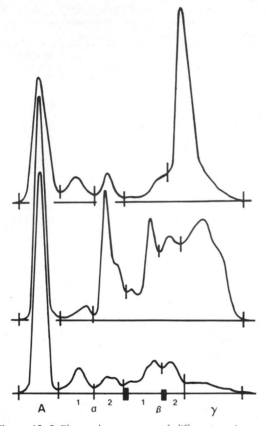

Figure 12-2 Electrophoretograms of different canine sera. **Top**: Monoclonal gammopathy (ehrlichiosis). **Middle**: Polyclonal gammopathy (blastomycosis, ehrlichiosis, and dirofilariasis). **Bottom**: Normal.

may involve only a physical examination to identify fleas and ticks or skin scrapings to detect mites. *Demodex canis* mites are usually detected easily, whereas *Sarcoptes scabiei* mites are often difficult to find. For canine heartworm disease, an enzyme-linked immunosorbent assay (ELISA) antigen test, Knott's test, and Difil test are appropriate screening procedures. Amicrofilaremic patients that show hyperglobulinemia with or without clinical signs of heartworm infection or other disease should have thoracic radiographs and serologic (ELISA) testing for *Dirofilaria immitis* antigen (see Chapter 15). In areas endemic for ehrlichiosis or Rocky Mountain spotted fever, titers are indicated (see Chapter 15), particularly if anemia, thrombocytopenia, and leukopenia are found. Testing for other infectious disorders (e.g., canine brucellosis, blastomycosis, histoplasmosis, coccidioidomycosis, or feline cryptococcosis) is dictated by the geographic location and other physical or radiographic abnormalities. The possibility of more than a single cause of hyperglobulinemia should always be taken into consideration. Gammopathies associated with immune-mediated disease and nonlymphocytic/plasmacytic neo-

beta or gamma region that is normally no wider than the albumin peak. Monoclonal immunoglobulin elevations are also called *paraproteins* or M proteins and are usually due to lymphocyte/plasma cell disorders such as multiple myeloma, macroglobulinemia, and lymphosarcoma (see Tables 12–2 and 12–6). Monoclonal or oligoclonal spikes can occasionally be due to infectious (e.g., ehrlichiosis, see Fig. 12–2) or idiopathic disorders. It is important to realize that both multiple myeloma and ehrlichiosis can have monoclonal electrophoretic patterns and bone marrow plasmacytosis. In ehrlichiosis, however, the typical electrophoretic pattern is often a monoclonal or oligoclonal pattern superimposed on or arising within a broader-based globulin peak. In contrast, monoclonal spikes associated with neoplastic disorders are most often accompanied by normal to decreased nonparaprotein globulin fractions.

A suggested diagnostic approach to patients with hyperglobulinemia is outlined in Figure 12–4. In dogs with hyperglobulinemia and severe pruritic dermatitis, diagnostic evaluation

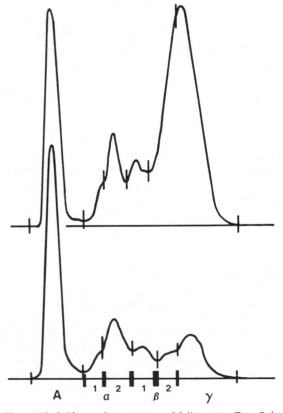

Figure 12-3 Electrophoretograms of feline sera. **Top**: Polyclonal gammopathy (feline infectious peritonitis). **Bottom**: Normal.

Table 12–5 SERUM IMMUNOGLOBULIN CONCENTRATIONS IN DOGS AND CATS

		Mean Concentration (mg/dl)			
		Puppy (2 weeks)	Puppy (2 months)	Adult Mongrel Dog	Adult Purebreed Dog	Adult Cat
IgA	Undetected	30	79	83	ND
IgG	56	143	1445	925	2400
IgM	73	118	45	156	ND

ND, not done.
(Data from Reynolds and Johnson, 1970; Reynolds et al., 1971; Heddle and Rowley, 1975; Schultz and Adams, 1978; Reimann et al., 1986.)

Table 12–6 INTERPRETATION OF ALTERED ELECTROPHORETIC FRACTIONS

Fraction Affected	Changes in Fraction	Associated Disease Condition
Albumin	Decrease	Cirrhosis, protein-losing enteropathy, severe starvation, neoplasia, renal (glomerular) loss
Alpha₁ (α₁)	Increase	
	Antitrypsin	Inflammation
	Glycoprotein	Chronic inflammation, malignancy, rheumatoid arthritis
	Fetoprotein	Hepatoma, naturally in newborns
	Decrease	
	LP-A	Hepatic syndrome*
	Gc globulin	Hepatic syndrome*
Alpha₂ (α₂)	Increase	
	Haptoglobin	Inflammation, chronic inflammation
	AP glycoprotein	Inflammation
	Acidic ceruloplasmin	Malignancy
	Macroglobulin	Hepatic syndrome,* nephrotic syndrome
	Unspecified proteins	Systemic mycotic diseases
	Decrease	
	Transferrin	Inflammation, nephrotic syndrome, malignancy
	HS glycoprotein	Carcinoma
	Gc globulin	Hepatic syndrome*
	Haptoglobin	Hepatic syndrome,* hemolytic anemia, hypohaptoglobulinemia (inherited)
Beta₁ (β₁)	Increase	
	LP-B	Nephrotic syndrome
	Decrease	
	C1r, C3, C4	Autoimmune diseases, systemic lupus erythematosus
	Hemopexin	Hemolytic anemia
	LP-B	Abetalipoproteinemia (inherited)
Beta₂ (β₂)	Increase	
	C-reactive protein	Acute inflammation
	IgM, IgA	Myeloma, hepatic syndrome*
	Unspecified	Systemic mycotic disease, protein-losing enteropathy
Gamma (γ)	Increase	
	C-reactive protein	Acute inflammation
	Immunoglobulins	Chronic or severe infection, hepatic syndrome,* myeloma
	Decrease	
	Immunoglobulins	Immunosuppression, immunodeficiency, hypogammaglobulinemia, newborn precolostral blood serum, failure of passive transfer of colostral antibodies

*Hepatic syndrome; any abnormalities of the liver that lead to decreased synthesis of some serum proteins, namely, α globulins.
LP-A, lipoprotein A (migrating in α globulin fraction); LP-B, lipoprotein B (migrating in β globulin fraction); Gc globulin, one of the α globulins that decreases with liver damage; Gc globulin migrates in the middle of α region; AP glycoprotein, one of the inflammatory α globulins; HS glycoprotein, human serum glycoprotein migrating in α region; C1r, C3, C4, components of the complement system; C-reactive protein, one of the acute phase proteins that rise first after antigenic or other inflammatory stimuli; IgM and IgA, immunoglobulins M and A.
(Data from Benjamin, 1978; Kaneko, 1980; Barta and Pourciau, 1984a.)

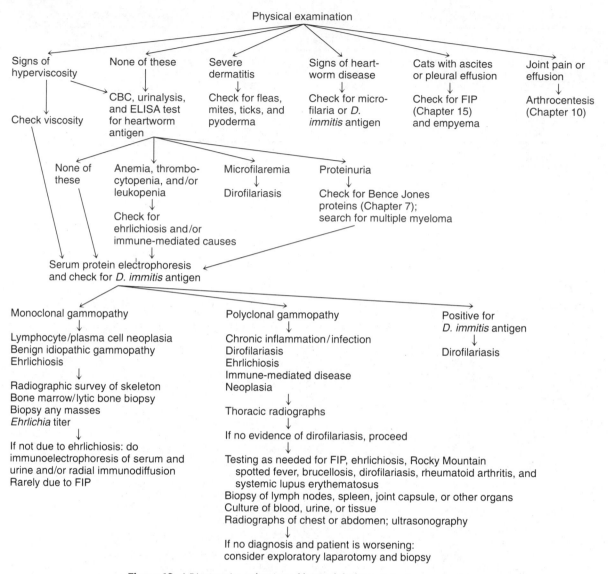

Figure 12–4 Diagnostic evaluation of hyperglobulinemia in dogs and cats.

plasia are usually mild and rarely require further evaluation of the gammopathy.

Despite the limitations of the test (see Chapter 15), an FIP titer may be considered in any cat with signs consistent with FIP. If an exudative effusion is present, fluid: serum gamma globulin ratios can be determined (see Chapter 15). Hyperglobulinemia can be due to dirofilariasis in cats, but the disease is much less common than in dogs. Hyperglobulinemia can also be present in chronic feline leukemia virus infections.

The concurrence of hyperglobulinemia with hemolytic anemia is an indication for performing a Coombs' test and antinuclear antibody (ANA). If joint pain, stiff gait, or increased joint fluid volume accompanies hyperglobulinemia, radiographs and joint fluid analysis (see Chapter 10) are indicated. Rheumatoid factor (RF), ANA, and rickettsial titers are indicated if the joint fluid is a nonseptic exudate.

If a diagnosis is not obtained at this stage, if a patient appears inappropriately ill, if the magnitude of the hyperglobulinemia seems excessive, or if any signs consistent with hyperviscosity are present (see Serum Viscosity), it is necessary to differentiate monoclonal from polyclonal gammopathies by serum protein electrophoresis. If a monoclonal gammopathy is detected in a patient with myeloma or lymphoma, immunoelectrophoresis or quantitation of immunoglobulins by RID identifies the class of immunoglobulin composing the paraprotein. These tests also detect nonparaprotein immunoglobulin deficiencies, which are common in patients with lymphocytic or plasmacytic neoplasias (see Causes of Hypoglobulinemia, next).

Polyclonal gammopathies may be caused by infectious, immune-mediated, or neoplastic disorders. If the cause of a polyclonal gammopathy cannot be established, thoracic and abdominal radiographs and ultrasonography are indicated to screen for occult neoplasia. Finally, exploratory laparotomy and biopsy may be indicated.

Monoclonal gammopathies are usually caused by lymphoproliferative (including plasma cell) neoplasia. The diagnostic evaluation of a monoclonal gammopathy should include skeletal radiographs, serum and urine immunoelectrophoresis, and bone marrow biopsy with cytologic and histologic evaluation. Diagnosis of multiple myeloma in dogs requires finding at least two of the following: lytic skeletal lesions, bone marrow plasmacytosis, Bence Jones proteinuria, or a monoclonal spike on serum protein electrophoresis. Skeletal lesions are uncommon in feline multiple myeloma. In areas endemic for ehrlichiosis, dogs with a monoclonal gammopathy should have an *Ehrlichia canis* titer performed. Ehrlichiosis commonly causes proteinuria and bone marrow plasmacytosis, closely resembling multiple myeloma. FIP rarely causes monoclonal spikes. Serum viscosity and the presence of cryoglobulins can be checked if indicated by clinical and laboratory abnormalities (see next sections).

Causes of Hypoglobulinemia ● Newborn animals are physiologically hypogammaglobulinemic and have serum total protein concentrations 60% to 80% of adult values. Congenital combined or selective immunodeficiencies occur but are rarely diagnosed, probably because immunodeficient puppies or kittens rapidly succumb to infections. In dogs, these infections are usually distemper or parvovirus, and they occur in the postnatal period after maternal immunity wanes. Immunodeficiency should be suspected when more than one pup in a properly cared-for litter dies of infection in the first 2 to 6 months of life. Minimal evaluation of these patients consists of a complete blood count (CBC), serum chemistry profile, serum protein electrophoresis, and immunoelectrophoresis. Immunoglobulin quantitation by RID is recommended for confirmation and characterization of the type of immunoglobulin deficiency present. Immunoglobulin quantitation techniques have the advantage of being more precise than the more qualitative methods (immunoelectrophoresis). More important, selective (single class or subclass) and partial immunoglobulin deficiencies may not be readily detectable using serum electrophoresis and immunoelectrophoresis alone. When a humoral immunodeficiency of any type is suspected, all the immunoglobulin classes (and IgG subclasses when available) should be quantitated. Humoral immunodeficiency is usually detected by finding decreased IgG and IgA and normal to decreased IgM concentrations. Selective IgA deficiency and transient hypogammaglobulinemia also occur in dogs. Dogs with selective IgA deficiency show chronic problems involving mucosal barrier immunity, especially small intestinal bacterial overgrowth. Serum electrophoresis in cases of selective or partial immunoglobulin deficiency may have normal results or even show polyclonal elevations in globulins as a whole. Immunoelectrophoresis of normal canine serum may show a low or absent stainable IgA precipitation band that can be due to IgA's relatively low concentration in serum normally or due to quality assurance problems involving antisera or technique. When selective IgA deficiency is suspected based on clinical signs, the best method for diagnosis is quantitative RID or rocket electrophoresis. IgA deficiency is sometimes accompanied by elevated levels of IgM. It is important to remember that the relationship between certain types of chronic inflammatory enteropathy, such as lymphocytic plasmacytic enteritis, and serum IgA deficiency is unclear at this time because both normal and abnormal values have been found (Williams, 1991). It is also likely that deficiency of local secretory IgA may not always be reflected by serum IgA levels. Finally, breed-specific normal ranges for immunoglobulin levels may provide a clearer picture of the role of selective IgA deficiency in chronic enteropathies.

The most common causes of hypoglobulinemia are acquired conditions including external blood loss and protein-losing enteropathy. Less common causes are protein-losing nephropathy and hepatic insufficiency (see Chapters 7 and 9). In patients with paraproteinemias (e.g., multiple myeloma, macroglobulinemia, or lymphosarcoma), the remainder of the immunoglobulins are usually depressed. A complement measurement and evaluations of lymphocyte and phagocyte functions may also be indicated for patients with suspected congenital immunodeficiency (see Testing for Cellular Functions in Immunity, later).

SERUM VISCOSITY

Rare Indications • Monoclonal gammopathy, hyperglobulinemic patients with signs of hyperviscosity (i.e., poor tissue perfusion, dilated retinal vessels, retinal hemorrhage or retinal detachment, renal disease, central nervous system dysfunction, and bleeding problems), or to monitor treatment of diseases causing hyperviscosity. Hyperviscosity may also be suspected on the basis of a high serum protein value (usually > 10 g/dl) or on the physical characteristics of the serum (i.e., viscous). Polycythemia should also be included as a cause of increased blood viscosity to be ruled out in patients showing clinical signs of hyperviscosity. Advantages: simple and diagnostically significant.

Analysis • Measured in 0.5 to 1.0 ml of serum with an Ostwald's viscosimeter or a 0.1-ml capillary pipette. The time for a given volume of serum to flow from the pipette is compared with that for the same volume of water.

Normal Values • Relative viscosity, 1.4 to 1.8. (Relative viscosity = flow time of serum [seconds] divided by flow time of water [seconds].)

Artifacts • Volume depletion causing increased serum protein concentration may increase serum viscosity, but it is unlikely to be of clinical significance. Markedly increased blood viscosity can be of laboratory importance because increased viscosity may interfere with tests that use flow-through devices (e.g., Coulter counters).

Drug Therapy That May Alter Serum Viscosity • Any drug that causes volume depletion can increase serum viscosity.

Causes of Serum Hyperviscosity • Because of the relatively large size of IgM, it has the greatest potential to cause hyperviscosity. IgA (which can exist as a polymer or dimer) and very high concentrations of IgG can also cause hyperviscosity. Clinically significant serum hyperviscosity is almost invariably caused by lymphocyte/plasma cell neoplastic disorders (e.g., multiple myeloma, macroglobulinemia, and lymphosarcoma; see Table 12–2). Hyperviscosity syndrome rarely occurs in monoclonal gammopathy caused by ehrlichiosis. A relative viscosity of four or greater is abnormal in humans and is probably abnormal for dogs.

The diagnostic approach is described in Figure 12–4 under "monoclonal gammopathy."

Because lymphosarcoma and plasma cell myeloma are the major causes of serum hyperviscosity, aspiration of bone marrow and lymph nodes is indicated. If results are equivocal, a core biopsy and histopathologic evaluation of bone marrow or lymph node are indicated. Cytologic or histologic evaluation of the spleen and liver can occasionally help to establish a diagnosis of lymphocytic or plasmacytic neoplasia when samples from lymph nodes, bone marrow, or solid masses are not diagnostic.

CRYOPRECIPITATION

Cryoglobulins are usually monoclonal or complexed immunoglobulins that reversibly precipitate or gel at low temperatures but dissolve when heated. Cryoglobulins are rarely found in multiple myeloma and macroglobulinemia in dogs.

Rare Indications • Paraproteins that precipitate or gel when blood or serum is refrigerated at 4° C. Such samples, though rare, can come to attention as a result of difficulty in obtaining accurate readings on flow-through autoanalyzers. Note: Cryoglobulins are not cold agglutinins (i.e., antibodies that bind antigen reversibly at temperatures < 37° C). Advantage: Detection of the presence of cryoglobulins is important because failure to detect them is a cause of false-negative test results for hyperglobulinemia or monoclonal paraproteinemia in patients who show clinical or laboratory evidence of hyperviscosity (see Indications for Serum Protein Electrophoresis and for Serum Viscosity).

Analysis • Measured in 1.0 ml of serum harvested from blood collected and maintained at 37° C through initial centrifugation for separation from clot and cells. Significant refrigeration-induced precipitation or gel formation followed by dissolution on rewarming is diagnostic of the presence of a cryoglobulin. Further characterization can be achieved by serum electrophoresis, immunoelectrophoresis, or immunoglobulin quantitation procedures performed under temperature-controlled conditions. Ideally, electrophoresis should be performed on serum samples both before and after cryoprecipitation, as well as on the redissolved cryoprecipitate.

Artifacts • Cryoglobulins are often discarded with the clotted cell fraction under routine processing conditions at room temperature or less (refrigerated samples). This can lead to spuriously lower values than the actual globulin content measured or failure to detect the presence of a gammopathy on electrophoresis. Cryoprecipitation can also cause erroneous CBC results in automated cell counters.

Causes of Cryoglobulinemia • Macroglobulinemia or multiple myeloma of the IgM and IgA classes may cause cryoglobulinemia in dogs. Finding cryoglobulinemia indicates diagnostic evaluation for lymphocyte/plasma cell neoplasia as described for monoclonal gammopathies. Nonimmunoglobulin cryoprecipitation (e.g., cryofibrinogenemia) has not been described in animals.

ANTINUCLEAR ANTIBODY

Occasional Indications • Multiple abnormalities suggestive of systemic lupus erythematosus (SLE). These commonly include symmetric dermatitis principally distributed on the head and mucous membranes, hemolytic anemia, thrombocytopenia, nonseptic polyarthritis, myositis, proteinuria, or fever of unknown origin. Less common signs are neurologic, cardiac, or pulmonary abnormalities. The test is also used to monitor patients being treated for SLE. Advantages: simple and indicative of immune-mediated disease when positive with a relatively high titer in conjunction with compatible clinical abnormalities. Disadvantage: not a disease-specific test (i.e., many diseases besides SLE may have a positive titer; Table 12–7).

Analysis • Measured in 0.5 ml of serum by indirect immunofluorescence testing (IIT). Dilutions of the patient's serum are incubated with specific tissue on a microscope slide. If present, ANAs bind to the nuclear substrates and are revealed by the fluorescein-labeled antiglobulin. The result should be reported as the highest dilution of a patient's serum that causes definite staining of nuclei. Several patterns of nuclear fluorescence are recognized: homogeneous (diffuse), rim (peripheral), speckled (fine or large speckles), and nucleolar.

Normal Values • Values vary among laboratories owing to different substrates, controls, and procedures used. Accuracy of the results requires procedural consistency and experience. Fetal and newborn sera give no staining of the nuclei. Titers of 1:5 to 1:10 are common in serum from nondiseased, mature animals tested using

Table 12–7 CAUSES OF INCREASED ANA TITER IN DOGS AND CATS

*Systemic lupus erythematosus (titer most consistently elevated in this disease)**
Skin disorders
  Pemphigus erythematosus, seldom pemphigus vulgaris†
  Discoid lupus
  Generalized demodicosis
  Fleabite hypersensitivity
  Plasma cell pododermatitis
Hematologic disorders
  Immune-mediated hemolytic anemia
  Immune-mediated thrombocytopenia
Cardiopulmonary disorders
  Bacterial endocarditis
  Dirofilariasis
Other disorders
  Cholangiohepatitis
  Feline leukemia virus infection
  Feline infectious peritonitis
  Rheumatoid arthritis
  Lymphocytic thyroiditis
  Various neoplasms
  Ulcerative autoimmune stomatitis†

*Moderate to high titers (80 to >160).
†Moderate titers (80 to 160).
ANA titer, if positive, in disorders without * or † is likely to be ≤40.
(Data from Muller et al., 1983; Scott et al., 1987a.)

monolayer cell cultures (Barta and Pourciau, 1984b) or mouse liver sections (Werner and Gorman, 1984). Definite staining of nuclei at 1:40 or greater (depending on the laboratory) is generally considered a significant positive titer for both of these substrates.

Drug Therapy That May Alter ANA Titer • Anything decreasing antibody synthesis (e.g., cytotoxic drugs or chronic or high-dose corticosteroid therapy) can decrease the titer. Positive ANA titers have been attributed to treatment with griseofulvin, hydralazine, procainamide, sulfonamides, and tetracyclines. Positive ANA titers can occur in cats treated with propylthiouracil or methimazole (Peterson et al., 1984, 1988). A proportion of these cats develop drug-induced immune-mediated hemolytic anemia and thrombocytopenia.

Artifacts • Falsely negative: use of fluorescein-labeled antiglobulin that is not species specific. Falsely negative or falsely positive: improper reagent preparation, storage, or application; inadequate controls.

Causes of Increased ANA Titer • A positive titer is not specific for any one disease because it can be increased in a number of infectious, inflammatory, and neoplastic disorders. A partial list of diseases in addition to SLE in which a positive

ANA titer can be found is given in Table 12–7. Normal dogs and cats can also have detectable ANA; however, these tend to be low titers. Positive titers that are obtained in disorders other than SLE are generally not markedly elevated; therefore, it is important to consider the values established by the laboratory for low, moderate, and high titers. Equally important is consideration of other clinical and clinicopathologic changes that are consistent with a diagnosis of SLE.

The suggested criteria for diagnosis of canine and feline SLE are a positive ANA titer plus one or more of the following: skin or oral cavity lesions with histopathologic and immunofluorescent changes consistent with SLE, polyarthritis, Coombs'-positive hemolytic anemia, thrombocytopenia, protein-losing nephropathy (with immunofluorescent changes consistent with SLE), myositis, or, particularly in cats, neurologic disturbances.

A positive ANA titer is the most important criterion for the diagnosis of SLE, providing that established clinical criteria are met and that exclusionary diagnoses are not made (e.g., feline leukemia virus [FeLV] or FIP, infection, cholangiohepatitis, rickettsial or systemic parasitic diseases). There are no well-established patterns of ANA fluorescence in dogs and cats that distinguish SLE from other (non-SLE) immune-mediated diseases or other conditions associated with some incidence of positive ANA titers (see Table 12–7). Although ANA titers in SLE are frequently higher than in other disorders, there can be some overlap. The magnitude of the titer does not parallel the severity of the disease in dogs and cats. However, periodic ANA titrations may prove useful in monitoring patients' progress on an individual basis.

A positive ANA titer is an indication for performing a battery of other tests to detect evidence of SLE or non-SLE disease: Dermatitis favoring the mucocutaneous junctions is an indication for biopsy, histopathologic examination, and direct immunofluorescent testing (DIT) (see Direct Immunofluorescent Testing); hemolytic anemia is an indication for an antiglobulin (Coombs') test (see Chapter 3) and tests for hemoparasites; swollen, painful joints are an indication for arthrocentesis and fluid analysis (see Chapter 10) as well as RF test; tests for antiplatelet or antimegakaryocyte antibody are indicated when thrombocytopenia exists without obvious cause (see Tests for Immune-Mediated Thrombocytopenia, later). A kidney biopsy may be useful if proteinuria is present.

LUPUS ERYTHEMATOSUS TEST (LE CELL TEST)

Occasional Indications • Suspected SLE (see Antinuclear Antibody, earlier). Advantages: highly specific; does not require species-specific reagents, therefore more widely available. Disadvantages: time-consuming and much less sensitive than the ANA test; requires very fresh blood sample.

Analysis • Depending on the laboratory, 3 ml of heparinized or clotted blood is used. Mechanical disruption followed by incubation of fresh blood from a patient with SLE leads to the formation of LE cells by opsonization of exposed dead cell nuclear material by ANA (LE cell factor) and uptake of this material into surviving phagocytic cells. These cells are found on cytologic examination of specially prepared smears. The formation of LE cells *in vivo* is rarely demonstrated in routinely stained bone marrow smears or in joint fluid from patients with polyarthritis (Color Plate 4A) but this finding is highly suggestive of SLE when present.

Artifacts • LE cells must be differentiated from "tart" cells, which are neutrophils that have phagocytosed intact nuclei. The LE cell test is complement dependent, and low concentrations of complement, excessive heparin, or failure to use freshly drawn blood may cause false-negative results.

Drug Therapy Causing False-Negative Results • Steroid therapy alters test results. The LE cell test is more sensitive to the effects of steroids than are ANA titers.

Causes of Positive LE Cell Preparations • A minimum of three to four LE cells on a slide is necessary for a diagnosis of SLE. The test should be performed at least three times before results are considered negative. As discussed, the test is relatively specific for SLE but is insensitive. Negative results are common in SLE patients positive for ANA by immunofluorescence. Such patients may lack the particular autoantibodies to histone-DNA involved in LE cell formation yet have other types of ANA detectable by immunofluorescence. Positive test results may rarely be obtained in other diseases (e.g., osteochondritis dissecans, nonimmunologic joint disease, neoplasia, and disseminated intravascular coagulation). If a positive LE cell preparation is obtained, an ANA titer and tests to obtain other evidence of SLE are indicated, as described earlier under Antinuclear Antibody. Currently, an ANA titer is the preferred screening test for SLE.

ANTIGLOBULIN (COOMBS') TEST
(see Chapter 3, Erythrocyte Disorders)

TESTS FOR IMMUNE-MEDIATED THROMBOCYTOPENIA (IMT)

Occasional Indications • Dogs and cats showing marked thrombocytopenia ($< 50,000/\mu l$), especially when associated with abnormal bleeding attributable to simple thrombocytopenia with or without qualitative platelet dysfunction. Typical hemorrhagic signs associated with deficient platelets are mucosal bleeding (epistaxis, hematuria, melena, and so on) and petechial, purpuric, or ecchymotic hemorrhages. Patients who manifest thrombocytopenia as a result of immunologic mechanisms can have autoantibodies (or cross-reactive antibodies) to platelets, high levels of platelet-associated antibodies (to drugs or other foreign antigens) or immune complexes, or infectious diseases involving organisms or parasites that directly infect platelets or megakaryocytes (e.g., *E. canis* or *Ehrlichia platys*, FeLV infection). At the present time there is no widely available test for making a diagnosis of IMT. The platelet factor 3 (PF-3) test, based on immunoinjury of donor platelets by a patient's test plasma, is no longer recommended to veterinarians because it is lacking in sensitivity, specificity, and reproducibility. Alternative tests involving various immunoassay techniques for measuring platelet-associated antibody or circulating antiplatelet antibody show promise but have yet to be sufficiently validated or widely offered for routine use. Currently, the most available test, called the *antimegakaryocyte antibody test*, is a direct immunofluorescence procedure (see Direct Immunofluorescent Testing, later) for detecting megakaryocyte-associated antibody. Megakaryocytes are the precursor hematopoietic cells that produce platelets in mammalian bone marrow.

Analysis • Air-dried, unfixed bone marrow smears or imprints are submitted. The laboratory procedure followed for antimegakarocyte antibody testing is essentially the same as that described in the later section on DIT. Advantage: A positive test result helps support a clini-

cal diagnosis of IMT. Disadvantages: The test is not specific for autoantibodies to megakaryocyte/platelet antigens and may therefore be positive in infectious causes of thrombocytopenia (some of which may have a significant immunoinjury component contributing to the thrombocytopenia). Data on sensitivity and specificity for this test are lacking. Some patients may lack megakaryocytes in the bone marrow, whereas blood-diluted marrow samples may fail to reveal megakaryocytes that are present.

Results • A positive antimegakaryocyte antibody test is highly supportive of a diagnosis of primary or secondary IMT and indicates that every effort should be made to rule out drug-induced or infectious processes commonly associated with thrombocytopenia (see Chapter 5). A negative antimegakaryocyte antibody test result does not rule out a diagnosis of IMT. Like the tests for ANA and RF, any test for platelet or megakaryocyte-associated antibodies must be interpreted in the context of other supportive clinical and laboratory findings including the elimination of other causes of thrombocytopenia, evidence of concomitant immune-medicated or autoimmune phenomena occurring in a thrombocytopenic patient, and, where appropriate, response to corticosteroid or combination immunosuppressant therapy.

RHEUMATOID FACTOR TEST

Occasional Indications • Dogs, particularly small breeds, suspected of having rheumatoid arthritis (RA), because of lameness, heat, swelling, or pain of multiple joints, particularly peripheral joints. Crepitation and joint laxity may be detected in chronic cases. Nonspecific signs include anorexia, fever, depression, and reluctance to move and may precede clinically or radiographically detectable evidence of joint disease. Disadvantage: insensitive (i.e., many false negatives) and not highly specific for RA in dogs because of relatively low titers.

Analysis • Serum, 0.5 ml, is submitted refrigerated but unfrozen. The commonly used Rose-Waaler test detects autoantibody (i.e., RF) reacting against a patient's own IgG. Canine rheumatoid factors are predominantly IgG but may also be mixed complexes of IgG, IgA, and IgM (Halliwell et al., 1989). Factors are detected by incubating rabbit IgG-sensitized sheep red blood cells (RBCs) with serial dilutions of the patient's serum (the rabbit Rose-Waaler test). If RF is present, agglutination occurs. Because canine sera often contain naturally occurring antibodies to sheep RBCs, a control must be performed with unsensitized sheep RBCs. If agglutination to an equal or higher dilution appears in the control, the natural antibodies must be absorbed from the sera before testing for RF. Latex agglutination tests for canine RF are not recommended because results are poorly reproducible and lack specificity. Latex agglutination test titers may differ substantially from those obtained by Rose-Waaler tests (Wood et al., 1980; Halliwell et al., 1989). Both tests are available through human laboratories; however, the proper test controls must be used.

Results • For the Rose-Waaler test in normal animals, the differential titer (the difference between the titers at which agglutination of unsensitized versus sensitized sheep RBCs occurs) should be < 8 (Barta, 1993a). A titer against sensitized RBCs that is not corrected for natural antibodies to sheep RBCs by measurement of the latter cannot be extrapolated based on the assumption that normal animals have a titer of 1:2 against sheep RBCs. Some normal animals have higher titers of naturally occurring antibodies to sheep RBCs. Some laboratories perform the Rose-Waaler test by preabsorbing all test sera with sheep RBCs. In this case, a titer of < 16 is expected in normal dogs (Halliwell et al., 1989).

Artifacts • RF, especially IgM, may be sensitive to freezing. This can lead to a false-negative result. Therefore, serum submitted for RF testing should not be frozen. In addition, canine RF tends to self-associate, forming multimeric complexes that significantly lower the detectable titer. Wide, sometimes negative, fluctuations in RF titer occur over time in individual canine RA patients, and these fluctuations do not appear to correlate with the clinical severity of the disease (Halliwell et al., 1989). False-positive results may be reported when the Rose-Waaler test is used if a patient's serum has antibodies against sheep RBCs at a titer above 1:2 and appropriate controls or absorption of these antibodies is not performed.

Causes of an Increased RF Titer • Because RF is an antibody against the Fc fragment of immunoglobulin molecules that become exposed only after the antibody binds to the antigen, any disease with a chronic appearance of immune complexes can eventually induce RF formation.

In the Rose-Waaler test, a differential titer of 1:8 and greater is positive for RF (Barta, 1993a). Between 40% and 75% of dogs with RA have a positive RF test result. Hence, a negative result does not rule out the disease (Gorman and Werner, 1986). The RF test is rarely positive in normal dogs and occasionally positive in some patients with SLE because RA may be a part of the SLE complex. The incidence of RF in other types of arthropathy and systemic diseases has not been adequately studied using the Rose-Waaler method, but other methods have shown some occurrence of RF (in titers comparable with RA patients) in other types of canine arthropathy (Carter et al., 1989). Therefore, a positive RF test result should never be interpreted as the sole criterion for a diagnosis of canine RA.

RA is a progressive erosive type of immune-mediated polyarthritis that must be differentiated from other types of erosive and nonerosive joint diseases, preferably before significant radiographically apparent joint destruction occurs. Unfortunately, no test for canine RF has proved highly reliable in making this distinction. Other routine tests indicated in making the diagnosis include radiographic joint surveys and synovial fluid analysis. Cases of septic polyarthritis often show erosive lesions favoring a distribution involving larger joints more severely, as well as evidence of sepsis on routine blood and synovial fluid examinations (see Chapter 10), including culture. In contrast, RA typically shows erosive radiographic lesions favoring the smaller peripheral joints before any progression to larger joints. However, radiographic lesions may be lacking or inconclusive early in the course of RA. Furthermore, there are no distinguishing cytologic features that can reliably differentiate between RA, SLE, and other types of immune-mediated joint disease for which similar findings of a purulent or chronic active inflammation without evidence of sepsis are expected. Histopathologic examination of synovium from affected joints remains the most reliable means of confirming a diagnosis of canine RA. Histopathologic examination has particular merit for making an early diagnosis and instituting therapy in patients lacking classic radiographic changes. An ANA titer is indicated and helps distinguish SLE from RA; the titer is usually positive in SLE but is occasionally positive in RA. The finding of both types of autoantibodies may represent the rare, combined occurrence of both SLE and RA, a so-called overlap syndrome, or merely the appearance of multiple autoantibodies in a patient with RA or SLE. In either case, it is the clinical criteria for each disease that must be met to make the diagnosis.

DIRECT IMMUNOFLUORESCENT TESTING

Immunofluorescent testing of tissues uses a fluorescent dye conjugated with an antibody (FITC-reagent) that detects antigen or immunoglobulin. The testing may be direct or indirect. In the direct test, tissues are assayed for deposits of immunoglobulins and complement.

Common Indications • Suspected autoimmune skin disease or diseases of internal organs (e.g., kidney) that may have an immunologic basis. In veterinary medicine, the test is used mainly on biopsy specimens of vesicular or bullous cutaneous lesions or of the renal cortex. Advantage: A definitive diagnosis or confirmation can occasionally be made. Disadvantages: Extreme care must be taken in tissue selection and preservation; the test result is markedly influenced by corticosteroids; requires a special fixative/transport medium or fresh, snap-frozen tissue.

Sample Preparation • In cutaneous diseases, it is imperative that early primary lesions (vesicles, bullae, or pustules) as well as a margin of uninvolved skin be obtained. Multiple specimens are recommended. Obtaining primary lesions may necessitate checking a patient several times daily to identify a suitable, newly erupting lesion. Ulcerated, crusted, or scarred lesions are worthless. Ideally, biopsy specimens should not be obtained from the planum nasale or foot pads if other primary lesions are available, because immunoglobulin deposition is noted at the basement membrane of these sites in 45% and 73%, respectively, of normal dogs (Scott et al., 1987a). The specimen is transported to the laboratory in a closed container with a saline-soaked gauze sponge or filter paper within 3 to 4 hours. Specimens that cannot be transported immediately should be kept cold but not frozen. Alternatively, the biopsy specimen may be preserved in Michel's fixative. Specimens are stable in the fixative at room temperature for up to 1 year or more (Ihrke et al., 1985). Specimens can also be quick-frozen in liquid nitrogen when this is available. Thick biopsy specimens could potentially be inadequately preserved, but skin samples taken with a 6-mm biopsy punch and cut in half are suitable. Biopsy specimens for

routine histopathology should be taken from the same, or at least a similar, lesion. Ideally, larger samples can be bisected to provide comparable lesional material for both tests. The biopsy specimen should not remain attached to the wall of the container, since this may cause inadequate preservation and false-negative results. It should be noted that more laboratories are offering immunohistochemical stains based on enzyme-labeled antisera. Laboratories offering this kind of immunostaining should be consulted for sample preparation.

Analysis • Sections of frozen tissue prepared in a cryostat are incubated with fluorescein-conjugated antibodies (FITC anti-whole immunoglobulin, IgG, IgM, IgA, or C3) and examined by fluorescent microscopy.

Normal Values • Healthy epidermis has no detectable deposits of immunoglobulins in the intercellular spaces or at the basement membrane. Nonspecific fluorescence of the stratum corneum should not be mistaken for deposits of immunoglobulins.

Artifacts • Biopsy of inappropriate lesions results in false-negative results. The pH of Michel's fixative should be between 7.0 and 7.2. Fixative with pH of 6.8 or less is associated with negative DIT even if other findings support a diagnosis of autoimmune skin disease (Scott et al., 1987a). Cutaneous bacterial infections may cause immunoglobulin deposits in pustules, which should not be mistaken for deposits typical of autoimmune disease. Proper FITC-reagent quality control and reader expertise are required for discrimination between artifactual, nonspecific fluorescence and true specific fluorescence.

Drug Therapy That May Affect Results • Corticosteroids and immunosuppressive drugs (e.g., cyclophosphamide) may cause negative results. If an animal is receiving short-acting corticosteroids, the drug should be withdrawn for at least 3 weeks before biopsy. A longer period (1–2 months) may be necessary if long-acting injectable corticosteroids have been used.

Causes of Positive DIT Staining • The major skin diseases in which DIT is useful, the site of deposition of immunoglobulin/complement, and other relevant laboratory features are listed in Table 12–8. It cannot be emphasized enough that DIT results must be interpreted in light of

Table 12–8 DIAGNOSTIC CRITERIA IN AUTOIMMUNE SKIN DISEASE OF DOGS AND CATS

Disease	Histopathology	Direct Immunofluorescence	Indirect Immunofluorescence	LE Cell Test (LE), Antinuclear Antibody (ANA)	Frequency Among Autoimmune Disorders
Pemphigus vulgaris	Suprabasilar acantholysis, cleft and vesicle formation	Intercellular substance. Dogs: IgG > IgA, IgM, C. Cats: Ig > C	Usually negative	Nearly always negative	Common
Pemphigus vegetans	Epidermal hyperplasia, papillomatosis, and intraepidermal eosinophilic microabscesses with acanthocytes	Intercellular substance	Unknown	Negative	Rare in dogs; Not found in cats
Pemphigus foliaceus	Intragranular to subcorneal acantholysis, cleft and pustule formation	Intercellular substance. Dogs: IgG ≫ IgA, IgM, C. Cats: Ig	Usually negative	Dog: Occasionally positive (low ANA titer). Cat: ANA and LE negative	Common
Pemphigus erythematosus	Intragranular to subcorneal acantholysis and pustule formation	Intercellular substance; Basement membrane zone. Dogs: IgG > IgA, IgM, C. Cats: Ig, C	Negative	LE: Negative. ANA: Dog: Occasionally positive. Cat: Negative	Rare
Bullous pemphigoid	Subepidermal vacuolar alteration and vesicle	Basement membrane zone. Dogs: IgG, IgA, C > IgM	Usually negative	Negative	Not found in cats
Discoid lupus	Hydropic and lichenoid interface dermatitis	Basement membrane zone. IgG, IgM, IgA, C	Unknown	LE: Negative. ANA: Usually negative	Common in dogs; Not found in cats
Systemic lupus erythematosus	Dogs: hydropic and lichenoid interface dermatitis or stomatitis	Basement membrane zone. Dogs: C > IgM, IgA > IgC. Cats: Ig	Unknown	LE: Usually negative. ANA: Nearly always positive	Common
Vasculitis	Leukocytoclastic vasculitis	Walls of dermal blood vessels. IgG, IgM, C > IgA	Negative	Negative	Not found in cats
Vogt-Koyanagi-Harada syndrome	Lichenoid interface dermatitis	Uncommon—basement membrane zone. IgG, IgA	Unknown	LE: Negative. ANA: May be positive	Rare
Linear IgA dermatitis	Subcorneal pustular dermatitis	Basement membrane zone. IgA > C	Unknown	Unknown	Rare

(Data from Scott et al., 1987a, b.) >, more common than.

clinical and histopathologic findings. Immuno-globulin deposits can occur in other skin disorders including mycosis fungoides, pyodermas, and acariasis. In these disorders, however, the staining is usually patchy and focal and present in pustules rather than in the adjacent tissues.

In DIT of renal tissue, fluorescence is detected in the majority of dogs with immune-mediated glomerulonephritis. The immuno-globulins are deposited around the glomerular membrane, showing a granular, multifocal, or segmental pattern of immunofluorescence. Staining may also occur in the mesangium, tubules, and vasculature. The staining is due to the presence of immune complexes containing IgG, IgM, C3, and less commonly IgA. Immune complex glomerulonephritis (ICG) is the most common cause of glomerular fluorescence in dogs and cats. The immunoglobulins are on the epithelial side of the basement membrane. A partial list of diseases associated with glomerulonephritis includes chronic inflammatory skin disease, neoplasia, SLE, peritonitis, pancreatitis, dirofilariasis, congenital renal disease, gastroenteritis, hypothyroidism, diabetes mellitus, pyometra, endocarditis, and FeLV infection. Cases of canine glomerulonephropathy in which predominantly or solely IgA deposits are found are rare, but such cases may represent an immune-mediated disorder similar to IgA nephropathy in humans (Harris et al., 1993). Idiopathic glomerulonephritis caused by autoantibody to glomerular basement membrane occurs in humans and has a distinctive linear pattern of fluorescence along the basement membrane. When this type of autoimmune glomerulonephritis occurs in conjunction with similar lesions of the pulmonary alveolar membranes, Goodpasture's syndrome is diagnosed. Although linear glomerular fluorescence has been described infrequently in canine glomerulonephropathy, attempts to link this finding with an autoantibody have not been successful.

It is important to interpret renal tissue immunologic findings with other clinical and pathologic data, particularly with the urinalysis to detect proteinuria, and with histopathologic findings to determine the severity and progression of the disease. Any immunoglobulin deposit at the basement membrane, however, indicates pathologic change.

INDIRECT IMMUNOFLUORESCENT TESTING

In the indirect test, serum is assayed for circulating autoantibodies to a specific tissue component such as cutaneous basement membrane, intercellular cement substance, or renal glomerular basement membrane. The ANA test is another example of IIT discussed in a previous section.

Rare Indications • As an adjunct test for suspected cases of pemphigus, bullous pemphigoid, or immune-mediated glomerulonephritis. Advantage: noninvasive method to detect circulating autoantibodies to tissue, especially when biopsy of these organs is problematic or nondiagnostic. Disadvantage: significantly less sensitive than DIT because a relatively large amount of antibody has to be present to be detected. This test is so rarely positive in confirmed cases of canine and feline autoimmune skin disease or immune-mediated glomerulonephritis that it cannot be recommended for routine diagnostic use.

Analysis • Measured in 0.5 ml of refrigerated or frozen serum. The serum is added to species-specific tissue sections, overlaid with fluorescein-conjugated antisera, and examined by fluorescent microscopy.

Normal Values • A normal skin biopsy specimen treated with normal animal serum and fluorescein-conjugated anti-Ig or anti-C3 shows no staining of the epithelium.

Artifacts • Nonspecific background and particulate fluorescence must be differentiated from specific fluorescence by using appropriate procedures for FITC-reagent preparation and quality control as well as serum controls.

Drug Treatment That May Alter Results • See Direct Immunofluorescent Testing, earlier.

Causes of Negative Indirect Immunofluorescence • Nearly all canine and feline patients with pemphigus, pemphigoid, or glomerulonephritis have negative IIT (see Table 12–8).

Causes of Positive Indirect Immunofluorescence • Positive results are uncommonly obtained with bullous pemphigoid, pemphigus foliaceus, and pemphigus vulgaris. The staining may occasionally be positive in some nonpemphigus diseases (e.g., demodicosis).

Limited investigations of autoantibodies to internal organs are promising, but their application in veterinary medicine is limited. Sera from patients with chronic thyroiditis may have antibodies to various thyroid antigens. Antibodies to thyroglobulin and microsomal antigen are most common, whereas antibodies to the colloidal antigen and cytotoxic antibodies to the cell surface are less common. Patients with idiopathic hypoadrenocorticism may have circulating antibodies to adrenal antigens, especially the microsomes. These antibodies stain the cytoplasm of cells in the adrenal cortex. In idiopathic hypoparathyroidism, the antibodies are directed against cytoplasmic antigens of parathyroid cells. Patients with insulin-dependent diabetes mellitus may have antibodies to pancreatic islet cells.

TESTING FOR CELLULAR FUNCTIONS IN IMMUNITY

Routinely available tests should be used to screen suspected cases of immunodeficiency. These tests include serial CBC examinations for establishing total lymphocyte and neutrophil numbers, as well as tests to evaluate serum immunoglobulins (see Causes of Hypoglobulinemia, earlier), including specific antibody titers to common viral vaccines such as distemper or parvovirus. Sustained lymphopenias well below $1000/\mu l$ are noted in some cases of severe combined immunodeficiency, and marked neutrophilias ($> 50,000/\mu l$) are often observed in neutrophil function or chemotactic disorders (see Chapter 4). Routine histologic evaluation of lymph node tissue taken in biopsy can also occasionally prove useful in pursuing a diagnosis of congenital or acquired immunodeficiency. Possible abnormal findings include depletion or altered distribution of B- or T-lymphocyte populations within the nodal architecture.

Techniques for the evaluation of cellular immune functions in small animals are well established, but their clinical implementation has been limited because of the small number of laboratories offering the service plus the need, in certain tests, to process samples within hours of collection. Tests for cellular immunity include lymphocyte blastogenesis (transformation), enumeration of T and B lymphocytes, neutrophil function, and evaluation of leukocytic/erythrocytic histocompatibility antigens. If cellular immunity needs to be evaluated, the veterinarian should contact a college of veterinary medicine to determine availability. Many researchers eagerly respond to the opportunity to study spontaneously arising congenital or familial disorders in the field.

Evaluation of Phagocytes

Clinically significant phagocytic function disorders tend to occur in purebreds (e.g., Irish setters and Weimaraners) or closely related crossbreds as a congenital or inherited defect. These animals show chronic or recurrent bacterial infections from a young age, along with markedly elevated neutrophil counts and general unthriftiness. Tests include phagocytic assays, bactericidal assays, chemotactic response, and testing for cell surface markers such as CD18 adhesion molecule.

Enumeration of Proportions of T and B Lymphocytes

Occasional Indications ● Poor response to vaccinations; chronic unresponsive infections; persistently elevated or decreased lymphocyte counts; distinguishing between neoplastic and reactive lymphoproliferation by evaluating clonality.

Analysis ● Studies are usually performed on peripheral blood lymphocytes but can also be performed on lymph node tissue obtained by biopsy. Consult individual laboratories for sample specification. The T and B cells differ in the composition of their surface molecules (markers or receptors). The surface receptors are detected by heterologous RBC rosetting (some T cells), peanut agglutinin (most T cells), specific antisera to immunoglobulin M (most B cells), specific antisera to T cells, or monoclonal antibodies to specific cell surface differentiation (CD) antigens. Advantage: Monoclonal antibodies detect specific subgroups of functionally distinct lymphocyte subpopulations. Disadvantages: Analysis of surface markers or binding of polyclonal antisera to T cells is not always accurate or yielding of a specific diagnosis; enumeration procedures for B and T cells do not assess their functional capabilities; limited availability in veterinary laboratories.

Normal Values ● Values for peripheral blood lymphocytes vary according to species, breed, and age, as well as the laboratory and the type of surface marker used. Numbers of canine T cells peak around 5 to 6 years of age. The proportion of B cells peaks at 1 to 2 years of age. Both types of cells decline with advancing age in mammalian species that have been studied.

Artifacts ● Proportions of T and B cells depend

on the procedure used and the subjective judgment of the evaluator. Proportions of patients' T and B cells must simultaneously be compared with normal, healthy, age-matched controls tested. Numbers obtained in different laboratories under different testing conditions should be compared with caution.

Causes of Altered Proportions of T and B Cells

● Inherited defects of the immune system, lymphosarcoma, lymphocytic leukemia, and some viral infections (especially retroviruses like FeLV, FIV, and other viruses infecting lymphoid cells) change the proportions of T and B cells. Limited data are currently available for interpretation of results in dogs and cats.

Evaluation of Lymphocyte Functions
In Vitro

Occasional Indications ● Poor vaccination response or recurrent infections. The lymphocyte transformation test is the most commonly used test for assessing the functional capability of lymphocytes. Disadvantages: the test is not readily available and is only a simulation of an *in vivo* situation; therefore, the results should be interpreted as an approximation only, not a true extrapolation.

Analysis ● The evaluation varies among laboratories but usually requires 10 to 20 ml of heparinized whole blood. Isolated lymphocytes are exposed to various substances that cause their activation and division, such as concanavalin A, phytohemagglutinin (both are T-cell mitogens), and pokeweed mitogen (a T-cell–dependent, B-cell mitogen). The proliferation response of stimulated cells is quantitated by their increased uptake of radionucleotide compared with control cells from healthy animals of the same species and similar age. The lymphocytes should be tested in both autologous and healthy homologous serum. A control with bovine fetal serum is usually included as well. These tests examine for intrinsic lymphocyte function defects as well as the presence of patient serum suppressive factors, which can be found in many acquired disease states.

Normal Values ● Values vary among laboratories. The degree of stimulation of lymphocytes in lymphocyte transformation tests is expressed in counts per minute (CPM), which reflect the extent of blastogenesis (mitogenesis), or in stimulation indices (SI), which reflect the increase in blastogenesis of stimulated cells over that detected in unstimulated cells.

Artifacts ● The stress of disease or of being examined in a veterinary clinic may decrease measured responsiveness of lymphocytes to mitogens.

Causes of Abnormal Response to Mitogens ● Inherited or acquired intrinsic lymphocyte immunodeficiencies result in decreased CPM and SI in cells grown both in autologous and in healthy control serum when compared with control animals. Animals with acquired immunodeficiency caused by suppressive humoral factors (e.g., dogs with pyoderma, disseminated fungal infections) have decreased CPM and SI only when cells are grown in autologous serum. Animals with leukemias can have increased CPM of unstimulated cells, which is comparable to CPM of normal stimulated cells, but a low SI. Younger animals have lower CPM and SI than do mature animals. Patients incubating infectious diseases may have transiently increased background CPM of unstimulated cells; however, this is usually less than that noted in animals with leukemia. If decreased response to phytomitogens is detected, repeated testing is recommended. Quantitative analysis of T and B cells, as well as of T-helper and T-suppressor cells, is indicated, if available.

Decreased blastogenesis may result from intrinsic cellular defects or from their environment (extrinsic, i.e., serum or plasma immunosuppressive factors). Determining whether lymphocyte ability to undergo blastogenesis is suppressed by intrinsic defects or by humoral suppressive factors helps to determine the probability of successful treatment. The severity of suppression detected *in vitro* reflects the *in vivo* situation. In general, animals with decreased mitogenic response mediated by humoral suppressor factors have a more favorable prognosis than do animals with suppressed blastogenesis due to cellular dysfunction. Detection and successful treatment of an underlying disease or infection causing extrinsic suppression can result in return to normal lymphocyte function *in vitro*.

Bibliography

Barta O: Rose-Waaler test. *In* Barta O (ed): Veterinary Clinical Immunology Laboratory. Blacksburg, BAR-LAB, Inc., 1993a, pp D2-7–D2-14.

Barta O, Arnold DE: Electrophoresis. *In* Barta O (ed): Veterinary Clinical Immunology Laboratory. Blacksburg, BAR-LAB, Inc., 1993b, pp C1-1–C1-17.

Barta O, Barta V: Antinuclear antibody (ANA) testing. *In* Barta O (ed): Veterinary Clinical Immunology Laboratory. Blacksburg, BAR-LAB, Inc., 1993c, pp D1-1–D1-11.

Barta O, Pourciau SS: Electrophoresis. *In* Barta O (ed): Laboratory Techniques of Veterinary Clinical Immunology. Springfield, Charles C Thomas, 1984a, pp 116–122.

Barta O, Pourciau SS: Antinuclear antibody (ANA) testing. *In* Barta O (ed): Laboratory Techniques of Veterinary Clinical Immunology. Springfield, Charles C Thomas, 1984b, pp 159–163.

Benjamin MM: Protein. *In* Outline of Veterinary Clinical Pathology. 3rd ed. Ames, Iowa State University Press, 1978, pp 108–115.

Breitschwerdt EB, Woody BJ, Zerbe CA, et al: Monoclonal gammopathy associated with naturally occurring canine ehrlichiosis. J Vet Intern Med 1987; 1:2–9.

Carter SD, Bell SC, Bari ASM, Bennett D: Immune complexes and rheumatoid factors in canine arthritides. Ann Rheum Dis 1989;48:185–195.

Cornelius LM: Abnormalities of the standard biochemical profile. *In* Lorenz MD, Cornelius LM: Small Animal Medical Diagnosis. Philadelphia, JB Lippincott, 1987, pp 539–591.

Duncan JR, Prasse KW: Proteins, lipids and carbohydrates. *In* Veterinary Laboratory Medicine. 2nd ed. Ames, Iowa State University Press, 1986, pp 105–120.

Fritzler MJ: Immunofluorescent antinuclear antibody test. *In* Rose NR, Friedman H, Fahey JL (eds): Manual of Clinical Laboratory Immunology. 3rd ed. Washington, DC, American Society of Microbiology, 1986, pp 733–739.

Gorman NT, Werner LL: Diagnosis of immune-mediated disease and interpretation of immunologic tests. *In* Kirk RW (ed): Current Veterinary Therapy IX. Philadelphia, WB Saunders, 1986, pp 427–435.

Halliwell REW, Werner LL, Baum DE, et al: Incidence and characterization of canine rheumatoid factor. Vet Immunol Immunopathol 1989;21:161–175.

Harris CH, Krawiec DR, Gelberg HB, Shapiro SZ: Canine IgA glomerulonephropathy. Vet Immunol Immunopathol 1993;36:1–16.

Heddle RJ, Rowley D: Dog immunoglobulins. Immunochemical characterization of dog serum, saliva, colostrum, milk and small bowel fluid. Immunology 1975;29:185–195.

Ihrke PJ, Stannard AA, Ardans A, Yaskulsi SG: The longevity of immunoglobulin preservation in canine skin using Michel's fixative. Vet Immunol Immunopathol 1985;9:161–170.

Kaneko JJ: Serum proteins and the dysproteinemias. *In* Kaneko JJ (ed): Clinical Biochemistry of Domestic Animals. 3rd ed. New York, Academic Press, 1980, pp 97–118 and Appendix VI.

Medleau L, Miller WH: Immunodiagnostic tests for small animal practice. Comp Cont Ed 1983;5:705–716.

Moore GE, Mahaffey EA, Hoenig M: Hematologic and serum biochemical effects of long-term administration of anti-inflammatory doses of prednisone in dogs. Am J Vet Res 1992;53:1033–1037.

Muller GH, Kirk RW, Scott DW (eds): Immunologic diseases. *In* Small Animal Dermatology. 4th ed. Philadelphia, WB Saunders, 1989, pp 427–574.

Peterson M, Hurvitz A, Leib M, et al: Propylthiouracil-associated hemolytic anemia, thrombocytopenia, and antinuclear antibodies in cats with hyperthyroidism. JAVMA 1984;184:806–808.

Peterson M, Kintzer PP, Hurvitz A: Methimazole treatment of 262 cats with hyperthyroidism. J Vet Intern Med 1988;2:150–157.

Reimann KA, Bull RW, Crow SE, et al: Immunologic profiles of cats with persistent naturally acquired feline leukemia virus infection. Am J Vet Res 1986;47:1935–1939.

Reynolds HY, Johnson JS: Quantitation of canine immunoglobulins. J Immunol 1970;105:698–703.

Reynolds HY, Dale DC, Wolff SM, et al: Serum immunoglobulin levels in Grey Collies. Proc Soc Exp Biol Med 1971;136:574–577.

Rice CE: Comparative serology of domestic animals. Adv Vet Sci Comp Med 1968;12:105–162.

Schultz RD, Adams LS: Immunologic methods for the detection of humoral and cellular immunity. Vet Clin North Am 1978;8:721–753.

Scott DW, Walton DK, Slater MR: Immune-mediated dermatoses in domestic animals: Ten years after. Part I. Comp Cont Ed 1987a;9:424–436.

Scott DW, Walton DK, Slater MR, et al: Immune-mediated dermatoses in domestic animals: Ten years after. Part II. Comp Cont Ed 1987b;9:539–554.

Speicher CE, Smith JW Jr (eds): Unexpected test results. *In* Choosing Effective Laboratory Tests. Philadelphia, WB Saunders, 1983, pp 299–355.

Table of Plasma Proteins. Mannheim, Germany, Institute Behring, undated.

Thomas LA, Brown SA: Relationships between colloid osmotic pressure and plasma protein concentration in cattle, horses, dogs and cats. Am J Vet Res 1992;53:2241–2244.

Turnwald GH, Barta O: Immunologic and plasma protein disorders. *In* Willard MD, Tvedten H, Turnwald GH: Small Animal Clinical Diagnosis by Laboratory Methods. 1st ed. Philadelphia, WB Saunders, 1989, pp 264–282.

Werner LL, Brown KA, Halliwell REW: Diagnosis of autoimmune skin disease in the dog: Correlation between histopathologic, direct immunofluorescent and clinical findings. Vet Immunol Immunopathol 1984;5:47–64.

Werner LL, Gorman NT: Immune-mediated disorders of cats. Vet Clin North Am 1984;14:1039–1064.

Williams DA: Gammopathies. Comp Cont Ed 1981;3:815–823.

Williams DA: Markedly subnormal serum cobalamin in Shar-Pei dogs with signs of gastrointestinal disease (abstract 78). J Vet Intern Med 1991; 5: 133.

Wood DD, Hurvitz AI, Schultz RD: A latex test for canine rheumatoid factor. Vet Immunol Immunopathol 1980;1:103–111.

Cheri A. Johnson

13 Reproductive Disorders

GENERAL DIAGNOSTIC APPROACH

Clinicopathologic testing of the reproductive system is often indicated in normal as well as abnormal animals. The reproductive system should be included in routine prepurchase and prebreeding examinations. Evaluation of the reproductive tract of normal animals is also indicated to optimize both conception rates and litter size, to aid pregnancy management, and to assess semen quality before freezing semen. Abnormalities that indicate the need for evaluation include infertility, discharges from the external genitalia, abnormal sexual behavior, and abnormal conformation of the genitalia. The most important diagnostic procedures for evaluation of the reproductive system of normal and diseased animals are the history, the physical examination, and vaginal cytology in females or semen evaluation in males.

The reproductive history should include methods used to screen for infectious diseases that affect reproduction (e.g., *Brucella canis* in dogs and viral rhinotracheitis in cats), medications known to affect reproductive function (e.g., glucocorticoids, thyroid hormones, gonadotropins, estrogens, progestins, androgens, or prostaglandins) and familial association with infertility. One should also ask about stressful activities such as travel, being shown, or hard work (e.g., racing, hunting, training, and so on).

For females, the history of estrous cycles should include the dates of the onset of each cycle, the physical and behavioral characteristics of the female during each cycle, and the duration of each estrous period. The breeding dates and method of insemination (i.e., natural or

273

artificial) should be recorded. The stud's reproductive performance with other bitches before and after breeding the bitch in question is important. The dates and methods of pregnancy examination and any signs of abortion should be noted. If pregnancy occurred, was parturition normal? What were gestation length and litter size?

For males, the history should investigate libido and mating ability. It should include the number of females bred and the conception rate. Breeding methods, such as natural or artificial insemination, frequency of use, and how insemination dates are chosen should be investigated. The reproductive performance of bitches before and after being bred to the male in question is important.

Physical examination of the male reproductive tract includes inspection of preputial and scrotal skin and the penis. Both testes, epididymides, and spermatic cords should be palpated. The prostate is palpated both rectally and transabdominally. Physical examination of the female includes inspection of the vulva and vestibule. The uterus is palpated transabdominally. The posterior vagina is palpated with a gloved finger. Rectal palpation of the vagina may also be helpful.

VAGINAL CYTOLOGY

Common Indications • Vaginal cytology is used to monitor the stages of the estrous cycle, to determine breeding and whelping management, to investigate abnormal estrous cycles, to investigate "mismating," and to determine the nature of vulvar discharges and other reproductive disorders. Vaginal cytology does not identify ovulation.

Technique • A saline-moistened cotton-tipped swab is inserted into the vagina, or saline is flushed into and aspirated from the vagina with a pipette. One should avoid the clitoris, the clitoral fossa, and the skin when obtaining the sample because these areas contain keratinized cells that confuse the interpretation. Next, the swabs are gently rolled onto slides, or drops of the saline aspirate are placed on slides. Slides are then fixed and stained as desired. New methylene blue (NMB), Wright-Giemsa, Wright's stain, trichrome stain, and modified Wright-Giemsa (Diff-Quick) are commonly used, but many other stains are equally acceptable. NMB may be used on wet or air-dried preparations. A drop of stain is placed on the cells on the slide, and a cover-

slip is used. Slides can be read immediately. Disadvantages of NMB staining are that red blood cells (RBCs) are not stained and that slides must be read immediately. Wright's, Wright-Giemsa, and trichrome stains require several different staining solutions. Instructions must be followed carefully for reproducible results. This makes them cumbersome, but all cell types are stained and slides can be stored. Diff-Quik stain is a reasonable compromise. Slides are fixed in methanol and then dipped in the two Diff-Quik solutions. Vaginal epithelial cells stain more slowly than do blood cells, so staining time may need to be increased beyond the manufacturer's recommendations. Slides can be stored for several days without a coverslip, although a coverslip prolongs storage time. A minimum of 100 epithelial cells are examined and tabulated.

Interpretation • The cell types of the vaginal epithelium have been described (Johnston et al., 1982; Olson et al., 1984). From the lamina propria to the epithelial surface, in order of increasing maturity, they are basal, parabasal, intermediate, superficial-intermediate, and superficial cells. The basal cells are on the basement membrane and are not exfoliated. Parabasal cells are small and round with a large nuclear:cytoplasmic ratio. Intermediate cells are round, are about twice the size of parabasal cells, and have a similar nucleus. Superficial-intermediate cells are larger, have angular borders, and are often folded. The nucleus is still large but beginning to show karyolysis. The superficial cells are angular, thin, and folded. The nucleus is pyknotic, or takes up no stain if very karyolytic.

Estrogen causes proliferation and maturation (cornification) of the vaginal epithelium. Therefore, vaginal cytology can be used to monitor the estrous cycle, especially the follicular phase of proestrus and estrus when estrogen is being produced by the ovarian follicles (Table 13–1). During proestrus, the parabasal, intermediate, and some superficial cells are exfoli-

Table 13–1 VAGINAL CYTOLOGIC FINDINGS DURING THE ESTROUS CYCLE

	Proestrus		Estrus		Diestrus
Parabasal	+		−		−
Intermediate	+		rare		+
Superficial-intermediate	+/−		+		+/−
Superficial	rare	−>	≥ 90%	−>	rare
RBCs	+		+/−		+/−
WBCs	+		−		+ +/+

ated. RBCs, white blood cells (WBCs), and bacteria are present. As estrus approaches there is a gradual increase in the maturity of the epithelial cells and a decrease in WBCs. During estrus, superficial cells are the predominant cell type, eventually accounting for > 90% of the exfoliated epithelial cells. RBCs are often present during estrus. Bacteria may be present. WBCs are absent during estrus unless there is concurrent inflammation.

Diestrus (luteal phase) is marked by an abrupt change: The less mature parabasal and intermediate cells outnumber the superficial cells. Sheets of epithelial cells are often noted at the onset of diestrus. WBCs almost always return at this time. RBCs and bacteria are often present. Thus, it is impossible to differentiate proestrus from diestrus based on a single vaginal smear. RBCs are often present in both. Fewer cells are exfoliated during anestrus. Parabasal and intermediate epithelial cells, with or without a few WBCs and bacteria, are present (see Table 13–1). Similar changes in vaginal cytology occur during the feline estrous cycle, except that RBCs and WBCs are uncommon.

Breeding and Whelping Management in Dogs

Determining the various stages of the estrous cycle can help determine optimal breeding dates in order to maximize conception and litter size and to predict whelping dates more closely. Maximal conception rates and litter size are obtained when normal bitches are bred on the first day of estrus and again 3 or more days later. Although it may not perceptibly change conception rates or litter size, breeding every other day is also acceptable, provided that breeding begins at the onset of estrus and covers at least 4 to 6 days (Table 13–2). Because ovulation occurs at variable and unpredictable times during behavioral or cytologic estrus and because canine sperm maintains its ability to fertilize for at least 4 to 6 days in the estrual tract, normal gestation length varies from 58 to 72 days after the first breeding date. When gestation length is calculated from the first day of cytologic diestrus, there is very little variation, with 93% of bitches whelping 57 days after the first day of diestrus. Calculating gestation length from cytologic diestrus, rather than breeding dates, is helpful in managing pregnancies.

Abnormal Cycles ● Proestrus plus estrus lasting longer than 3 weeks in a bitch is considered

Table 13–2 CANINE BREEDING MANAGEMENT

1. Choose only healthy, *Brucella canis*–negative, normal animals for breeding.
2. Identify the first day of estrus.
   Begin early (day 3) in season (proestrus).
   Check the bitch every other day by behavioral (tease with experienced stud) and/or vaginal cytology examination.
   (Note: Breeding a predetermined number of days after onset of proestrus is not optimal management).
3. Breed on the first day of estrus.
4. Breed once again 3 or more days later.
   (Note: Breeding every other day for at least three times is also acceptable.)
   (Note: Progesterone can be used to more accurately predict ovulation and determine breeding dates.)
5. Pregnancy examination is indicated 20 to 30 days later.
   If pregnant, discuss pregnancy and parturition management.
   If not pregnant, determine serum progesterone to assess ovulation and luteal function.

prolonged. Because the time of ovulation during an abnormal cycle is unknown, breeding should continue every 2 to 4 days throughout the prolonged estrus unless progesterone is being monitored to predict ovulation (see Progesterone, later in this chapter). Persistent estrus is uncommon in bitches and queens. The most common cause of "abnormal cycle" in bitches is usually owner impatience (i.e., the bitch is normal), and in a queen it is usually the cat's normal, frequent cycles. Causes of persistent estrus include ovarian cysts, ovarian neoplasia, and exogenous estrogen administration. Conversely, some bitches are thought to have no apparent external or behavioral signs of proestrus or estrus. This so-called silent heat might be identified prospectively by frequent (every 1–2 weeks) examination of vaginal cytology or retrospectively by determining serum concentrations of progesterone. Progesterone concentrations of > 2 ng/dl (3 nmol/L) denote luteal function, which normally occurs during the 60 days after estrus in bitches.

Mismating ● Vaginal cytology may help determine if a bitch has recently been bred, since sperm heads (not intact sperm) are detected in vaginal smears from 68% of bitches bred 24 hours earlier and from 50% of bitches bred 48 hours earlier. Absence of sperm does not rule out the possibility of recent copulation. Vaginal cytology is indicated before administration of estrogens (i.e., mismating shot). If the cytologic appearance is that of diestrus, estrogens are contraindicated because pyometra occurs in 25% of bitches given estradiol cypionate (ECP) during diestrus (Bowen et al., 1985). Note: Administration of ECP to any bitch is not recommended. It may produce mild to fatal bone marrow suppression.

VULVAR DISCHARGES AND OTHER DISORDERS

The nature of a vulvar discharge is best determined by vaginal cytology (Olson et al., 1984b). One must first differentiate normal from abnormal discharges and then identify the cause. The cytologic examination should be systematic. The morphologic characteristics and numbers of vaginal epithelial cells, RBCs, WBCs, and bacteria are noted, as is the presence of other elements such as neoplastic cells, mucus, debris, uteroverdine, endometrial cells, or macrophages. Many reproductive disorders are reflected by abnormal vaginal cytology, even in the absence of a detectable vulvar discharge.

Hemorrhage ● RBCs are common in normal and abnormal vulvar discharges (Table 13–3), and their significance is determined by accompanying cells. Mature (cornified) epithelial cells with RBCs are expected during normal proestrus and estrus but may also be present because of exogenous estrogens or ovarian pathology. RBCs mixed with mucus are found in the normal postpartum vaginal discharge, lochia. When the cytologic appearance is that of peripheral blood plus noncornified epithelial cells, a cause of hemorrhage should be sought. These causes include subinvolution of placental sites, vaginal laceration, uterine and vaginal neoplasia, uterine torsion, and coagulopathies.

When hemorrhage is present, a review of the history and physical findings is indicated. Subinvolution of placental sites is a postpartum disorder characterized by a bloody discharge that persists for 8 to 12 weeks. It occurs most often in primiparous bitches that are otherwise

healthy. The blood loss is rarely significant. The diagnosis is based on the historical, physical, and cytologic findings. The diagnosis could be confirmed by histopathologic examination of placental sites, but confirmation is rarely necessary. Vaginal lacerations are relatively uncommon. They may occur as a result of breeding trauma, dystocia, obstetric procedures, or vaginoscopy. When vaginal laceration is suspected, the next diagnostic procedure should be endoscopy while the patient is anesthetized.

Hemorrhagic vulvar discharge, with or without an obvious mass, is the most common sign of uterine and vaginal leiomyoma in bitches and queens. Leiomyomas are the most common tumors of the uterus and vagina in small animals. Leiomyomas do not readily exfoliate; therefore, neoplastic cells are rarely found on cytologic preparations. When neoplasia is suspected, the next diagnostic procedure should be careful digital palpation of the vagina and transabdominal palpation of the uterus. Next, radiography/ultrasonography can evaluate the uterus, and endoscopy can evaluate the vagina.

Uterine torsions usually occur in gravid females, near term. Abdominal pain is the most prominent finding, but a hemorrhagic discharge is usually found. When uterine torsion is suspected, the next diagnostic procedure should be radiology/ultrasonography of the uterus. Rarely, vulvar bleeding may be the only sign of a bleeding disorder. Other, more common causes of vulvar bleeding should be ruled out first (see Table 13–3). Then, if a bleeding disorder is suspected, evaluation of platelet numbers and function, plus the coagulation system (see Chapter 5), is indicated.

Bleeding can accompany any inflammatory process. When the number of WBCs obviously exceeds that of peripheral blood, the cause of the WBCs (i.e., inflammation) rather than the RBCs (i.e., hemorrhage) should be determined. It is worth emphasizing that the presence of a bloody vulvar discharge, even when associated with attraction of male dogs, does not always represent proestrus or estrus (see Table 13–3).

Purulent/Septic Discharge ● WBCs, with or without bacteria, suggest inflammation. They are normally found in large numbers during the first 1 to 2 days of diestrus and in lesser numbers in normal lochia. Septic or purulent vulvar discharges may originate from the vulva, vestibule, vagina, or uterus. Because of markedly different prognoses, the source of a septic/purulent exudate must be determined. Vaginoscopy is indicated next. If vulvitis or vaginitis is the cause, physical evidence of inflammation (e.g., hyper-

Table 13–3 CAUSES OF HEMORRHAGIC VULVAR DISCHARGE IN THE BITCH AND QUEEN

With Cornified (Mature) Epithelial Cells
 Normal proestrus, estrus, or early diestrus
 Ovarian pathology (i.e., cystic follicles or functional ovarian tumor)
 Exogenous estrogen
Without Cornified (Mature) Epithelial Cells
 Normal lochia
 Subinvoluted placental sites
 Vaginal laceration
 Neoplasia of vagina or uterus
 Uterine torsion
 Bleeding disorder

emia, edema, pain, mucosal lesions, and so on) should be noted.

However, finding vaginitis does not rule out concurrent uterine pathology (Fig. 13–1). If endoscopy suggests a uterine source of the discharge or if endometrial cells are found during cytologic evaluation, uterine involvement is suspected and abdominal radiography or ultrasonography is indicated. Knowledge of the stage of the estrous cycle is essential for evaluating uterine pathology. During the luteal phase (diestrus), a septic or purulent discharge can occur because of cystic endometrial hyperplasia-pyometra, pregnancy with concurrent uterine or vaginal infection, or impending abortion. If the discharge occurs postpartum, postabortion, or otherwise during anestrus, metritis or uterine stump granuloma/abscess should be considered. Predisposing causes of metritis such as retained placenta, retained fetus, abortion, or obstetric procedures should be sought (see Fig. 13–1).

Neoplastic Cells • Fine-needle aspiration of vaginal and vulvar masses is indicated. Vaginoscopy may be used to evaluate the extent of involvement and the external urethral orifice. Transmissible veneral tumors (TVTs) exfoliate readily. Most often bitches with TVTs are examined because of a mass protruding from the vulva (see Chapter 16). Urethral transitional cell carcinomas and vaginal squamous cell carcinomas may also be identified by vaginal cytology. Rarely, mammary gland adenocarcinoma and lymphosarcoma involve the external genitalia. If cytology does not provide a definitive diagnosis of neoplasia, incisional biopsy is indicated. Additional diagnostic tests for staging the disease are dictated by the tumor type.

Mucus • This is the predominate component of lochia. It may also occur during normal late pregnancy and possibly in scanty amounts during the nonpregnant, luteal phase (diestrus). No further testing of these animals is necessary. Cervicitis and mucometra could also be associated with a mucoid discharge. Endoscopy or abdominal radiology/ultrasonography may be helpful in identifying these latter disorders. Some bitches with scanty mucoid vulvar discharge are apparently normal (Table 13–4).

Mibolerone or testosterone administration and intersex conditions may cause a slight mucoid discharge. History should reveal drug administration. Clitoral enlargement is often present. The vagina may end blindly in some intersex animals. Measuring testosterone before and after human chorionic gonadotropin (hCG) administration (see Testosterone, later in this chapter) and finding a significant difference suggest functional testicular tissue in suspected intersex animals. These patients may also be karyotyped, but exploratory laparotomy may be the most cost-effective diagnostic and therapeutic approach for an intersex animal.

Uteroverdine • This dark green blood pigment is normally found in the placenta. Its presence in a vulvar discharge implies placental separation. This is normal during labor. In the absence of obvious labor, uteroverdine may be found in animals with dystocia and during or after abortion. If the history and physical examination do not differentiate these causes, ab-

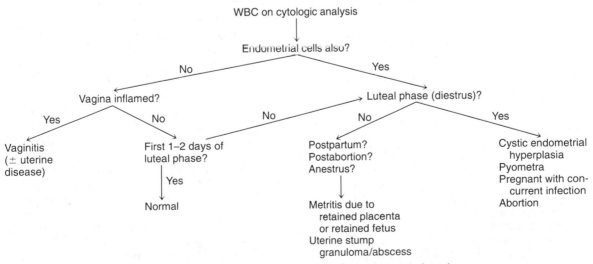

Figure 13–1 Diagnostic considerations for purulent/septic vaginal cytology.

Table 13–4 CAUSES OF MUCOID VULVAR DISCHARGE

Normal
  Lochia
  Late pregnancy
  Luteal phase (diestrus)
Androgenic stimulation
  Endogenous (intersex)
  Exogenous (mibolerone, testosterone)
Cervicitis
Mucometra
Idiopathic (?)

dominal ultrasonography is indicated. The presence of fetuses and their viability can also be determined by ultrasonography.

MAMMARY GLANDS

Disorders of the mammae are usually reflected by abnormal size of the glands or abnormal secretions from one or more glands. The most common cause of mammary gland enlargement and secretion is lactation, which may or may not be normal. Mastitis, hyperplasia, and neoplasia of the mammary glands are also common in dogs and cats.

Galactorrhea ● Inappropriate lactation that is not associated with pregnancy and parturition is common in bitches with false pregnancy and occasionally occurs in false-pregnant queens. False pregnancy occurs at the end of the luteal phase, which is approximately 60 days after estrus in a bitch and approximately 40 days after induced ovulation (without conception) in a queen. Galactorrhea may also occur after withdrawal of progesterone stimulation, such as oophorectomy during diestrus or discontinuation of an exogenous progestin (e.g., megestrol). The diagnosis of galactorrhea is established by historical and physical findings. This disorder resolves spontaneously but rarely persists for months in some bitches (Chastain and Schmidt, 1980). Testing is usually unnecessary, but because it has been associated with hypothyroidism, thyroid function testing is reasonable in bitches with protracted galactorrhea.

Mastitis ● A bacterial infection of one or more lactating mammary glands, mastitis is most common in postpartum bitches. It rarely occurs in false-pregnant lactating bitches or in postpartum queens. The diagnosis is based on the history of recent parturition and finding warm, swollen, painful glands with purulent milk. If the milk is not visibly abnormal, cytology of the milk or a mammary aspirate shows purulent or septic inflammation. Galactostasis, or accumulation and stasis of milk, can also cause warm, swollen, painful glands, but there is no bacterial infection and the milk is cytologically normal. Galactostasis is most common during weaning.

Mammary Hypertrophy ● Mammary hypertrophy (mammary hyperplasia, fibroadenomatous change, fibroadenomatosis, fibroadenoma) occurs more often in cats than in dogs. It is characterized by rapid, abnormal mammary growth, which has a temporal association with progestational stimulation. Mammary hypertrophy occurs during the luteal phase of the estrous cycle of intact bitches and queens. It has also been reported in neutered queens and toms that have been treated with progestins (e.g., megestrol acetate [Ovaban]). If the history confirms progesterone stimulation, then mammary hypertrophy is suspected. If in doubt, biopsy is indicated because the other diagnostic consideration is neoplasia.

Mammary Neoplasia ● Mammary neoplasia is common in middle-aged to older female dogs and cats. Any mammary growth in male or neutered animals or intact anestrous females should be considered neoplastic until proven otherwise. Fine-needle aspiration of the mass is easily performed; however, cytologic findings must be interpreted cautiously (see Chapter 16). Excisional biopsy is the diagnostic method of choice.

SEMEN EVALUATION

Common Indications ● Semen evaluation is indicated whenever there is a question of male infertility (Fig. 13–2) and as a routine part of a prebreeding examination (Johnston et al., 1982). Cytologic examination of the ejaculate is also used to evaluate diseases of the prostate, testes, and epididymides.

Technique ● Semen is collected by manual stimulation of the dog's penis through the prepuce or an artificial vagina. Most dogs with previous breeding experience can be collected without a teaser bitch. Inexperienced or timid males may need a bitch in estrus in order to ejaculate. A docile anestrous bitch may also work as a teaser. The presence of an estrual bitch may improve the quality of the ejaculate. Use of the synthetic pheromone methyl-*p*-hydroxy benzoate (Sigma Chemical) may also be helpful. The collection

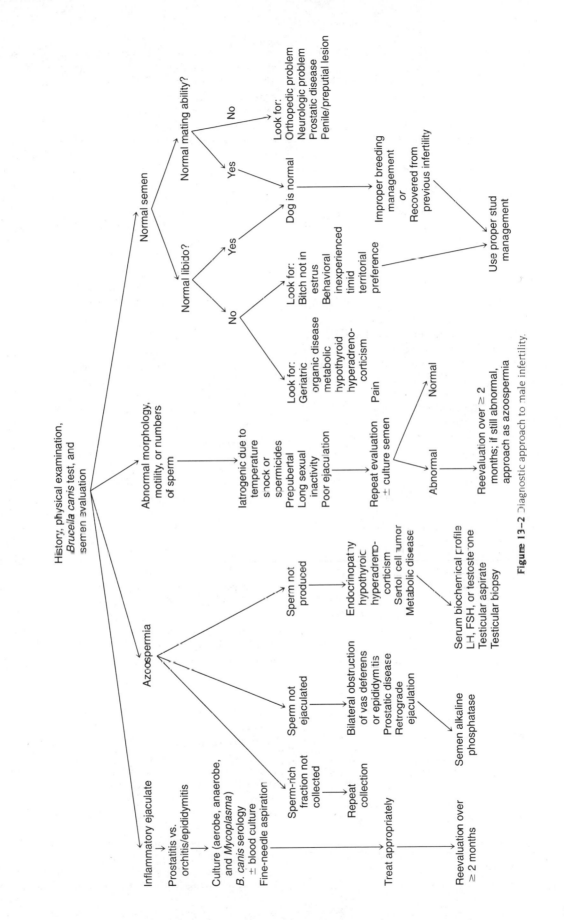

Figure 13-2 Diagnostic approach to male infertility.

area should be quiet and free from distractions and should have a nonskid floor.

Care should be taken when handling the semen sample. All equipment should be clean and free from chemical contaminants (e.g., water and excessive lubricant) that may affect sperm viability. The sample should be protected from temperature shock. Dog semen can be handled at room temperature for approximately 15 minutes without adverse effect. Nevertheless, the sample should be processed promptly. Slides and coverslips should be maintained at 37° C. The semen sample is evaluated for volume and color, plus concentration, motility, and morphology of spermatozoa (Table 13–5).

Volume • The volume is read directly from the calibrated centrifuge tube into which the sample was collected. Canine semen is ejaculated in three fractions. The first fraction is clear, and the volume is usually several drops. Some individuals may have as much as 2 ml of this presperm fraction. The sperm-rich fraction is the second fraction. The volume varies from 0.5 to 5 ml. The third fraction is prostatic fluid, which is the largest fraction of the canine ejaculate. More than 20 ml of prostatic fluid may be collected. Normal prostatic fluid is clear and easily differentiated from the milky sperm-rich fraction. For routine semen evaluation, it is necessary to collect only enough prostatic fluid to ensure that the entire sperm-rich portion has been ejaculated.

The total volume varies with technique, frequency, age, and the amount of prostatic fluid collected. Young dogs tend to have less volume than mature dogs. Volume is not correlated with fertility unless the dog fails to ejaculate.

Color • The color is evaluated by direct visualization. Normal canine semen is usually the color of skim milk. An abnormally colored sample should be closely examined for the presence of foreign matter. Any contaminant may adversely affect sperm viability and concentration. A yellow appearance may represent urine contamination. To avoid urine contamination of subsequent samples, dogs should not be allowed to micturate immediately before semen collection. Rarely, certain abnormal individuals urinate during ejaculation; they are usually infertile. Blood colors the sample pink or red. Blood is usually of prostatic origin or from penile abrasions. The later can be ruled out by prompt visual inspection of the penis.

Inflammatory cells may cause the sample to appear flocculated or yellow-green. These cells can originate anywhere in the urinary or reproductive tracts. When an inflammatory ejaculate is obtained, it should be cultured for bacteria and *Mycoplasma* sp. Dogs should be tested for *Brucella canis* infection (see Chapter 15).

Concentration • The volume, and thus the concentration, of the ejaculate is principally influenced by the sperm-free prostatic fluid. Therefore, the number of spermatozoa is reported as the total sperm per ejaculate rather than sperm per milliliter. The sample is diluted before counting using standard hematology dilution methods (see Chapter 2). The easiest to use are the Unopette pipettes. Either the RBC or the WBC/platelet Unopette may be used for canine semen. The RBC pipette dilutes the sample 1:200. The WBC/platelet pipette dilutes the sample 1:100. Dilution may be unnecessary for oligospermic samples. The number of sperm per milliliter is then multiplied by the number of milliliters collected to give the number of sperm per ejaculate. Values of 200 to 500 × 10^6 sperm per ejaculate are considered normal; however, numbers > 500 × 10^6 are common. There is considerable breed variation, because the spermatogenic potential increases with testicular size (Olar et al., 1983).

Motility • A drop of semen is placed on a warm slide (37° C), covered with a warm coverslip, and allowed to sit on the slide warmer for 15 to 30 seconds. It is then examined microscopically for progressive motility. Spermatozoa should move in a rapid, steady, forward manner, straight across the field. Dead sperm may be moved back and forth by live sperm, especially in a concentrated sample. This passive movement should not be mistaken for active motility. A concentrated sample should be diluted with an equal volume of 0.9% saline (37° C). One hundred sperm are examined, and the per cent having progressive motility is estimated. Dogs

Table 13–5 CHARACTERISTICS OF NORMAL CANINE SEMEN

Fraction	Volume	Color
Presperm	Drops (rarely several milliliters)	Clear
Sperm-rich	0.5–5.0 ml	Cloudy white, opalescent
Prostatic fluid	1–20 ml	Clear

Total sperm/ejaculate = 200 × 10^6 to > 500 × 10^6.
Motility ≥ 80% progressively motile.
Morphology ≤ 25% abnormal.

with good fertility usually have $> 80\%$ motility. It is unusual to have $> 95\%$ progressive motility. Wave patterns such as those seen in bull semen are rarely seen in canine semen because the concentration of sperm is too low.

The per cent motility and the quality of the motility can be diminished by exposure to heat or cold, excessive lubricant, water, urine, and inflammatory cells. Motility of sperm ejaculated after a long sexual rest may be lower. Semen that has been chilled or frozen usually does not regain its original motility when it is warmed. In chilled semen, the per cent of motile sperm is usually the same; however, the individual spermatozoa tend to move slowly. In semen that has been frozen then thawed, both the per cent and the speed of motility are usually lower.

Morphology • Phase contrast light microscopy is an ideal method for evaluation of sperm morphology, but it has limited availability. Several different stains may be used to evaluate the morphologic characteristics of sperm. Unfortunately, some stains cause morphologic defects (most commonly bent tails) in canine sperm. The stain-induced morphologic defects may reflect inappropriate osmolality or pH. The most common stains contain eosin-nigrosin. An inexpensive stain is Pelican india ink, which is available from art stores. One drop of stain is mixed with one drop of semen on a slide. This fluid is then drawn across the slide with the edge of a second slide to make a thick smear (similar to how a blood smear is made). Several smears can be made from the original drops. These are allowed to dry and are then examined microscopically under oil immersion. Samples may also be stained with NMB or Wright's stain.

A minimum of 100, but preferably 200, spermatozoa are examined and classified as being normal or as having some abnormality. The presence of more than one abnormality in one spermatozoan is classified according to the most severe abnormality. Abnormalities affecting the size and shape of the sperm head, acrosome, and midpiece and proximal droplets are usually considered most severe. Loose or detached heads that are otherwise normal, as well as bent tails, are considered less severe; however, they are often the first abnormalities noticed after testicular insult. The correlation between morphologic characteristics and fertility has not been evaluated in dogs or cats.

Primary abnormalities are usually attributed to abnormal spermatogenesis in the testicle, whereas secondary abnormalities are usually attributed to errors in the maturation process in the epididymis or sample handling. This may be inaccurate in some cases. Therefore, it is best to describe the abnormalities (i.e., bent tail or large head) rather than merely to classify them as primary or secondary. In this way, comparison with future samples may be more accurate. Dogs with good fertility usually have no more than 20% to 25% abnormal sperm. Abnormalities due to improper sample handling should disappear in subsequent, properly handled samples. The most common iatrogenic change in canine semen is bent tails.

During the morphologic examination, the presence of other cell types or foreign matter should be recorded. RBCs denote hemorrhage, whereas WBCs imply an inflammatory process somewhere in the urogenital tract. Some epithelial cells are normally present in canine semen, and their number increases after a long sexual rest. If excessive numbers of cells other than spermatozoa are found, their source should be investigated. These cells are most easily evaluated if stains such as Wright's stain are used. Crystals are a common type of foreign matter. They may be found in samples contaminated with urine or talc.

Seminal Alkaline Phosphatase

Alkaline phosphatase is produced by the canine epididymis and is found in high concentrations (i.e., > 1000 IU/dl) in normal ejaculates. Determination of seminal plasma alkaline phosphatase is helpful in evaluating azoospermic semen samples. The sample is centrifuged as for serum (e.g., 3000 rpm for 10 minutes), and the supernatant seminal plasma is harvested. The centrifugation may need to be modified according to the viscosity of the sample, but canine semen is rarely more viscous than serum. The concentration of alkaline phosphatase in the seminal plasma is then determined in the same manner as for serum alkaline phosphatase (see Chapter 9). If the sperm-rich fraction was not contained in the semen sample because of incomplete ejaculation or because of bilateral obstruction to outflow, seminal alkaline phosphatase will be low (i.e., < 100 IU/dl). If the sample has high alkaline phosphatase but no spermatozoa, failure of testicular spermatogenesis is suggested. Azospermic animals with seminal alkaline phosphatase in the midrange require additional testing.

Interpretation • The semen sample does not reflect testicular or epididymal function on the day the sample is collected. Spermatogenesis requires approximately 60 days in dogs. The length of the spermatogenic cycle in cats is unknown. To help establish a prognosis or resolve doubt about the cause of an unsatisfactory sample, the dog should be reevaluated several times over a period of at least 2 months. A dog's age, breed (testicle size), and frequency of use must be considered before the sample is pronounced "satisfactory" or "unsatisfactory." The presence of semen of satisfactory quality is not proof of fertility. A male must also have normal libido and mating ability (see Fig. 13–2). Likewise, the presence of unsatisfactory semen does not necessarily signify sterility, unless there is azoospermia or complete necrospermia (i.e., dead spermatozoa).

PROSTATE

Prostatic disease is common in older male dogs. Benign prostatic hyperplasia, bacterial prostatitis, prostatic abscess, prostatic and paraprostatic cysts, and prostatic neoplasia may occur. The history and physical examination (especially rectal palpation) often localize a disease process to the prostate, but additional tests are necessary to differentiate between the various causes. Prostatic fluid is the third and largest fraction of the canine ejaculate; therefore, evaluation of ejaculated prostatic fluid has been advocated for the diagnosis of prostatic disease (Barsanti and Finco, 1984; Barsanti et al., 1983; Thrall et al., 1985). Prostatic massage, fine-needle aspiration, and biopsy of the prostate can also be performed, but ejaculation is less invasive and more easily performed if a dog is willing and able to ejaculate.

The results of cytologic examination of the ejaculate correlate well with histopathologic examination of biopsy specimens, except for prostatic neoplasia. Neoplastic cells are rarely found in the ejaculate of dogs with prostatic neoplasia. Hemorrhage is the most frequent cytologic abnormality in semen from dogs with prostatic hyperplasia. Inflammation is the most frequent cytologic abnormality in semen from dogs with chronic bacterial prostatitis. Because prostatic fluid normally refluxes into the urinary bladder, urinary tract infection frequently develops in animals with chronic bacterial prostatitis. When urinary tract infection exists concurrently with bacterial prostatitis, cytologic examination of semen is a more accurate diagnostic method for prostatitis than prostatic massage (Barsanti et al., 1983). If cytologic examination of semen or prostatic massage specimens yields equivocal results, percutaneous fine-needle aspiration or biopsy of the prostate (preferably with ultrasonographic guidance) should be considered. Radiology and ultrasonography also provide useful information. Biochemical evaluation of canine prostatic fluid has not been helpful in differentiating various prostatic diseases.

TESTES AND EPIDIDYMIDES

The most important diagnostic procedure for evaluation of the testes and epididymides is physical examination, but semen evaluation is also useful. For example, as early as 5 weeks after infection with B. canis, abnormal sperm are ejaculated (George et al., 1979). Abnormalities include deformed acrosomes, swollen midpieces, and retained protoplasmic droplets. By 15 weeks after infection, bent tails, detached heads, and head-to-head agglutination are also found. Between 8 and 35 weeks after B. canis infection, clumps of inflammatory cells are found in semen. These include neutrophils and macrophages, with phagocytosis of sperm. With chronic infection (60–100 weeks), fewer inflammatory cells are found. When testicular atrophy occurs as a result of B. canis infection, azoospermia is likely. Any dog with infertility or inflammatory cells in the semen should be evaluated for B. canis with serology and microbiology.

Fine-needle aspiration of the testes can easily be performed using a 25-gauge needle. This technique is especially helpful in evaluating focal lesions such as a palpable testicular mass. It may also be done to demonstrate the presence of spermatogenesis. Aspiration of the epididymides causes more discomfort and may be associated with the formation of granulomas.

ENDOCRINE EVALUATION

The most important diagnostic methods for evaluation of the hypothalamic-pituitary-gonadal axis are the history and physical examination. Historical findings of normal libido and mating behavior in males and females, normal cyclicity in females, and a physically normal reproductive tract suggest a normal hypothalamic-pituitary-gonadal axis. This can be substantiated by demonstrating normal end products of that axis: normal semen in males and normal ovulations in females. There are no noninvasive procedures that prove that ovulation occurred. However, luteal function is demonstrated by finding high serum concentrations of progesterone, which strongly suggest that ovulation did occur.

The gonadotropins luteinizing hormone (LH) and follicle-stimulating hormone (FSH) and the gonadal steroids estradiol, progesterone, and testosterone can be measured using radioimmunoassay (RIA). Normal ranges vary considerably from laboratory to laboratory. Because reproductive hormones all are released in pulsatile or cyclic manners, the results must be interpreted in conjunction with each other and the reproductive history. Serial samples (e.g., every 15–30 minutes for 2 hours) or determinations of serum concentrations before and after administration of trophic hormones is preferable to single, random sampling (Shille and Olson, 1989).

Progesterone

Occasional Indications • Progesterone can be used to help predict ovulation in bitches because luteinization begins as a preovulatory event in the canine species. The transition of progesterone concentration from anestrus levels (< 2 ng/ml) to > 2 ng/ml (3 nmol/L) is approximately coincident with the LH surge. Ovulation follows the LH surge by about 2 days. The oocyte completes its development and is ready for fertilization approximately 2 days after ovulation. Therefore, insemination is recommended 3 to 4 days after the transition from anestrous progesterone to concentrations > 2 ng/ml. Finding progesterone concentrations > 5 ng/ml implies that ovulation has already occurred.

Sample • Check with the laboratory (serum or plasma). Heparinized and EDTA plasma yield similar results to serum. RIA and ELISA methodologies used.

Artifactual Changes • Storage on RBCs or at room temperature can decrease concentrations. Unaffected by lipemia, icterus (bilirubin < 20 mg/dl), or hemolysis when RIA is used for determination. RIAs are highly specific for progesterone but may have slight cross-reactivity with other steroids such as deoxycorticosterone, deoxycortisol, dihydroprogesterone, or 5 β-pregnan-3,20-dione. This assay should not cross-react with androstenediol, corticosterone, cortisol, estradiol, testosterone, or pregnenolone. Cross-reactivity may vary with specific assay systems.

Administration of radioactive compounds or exogenous progestins may affect the RIA directly. Exogenous progestins are likely to suppress endogenous progesterone via negative feedback. The enzyme-linked immunosorbent assay (ELISA) progesterone determination* has been shown to be approximately 85% accurate when compared with RIA (Hegstad, 1989).

Interpretation • The importance of using all the data rather than one parameter alone can be illustrated with progesterone. The finding of progesterone concentrations > 2 to 5 ng/dl suggests luteal function, which in turn implies but does not prove that ovulation occurred. In a bitch, luteal function normally lasts for approximately 65 days after estrus, whether or not pregnancy occurs (Concannon, 1986). A queen, on the other hand, has a luteal phase with increased progesterone only if ovulation is induced. If pregnancy does not occur after ovulation, luteal function persists for approximately 40 days in queens, whereas if pregnancy does occur, progesterone remains > 2 ng/ml to term (Verhage et al., 1976). Serum concentrations of progesterone are highest approximately midway through the luteal phase, at which time it may be > 50 ng/ml (> 75 nmol/L), depending on the laboratory. At all times of the normal estrous cycle other than the luteal phase, progesterone concentrations are < 2 ng/dl because there is no functional luteal tissue. Therefore, finding serum concentrations of < 2 ng/dl in a clinical patient may denote normal anestrus, failure to ovulate, or failure to maintain normal luteal function, depending on the stage of the cycle the sample was obtained (Fig. 13–3).

Testosterone

Occasional Indications • May be useful for evaluating suspected cryptorchid or intersex animals.

Sample • Check with a laboratory. EDTA plasma may yield lower results than heparinized plasma or serum. RIA used for determination.

Artifactual Change • Storage on RBCs or at room temperature can decrease concentrations. Unaffected by bilirubinemia (< 20 mg/dl), hemolysis, and lipemia. RIA is highly specific for testosterone; however, there may be important cross-reactivity with dihydrotestosterone, 19-nortestosterone, 11-ketotestosterone, methyltestosterone, and 11-β-hydroxytestosterone. Cross-reactivity with aldosterone, corticosterone,

---

*International Canine Genetics, Malvern, PA.

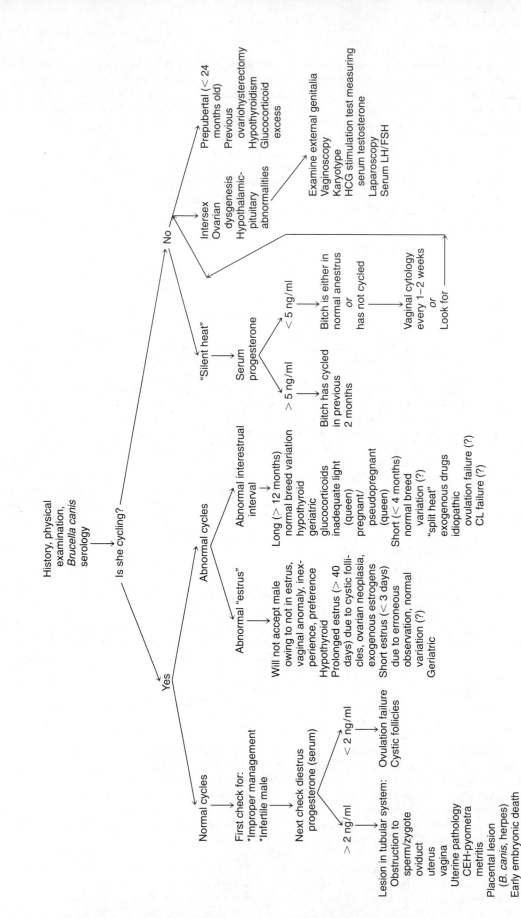

Figure 13-3 Diagnostic approach to infertility in a bitch.

cortisol, cortisone, estradiol, and progesterone should be insignificant. Cross-reactivity may vary with the specific assay system.

Administration of radioactivity and exogenous testosterone or drugs metabolized to testosterone, methyltestosterone, or other cross-reacting androgens listed earlier may affect the RIA directly. Exogenous androgens are likely to suppress endogenous testosterone via negative feedback.

Interpretation ● Serum concentrations of testosterone fluctuate greatly within and among individual males. These "spikes" in the serum testosterone concentration occur about every 30 to 90 minutes, depending on the species. Determination of testosterone on a single, random occasion has no diagnostic value because normal, fertile males (cats) may have undetectable amounts at given times during the day. Testosterone is determined before and after administration of hCG or gonadotropin releasing hormone (GnRH). A substantial increase in testosterone signifies the presence of testicular tissue. A widely accepted protocol for hCG or GnRH stimulation testing in dogs and cats has not been established; therefore, consultation with the laboratory performing the testosterone determination is recommended to determine the dose of hCG or GnRH to administer to the patient.

Luteinizing Hormone

Rare Indications ● To evaluate pituitary responsiveness.

Sample ● Serum must be promptly removed from RBCs and kept frozen until assayed because LH is labile, especially at room temperature. LH can be measured before and 10 minutes after GnRH administration (250 ng/kg, intravenously in dogs). RIA used for determination.

Artifactual Change ● There is cross-reactivity between the LH assay and pregnant mare serum gonadotropin (PMSG) but not with hCG. Hemolysis, icterus, and lipemia do not interfere with the assay.

Interpretation ● Determination of basal LH alone is not helpful except to assess an absence of gonadal hormone negative feedback. LH concentrations increase above the ranges of sexually intact animals within days of gonadectomy

in males and females. Some dogs with testicular failure have also been found to have increased levels of LH.

Estradiol

Sample ● Serum is used. Storage on RBCs and at room temperature may decrease the concentration. RIA is used for determination.

Artifactual Changes ● There is insignificant cross-reactivity between the RIA for estradiol-17β and other endogenous steroid hormones except estriol and estradiol-17α. Administration of radioactivity and exogenous estrogens may directly affect the assay. Cross-reactivity may vary with the assay system.

Interpretation ● Estradiol assays are available but have not been particularly useful for evaluating dogs and cats because normal serum concentrations in these species are at or below the level of detection for the assays. Therefore, normal and abnormal conditions cannot always be differentiated.

Miscellaneous

Assays for FSH are not readily available at this time.

ANCILLARY TESTS

Animals suspected of having intersex conditions or abnormal gonadal development may be karyotyped. If infectious diseases are suspected, microbiology and serology are indicated. Fine-needle aspirates are easily obtained from the testes, epididymides, and prostate, as well as from vaginal lesions. Biopsy specimens can be obtained from any part of the reproductive tract, although gonadal biopsy might have deleterious effects on remaining normal tissue.

Complete Blood Count

Hematologic abnormalities are not specific for any disease process; however, several reproductive disorders cause characteristic changes in the hemogram. The packed cell volume (PCV) and hemoglobin concentrations of pregnant bitches and queens decline after about day 20 of gestation. They continue to decline until parturition, when PCVs of 30.6% ± 0.8 can be expected in bitches (Concannon, 1986). WBC counts of pregnant animals may be slightly increased because of a mature neutrophilia. Dogs are very sensitive to the toxic effects of estrogens on bone marrow stem cells. Thrombocytopenia and anemia can occur when pharmacologic doses of estrogens are administered and also because of estrogen-producing Sertoli cell tumors.

Changes in the leukogram are uncommon with reproductive disorders unless an overt "abscess" exists. Neutrophilic leukocytosis with a left shift, variable degrees of neutrophil toxicity, and monocytosis are common in animals with mastitis, metritis, and prostatic abscesses. The leukogram of animals with pyometra is variable, although leukocytosis with a left shift is most often present. Profound leukocytosis (100,000–200,000/mm³) with a left shift may be present in animals with a closed-cervix pyometra. Conversely, a leukopenia with a degenerative left shift may be found in animals with severe sepsis due to pyometra or prostatic abscessation.

References

Barsanti JA, Finco DR: Evaluation of techniques for diagnosis of canine prostatic disease. JAVMA 1984; 185:198–200.

Barsanti JA, Prasse KW, Crowell WA, et al: Evaluation of various technique for diagnosis of chronic bacterial prostatitis in the dog. JAVMA 1983; 183:219–224.

Bowen RA, Olson PN, Behrendl MD, et al: Efficacy and toxicity of estrogens commonly used to terminate canine pregnancy. JAVMA 1985; 186:783–788.

Chastain CB, Schmidt B: Galactorrhea associated with hypothyroidism in intact bitches. JAAHA 1980; 16:851–854.

Concannon PW: Canine pregnancy and parturition. Vet Clin North Am Small Anim Pract 1986; 16:453–476.

George LW, Duncan JR, Carmichael LE: Semen examination in dogs with canine brucellosis. Am J Vet Res 1979; 40:1589–1595.

Hegstad RL: Use of a rapid qualitative ELISA technique to determine serum progesterone concentrations in the bitch. Proceedings, Society of Theriogenology, Coeur d'Alene, ID, September 1989, pp 277–287.

Johnston SD, Larsen RE, Olson PS: Canine theriogenology. J Soc Theriogenol 1982; 2:51–109.

Olar TT, Amann RP, Pickett BW: Relationships among testicular size, daily production and output of spermatozoa, and extragonadal spermatozoal reserves in the dog. Biol Reprod 1983; 29:1114–1120.

Olson PN, Thrall MA, Wykes PM, et al: Vaginal cytology. Part I. A useful tool for staging the canine estrous cycle. Comp Cont Ed 1984a; 6:288–297.

Olson PN, Thrall MA, Wykes PM, et al: Vaginal cytology. Part II. Its use in diagnosing canine reproductive disorders. Comp Cont Ed 1984b; 6:385–390.

Shille VM, Olson PN: Dynamic testing in reproductive endocrinology. In Kirk RW: Current Veterinary Therapy X. WB Saunders, Philadelphia, 1989, p 1282.

Thrall MA, Olson PN, Freemyer FG: Cytologic diagnosis of canine prostatic disease. JAAHA 1985; 21:95–102.

Verhage HG, Beamer NB, Brenner RM: Plasma levels of estradiol and progesterone in the cat during polyestrus, pregnancy and pseudopregnancy. Biol Reprod 1976; 14:579–585.

Joane Parent

14 Neurologic Disorders

DIAGNOSTIC APPROACH

The neurologic examination is the first and most important step toward a diagnosis. The objective is to localize the lesion, trying to account for all of the abnormalities with one lesion. If this is not possible, then a multifocal or diffuse disease is diagnosed. Clinicians should follow a routine when performing the examination to avoid missing any steps. A neurologic examination sheet should be used, allowing a more objective subsequent reevaluation (Table 14–1).

The following are general guidelines regarding lesion localization. Abnormal mental status suggests an intracranial lesion. The lesion is in the thalamocortex if there is behavioral change or seizure activity, or in the brainstem (i.e., midbrain, pons, medulla) if there is altered consciousness (depression, stupor, coma). Evaluation of the gait and posture may detect ataxia. Ataxia, deviation of the animal's body from the main axis (i.e., the vertebral column), can be caused by a lesion in the cerebellum, vestibular system, or ascending proprioceptive pathways. Vestibular ataxia causes concomitant head tilt. Cerebellar disorders cause ataxia in all limbs if the lesion is bilateral, or on the ipsilateral side if it is unilateral. There will be no proprioceptive deficits because ascending proprioceptive pathways to the cortex are intact, plus strength is preserved because descending motor pathways from the cortex to the lower motor neurons are intact. These animals are characteristically bouncy and spastic when ambulating. Proprioceptive ataxia due to involvement of ascending proprioceptive pathways is accompanied by inherent weakness from paralleled involvement of the descending motor pathways. Although weakness is not always obvious, lethargy and heaviness accompany the gait. By process of elimination, proprioceptive ataxia can be more easily diagnosed.

Cranial and spinal nerve deficits are valuable

Table 14-1 NEUROLOGIC EXAMINATION

MENTAL STATUS:

GAIT & POSTURE:

CRANIAL NERVE REFLEXES

II (Optic nerve & visual pathways)
Menace   L   R
Funduscopy   L   R

III (Oculomotor)
Resting pupil size:
• PLR: L   R
• Strabismus

IV (Trochlear)
Strabismus

V (Trigeminal)
Motor: Mandibular
Sensory: • Ophthalmic
         • Maxillary
         • Mandibular

VI (Abducent)
Strabismus

VII (Facial)
   L   R

VIII (Vestibular)
—Head tilt
—Nystagmus:
physiologic
abnormal: resting:
            positional:

IX, X (Glossopharyngeal, vagus)
Larynx-pharynx
XII (Hypoglossal)

SPINAL REFLEXES

1. Extensor (radial nerve)   L   R

2. Flexor   LF   RF
           LH   RH
   Crossed Extensor:
3. Patellar   L   R
4. Perineal   L   R
5. Muscle tone:

POSTURAL REACTIONS

1. Hopping   LF   RF
             LH   RH
2. Proprioceptive positioning
             LF   RF
             LH   RH

PAIN PERCEPTION

ASSESSMENT OF EXAM:

---

for localizing lesions within the neuraxis—the cranial nerves for the brainstem and the spinal nerves for the spinal cord. Counting mentally from 2 to 12 is the best way not to overlook cranial nerves while performing an examination. The funduscopic examination is a vital part. Because the optic nerve is a direct projection of brain tissue, the eyes may be involved by extension of a disease process (e.g., feline infectious peritonitis, canine distemper, and so on). Postural reactions are nonlocalizing by themselves but add information about severity of the lesion. With thalamocortical disease, these reactions may be absent contralateral to the lesion, despite the appearance of a normal gait. Pain perception is important for prognostication. Based on localization of the lesion, a differential diagnosis is generated. This in turn dictates the tests to be performed.

The information gathered from the neurologic examination is combined with the history, signalment, and physical examination findings. In some cases, the history is invaluable in establishing the diagnosis (road accident, known exposure to toxin, and so on). The signalment is important because many neurologic disorders

have a breed predisposition or a genetic cause (e.g., intervertebral disk disease of dachshunds, cervical vertebral instability of Dobermans, idiopathic epilepsy of German shepherds, and so on). Therefore, it is worthwhile to check a recent neurology text when an unusual breed is presented with deficits.

The physical examination plus the hematology findings (complete blood count [CBC]), biochemical profile, and urinalysis reveal if the disorder is restricted to the nervous system or involves other systems. It also evaluates the general health status of a patient before more specific testing is done, because many tests require general anesthesia. When the nervous system is affected secondary to a metabolic or toxic disorder, the abnormalities are usually generalized and symmetric in character (e.g., polyneuropathies, generalized seizure activity).

The cerebrospinal fluid (CSF) analysis is typically the most valuable and most readily available test for intracranial disease. Computed tomography (CT) and magnetic resonance imaging (MRI) are useful when a space-occupying lesion is suspected; however, they are expensive and not always available. For spinal cord disorders, survey radiographs, CSF analysis, and myelography are usually indicated. When the disorder affects the peripheral nervous system, fascicular nerve and muscle biopsies are often the most useful tests. Electrodiagnostics are more rewarding for peripheral nervous system lesions than for central nervous system (CNS) disorders. For CNS lesions, these tests are useful for prognostication and evaluation of response to treatment.

CEREBROSPINAL FLUID ANALYSIS

Frequent Indications • The CSF analysis is for the CNS what the CBC is for other systems. Every time a CNS disorder is suspected, a CSF analysis is warranted. It is unusual for primary CNS inflammatory diseases to cause changes in the CBC or serum biochemical profile. If abnormalities are noted in a CBC or profile, a multisystemic disorder has probably seeded the CNS secondarily. CSF analysis is indicated even if the CBC and profile are normal. Repeated CSF analysis can be helpful to evaluate response to treatment or to obtain baseline data before discontinuation of treatment. Although this procedure requires general anesthesia, CSF is the only readily accessible tissue that evaluates current CNS status. It is good practice to collect and analyze CSF obtained at the time of myelographic contrast agent injection.

Contraindications • Whenever the neurologic examination suggests increased intracranial pressure or tentorial herniation (as illustrated by altered consciousness, head pressing, anisocoria), obtaining CSF may precipitate or aggravate tentorial herniation. In such patients, CT or MRI should be performed first, if possible. If CT and MRI are not available, such patients should be handled as if increased intracranial pressure is present. Premedication with dexamethasone (0.25 mg/kg) to decrease the CSF production, followed by isoflurane anesthesia with hyperventilation to lower the partial pressure of carbon dioxide, minimizes risks. Monitoring blood gases ensures that the ventilation is adequate. Dexamethasone given 10 to 20 minutes before anesthesia does not alter the CSF cell count or protein concentration. Intravenous mannitol infusion can also be used to decrease intracranial pressure.

Technique for Collection • CSF is collected from the cerebellomedullary cistern. The anatomic landmarks are well known for that site, and

there tends to be less blood contamination than with lumbar puncture. The animal is anesthetized using gas anesthetic and positioned in right lateral recumbency for a right-handed clinician or left lateral recumbency for a left-handed clinician.* The patient's head and neck are brought to the edge of the table (to allow free hand motion for the clinician during collection), and the neck is flexed toward the chest. The point of insertion is at the crossing of two imaginary lines, one pulled between the *anterior* border of the wings of the atlas and the other from the occipital crest to meet the first line at a 90° angle. A 20- to 22-gauge 1½-inch spinal needle is used. The needle is inserted perpendicular to the skin. The lateral side of the hand used to insert the needle is supported by the patient's head so that the insertion is carefully controlled. When the subarachnoid space is entered, a sudden decrease in the resistance to the needle is felt. During the procedure, the stylet may be removed several times to ascertain if this space has been entered. Once the subarachnoid space has been entered, the collection is done by free flow into a red-top tube, and the sample (1 ml) is submitted for analysis. A red-top tube is preferred over an EDTA tube because there are usually no coagulation factors in the CSF, and EDTA increases the measured protein concentration while diluting a sample that is already low in cells.

Difficulties Related to the Collection • If the spinal needle is inserted into the spinal cord or caudal brainstem, mild to severe neurologic abnormalities (including death) may result. In mild cases, the animal recovers from anesthesia with body curvature, tetraparesis, and ataxia that are more pronounced on the side of the lesion. Nystagmus is often present. In severe cases, the animal has to be ventilated after the collection and may be severely tetraparetic, unable to get up or to lift its head during recovery. In a few patients, unassisted breathing does not return.

Practicing collection shortly after death in dogs and cats selected for euthanasia is a way of gaining experience. Because of reflux of blood into the cranial vault after heart arrest, the CSF pressure is maintained for many minutes after death. If a clinician does not collect CSF and analyze it a few times each month, the test is better left to a referral center where it is routinely performed.

---

*An assistant is required to firmly hold the patient's head and neck.

Analysis • Routine CSF evaluation includes appearance, red blood cell (RBC) and nucleated cell counts, cytology, and protein concentration. Ideally, the laboratory performing the analysis should be located close enough so that the sample can be analyzed within an hour of collection. The laboratory should be experienced in handling CSF. These drawbacks make it necessary for many private practices to develop an in-house system. Appearance, CSF cell counts, cellular sedimentation, and a protein estimate all can be performed in-house. The slide and leftover CSF are then sent to a laboratory for cytologic evaluation and protein quantitation.

Appearance • Normal CSF is colorless and clear. Discoloration corresponds to the number of RBCs or nucleated cells present. A visible discoloration is evident when at least 700 RBCs/μl or 200 nucleated cells/μl are present (Rand et al., 1990b). The most common source of RBCs is blood contamination during collection. When this occurs, the clinician can often see a swirl of blood surrounded by clear CSF during sampling. Centrifugation of the sample helps in differentiating between blood contamination and previous hemorrhage. Discoloration that persists after centrifugation suggests previous hemorrhage, whereas iatrogenic blood contamination has a clear supernatant. Centrifugation should be done after cell counts and cytology have been completed because centrifugation destroys the cells. Anticoagulants are usually unnecessary because CSF does not normally have coagulation factors. If the sample appears frankly turbid, an EDTA anticoagulated sample may also be taken to aid in cytologic evaluation.

Cell Counts • The CSF cell counts are performed using a Neubauer's hemocytometer chamber. Each side of the hemocytometer chamber is charged with one drop of *fresh undiluted* CSF. After the cells are allowed to settle for 10 minutes, all the cells on each side of the chamber are counted. The average of the two sides is calculated and then multiplied by 1.1 to produce the number of cells $\times$ 10^6/L of CSF. It is imperative to count RBCs and nucleated cells separately so blood contamination can be evaluated.

Cytology • The CSF nucleated cell count is normally very low; therefore, it is necessary to concentrate the cells. Centrifugation destroys the cells. Two concentration techniques are commonly used: the cytocentrifugation technique

for commercial laboratories and the sedimentation technique for in-house use. Cytocentrifugation requires relatively expensive equipment,* has an average cell retrieval of approximately 15%, and maintains excellent cellular morphology. It is important for the commercial laboratory to fill the cytocentrifuge chambers carefully using the same amount of CSF each time so an estimate of cellular retrieval for quality control is possible. The sedimentation preparation is inexpensive, can be done in-house, and has a cell retrieval of approximately 25% (Jamison and Lumsden, 1988). The apparatus consists of a 15-mm-diameter plastic cylinder† fixed to a glass slide with petroleum jelly. One-half milliliter of CSF is pipetted into the chamber (Fig. 14–1), and the cells are allowed to sediment for half an hour. The supernatant is then aspirated with a Pasteur's pipette, the cylinder removed, the edge of the remaining fluid gently blotted while the slide is tilted slightly, and the adherent cells quickly air dried by waving the slide vigorously. The cytology is done in-house if the expertise is available. If not, the unstained slide is sent to a clinical pathologist experienced in CSF cytology for differential cell count.

Protein Concentration • Protein concentration can be estimated at the time of collection using a

---

*Shandon-Elliot Cytocentrifuge, Southern Instruments Ltd., Surrey, England.
†Culturette Tube, Fisher Scientific, 184 Railside, Don Mills, Ontario, Canada.

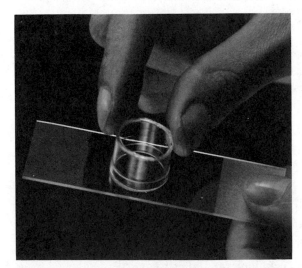

Figure 14–1 A microscope slide with a plastic well attached for the purpose of allowing cells in CSF to sediment to the slide for cytologic evaluation.

urinary dipstick.* The readings are negative, trace, 30 mg/dl, 100 mg/dl, and 500 mg/dl. The results are reliable below 30 mg/dl and at 100 mg/dl or above. However, when the results fall around 30 mg/dl, mild to moderate increases (33–60 mg/dl) in protein concentration may be missed and read as normal (Jacobs et al., 1990). This estimate should always be followed by a quantitative analysis done at a reputable laboratory.

Great care must be given to CSF analysis. The collection cannot be easily repeated because it necessitates general anesthesia, is sometimes hazardous for the patient, and is expensive for the client. Great care must be exercised to maximize the reliability of the results.

Normal Values • The reference ranges for canine and feline CSF are presented in Table 14–2. The laboratory report should include the gross appearance of the fluid, RBC and nucleated cell counts, the total number of cells counted on the slide preparation, the differential cell count, and the protein quantitation. The clinical pathologist should include an absolute count of the cells present on the slide preparation. Both concentration techniques result in loss of a large number of cells, cytocentrifuge causing twice as much loss as sedimentation. When a nucleated cell count is observed, often only a few cells are present. In our laboratory, we usually request two cytocentrifuge preparations from the same CSF sample and combine the evaluations of the two preparations to improve the reliability of the results. For example, a differential cell count of 75% neutrophils is meaningless if only four cells were present on the slide preparation.

---

*Chemstrip 9, Boehringer Mannheim LTD, Laval, PQ, Canada.

Table 14–2 REFERENCE RANGES FOR FELINE AND CANINE CEREBROSPINAL FLUID

	Feline*	Canine†
WBCs (× 10⁶/L)	≤2	≤3
RBCs (× 10⁶/L)	≤30	≤30
Cytology (%)		
• Monocytoid cells	69–100	87
• Lymphocytes	0–27	4
• Neutrophils	0–9	3
• Eosinophils	0	0
• Macrophages (large foamy mononuclear cells)	0–3	6
• Protein (mg/dl)	≤36	≤33

*(Data from Rand et al., 1990b.)
†(Data from Jamison, 1992a.)

Difficulties Related to Analysis • The major drawback of the CSF analysis is that the sample must be processed within 1 hour of collection. Few veterinary hospitals can get the sample to a laboratory so that it is analyzed within that hour. Furthermore, many laboratories do not have stringent procedures for handling CSF. For example, some laboratories do not perform cytology if the nucleated cell count is < 5 to 10 cells × 10⁶/L, even though the cytology may be abnormal despite a normal cell count. With normal cell counts, an absolute nucleated cell count of a few to 50 cells is to be expected on two cytocentrifuge preparations (using 200 μl of CSF per preparation). With nucleated cell counts of ≥ 2 cells × 10⁶/L, more than 50 cells should consistently be present on the cytology slides. The sedimentation technique, although not providing as good a cellular morphology as cytocentrifugation, allows better cell retrieval. Rapid drying of the slide and protection from heat and moisture are essential for preservation of cellular morphology. The *unstained* slide is sent to a clinical pathologist experienced with CSF. The CSF left after sedimentation and cellular counts is sent for quantitative analysis of protein concentration.

Effects of Drug Therapies • Steroids reduce the nucleated cell count, the neutrophil and lymphocyte counts, and the protein concentration (Jamison, 1990b), regardless of the ongoing disease process. If at all possible, the CSF analysis should be done before steroid treatment (except as noted earlier under Contraindications).

Blood Contamination • An RBC count > 30 × 10⁶/L represents contamination with blood. It has been found, at least in cats, that the RBC count is significantly correlated with the nucleated cell count and the neutrophil percentage (Rand et al., 1990b). An increase of one leukocyte for every 100 RBCs was observed with RBC counts of 30 to 1700 × 10⁶/L. With these counts, 0 to 67% neutrophils were present on cytology. The eosinophil percentage increased from 0 to 15% on these same samples. Although blood contamination can be unavoidable, it is important to consider it during interpretation. It may significantly alter other measured CSF variables. When the blood contamination is > 1700 cells × 10⁶/L, the analysis cannot be relied on.

CSF Interpretation • Table 14–3 presents a summary of canine and feline CSF analysis results according to specific disease entities. Although

Table 14-3 CANINE AND FELINE CEREBROSPINAL FLUID ANALYSIS IN VARIOUS CONDITIONS

	Appearance	RBCs/ μl*	WBCs/ μl	Protein (mg/dl)	Pándy	Cytology
Normal	Clear, colorless	0	<5	<30	−	Mononuclear
Degenerative	Clear, colorless	N	N	↑ to ↑↑	+/−	Mononuclear
Neoplastic	Clear, colorless	N to ↑	N to ↑	N to ↑↑	+/−	Rarely see tumor cells
Inflammatory						
Bacterial	Hazy to cloudy	N to ↑↑	↑↑ to ↑↑↑	↑↑ to ↑↑↑	+	Neutrophils early, mixed population later
Viral	Clear, colorless	N	N to ↑↑	N to ↑↑	+/−	Mononuclear
Feline infectious peritonitis	Hazy to cloudy	N to ↑↑↑	↑↑ to ↑↑↑	↑↑ to ↑↑↑	+	Mixed mononuclear and neutrophils
Fungal	Clear to cloudy	N to ↑↑	↑ to ↑↑↑	↑ to ↑↑↑	+	Neutrophils early, mixed population later
Protozoal	Clear	N to ↑	↑ to ↑↑	↑↑ to ↑↑↑	+	Mixed
Parasitic	Clear to xanthochromia	N to ↑↑	↑↑ to ↑↑↑	↑↑ to ↑↑↑	+	Mixed with eosinophils
Rickettsial	Clear, colorless	N to ↑	N to ↑↑↑	N to ↑↑↑	+/−	Mononuclear; neutrophils with Rocky Mountain spotted fever
Granulomatous meningo-encephalitis	Clear to cloudy	N to ↑↑	↑↑ to ↑↑↑	↑ to ↑↑	+	Mononuclear
Traumatic	Xanthochromia	↑↑↑	N to ↑	N to ↑	+/−	Blood contamination
Vascular (ischemia)	Clear, colorless	N	N	N to ↑	+/−	Mononuclear

*RBC count must always be considered in light of possible iatrogenic contamination.
N, normal; + positive; − negative; ↑, slight increase; ↑↑, moderate increase; ↑↑↑, marked increase; mixed, mixed population of mononuclear and polymorphonuclear cells.

tables help ensure that all diseases have been considered, they are not always helpful in establishing a final diagnosis because overlaps exist. The CSF of many diseases has been described, but rarely is consideration given to whether steroid treatment has preceded CSF collection. Furthermore, the time between collection and postmortem study is seldom reported; therefore, we have poor knowledge of the correlation between postmortem anatomopathologic diagnosis and CSF analysis. The following guidelines should help veterinary clinicians reach a decision for managing patients.

At the time of CSF analysis, the signalment, onset of clinical signs, physical examinations, lesion localization, hematology, and biochemical profile are known. If abnormalities are noted on the physical examination or blood studies, the disorder is likely multisystemic, and investigating that abnormality may be diagnostically rewarding. Thrombocytopenia associated with a CNS disorder may lead to a diagnosis of *Ehrlichia canis* (see Chapter 15). A nonregenerative anemia in a young dog with a poor appetite and neurologic signs suggests an infectious disorder; appropriate titers may be considered (see Canine Distemper, Chapter 15).

If, however, the findings on the physical examination and the blood studies are normal, the disease is limited to the CNS, and then the CSF analysis becomes very specific in suggesting a diagnosis. Because CSF is contained between meningeal layers, analyzing it is more rewarding when the meninges are involved. Deep parenchymal disease may lead to very few abnormalities (if any), especially when the clinical syndrome is mild and acute. Neutrophils are the first cells on site in an inflammatory response. The more neutrophils present, the more active the inflammatory process. Chronic idiopathic inflammatory CNS disease is common and may hide multiple causes. Many of these diseases are responsive to steroids. Before diagnosing such a syndrome, especially in dogs younger than 2 years and in the elderly, the possibility of an infectious disorder should be considered and ruled out. If the cytology primarily reveals neutrophils, an infectious disease must be included in the differential diagnosis. Infectious diseases characteristically do not clinically wax and wane; a patient steadily deteriorates, and evidence of the infection might be noted on the physical examination (e.g., fever) or blood tests. In idiopathic CNS diseases that may be immune mediated, the cytologic picture can also be primarily neutrophilic. In these idiopathic syndromes, the clinical picture varies and transient periods of remission may be erroneously attributed to medical treatments. Neutrophilic pleocytosis is frequently observed with canine meningioma.

Small lymphocytes take more time to appear and represent an antigenic response. Predominantly lymphocytic cytology is seen with immune-mediated diseases, chronic inflammatory diseases, and the recovery period of self-limiting inflammatory diseases. The higher the small lymphocyte count, the more likely the syndrome is to respond to steroids. Macrophages are "cleaning-up" cells. An almost pure population of macrophages denotes a degenerative disease. Cellular storage diseases, posttraumatic head injury, and chronic encephalopathy are examples of such degenerative problems. A mixed population of neutrophils, lymphocytes, macrophages, and other mononuclear cells suggests a chronic active inflammatory disease with antigenic response, such as granulomatous meningoencephalomyelitis. Eosinophils are normally not present in the CSF. A primarily eosinophilic pleocytosis is probably due to an allergic syndrome, whereas lesser numbers may indicate neoplasia or parasitic infiltration (Smith-Maxie et al., 1989).

A few patterns of CSF response are noteworthy. A lack of cellularity is typically associated with CNS cryptococcosis (see Chapter 15). Neutrophils are commonly absent in encephalitis due to canine distemper and E. canis. Neutrophilic pleocytosis results from canine meningiomas. Neoplastic cells are extremely rare in primary CNS neoplasms of cats and dogs.

Because the albumin and most of the protein in CSF originate from the blood, protein increases in the CSF are indicative of a blood-brain barrier breakdown. Local synthesis of immunoglobulins cannot, however, be ruled out. Until the repeatability of the techniques and results for CSF protein electrophoresis and immunoglobulins are established between laboratories, we will not be able to differentiate transudation from local synthesis (Rand et al., 1990a; Jamison, 1992a).

Other Measured CSF Variables • Measurements of glucose, lactate dehydrogenase (LD), creatine kinase (CK), and aspartate transaminase (AST) in the CSF currently have limited usefulness. Until we can measure specific CNS isoenzymes, the CSF fluid is better used for routine tests. Measurement of intracranial pressure also has limited value. However, measurement of CSF immunoglobulins seems promising. Once the techniques become readily available, the IgG index (CSF [IgG]/serum [IgG] × serum [albumin]/CSF [albumin]) may enable clinicians to differentiate transudation of serum protein into CSF versus local synthesis of immunoglobulins.

Bacterial culture of the CSF is rarely rewarding, even when bacteria are seen on the cytology. The CSF would be better used for measurement of the routine parameters.

NEUROIMAGING

Spinal radiographs (survey and myelography) for diseases of the vertebral column and spinal cord and CT/MRI for diseases of the brain are diagnostically the most useful studies. Bullae radiographs are helpful in the diagnosis of middle/inner ear diseases. Skull radiographs are advised when CT and MRI are unavailable. Although they rarely lead to a diagnosis, they are inexpensive and may detect bony skull involvement, intracranial dense space-occupying lesions, and in some cases distortion of the cerebellar tentorium.

The quality of the radiographs, adequate preparation of the animal, and the position of the animal are important when performing and interpreting radiographs. Neuroradiography should be done with the animal under general anesthesia. It is a waste of time and money to attempt spinal radiographic study of an animal with manual restraint or sedation alone, especially if it is painful. As an example, in intervertebral disk disease, the relaxation provided by sedation is never adequate to relieve the muscle spasms present at the diseased site. The position of the animal is also of crucial importance. The animal must be in perfect lateral recumbency. Ribs in superposition is the checkpoint. The vertebral column must be parallel to the table throughout its length. The checkpoint is to make sure that the ends of the vertebrae are not visible, which would denote a curvature in the dog's body. Foam pads are often necessary to ensure a perfectly straight spine.

In the cervical area, the C4–5 intervertebral space is often erroneously read as abnormal. A dog's head and thorax are of different sizes. If appropriate padding is not used, an upward concavity of the spine results. Two lateral views should be taken: upper and lower cervical. For the upper cervical ventrodorsal view, the animal should be extubated. For thoracolumbar (T3–L3) study, three lateral views are necessary: thoracic, thoracolumbar, and lumbar. For lumbosacral study, a cone-down of the area is done. The ventrodorsal views are matched with the lateral views. The same views are repeated for the myelographic study with a cone-down of the suspicious area. In most cases of thoracolumbar disk disease (if not all), the diseased site is observable on survey radiographs. The myelogram provides information on the extent of spinal cord involvement and on the lateralization of the lesion. This dictates the surgical approach.

Myelography should be left to an experienced clinician in the facility where the animal is scheduled for neurosurgery. For lesions below

T1, the contrast injections are done at the L5–6 intervertebral space. Cervical injections are used for cervical lesions. Poor technique and positioning are the most common causes of misdiagnosis in spinal column diseases.

Bullae series are not very rewarding in the diagnosis of middle/inner ear diseases. Only advanced or severe changes can be observed on radiographs. Destructive bony lesions (infectious, neoplastic) of the tympanic bullae and narrowing of the external canals with and without calcifications are obvious. Most times only a subtle increase in density between tympanic bullae is noted. Textbooks advocate five views: lateral, dorsoventral, two obliques, and an open mouth. The latter three are the most useful. MRI is preferable if available. Extubation should also be done for the dorsoventral view of the skull. If a space-occupying lesion is suspected, we advise two lateral views of the skull: right and left sided.

ELECTRODIAGNOSTICS

Very few veterinary practices can justify the purchase of electrodiagnostic equipment. Electromyography is the most widely used of these tests and probably the most useful. Surgical facilities may benefit from having this equipment in-house. The diagnostic workup of myopathies, neuropathies, neuromuscular diseases, nerve sheath tumors, nerve entrapment, and cauda equina syndrome is enhanced by the use of electromyography, nerve conduction velocities, and repetitive nerve stimulations. In some cases, electromyography helps in lesion localization; in other cases, it offers an evaluation of the function versus the anatomopathologic evaluation that muscle/nerve biopsies provide.

Brainstem auditory evoked responses (BAER), visual evoked potentials, and somatosensory evoked potentials assess the ascending pathways. BAER is the most useful diagnostically. It is used as an objective screening test in animals suspected of having congenital nerve deafness. It also aids in the diagnosis of vestibular syndromes. By allowing evaluation of the cochlear part of the vestibulocochlear nerve, it helps diagnose idiopathic peripheral vestibular disorders when only the vestibular part of the nerve is affected. BAER also offers a noninvasive way to evaluate the brainstem. It is particularly helpful in evaluating response to treatment in animals that previously had a BAER. Electroencephalography has been poorly used in veterinary medicine; its usefulness has been controversial.

CREATINE KINASE

Infrequent Indications • Suspected muscle disorder. Patients have generalized weakness but no ataxia. The weakness is displayed by a stiff, short-stride gait. The spinal reflexes in most cases are present but may be significantly decreased if the muscle disorder is severe. In slowly progressive cases, generalized muscle wasting may be the only abnormality. Advantage: The test is specific for skeletal muscle disease. Disadvantage: It is a sensitive indicator of muscle damage but has poor specificity for disease processes (Cardinet, 1989). Minor muscle injury due to intramuscular injections, restraint, and physical activities may increase serum CK activity.

Analysis • Storage of serum sample at any temperature results in a loss of CK activity. The method of choice for analysis adds a reducing agent to the incubation medium to reactivate the CK activities lost during storage. The normal values are "activated" values. If serum is not assayed immediately, it should be refrigerated. Avoid exposure to bright light. If samples are to be shipped or stored for longer than 2 days, they should be frozen.

Normal Values • As with other enzymes, these vary between laboratories, depending on technique and units used. At my laboratory, the high end of the reference range is ≤ 460 U/L for dogs and ≤ 580 U/L for cats.

Danger Values • None.

Artifacts • There are no interferences in recovery of values from hemolysis up to 1000 mg/dl of hemoglobin. Recovery is unaffected by lipemia.

Causes of Increased CK • Many laboratories include CK in their standard biochemical profile. As a result, more problems are associated with the interpretation of an increased CK than with inappropriate request of the test. CK is such a sensitive indicator of muscle damage that only large increases (≥ 10,000 U/L) or persistent increases, even if moderate (> 2000), generally are of clinical significance. Mild increases are observed with restraint, physical activity, intramuscular injections, prolonged recumbency, and muscle biopsies or operations. Moderate increases occur with trauma, convulsions, continuous trembling/shivering, and some neuropathies. Large increases are primarily observed with myositis. Feline obstructive urethral syndrome (CK is present in the urinary bladder) and muscle ischemia secondary to status epilepticus are occasionally observed with CK > 10,000 U/L. Because the half-life of CK is short, the test should always be repeated to determine if an increased activity persists. Persistent elevations are indicative of active myonecrosis and should be monitored diagnostically with electromyography (if available) and muscle/nerve biopsies.

Significant muscle disease may exist without concomitant presence of CK elevation. CK increases as a result of myonecrosis. If degenerative pathology predominates, CK may only be mildly elevated.

Myositis is uncommon. The causes can be infectious (e.g., *Neospora caninum*, *Toxoplasma gondii*), immune mediated (e.g., masticatory myositis, polymyositis), toxic (e.g., monensin poisoning), endocrine (e.g., hypothyroidism, hyperadrenocorticism), congenital (e.g., muscular dystrophy), nutritional (e.g., vitamin E or selenium), or exertional (e.g., exertional myopathy). Physical examination and blood studies help in differentiating between the causes. Histochemical analysis of muscle biopsy specimens is useful in defining myopathies. The laboratory processing the samples should be contacted ahead of time, and their protocol for storing and shipping the samples be adhered to rigidly.

ACETYLCHOLINE RECEPTOR ANTIBODY

Occasional Indications • Exercise-induced weakness, generalized weakness that worsens with exercise, and megaesophagus with or without concomitant presence of pharyngeal weakness and weak palpebral reflexes. Advantage: The test is fairly specific for myasthenia gravis. Disadvantage: Some dogs with myasthenia gravis are seronegative (i.e., have no detectable antibody against acetylcholine receptors) (Shelton et al., 1990).

Analysis • One milliliter of serum is necessary. The sample is sent on dry ice by an overnight carrier. See Appendix I for availability.

Normal Values • Values vary with laboratories.

Danger Values • None.

Drug Therapy That May Alter Results • In principle, steroids and other immunosuppressive drugs may lead to false-negative results.

Cause of Increased Titers • Myasthenia gravis. Two acquired forms of myasthenia gravis have been recognized: a generalized form and a restrictive form in which only the esophagus or pharynx is implicated. Repetitive nerve stimulation studies are also diagnostic but are often unavailable. Administration of edrophonium chloride, a short-acting acetylcholinesterase inhibitor, can be used as a diagnostic tool for myasthenia. However, most weak animals become stronger after administration of the drug, meaning that false-positive reactions are numerous.

Acknowledgment: The author would like to express his thanks to Dr. Patricia J. Luttgen for her permission to use certain material in this chapter.

Bibliography

Cardinet GH: Skeletal muscle function. *In* Kaneko JJ (ed): Clinical Biochemistry of Domestic Animals. 4th ed. Academic Press, San Diego, 1989, pp 481–486.

Jacobs RM, Cochrane SM, Lumsden JH, Norris AM: Relationship of cerebrospinal fluid protein concentration determined by dye-binding and urinary dipstick methodologies. Can Vet J 1990;31:587–588.

Jamison EM: Chapter one: Reference values for cerebrospinal fluid in healthy dogs, DVSc Thesis, University of Guelph, Ontario, Canada, 1992a.

Jamison EM: Chapter two: Cerebrospinal fluid analysis in dogs with inflammatory central nervous system disease treated with corticosteroids, DVSc Thesis, University of Guelph, Ontario, Canada, 1992b.

Jamison EM, Lumsden JH: Cerebrospinal fluid analysis in the dog: Methodology and interpretation. Semin Vet Med Surg (Small Anim) 1988;3:122–132.

Rand JS, Parent J, Jacobs R, Johnson R: Reference intervals for feline cerebrospinal fluid: Biochemical and serologic variables, IgG concentration, and electrophoretic fractionation. Am J Vet Res 1990a;51:1049–1054.

Rand JS, Parent J, Jacobs R, Percy D: Reference intervals for feline cerebrospinal fluid: Cell counts and cytologic features. Am J Vet Res 1990b;51:1044–1048.

Shelton GD, Willard MD, Cardinet GH, Lindstrom J: Acquired myasthenia gravis: Selective involvement of esophageal, pharyngeal and facial muscles. J Vet Intern Med 1990;4;281–284.

Smith-Maxie LL, Parent J, Rand JS, Norris AM: Cerebrospinal fluid analysis and clinical outcome of eight dogs with eosinophilic meningoencephalomyelitis. J Vet Intern Med 1989;3:167–174.

Michael R. Lappin
Grant H. Turnwald

15 Microbiology and Infectious Diseases

Infectious agents may be identified directly by cytologic analysis, histopathologic evaluation, culture, viral isolation, or antigen detection. Detec- tion of antibodies against infectious agents can provide indirect evidence of prior exposure or current infection. This chapter describes methods for obtaining specimens, outlines currently used testing procedures for the more common infectious diseases, and discusses interpretation of results from the various procedures and tests.

The assistance of Hollis Utah Cox, DVM, PhD, and Alma F. Roy, BS (MTASCP), with the culture and sensitivity section is acknowledged.

WHEN TO SUSPECT VIRAL / BACTERIAL /FUNGAL / RICKETTSIAL AGENTS

Infectious diseases should be considered on the differential list for most problems affecting dogs and cats, especially those with fever or other clinical signs of inflammation. Historical findings, physical examination findings, and findings on routine clinical pathologic testing are generally not pathognomonic for an infectious cause but help a veterinary clinician rank differentials and develop a logical diagnostic plan.

First of all, historical findings can increase the degree of suspicion for infectious diseases. Exposure to other infected animals or contaminated fomites is important for agents with direct transmission, such as those inducing respiratory tract disease (e.g., feline herpesvirus; canine bordetellosis) or gastroenteritis (e.g., canine and feline giardiasis; canine and feline parvovirus infection). Potential exposure to vectors (e.g., mosquitoes for dirofilariasis; ticks for Lyme borreliosis [*Ixodes* spp], ehrlichiosis [*Rhipicephalus sanguineus*], Rocky Mountain spotted fever [RMSF; *Dermacentor* spp.], babesiosis [*R. sanguineus*]) or appropriate travel history (e.g., coccidioidomycosis in the Southwest; RMSF in the Southeast; blastomycosis in the Mississippi, Missouri, and Ohio River valleys) can also suggest an infectious cause of clinical signs of disease. Vaccination history, deworming history, and the determination of whether other animals or people in the environment of an infected animal are also affected can aid in ranking infectious diseases on a differential diagnoses list.

Second, physical examination findings can suggest an infectious cause. Fever can be induced by infectious agents. Lymphadenopathy characterized cytologically as reactive lymphoid hyperplasia can be induced by infectious agents. Hepatosplenomegaly occurs as a result of the immunologic stimulation induced by chronic intracellular infections such as ehrlichiosis or brucellosis. Endogenous uveitis commonly occurs after infections by feline leukemia virus (FeLV), feline immunodeficiency virus (FIV), *Toxoplasma gondii,* and systemic mycoses. Mucopurulent discharges can suggest primary or secondary bacterial infections. Certain infectious diseases cause specific physical examination abnormalities such as dendritic ulcers (feline herpesvirus), chorea mycolonus (canine distemper virus), and testicular swelling and pain (canine brucellosis).

Finally, clinical pathologic abnormalities can suggest disease due to infectious agents. Neutrophilic leukocytosis, particularly if found concurrently with a left shift or degenerative neutrophils, is suggestive of inflammation induced by infectious agents. Monocytosis can be induced by persistent infection with a number of intracellular agents resulting in persistent infection. Polyclonal (e.g., multiple infectious etiologies) or monoclonal gammopathies (e.g., usually induced by neoplasia; rarely associated with canine ehrlichiosis) may suggest chronic immune stimulation. Neutrophils in aqueous humor, cerebrospinal fluid (CSF), synovial fluid, or urine may indicate inflammation induced by infectious diseases.

CYTOLOGY

Common Indications ● Cytologic examination of exudates, blood film, tissue imprint, aspiration biopsy, or wet mount of hair is indicated when bacterial and fungal diseases (and occasionally rickettsial and viral diseases) are suspected. Advantages: inexpensive, readily available, and may allow rapid confirmation and identification of an infectious agent. Disadvantages: Infectious agents cannot always be found, even though they may be responsible for the clinical signs of disease (e.g., ehrlichiosis, L-form bacterial infections); sometimes a presumptive cytologic diagnosis must be confirmed by other methods (e.g., histopathology); and cytology is of limited value in detecting viral inclusions except in acute canine distemper and feline viral respiratory diseases.

Specimen Procurement and Analysis

See also Chapter 16, Cytologic Techniques and Cytologic Conclusions.

Bacterial Diseases ● Discharges from animals with suspected bacterial disease should be placed on a microscope slide, air dried, fixed, and stained with both Gram's and Romanovsky's-type stains (see Chapter 16). The examination is started on low power (10 ×), with oil immersion (100 ×) used for inspection of bacterial morphologic features (i.e., rods or cocci) and Gram's stain characteristics (i.e., gram positive [blue] or gram negative [pink]). The primary disadvantage of Gram's staining is that gram-negative bacteria may be difficult to find because background material stains pink. It is easier to find bacteria (dark blue stain) and easier to study morphologic detail of other cells (i.e., inflammatory cells) using Romanovsky's-type stains. Gram's stain demonstrates the gram-positive, branching filaments of *Actinomyces* spp. and *Nocardia* spp. (Color Plate 4E). Acid-fast stains can be used for *Mycobacterium* spp. and to help differentiate *Nocardia* spp. (acid-fast) from *Actinomyces* spp.

Mixed bacterial populations identified in exudates can indicate anaerobic bacterial involvement (Dow and Jones, 1987). Anaerobic bacteria can produce lecithinase, which can destroy neutrophils; thus, cytology of thin exudates with many bacteria but few neutrophils may suggest anaerobic bacterial infection.

Some bacteria have characteristic morphologic features. Large rod-form bacteria containing spores found on fecal cytology of dogs or cats with diarrhea suggest *Clostridium perfringens* (see Chapter 9). Bipolar-staining, gram-negative coccobacilli found in aspirates of inflamed cervical lymph nodes from cats in the Southwest or West suggest *Yersinia pestis* (Macy and Gasper, 1990). Spirochetes found on fecal cytology of animals with diarrhea suggest campylobacteriosis (Fox, 1990).

To demonstrate inclusion bodies in acute feline chlamydial conjunctivitis, conjunctival scrapings are obtained with a flat spatula, smeared on a slide, stained with Romanovsky's-type stains, and examined for intracytoplasmic aggregations of *Chlamydia* spp.

Morulae of *Ehrlichia* spp. are rarely seen in the cytoplasm of mononuclear cells (*Ehrlichia canis*), neutrophils (*Ehrlichia ewingii*), or platelets (*Ehrlichia platys*). *Haemobartonella* spp. and *Babesia* spp. can sometimes be seen infecting canine or feline erythrocytes.

Fungal Diseases ● For identification of dermatophytes, hairs are plucked from the periphery of a lesion, placed on a microscope slide, and covered with 10% to 20% potassium hydroxide to clear debris. The slide is then heated (not boiled) and examined under the 10 × or 40 × objective to search for hyphae, spores, conidia, budding yeasts, and fungus-induced damage (e.g., broken hair shafts). The 40 × objective is used to identify arthrospores (dense aggregates of spherical structures that may cover the hair shaft [Color Plate 2C]). However, failure to find arthrospores by this method does not rule out dermatomycosis. Culture is more sensitive for diagnosis of dermatophytosis (see Fungal Culture, later).

Wet mount preparations may be used when looking for fungi other than dermatophytes (see Chapter 16, Selected Etiologic Agents). Blue-black Parker's ink may also be added to the wet mount to aid in outlining the fungus. India ink (one drop of ink plus one drop of water) demonstrates encapsulated yeasts (*Cryptococcus neoformans*) and is of most use in central nervous system (CNS) infection. Romanovsky's-type stains are useful in identifying yeasts such as *Blastomyces dermatitidis*, *Histoplasma capsulatum*, or *Coccidioides immitis* in exudates, lymph node aspiration cytology, or transtracheal aspiration cytology.

Potassium hydroxide should not be mixed with india ink because it causes the carbon particles in the ink to precipitate. False "halos" may appear around leukocytes and debris when they are first stained with india ink, but these disappear in about 30 minutes.

Cutaneous Parasitic Diseases ● For demonstration of *Cheyletiella* spp., a piece of transparent adhesive tape is gently pressed against areas with crusts or dandruff and then placed on a microscope slide. After the tape test, the hair is clipped, mineral oil is placed on the skin as well as on a microscope slide, and the skin is scraped using a blunt number 10 scalpel blade. For skin scrapings to look for *Demodex* spp., the skin should be immobilized and mites expressed from follicles by pinching and scraping the extruded material. For scrapings to look for *Sarcoptes* spp. or *Cheyletiella* spp., the scraping is continued more superficially (induce a mild capillary ooze) over a larger surface area. After transfer of the scraping, the microscope slide field is scanned at 10 × for mites.

Viral Diseases ● In dogs, blood smears can be examined for distemper virus inclusions in lymphocytes, neutrophils, and erythrocytes (Color Plates 1D and 1E).

CULTURE AND ANTIMICROBIAL SUSCEPTIBILITY

Common Indications ● Culture and antimicrobial susceptibility is indicated in most suspected bacterial diseases, especially when clinical syndromes have been resistant to medications. Remember that skin and mucosal surfaces have a resident microflora (Table 15–1); therefore, care must be taken to avoid contamination. Advantages: usually allows the most effective treatment to be administered. Disadvantages: requires time for agents to grow; some organisms

Table 15–1 NORMAL BACTERIAL FLORA AT VARIOUS SITES IN DOGS AND CATS

Integument
Skin
  Aerobes
    Micrococcus spp.
    Staphylococcus spp.
    Streptococcus spp.
    Gram-negative rods including
      Pasteurella spp.
    Diphtheroids
  Anaerobes
    Clostridium spp.
  Ear
    Aerobes
      Staphylococcus spp.
      Corynebacterium spp.
      Streptococcus spp.
      Coliforms
      Bacillus spp.
    Yeast
      Malassezia spp.

Respiratory System
Nasal cavity, pharynx
  Aerobes
    Staphylococcus spp.
    Streptococcus spp.
    Neisseria spp.
    Corynebacterium spp.
    Escherichia coli
    Lactobacillus spp.
    Proteus spp.
  Anaerobes
    Clostridium spp.
    Bifidobacterium spp.
    Propionibacterium spp.
    Fusobacterium spp.
    Bacteroides spp.
  Trachea
    Streptococcus spp.
    Staphylococcus spp.
    Pasteurella spp.
    Klebsiella spp.
    Corynebacterium spp.

Eyes
Cornea and conjunctiva
  Aerobes
    Staphylococcus spp. (coagulase
      positive and negative)
    Nonhemolytic, alpha- and
      beta-hemolytic
      streptococci
    Bacillus spp.
    Pseudomonas spp.
    E. coli
    Corynebacterium spp.
    Neisseria spp.
    Moraxella spp.

Gastrointestinal Tract
Oral cavity and feces
  Aerobic
    Gram + *Streptococcus* spp.
            Staphylococcus spp.
            Bacillus spp.
            Corynebacterium spp.
    Gram − Enterobacteriaceae (especially *E. coli*,
              Enterobacter spp. and
              Klebsiella spp.)
            Pseudomonas spp.
            Proteus spp.
            Neisseria spp.
            Moraxella spp.
  Anaerobic
    Gram + *Clostridium* spp.
            Lactobacillus spp.
            Propionibacterium spp.
            Bifidobacterium spp. (feces)
    Gram − *Bacteroides* spp.
            Fusobacterium spp.
            Veillonella spp.
    Other   Spirochetes
            Mycoplasma spp.
            Yeasts

Genitourinary Tract
Distal urethra and prepuce
  Gram + *S. aureus*
          S. epidermidis
          Streptococcus spp.
          Mycoplasma spp.
          Bacillus spp.
          Corynebacterium spp.
  Gram − *Flavobacterium* spp.
          Haemophilus spp.
          Moraxella spp.
          Pasteurella spp.
          Klebsiella spp.

(Data compiled from Lorenz MD: Integumentary Infections; Thayer GW: Infections of the respiratory system; Martin CE: Ocular infections; Greene CE: Gastrointestinal, intraabdominal and hepatobiliary infections; Barsanti JA: Genitourinary tract infections. In Greene 1984; McKiernan et al. 1984; Cox et al. 1988.)

are fastidious or have special culture requirements; expense; and it is easy to contaminate or inactivate cultures, rendering results worthless.

Bacterial Culture

Specimen Procurement

Integument and Ear • In superficial pyoderma, hair is clipped from the surrounding area but disinfection is not attempted. A pustule is ruptured with a sterile fine-gauge needle, and a swab of the pus is obtained for culture.

In deep pyoderma, hair surrounding the lesion is clipped and the area is disinfected with an antiseptic (e.g., Novalsan). The lesion is squeezed to express exudate, which is collected on a swab. Gloves should be worn.

For culture of ears, a sterile otoscope cone is inserted to the level of the horizontal canal and the ear is swabbed through the cone. When middle ear infection is suspected, the animal is anesthetized and material for culture is retrieved by myringotomy using a sterile CSF needle placed through a sterile otoscope cone and used to penetrate the tympanum.

Respiratory System • Lower airway specimens are best obtained by transtracheal aspiration or bronchoalveolar lavage during bronchoscopy. Fine-needle pulmonary aspiration biopsy can also be used but has more risk for a patient (see Chapter 11). Bacteria can be isolated from the trachea in at least 35% of clinically healthy dogs (McKiernan et al., 1984). These are probably transient; common isolates are listed in Table 15–1. Because many of the organisms isolated from normal dogs have also been associated with lower respiratory tract inflammation, all transtracheal aspiration samples should be evaluated by culture, antimicrobial susceptibility, and cytology. Bacteria should not be considered significant unless accompanied by neutrophilic inflammation. *Mycoplasma* spp. have been isolated in pure culture from the lower airways of dogs with clinical signs of respiratory disease (Jameson et al., 1993). Culture for *Mycoplasma* spp. should be performed on all transtracheal aspiration samples; these samples need to be transported to the laboratory in Amies' medium or modified Stuart's bacterial transport medium. *Mycoplasma* spp. culture should be specifically requested.

Nasal specimens are best obtained from nasal lavage, core biopsy, or by passing a swab through a sterile otoscope cone (see Chapter 11). Pharyngeal specimens are best obtained by a guarded swab taken during pharyngoscopy. However, nasal and pharyngeal cultures are rarely useful because of the extensive normal flora in the nasal cavity and nasopharynx.

Gastrointestinal Tract • Primary bacterial gastroenteritis occasionally occurs in dogs and cats. *Salmonella* spp., *Campylobacter* spp., and *C. perfringens* are three of the most important genera. However, these organisms can also be isolated from normal animals. *Salmonella* spp. and *Campylobacter* spp. can cause small or mixed bowel diarrhea; *C. perfringens* is usually associated with large bowel diarrhea. Approximately 2 to 3 g of fresh feces should be submitted to the laboratory for optimal results. If a delay in transport of feces to the laboratory is expected, consult your laboratory for appropriate transport media. Because these organisms have special culture requirements, the laboratory must be notified of the suspected pathogen.

Genitourinary Tract • Urine obtained by cystocentesis is preferred for urine culture. If a patient is severely thrombocytopenic ($< 20,000/\mu l$) or if cystocentesis cannot be performed, catheterization or a midstream voided sample are alternate collection methods. Quantitative culture is indicated. Isolation of bacteria should always be assessed concurrently with the urine sediment. Rarely, difficult-to-diagnose urinary tract infections require maceration and culture of a bladder wall biopsy specimen. Calculi should be crushed with a sterile mortar and pestle and cultured.

Culture of the third fraction of an ejaculate (preferred) or prostatic massage is recommended for prostatic culture. Culture of the second fraction of an ejaculate is recommended for testicular culture. Culture of prostatic or testicular material retrieved by aspiration or biopsy can also be performed. Prostatic massage and closed prostatic aspiration or biopsy should be avoided in dogs with suspected prostatic abscesses. Obtaining distal urethral specimens for quantitative culture before and after ejaculation may help avoid confusion due to urethral contamination. Culture for *Mycoplasma* spp. or *Candida* spp. should be performed if pyuria is identified in the absence of calculi, masses, and aerobic bacteria. Anaerobic culture of urine or prostatic fluid is rarely indicated.

Central Nervous System • Bacterial infection of the canine and feline CNS is uncommon. Even when infection is present, low numbers of organisms make culture a low-yield procedure. However, if increased neutrophils and increased protein are detected in CSF (see Chapter 14), aerobic and anaerobic bacterial culture as well as antimicrobial susceptibility testing is indicated. CSF should be placed in transport media* and delivered to the laboratory as soon as possible. Aerobic bacterial culture should be performed on all animals with suspected bacterial infection of the CNS; anaerobic culture should be performed on all animals with potential mass lesions consistent with abcessation.

Musculoskeletal System • There are no normal flora in the tissues of the musculoskeletal system. All dogs with radiographic evidence of diskospondylitis should be evaluated for *Brucella canis* infection serologically (see Serologic Tests for Bacterial Infections). Intervertebral joints are generally not cultured except when decompressive spinal surgery is required. Most cases of diskospondylitis develop after hematogenous spread of bacteria from an extravertebral source. Blood and urine are commonly cultured from patients with diskospondylitis; *Staphylococcus* spp. are commonly involved.

Dogs or cats with suppurative arthritis with or without cytologic visualization of bacteria should have synovial fluid cultured for aerobes and *Mycoplasma* spp. (see Chapter 10). The likelihood of positive culture results increases if the synovial fluid is septic or contains degenerative neutrophils. L-form bacteria usually give negative culture results. Synovial biopsy for culture and histopathologic evaluation for L-form bacteria is indicated in some cases. *Borrelia burgdorferi* is almost never isolated from joints of dogs with Lyme disease.

In osteomyelitis, culture of fistulous tracts is inferior to culture of affected bone. Culture for infectious myositis is seldom performed unless an anaerobic infection (e.g., *Clostridium* spp.) is suspected based on foul odor, subcutaneous emphysema, or empyema. Other infectious myopathies (e.g., toxoplasmosis and leptospirosis) are better evaluated by serologic testing.

Cardiovascular System • Blood cultures are indicated in suspected bacterial endocarditis or septicemia. A large vein, prepared surgically with sequential iodine and alcohol scrubs, is used for three blood culture specimens obtained during a febrile episode over a 24-hour period in dogs with suspected endocarditis (Calvert and Dow, 1990). Culture of less than three specimens sig-

nificantly decreases the chance of positive results. At least 5 ml of blood is placed into each of two blood culture bottles* or Vacutainers containing culture media.† One is vented (i.e., aerobic), and one is unvented (i.e., anaerobic). Clotted blood or blood containing EDTA or citrate is unacceptable because it decreases isolation of organisms. Patients that are receiving antibiotics or that have recently been exposed to antibiotics require use of an antibiotic removal device.‡ If a patient is critically ill owing to probable sepsis, three cultures should be obtained over 1 to 3 hours before antimicrobial therapy is instituted.

Body Cavities • The site of skin puncture should be prepared as for blood culture. If pyothorax or peritonitis seems likely but fluid cannot be aspirated, lavage (see Chapter 10) is indicated. Because mixed infections are common, aerobic and anaerobic cultures should be performed

Eye • Conjunctival culture should be performed before topical anesthesia by rolling a moistened sterile swab over the conjunctiva. Ocular paracentesis is necessary for intraocular culture. Readers are referred elsewhere for a description of technique (Martin, 1990).

Specimen Transport • For aerobic culture, no special transport medium is required if the swab remains moist and can be inoculated onto the culture medium within 3 hours. However, swabs containing liquid or gel transport media§ are frequently used. Routine cultures can be safely stored in transport media at room temperature for up to 4 hours. After this time, overgrowth is a potential problem because of various growth rates of different organisms. Refrigerated, routine specimens can be stored in transport media for at least 2 days, and the majority can be frozen before culture. Tissue samples can be refrigerated for up to 2 days. Fluids (e.g., urine) can be safely stored at room temperature for 1 to 2 hours, refrigerated for 24 hours, and refrigerated in transport media for 72 hours (Jones, 1990). However, quantitative culture is not accurate for fluids stored in transport media because of artifactual dilution.

For anaerobic culture, fluid should be aspi-

---

*Vacutainer culture tube system, Becton-Dickinson Co., Rutherford, NJ 07070.

---

*Tryptic soybroth, Difco Labs, Detroit, MI 48232.

†Vacutainer culture tube system, Becton-Dickinson Co., Rutherford, NJ 07070.

‡Antibiotic removal device, Marion Scientific Corp., Kansas City, MO 64114.

§Culturette, American Scientific Products, McGaw Park, IL 60085.

rated into a syringe, the needle capped with a rubber stopper, and the sample inoculated onto culture medium within 10 minutes of collection. A transport medium* is available, but it is not ideal for fastidious *Bacteroides* spp. and *Fusobacterium* spp. With these limitations, samples can be stored refrigerated for 2 days in a transport medium.

Analysis ● Blood agar plates grow almost all routine bacterial pathogens. A biplate containing blood agar and MacConkey's agar is frequently used. The common anaerobic culture medium is thioglycolate. The decision to perform in-office testing instead of using a commercial laboratory is based on case load and available equipment. With the exception of blood and feces, the majority of culture procedures can be performed in-office. Readers are referred elsewhere for details of equipment and operation of an in-office microbiology laboratory (Hirsh and Ruehl, 1986).

Sensitivity Testing ● Sensitivity testing gives an *in vitro* estimation of the suitability of a given concentration of an antimicrobial agent. Two techniques are used, the dilution test and the disk diffusion test.

Dilution Test ● This test is quantitative and determines the least amount of antimicrobial needed to prevent growth of a microorganism (minimum inhibitory concentration [MIC]). Quantitative susceptibility testing is indicated when antimicrobial dosage schedules need to be monitored closely, as with gentamicin, or when disk test results are inapplicable, equivocal, or unreliable (e.g., slow-growing organisms, confirmation of susceptibility to the polymyxins, confirmation of susceptibility or resistance to given doses of aminoglycosides). Other indications include anaerobes and testing for synergism or antagonism between antimicrobials. Advantages: may show that certain drugs will be efficacious despite contrary results by the disk diffusion test (e.g., antibiotics that are concentrated in urine). Disadvantages: expense, inability to perform in-office, and need to determine if required concentrations of a certain antibiotic are feasible. Ideally, blood concentrations of drugs should be more than four times the MIC, and urine concentrations 10 to 20 times the MIC. MIC sensitivity for topically administered antimicrobials is seldom done because these methods are based on blood or urine concentrations.

Disk Diffusion Test ● This is the most widely used method in clinical practice (the Kirby-Bauer technique). A zone of inhibition of bacterial growth is noted around a disk containing a fixed amount of antibiotic. The procedure is qualitative and allocates organisms to the sensitive (susceptible), intermediate (indeterminate), or resistant category. Advantages: simplicity and suitability for most routine cultures; can be done in-office; and applicability for rapidly growing organisms (e.g., Enterobacteriaceae and *Staphylococcus aureus*). Disadvantages: not suitable for slow-growing organisms and anaerobes; inaccuracy in predicting susceptibility of poorly diffusing antibiotics (e.g., polymyxins); factors that influence the test (e.g., pH and thickness of the medium, concentration of organisms, and incubation time) must be standardized.

Artifacts ● Artifacts result from improper sample collection (i.e., the wrong sample or contamination), improper sample transport, failure to notify the laboratory of suspected pathogens (e.g., *Salmonella* spp., anaerobic bacteria, *Campylobacter* spp., and *Mycoplasma* spp.), recent antibiotic treatment, and culture for a secondary rather than a slow-growing primary pathogen (i.e., insufficient duration of culture). Failure to grow fastidious anaerobes may be due to short, seemingly insignificant exposure to oxygen or failure to use prereduced culture media.

Interpretations ● Recognizing normal flora (see Table 15–1) is necessary to interpret cultures properly. Preliminary identification is expected in 18 to 24 hours, and antibiotic sensitivity is reported in 36 to 48 hours. Most aerobic and facultative organisms are identified within 5 days; identification of anaerobic organisms or *Mycoplasma* spp. may require an additional 2 to 3 days.

Bacterial pathogens commonly isolated from various body systems are listed in Table 15–2. Note the overlap between resident and pathogenic organisms.

Staphylococcus intermedius is the major pathogen isolated from the skin of dogs with pyoderma. Gram-negative organisms are likely to be contaminants in superficial pyoderma and secondary to *S. intermedius* in deep pyoderma.

Primary bacterial rhinitis is rare in dogs and cats. Primary bacterial pneumonia can result from *Bordetella bronchiseptica* or *Mycoplasma* spp., whereas other organisms are usually secondary to viral infections or aspiration.

Bacterial growth from urine obtained by cy-

*Anaerobic culturette, Marion Scientific Corp., Kansas City, MO 64114.

Table 15-2 BACTERIA COMMONLY ISOLATED FROM VARIOUS SITES IN INFECTIOUS
DISORDERS IN DOGS AND CATS

Integument
Pyoderma
 Staphylococcus aureus/intermedius
 Proteus spp.
 Pseudomonas spp.
 Escherichia coli (usually secondary to staphylococci)
Ear
 Malassezia spp.
 Pseudomonas spp.
 S. aureus/intermedius
 Proteus spp.

Respiratory System
Pneumonia
 Pseudomonas spp.
 E. coli
 Klebsiella spp.
 Pasteurella spp.
 Bordetella spp.
 Staphylococcus spp.
 Streptococcus spp.
 Mycoplasma spp.
Pleural cavity
 Nocardia spp.
 Actinomyces spp.
 Pasteurella spp.
 Anaerobes

Gastrointestinal Tract
Intestine
 Salmonella spp.
 E. coli
 Campylobacter spp.
 Clostridium perfringens, type A

Musculoskeletal System
Polymyopathy
 Leptospira spp.
Appendicular osteomyelitis
 S. aureus
Vertebral osteomyelitis
 S. aureus/intermedius
 Beta-hemolytic streptococci
 Brucella canis

Genitourinary Tract
 E. coli
 Proteus spp.
 Klebsiella spp.
 S. aureus/intermedius

Eye
Conjunctiva and cornea
 S. aureus (coagulase positive and negative)
 Streptococcus spp.
 S. epidermidis
 E. coli
 Proteus spp.
 Bacillus spp.

Cardiovascular System
Aerobes
 S. aureus
 Beta-hemolytic streptococci
 E. coli
 Klebsiella spp.
 Pseudomonas spp.
 Proteus spp.
 Salmonella spp.
Anaerobes
 Bacteroides spp.
 Fusobacterium spp.
 Clostridium spp.

(Data compiled from (1) Lorenz MD: Integumentary infections; Thayer GW: Infections of the respiratory system; Greene CE: Gastrointestinal, intraabdominal and hepatobiliary infections; Kornegay JN: Musculoskeletal infections; Barsanti JA: Genitourinary tract infections; Martin CE: Ocular infections; Calvert CA: Cardiovascular infections. In Greene CE [ed]: Clinical Microbiology and Infectious Diseases of the Dog and Cat. Philadelphia, WB Saunders, 1984; Berg et al. Identification of the major coagulase-positive *Staphylococcus* sp of dogs as *Staphylococcus intermedius*. Am J Vet Res 1984;45:1307–1309; Calvert and Greene: Bacteremia in dogs: Diagnosis, treatment, and prognosis. Comp Cont Ed Pract Vet 1986;8:179–187, 1986.)

tocentesis is significant, since the bladder is normally sterile. Urine cultures are, however, best interpreted in conjunction with a urinalysis. If growth occurs despite absence of significant pyuria (see Chapter 7), sample contamination, improper sample transport, or diseases causing immune suppression (e.g., hyperadrenocorticism; diabetes mellitus; FIV infection) must be considered. In quantitative culture of urine obtained by catheterization or midstream voiding, 100,000 colonies/ml or greater is significant. In samples of prostatic fluid obtained by ejaculation, infection is diagnosed if the specimen con-

tains ≥ 100 times more bacteria than the urethral sample (Ling et al., 1983); however, culture of prostatic aspirates may be more accurate (Ling et al., 1990).

Blood cultures can be difficult to interpret. False-positive results are due to contamination with normal cutaneous microflora including *Corynebacterium* spp., *Bacillus* spp., coagulase-negative staphylococci, anaerobic diphtheroids, streptococci, and *Clostridium* spp. Isolation of the same organism from at least two cultures strongly suggests it to be pathogenic, whereas growth in only one culture is less certain unless it is a pathogenic bacterium that is unlikely to be a contaminant.

CSF is normally sterile; any growth in an aseptically obtained sample is significant.

Fungal Culture

Specimen Procurement • For dermatophyte culture, hair is clipped from the lesion periphery; the hair shafts are plucked with forceps and cultured on dermatophyte test medium (DTM)* or Derm Duet.†

Subcutaneous and deep fungal infections are best diagnosed by cytologic or histopathologic evaluation. If organisms cannot be identified, cutaneous lesions can be cultured, but these are rarely useful owing to overgrowth by resident bacteria and fungi. The lesion is prepared as for dermatophytes, and a swab is cultured onto Sabouraud's and Mycose medium.

Interpretation • Saprophytic fungi isolated from the skin may include *Alternaria* spp., *Cladosporium* spp., *Aspergillus* spp., and *Fusarium* spp. The most common dermatophytes in dogs and cats are *Microsporum canis, Microsporum gypseum,* and *Trichophyton mentagrophytes.* Dermatophytes usually cause red discoloration of DTM after 4 to 5 days; saprophytic fungi usually cause red agar after 12 to 14 days. Therefore, it is important to check the medium daily. The diagnosis should be confirmed by cytologic examination of the fungi.

Systemic and subcutaneous fungi may require culture up to 2 weeks on Sabouraud's medium for growth.

SEROLOGIC TESTS FOR FUNGAL INFECTION

Blastomycosis (*Blastomyces dermatitidis*)

Occasional Indications • Dogs that are from endemic areas and that have fever, weight loss, pulmonary interstitial disease, lymphadenopathy, uveitis/blindness, ulcerative or draining skin lesions, undiagnosed prostatic or testicular disease, intracranial disease, osteomyelitis, or rarely renal disease can be serologically screened for antibodies against *B. dermatitidis* if

---

*DTM, Pitman Moore, Mundelein, IL 60060.
†Derm Duet, Bacti Laboratories, Mountain View, CA 94042.

the organism is not demonstrated by cytology, histopathology, or culture.

Analysis, Artifacts, and Interpretation • Circulating antibodies are detected in serum by agar gel immunodiffusion (AGID), counterimmunoelectrophoresis (CIEP), and enzyme-linked immunosorbent assay (ELISA) (Legendre, 1990).

False-negative results can occur in animals with peracute infection or in advanced cases that overwhelm the immune system. The sensitivity (i.e., ability to identify infected animals) and specificity (i.e., ability to identify noninfected animals) of the AGID and CIEP are > 90%. A titer $\geq$ 1:8 in the ELISA had a sensitivity of 100% and a specificity of 97% in one study (Turner et al., 1986). Antibody titers do not always revert to negative after successful treatment.

Definitive diagnosis requires identification of the yeast by cytology, histopathology, or fungal culture. Impression smears from skin lesions and aspirates from enlarged lymph nodes frequently reveal organisms; recovery of organisms from transtracheal aspiration, pulmonary aspiration biopsy samples, or urine is less consistent. Culture requires 10 to 14 days and is of lower yield than cytology or biopsy. Diffuse nodular pulmonary interstitial lung disease and hilar lymphadenopathy are commonly seen on thoracic radiographs. Positive serologic results combined with appropriate clinical signs and radiographic abnormalities allow presumptive diagnosis if the organism cannot be demonstrated.

Histoplasmosis (*Histoplasma capsulatum*)

Rare Indications • Dogs or cats with weight loss, pulmonary interstitial disease, uveal disease, diarrhea, or lymphadenopathy can be serologically screened for antibodies against *H. capsulatum* if the organism is not demonstrated by cytology, histopathology, or culture.

Analysis, Artifacts, and Interpretation • Circulating antibodies are detected in serum by complement fixation (CF) and AGID.

Significant CF titers vary by the laboratory. The presence of a positive antibody titer confirms exposure but not clinical illness due to infection. If paired samples are obtained several weeks apart in patients with acute histoplasmosis, a four-fold increase in titer is expected (Barsanti, 1984). This may not occur in chronic cases. The CF test has poor sensitivity and poor specificity and cross-reacts with antibodies to other fungi and undetermined antigens. AGID has questionable clinical usefulness, since titers persist > 1 year after resolution of disease in some animals. These tests are even less rewarding in cats.

Definitive diagnosis requires demonstration of the organism by cytology (Color Plate 2E), biopsy, or culture. The organism is more difficult to demonstrate than is *B. dermatitidis*; however, cytologic examination of rectal scrapings in patients with colonic histoplasmosis is often diagnostic. Fine-needle aspiration of other organs may demonstrate the organism. In most cats with systemic histoplasmosis, the organism is identified on bone marrow cytology. Thoracic radiographs are indicated if pulmonary histoplasmosis is suspected; a nodular interstitial pattern is expected. Culture of *H. capsulatum* is of lower yield than biopsy. Serologic diagnosis is unreliable and is used only to establish a presumptive diagnosis when the organism cannot be demonstrated by cytology, histopathology, or culture but other abnormalities are suggestive of the disease.

Crytococcosis (*Cryptococcus neoformans*)

Occasional Indications ● Cats and rarely dogs with undiagnosed infections of the respiratory tract (especially nasal), CNS, eye (especially uveal tract), and skin (especially nodular or ulcerative lesions) can be screened for *C. neoformans* antibodies or antigens if the organism is not demonstrated by cytology, histopathology, or culture.

Analysis, Artifacts, and Interpretation ● Measurement of antibodies against *C. neoformans* is not clinically useful. Cryptococcal antigen is detected in serum, aqueous humor, or CSF using latex agglutination (LA). See Appendix I for availability of testing.

Negative serum LA titers may occur in early disease or uncommonly in chronic low-grade infections, in chemotherapy-induced remission, or in nondisseminated disease. The specificity of the serum LA is high. A titer of > 1:1 in serum or CSF is positive; very high titers are commonly detected (Medleau et al., 1990). Decreases in serum titer parallel response to therapy, and a fourfold decrease in titer demonstrates successful response to chemotherapy, although low-grade persistent titers occur in some animals after apparently successful clinical responses. Cryptococcal encephalitis may cause a positive CSF LA titer despite a negative serum LA.

Definitive diagnosis is based on cytologic, histopathologic, or culture demonstration of the organism or a positive LA test result. Cytologic analysis is commonly positive since there are usually numerous yeasts in affected tissues (i.e., nasal and cutaneous lesions, aqueous and vitreous humor). CSF may contain the yeast, but concentration techniques (i.e., Cytospin) should be used. Gram's staining or india ink is used; some consider Gram's stain to be more definitive. Lymphocytes, fat droplets, and ink particles may resemble the organism if ink is used and budding is absent. This confusion is lessened if the preparation sits for 30 minutes before examination. Large numbers of organisms are usually seen, despite little or no inflammation. Culture is seldom necessary. Serologic testing is used if the yeast cannot be demonstrated cytologically or to monitor response to treatment.

Coccidioidomycosis (*Coccidioides immitis*)

Occasional Indications ● Dogs that are from endemic areas and that have pulmonary interstitial disease, fever of undetermined origin, hilar lymphadenopathy, osteomyelitis, uveitis, pericarditis, and nodular or ulcerative skin lesions can be serologically screened for antibodies against *C. immitis* if the organism is not demonstrated by cytology, histopathology, or culture. The disease is rare in cats.

Analysis, Artifacts, and Interpretation ● Circulating antibodies are detected in serum by CF, AGID, and tube precipitin (TP) tests. TP detects IgM antibodies; CF and AGID detect IgG antibodies (Barsanti and Jeffrey, 1990). See Appendix I for availability of testing.

False-negative results in the TP occur in early infections (< 2 weeks), chronic infection, rapidly progressive acute infection, and primary cutaneous coccidioidomycosis. False-positive results of the CF test occur as a result of anticomplementary serum, which may be due to bacterial contaminants or immune complexes. Finally, cross-reactions in patients with histoplasmosis and blastomycosis may occur with all tests. See Table 15–3 for interpretation of CF and TP tests. After resolution of disease, CF titers decrease over weeks to months but remain positive at a low titer (e.g., 1:32).

Table 15–3 INTERPRETATION OF SEROLOGIC TESTING FOR COCCIDIOIDOMYCOSIS

Complement Fixation Test Results	Precipitin Test Negative	Precipitin Test Positive
Negative	No infection Rapidly fatal fulminating infection in severely immunocompromised animal Early infection: repeat test in 2 weeks to detect positive precipitin test results	Early infection: probably pulmonary; precipitin test results are positive 2 weeks postexposure and become negative after 4 to 5 weeks
Positive	Past exposure or disease, long-standing residual titer (weak CF titer, 1:4) Later infection: precipitin titer frequently decreases after 5 to 6 weeks	Early active infection: the greater the titer, the more likelihood of dissemination Chronic infection: occasionally, positive precipitin tests occur later in disseminated disease

(Data from Bartsch RC: Southwestern Veterinary Diagnostics, Phoenix, Arizona, 1988.)
From Barsanti and Jeffrey (1990).

Definitive diagnosis requires demonstration of the organism on smears, aspirates, histopathologic evaluation, or culture. The organism is often difficult to demonstrate. Wet mount examination of unstained or stained (periodic acid–Schiff) smears or aspirates is more suitable than are dry mounts, which may distort the spherules. Common thoracic radiographic findings are mixed interstitial/bronchial/alveolar pulmonary patterns. Hilar lymphadenopathy is also common. Serologic tests and radiographic signs allow tentative diagnosis if the organism cannot be demonstrated.

Aspergillosis (Aspergillus fumigatus)

Occasional Indications • Dogs and cats with nasal or pulmonary disease can be serologically screened for antibodies against *A. fumigatus*. Results are interpreted with those from cytology, radiology, histopathology, and culture.

Analysis, Artifacts, and Interpretation • Circulating antibodies are detected in serum by AGID, CIEP, and ELISA (Sharp, 1990).

The presence of serum antibodies can represent exposure or infection. Many dogs with nasal aspergillosis are falsely negative. Owing to persistence of titers in some treated dogs ($\geq$ 12 months), monitoring for serologic response to therapy is of dubious benefit.

Radiographic demonstration of nasal turbinate destruction suggests aspergillosis or nasal neoplasia. Cytologic analysis (Color Plate 2D) and culture of canine nasal exudate alone are not diagnostic of infection because fungal elements may be sparse or nondetectable in affected dogs while being found by cytologic analysis or culture from noninfected dogs (including dogs with nasal tumors). The organism is sometimes difficult to culture from an aspergilloma (fungal ball). Nasal lavage is a low-yield procedure for demonstration of the organism. Nasal biopsy is suggested (see Chapter 11). Definitive diagnosis should be based on demonstration of histopathologic evidence of tissue invasion or an aspergilloma combined with serologic and culture evidence of infection or serologic and radiographic evidence of infection. In the rare case of disseminated disease, cytologic evaluation of aspirates of affected tissue may be useful. If the organism cannot be demonstrated by biopsy samples obtained through the nares, positive serologic tests may support exploratory surgery.

SEROLOGIC TESTS FOR RICKETTSIAL INFECTIONS

Ehrlichiosis (Ehrlichia canis)

Common Indications • Serologic testing for ehrlichiosis is indicated for dogs from endemic areas or those having an appropriate travel history and thrombocytopenia, anemia, leukopenia, hyperglobulinemia, proteinuria, polyarthritis, fever, lymphadenopathy, hepatosplenomegaly, or inflammatory CNS disease. There is often no history of tick exposure.

Analysis, Artifacts, and Interpretation • Circulating antibodies are detected in serum by indirect immunofluorescent antibody assay (IFA); they do not cross-react with *Rickettsia rickettsii* or *E. platys* antigens (Troy and Forrester, 1990). *Ehrlichia equi* (Lewis et al, 1975), *Ehrlichia risticii* (Holland CJ: Personal communication, 1993), and *E. ewingii* (Anderson et al., 1992) can also cause disease in dogs. Cross-reactivity of antibodies against these agents with *E. canis* antigen is variable, and infected dogs can be serologically negative. Specific serologic tests are available for the detection of specific antibodies against specific species in canine serum. See Appendix I for availability of testing.

Definitive diagnosis of *E. canis* infection requires demonstration of morulae (clusters of the organism) in leukocytes or an IgG antibody titer ≥ 1:20. Morulae are rarely found on routine blood smear or bone marrow aspiration cytology unless the dog has been immunosuppressed. Antibodies against *E. canis* can be detected as early as 7 days after inoculation and are usually positive by 20 days after inoculation. Antibody titers continue to increase for weeks to months after inoculation in untreated, experimentally infected dogs (Buhles et al., 1974). An *E. canis* titer of 1:10 is suspicious and should be rechecked in approximately 21 days, whereas a titer of 1:20 or higher is diagnostic. Because most dogs infected with *E. canis* ultimately develop a chronic phase of disease, all seropositive dogs should be treated even if currently subclinically affected. Titers remain increased in untreated dogs, with the titer magnitude closely correlating with duration of infection. Positive titers revert to negative 3 to 9 months after resolution of infection; persistence of titers for 9 months or longer can suggest a carrier state (Greene, 1986). Positive antibody titers have been detected for up to 31 months after therapy in some naturally infected dogs (Perille and Matus, 1991).

Ehrlichia spp. can be isolated by tissue culture of heparinized infected canine blood or bone marrow aspiration samples but is of limited availability, expensive, and of low yield since the organism is difficult to culture. Bone marrow plasmacytosis is consistent with ehrlichiosis but not diagnostic of it. Some infected dogs are Coombs' positive. Both monoclonal (IgG) and polyclonal gammopathies occur with chronic phase ehrlichiosis.

Infectious Cyclic Thrombocytopenia (*Ehrlichia platys*)

Occasional Indications ● Serologic testing for *E. platys* infection is indicated for dogs that have thrombocytopenia or endogenous uveitis and that live in endemic areas or have an appropriate travel history.

Analysis, Artifacts, and Interpretation ● Circulat-

ing IgG antibodies against *E. platys* are detected in serum by IFA. Antibodies against *E. platys* do not react with *E. canis* antigens. See Appendix I for availability of testing.

The cutoff for a positive IgG antibody titer varies by the laboratory. Experimentally infected dogs become antibody positive 13 to 19 days after infection (French and Harvey, 1983). Low antibody titers in suspected clinical cases should be rechecked after 21 days. Because many dogs are subclinically infected, positive antibody titers do not prove clinical disease. Definitive diagnosis requires demonstration of the organism within platelets (difficult owing to cyclic parasitemia).

Rocky Mountain Spotted Fever (*Rickettsia rickettsii*)

Occasional Indications ● Serologic testing for RMSF is indicated for dogs that are from endemic areas or that have an appropriate travel history and acute onset of fever, lymphadenopathy, petechiae, neurologic signs, stiff gait, peripheral edema, respiratory distress, or scleral congestion. There is often no history of tick exposure. Exposed dogs either develop acute disease with approximately a 14-day clinical course or they are subclinically infected (Greene and Breitschwerdt, 1990). The primary tick vectors are active from spring to fall in most regions of the United States; therefore, RMSF should only be considered a principal differential diagnosis for clinically ill dogs during this time span.

Analysis, Artifacts, and Interpretation ● Antibodies against *R. rickettsii* can be measured in canine serum by IFA, ELISA, and LA (Greene et al., 1993). See Appendix I for availability of testing.

IgM and IgG antibodies against RMSF can be detected by ELISA or IFA. LA is not antibody class specific. Cutoffs for positive antibody titers as well as specificity and sensitivity vary by the assay (Greene et al., 1993). After experimental inoculation, IgM antibodies can be detected by IFA by day 9, peak by day 20, and are negative by day 80 after inoculation (Breitschwerdt, 1992). In dogs with clinical illness due to RMSF, IgM antibody titers are generally positive. Because IgM has short duration in serum, false-negative results may occur with IgM testing. False-positive results are most common in the IgM ELISA. Positive IgG titers are detectable 20 to 25 days after infection. Serum samples with IgG titers ≥ 1:64 are generally considered positive. If IgG or IgM antibodies are not detected in a patient with clinical and laboratory evidence of RMSF, a convalescent IgG titer 2 to 3 weeks later is recommended. Timing of the second titer is not critical because IgG antibody titers do not decrease for at least 3 to 5 months after infection (Greene and Breitschwerdt, 1990). Documentation of seroconversion or a fourfold increase in IgG titer is consistent with recent infection.

Most dogs exposed to *R. rickettsii* are subclinically infected; therefore, the presence of antibodies in serum only denotes exposure, not clinical illness. Cross-reaction in the serologic tests occurs when antibodies against other spotted fever rickettsiae (e.g., *Rickettsia montana, Rickettsia rhipicephali, Rickettsia belli,* and some typhus group rickettsiae) are present; thus, a positive antibody titer does not document exposure to *R. rickettsii.* However, extremely elevated antibody titers (> 1:256) are most consistent with exposure to *R. rickettsii.* A diagnosis of clinical RMSF in dogs should be based on appropriate clinical, historical, and laboratory evidence of disease combined with positive serologic testing and response to therapy. Infection can also be confirmed in clinically ill dogs by documenting the organism in endothelial cells using direct fluorescent antibody staining (Davidson et al., 1989).

Clinical signs of *E. canis* infection and RMSF are similar, but anemia and leukopenia are more common in ehrlichiosis, whereas leukocytosis is more common in RMSF. Platelet counts tend to be lower in ehrlichiosis. Hyperglobulinemia occurs only in chronic phase ehrlichiosis, not in RMSF.

SEROLOGIC TESTS FOR BACTERIAL INFECTIONS

Leptospirosis (*Leptospira* spp.)

Occasional Indications • Serologic testing for antibodies against *Leptospira* spp. should be considered in dogs with undiagnosed fever, ecchymoses, vomiting, diarrhea, muscle pain, uveitis, coughing, respiratory distress, renal pain, anemia, thrombocytopenia, hyponatremia, hypokalemia, hyperphosphatemia, hypoalbuminemia, hypocalcemia, azotemia, or increased liver enzymes. Pathogenic serovars in dogs include *Leptospira canicola, Leptospira icterohaemorrhagiae, Leptospira grippotyphosa,* and *Leptospira pomona* (Rentko and Ross, 1992).

Analysis, Artifacts, and Interpretation • Circulat-

ing antibodies are detected in serum by the microscopic agglutination test (MAT), ELISA (IgM and IgG), and microscopic microcapsular agglutination test (MCAT). The primary disadvantage of serologic testing is that it is difficult to determine whether positive titers are due to active infection, previous infection, or vaccination. See Appendix I for availability of testing.

The IgM ELISA and MCAT are most likely to detect recent infection (Greene and Schotts, 1990). Titers detected by the IgM ELISA are positive by 1 week after inoculation, peak at 14 days after inoculation, and then decline. Acutely infected dogs are often IgM ELISA positive, MAT negative. Dogs with suggestive clinical signs of disease but negative MAT results should be retested in 2 to 4 weeks; development of a positive titer confirms recent infection. Titers detected by the IgG ELISA are generally positive by 2 to 3 weeks after inoculation, with peak values reached by 1 month after inoculation. A fourfold increase in antibody titer over 2 to 4 weeks confirms recent infection. Vaccination can induce positive MAT titers. Vaccination generally leads to high IgG ELISA titers with low to negative IgM ELISA titers; therefore, ELISA appears to be superior to MAT for differentiation of antibodies induced by natural infection from those due to vaccination (Greene and Schotts, 1990).

Definitive diagnosis requires demonstration of the organism by urine darkfield microscopy, phase contrast microscopy, or culture. However, examination of urine for leptospires is a low-yield procedure. Alternately, demonstration of spirochetes by histopathologic evaluation of renal tissue leads to a presumptive diagnosis, which may be confirmed by culture of the tissue. In acute disease, leptospiremia occurs for a few days to 2 weeks after infection, during which time the organism may sometimes be cultured from blood. Urine can be cultured, but repeated culture may be needed owing to intermittent shedding. The combination of seroconversion, IgM antibodies, or increasing antibody titers with appropriate clinical pathologic abnormalities and clinical findings is suggestive of clinical leptospirosis.

Brucellosis (*Brucella canis*)

Occasional Indications • Dogs with reproductive tract abnormalities, lymphadenopathy, diskospondylitis, or uveitis should be screened for antibodies against *B. canis.*

Analysis, Artifacts, and Interpretation • Circulat-

Table 15–4 COMPARISON OF DIAGNOSTIC SEROLOGIC PROCEDURES FOR CANINE BRUCELLOSIS

Procedure	Earliest Titer (Weeks After Inoculation)	Advantages	Disadvantages
Rapid slide agglutination test (RSAT)	1–2	Quick, very sensitive, few false negatives	Many false positives, low specificity, cross-reactions with other infections
Mercaptoethanol (2-ME) RSAT	3–4	Same as RSAT except increased specificity	Longer time required for patient to produce positive reaction compared with RSAT
Tube agglutination test (TAT)	3–6	Allows semiquantitative determination	False positives similar to RSAT
Mercaptoethanol (2-ME) TAT	5–8	Same as TAT except increased specificity	Longer time required for patient to produce positive titers compared with TAT
Agar gel immunodiffusion (AGID)			
Cell wall (somatic) antigen	5–10	More specific than agglutination tests	Complex procedure
Internal (cytoplasmic) antigen	1	Most sensitive test, detects abacteremic (early acute and later chronic) cases when other tests are equivocal or negative	Cross-reacts with other *Brucella* infections, complex procedure

(Adapted from Carmichael LE, Greene CE: Canine brucellosis. In Greene CE [ed]: Infectious Diseases of the Dog and Cat. Philadelphia, WB Saunders, 1990, pp 573–584.)

ing antibodies are detected in serum by rapid slide agglutination test (RSAT), tube agglutination test (TAT), AGID, and ELISA (Carmichael and Greene, 1990). See Appendix I for availability of AGID testing.

Up to 65% of positive RSATs are false, caused by cross-reactions to *Brucella ovis*, *B. bronchiseptica*, *Pseudomonas* spp., *Moraxella* spp., or *Actinobacillus equuli*. False-negative RSATs are rare (< 1%). Addition of 2-mercaptoethanol (2-ME) eliminates heterologous IgM agglutinins responsible for most false-positive RSAT reactions and is also used in the TAT. The 2-ME RSAT can be used as an in-house screening procedure.* The 2-ME TAT is the test most widely used in diagnostic laboratories. False-positive reactions in the 2-ME TAT may be due to autoagglutination in hemolyzed samples. False-negative reactions in the 2-ME TAT may occur in chronically infected dogs, especially males. Tetracycline therapy decreases the 2-ME TAT titer to insignificant values after 2 weeks of therapy. AGID can be performed using cell wall antigens or cytoplasmic antigens. Advantages and disadvantages of the various tests are listed in Table 15–4.

The minimal time between infection and a positive test result varies with the test (see Table 15–4). Use of 2-ME in the RSAT and TAT increases specificity but prolongs the time before

a positive result may be obtained. TAT titers from different laboratories cannot be meaningfully compared; however, a titer of 1:50 to 1:100 is generally suspicious, whereas a titer of 1:200 or higher is usually positive and correlates with isolation of *B. canis* from blood culture (Carmichael and Greene, 1990). After cessation of bacteremia, titers rapidly decrease to < 1:200 within a few weeks and remain low (1:25–1:50) for 6 months or longer.

In the AGID, antibodies to external antigens persist for a few weeks, whereas antibodies to internal (cytoplasmic) antigens persist up to 12 months after cessation of bacteremia. Although these animals are abacteremic, *B. canis* can be isolated from selected organs (e.g., epididymis and prostate).

Definitive diagnosis requires isolation of *B. canis*, although this is not always achieved. A suggested approach is outlined in Figure 15–1. Because of its sensitivity early in the disease, 2-ME RSAT is indicated as the initial screening test. If the 2-ME RSAT is positive, a 2-ME TAT should be performed. If the 2-ME RSAT is negative in a dog strongly suspected of having brucellosis, it should be repeated in 4 weeks to preclude the possibility of early infection. If the 2-ME TAT is positive, a tentative diagnosis of brucellosis is made, and one should attempt to culture the organism or perform AGID testing. Although blood culture is ideal, it is inconvenient and expensive. Culture of urine or an ejaculate may also be performed in males. Growth

*D-TEC CB Canine brucellosis antibody test kit, Synbiotics Corp., San Diego, CA 92127.

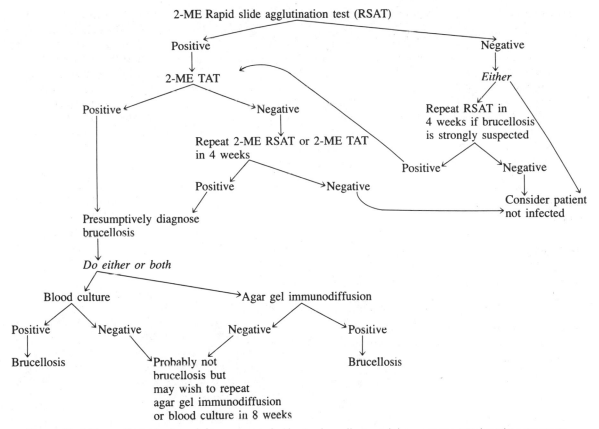

Figure 15–1 Diagnostic evaluation of dogs suspected of having brucellosis and dogs entering into breeding programs.

usually occurs within 7 days, but cultures should be held for 3 to 4 weeks before being discarded. At least three cultures from specimens obtained several days apart are recommended.

AGID for both internal and external antigens is a reasonable alternative to culture, because AGID has the best correlation with growth of *B. canis* from abacteremic patients.

Borreliosis (Lyme Disease; *Borrelia burgdorferi*)

Occasional Indications • Dogs that are from areas endemic for *Ixodes* ticks or that have an appropriate travel history with fever, lameness, or nonseptic, suppurative polyarthritis should be screened for antibodies against *B. burgdorferi*. Serologic testing should be considered in dogs with CNS disease, renal disease, and myocardial disease.

Analysis, Artifacts, and Interpretation • Circulating antibodies are detected in serum by IFA, ELISA, and Western immunoblot (Lindenmayer et al., 1990). See Appendix I for availability of testing.

Both IgM and IgG antibodies against *B. burgdorferi* can be detected in canine serum. Titers considered significant vary by laboratory and assay. Both antibody classes can persist in serum for months after exposure. ELISA techniques are considered more sensitive and specific than IFA. Cross-reactivity with *B. burgdorferi* antigens used in the IFA and ELISA occurs with other spirochetes, including *Leptospira* spp. and *Borrelia hermsii*; thus, a positive titer does not document exposure to *B. burgdorferi*. Some nonpathogenic strains of *B. burgdorferi* induce antibody production but not clinical disease (Breitschwerdt, 1992). Some dogs with acute Lyme disease are seronegative on initial testing; documentation of an increasing antibody titer can suggest recent exposure. However, healthy dogs develop the same antibody responses as clinically ill dogs. Because of these factors, interpretation of serum antibodies is difficult. The presence of antibodies against *B. burgdorferi* antigens in serum only documents exposure to *B. burgdorferi* or a similar antigen, not clinical disease. Antibody titers ≥ 1:1000 have been detected in clinically normal dogs. Detection of a greater concentration of antibody in CSF than in serum occurs in some dogs with suspected neurologic disease secondary to Lyme disease (Feder et al., 1991).

Definitive diagnosis requires demonstration of the organism by culture, histopathologic evaluation of tissue, or polymerase chain reaction (Wasmoen et al., 1992). A presumptive diagnosis of clinical Lyme disease in dogs can be based on appropriate clinical, historical, and laboratory evidence of disease combined with positive serologic testing and response to therapy.

Tularemia (Rabbit Fever) (*Francisella tularensis*)

Rare Indications • Testing for tularemia should be considered in cats and dogs that are from endemic areas and that develop fever, lymphadenopathy, weight loss, or oral ulceration, particularly if there is known tick exposure, rabbit ingestion, or potential for human infection. Tularemia is a direct zoonosis from clinically ill cats to people.

Analysis, Artifacts, and Interpretation • Antibodies are measured in serum by TAT (Rohrbach, 1988). Cross-reactivity with *Brucella abortus* and certain strains of *Proteus vulgaris* has been documented with human serum. See Appendix I for availability of testing.

Time between acquisition of infection and a positive titer is not known. A single titer of 1:80 or higher or a fourfold increase in titer between acute and convalescent sera (3 weeks later) is presumptive evidence of infection.

Definitive diagnosis is obtained by isolation of the bacterium in a culture of a blood specimen or by identification in tissue by immunofluorescence.

SEROLOGIC TESTS FOR PROTOZOAL INFECTIONS

Toxoplasmosis (*Toxoplasma gondii*)

Occasional Indications

Healthy Cats • *T. gondii*-specific antibodies and antigens form in the serum of both healthy and diseased cats and do not directly correlate with clinical toxoplasmosis. There is no available serologic test that predicts when a seropositive cat sheds oocysts. A seropositive, oocyst-negative cat is not likely to shed the organism again even if exposed. Seronegative cats are likely to shed the organism if exposed.

Clinically Ill Dogs and Cats • Serologic tests for toxoplasmosis should be considered in cats with endogenous uveitis, fever, muscle disease, icterus, pancreatitis, apparent inflammatory bowel disease that fails to respond to immunosuppressive therapy, CNS disease, and respiratory disease. Serologic tests for toxoplasmosis should be considered in dogs with fever, muscle disease, CNS disease, and respiratory disease. Dogs develop clinical toxoplasmosis less commonly than cats.

Analysis

Serum Antibody Testing • Antibodies against *T. gondii* can be detected with multiple techniques including ELISA, IFA, Western blot immunoassay, Sabin-Feldman dye test, and various agglutination tests (Lappin, 1993). Agglutination tests and ELISA are the techniques available in most commercial laboratories for use with canine and feline serum. Little is known about *T. gondii*-specific immune responses of dogs. See Appendix I for availability of testing.

T. gondii-specific IgM is detectable in serum by ELISA in approximately 80% of subclinically ill cats within 2 to 4 weeks after experimental induction of toxoplasmosis; these titers generally are negative within 16 weeks after infection. IgM titers > 1:256 have only been detected within the first 12 weeks after experimental induction of toxoplasmosis. Detectable IgM titers were present in the serum of 93.3% of the cats in a study of clinical toxoplasmosis; IgG titers were detected in 60% (Lappin et al., 1989). Some clinically ill cats have IgM titers > 1:256 that persist for > 12 weeks. Persistent IgM titers (> 16 weeks) have commonly been documented in cats coinfected with FIV and in cats with ocular toxoplasmosis. After repeat inoculation with *T. gondii*, primary inoculation with the Petaluma isolate of FIV, and administration of glucocorticoids, some cats with chronic toxoplasmosis have short-term recurrence of detectable IgM titers (Lappin, 1993). Healthy and clinically ill dogs occasionally develop detectable IgM titers. The kinetics of IgM titers in dogs after infection is unknown.

After experimental induction of infection in subclinically ill cats, *T. gondii*-specific IgG can be detected by ELISA in serum in the majority of cats within 4 weeks after infection. Positive IgG antibody titers generally last for years after infection. It has been suggested that single high IgG titers suggest recent or active infection. The author has demonstrated IgG antibody titers > 1:16,384 in subclinically ill cats up to 5 years after experimental induction of toxoplasmosis. Thus, the presence of a positive IgG antibody titer in a single serum sample denotes only exposure, not recent or active disease. The demonstration of an increasing IgG titer can document recent or active disease. Unfortunately, in experimentally infected cats, the time span from the first detectable positive IgG titer to the maximal IgG titer is approximately 2 to 3 weeks, leaving a very narrow window for the documentation of an increasing titer. Many cats with clinical toxoplasmosis have chronic low-grade clinical signs and may not be evaluated serologically until their IgG antibody titers have reached their maximal values. In humans with reactivation of chronic toxoplasmosis, IgG titers only rarely increase. It appears that this occurs in cats as well.

Several agglutination tests have been evaluated using cat serum. An LA* and an indirect hemagglutination assay (IHA)† are available commercially. These assays are not species specific and potentially detect all classes of immunoglobulins directed against T. gondii in serum. Unfortunately, the LA and IHA rarely detect antibody in feline serum samples positive only for IgM as determined by ELISA.

Serum Antigen Testing • T. gondii-specific antigens can be detected in serum from cats and dogs using ELISA (Lappin, 1993). After experimental induction of toxoplasmosis, most subclinically ill cats develop circulating antigenemia within 4 weeks after inoculation. Circulating antigenemia can be detected intermittently in some cats for months to years after infection. It has been hypothesized that these antigens are intermittently released from tissue cysts. Cats with clinical feline toxoplasmosis occasionally develop antigenemia without the presence of serum antibodies. Cats suspected of having clinical toxoplasmosis but seronegative for antibodies should be serologically screened for antigens. See Appendix I for availability of testing.

Aqueous Humor and CSF Antibody Measurement • Local production of T. gondii-specific antibodies and immune complexes in CSF and aqueous humor has been documented in experimentally inoculated, subclinically ill cats and in cats and dogs with clinical signs of disease referable to toxoplasmosis. The majority of cats with uveitis and evidence of local production of T. gondii-specific antibodies in aqueous humor have responded to the administration of anti-Toxoplasma drugs (13 of 15 cats), suggesting that

aqueous humor antibody testing can aid in the diagnosis of clinical ocular toxoplasmosis in cats (Lappin et al., 1992). See Appendix I for availability of testing.

Fecal Examination • Demonstration of oocysts in feces can be made after flotation using a number of solutions with a specific gravity of 1.15 to 1.18. Sugar solution centrifugation is believed to be the optimal technique. Oocysts of T. gondii are 10×12 μm in diameter, approximately one eighth the size of Toxocara cati eggs. Focusing on only one plane of the microscope slide or coverslip can result in oocysts being overlooked. The oocysts cannot be distinguished grossly from Hammondia hammondi or Besnoitia darlingi, which are nonpathogenic coccidians infecting cats. Sporulated oocysts isolated from feces can be inoculated into mice or onto tissue cultures for definitive identification. Because oocyst shedding has rarely been documented in cats with subfatal, clinical toxoplasmosis, the diagnostic utility of fecal examination is limited. However, cats with clinical signs referable to T. gondii should have feces evaluated because of the potential zoonotic risk.

Interpretation

Exposure to T. gondii is suggested by the presence of antibodies or antigens in serum, aqueous humor, or CSF. Recent or active toxoplasmosis is suggested by the presence of an IgM titer > 1:64, a fourfold or greater increase in IgG titer, and the presence of T. gondii-specific antigens without antibodies in serum or the documentation of local antibody production in aqueous humor or CSF. Because T. gondii-specific antibodies and antigens can be detected in the serum, CSF, and aqueous humor of subclinically ill cats as well as those with clinical signs of disease, it is impossible to make an antemortem diagnosis of clinical toxoplasmosis based on these tests alone. The antemortem diagnosis of clinical toxoplasmosis can be tentatively based on the combination of:

Demonstration of serologic evidence of infection
Clinical signs of disease referable to toxoplasmosis
Preclusion of other common causes
Positive response to appropriate treatment

Neosporosis (*Neospora caninum*)

Rare Indications • *Neospora caninum* serology can be performed in dogs with clinical evidence of

*Toxotest-MT, Eiken Chemical Co., Tanabe USA, Inc., San Diego, CA 92111.
†TPM-Test, Wampole Laboratories, Cranbury, NJ 08512

polyradiculomyositis, including progressive ascending rigid paralysis beginning in the rear limbs, dysphagia, muscle atrophy, and rarely myocardial dysfunction.

Analysis, Artifacts, and Interpretation • Circulating antibodies are detected in serum by indirect fluorescent antibody assay (IFA). See Appendix I for availability of testing.

Immunoglobulin G antibody titers ≥ 1:100 are consistent with infection by *N. caninum* (Lindsay DS: personal communication, 1993). Since the organism is a tissue protozoan, seropositivity may correlate with permanent infection. The presence of antibodies against *N. caninum* in serum only documents infection, not clinical disease caused by infection. A presumptive diagnosis of neosporosis can be made by combining appropriate clinical signs of disease and positive serology with the exclusion of other etiologies inducing similar clinical syndromes, in particular, *T. gondii*. Seropositive bitches that have whelped clinically affected puppies can repeat transplacental infection (Dubey, Koestner, and Piper, 1990).

Definitive diagnosis is based on demonstration of the organism in tissues. The organism can be differentiated from *T. gondii* structurally and by immunohistochemistry (Lindsay and Dubey, 1989).

Babesiosis (*Babesia canis*, *Babesia gibsoni*, and *Babesia vogeli* in Dogs; *Babesia cati*, *Babesia felis*, *Babesia herpailuri*, and *Babesia pantherae* in Cats)

Rare Indications • *Babesia* serology is indicated in dogs from endemic areas or with an appropriate travel history together with fever, anemia, icterus, splenomegaly (acute babesiosis), or intermittent fever and weight loss (chronic babesiosis). The species infecting cats are not found in the United States. Babesiosis rarely causes anemia in cats.

Analysis, Artifacts, and Interpretation • Circulating antibodies are detected in serum by IFA. See Appendix I for availability of testing.

In most laboratories, titers > 1:40 are considered positive (Breitschwerdt, 1992). Experimentally infected dogs develop detectable IgG titers approximately 3 weeks after infection. False-negative results can occur in immature dogs. Antibodies against *B. gibsoni* and *B. canis* may or may not cross-react, depending on the antigen

source used by a particular laboratory. Some dogs with babesiosis due to *B. gibsoni* are seronegative on IFA using *B. canis* antigen (Holland CJ: Personal communication, 1993). An IFA is available using *B. gibsoni* antigens (see Appendix I). Dogs that are suspected of having babesiosis and that are seronegative for *B. canis* should be screened for antibodies against *B. gibsoni*. It is important to determine which species is involved in a clinical case, because response to treatment varies. Duration of positive titers after resolution of disease is unknown. In untreated experimentally infected dogs, titers remain high for at least 6 months. Untreated, seropositive dogs should be considered carriers of the infection.

Definitive diagnosis requires demonstration of the organism on Giemsa's-stained blood smears, which are best found in blood (particularly in acute disease) from a microcapillary system (e.g., ventral surface of the ear or the toenail). In chronic disease or asymptomatic carriers, demonstration of organisms is unreliable, and a tentative diagnosis is made on the basis of clinical signs and a positive titer. Dogs with babesiosis are often Coombs' positive (see Chapter 3).

Trypanosomiasis (Chagas' Disease; *Trypanosoma cruzi*)

Rare Indications • Serologic testing for trypanosomiasis should be considered in dogs that are from endemic areas and that have generalized lymphadenomegaly, neurologic signs, or myocardial dysfunction, in particular, second- or third-degree heart block or ventricular tachycaridia.

Analysis, Artifacts, and Interpretation • Circulating antibodies are detected in serum of dogs most commonly by IFA (Barr, 1990) and ELISA (Barr et al., 1991). See Appendix I for availability of testing.

Dogs are generally seropositive 4 weeks after infection. A positive titer only documents exposure to the organism, not clinical disease induced by infection. Positive titers vary by the assay.

Definitive diagnosis requires demonstration of the organism on blood smear, lymph node impression, or buffy coat–plasma interface smear. *T. cruzi* is occasionally found in canine peripheral blood without demonstrable organisms in tissue. A standard workup for myocardial disease including chest radiographs, electrocardiogram, electrolytes, and echocardiography (if available) is indicated. Alternatively, *T. cruzi* amastigotes can be demonstrated in tissues.

SEROLOGIC TESTS AND IDENTIFICATION TECHNIQUES FOR VIRAL INFECTIONS

Feline Leukemia Virus

Common Indications ● Because of the diverse manifestations of FeLV infection, testing is indicated in essentially all clinically ill cats, especially those with evidence of infectious, neoplastic, reproductive, immunologic, or hematologic disease, as well as in clinically normal cats exposed to FeLV-positive cats.

Analysis, Artifacts, and Interpretation ● Viral antigen (p27) is detected by IFA in neutrophils and platelets from blood or bone marrow or in serum, saliva, or tears by ELISA. In-office ELISA tests for p27 in serum that are currently available include the microwell type* or the membrane filter type.† Saliva‡ and tears can also be tested. A serum ELISA combination test§ for FeLV and FIV is available. Antibody titers to FeLV envelope antigens (neutralizing antibody) and against virus-transformed tumor cells (FOCMA antibody) are available. The prognostic significance of results from these tests is unknown at this time. See Appendix I for availability of testing.

There are six stages of FeLV infection (Zenger and Wolf, 1992). Stages 1 through 3 are dissemination stages; bone marrow infection occurs in stage 4. Infected neutrophils and platelets are released from the bone marrow in stage 5, and virus appears in systemic epithelial tissues (including salivary glands and tear glands) during stage 6. ELISA can detect p27 antigen in serum during stages 2 through 6; p27 in cells is not detected by the IFA until stages 5 and 6. Tears and saliva are not positive for p27 until stage 6. Thus, the serum ELISA is the first assay to become positive after infection. Positive serum test results occur anywhere between 2 and 30 weeks (generally 2–8 weeks) after infec-

tion. There is generally a delay of 1 to 2 weeks after the onset of viremia before ELISA tear and saliva tests become positive.

Seropositivity can be detected by serum ELISA before a cat develops persistent infection (stages 4–6); thus, some cats revert to negative results after the development of neutralizing antibodies. Seropositive results by serum ELISA in all healthy cats should be confirmed by IFA or retesting by ELISA in 4 to 6 weeks. Some ELISA-positive cats that revert to negative have become latently infected. The majority of latently infected cats are negative on all testing, but the virus can be isolated from the bone marrow. False-positive ELISA results can develop secondary to poor laboratory technique. False-negative ELISA using tears or saliva occurs in cats in stages 1 through 5.

A positive IFA test has 99% correlation with virus isolation. False-negative reactions may occur when leukopenia or thrombocytopenia prevents evaluation of an adequate number of cells. False-positive reactions rarely occur from nonspecific staining of eosinophils. A positive IFA indicates that the cat is viremic and contagious. The viremia may be transient or sustained. Unless the IFA test is done during a transient infection, the animal will likely (> 95%) remain positive for life (Loar, 1988).

Virtually all IFA-positive cats are also ELISA positive. The rare combination of IFA-positive and ELISA-negative results suggests technique-related artifact. A negative ELISA is approximately 100% correlated with negative IFA and an inability to isolate FeLV. Cats that are ELISA positive but IFA negative are termed *discordant*. Discordant results are usually due to false-positive ELISA results, false-negative IFA results, or transient stage 2 to 3 infection. A suggested approach to discordant cats is given in Figure 15–2.

There is no reliable means of identifying latent FeLV infections other than virus isolation (see Appendix I) or polymerase chain reaction. A latently infected cat may become viremic (IFA and ELISA positive) after administration of corticosteroids or after extreme stress.

Feline Immunodeficiency Virus

Common Indications ● Cats with chronic weight loss, fever, rhinitis, conjunctivitis, gingivitis, dermatitis, diarrhea, uveitis, recurrent abscessation, clinical toxoplasmosis, any chronic infectious disease, chronic renal failure, or lymphadenopathy should be evaluated for FIV infection.

---

*Virocheck FeLV, feline leukemia virus antigen test kit, Synbiotics Corp., San Diego, CA 92127.

†Cite feline leukemia virus test kit, IDEXX Corp., Portland, ME 04101. UNI-TEC FeLV, feline leukemia virus antigen test kit, Synbiotics Corp., San Diego, CA 92127.

‡Assure/FeLV, Wand format, stat Feline leukemia virus antigen test kit, Synbiotics Corp., San Diego, CA 92127.

§Cite Combo, IDEXX Corp., Portland, ME 04101.

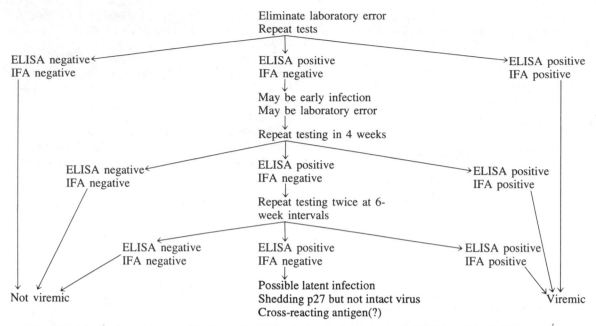

Figure 15–2 Evaluation of the cat with "discordant" feline leukemia virus test results (ELISA positive but IFA negative).

Analysis, Artifacts, and Interpretation ● IgG antibodies are detected in serum by ELISA, IFA, and Western blot immunoassay. Antibody testing is performed by a number of commercial laboratories (see Appendix I). An in-office ELISA* is available for FIV or FIV and FeLV combined.†

Seroconversion occurs 5 to 9 weeks after inoculation in experimentally infected cats (Yamamoto et al., 1988). Seropositive cats are likely infected with FIV for life. False-positive reactions are common using ELISA (Hardy and Zuckerman, 1991). It is recommended that positive ELISA results be confirmed using Western blot immunoassay. The presence of antibody in serum only confirms infection, not clinical illness due to FIV. Virus isolation is available in some laboratories (see Appendix I). Kittens can have detectable colostrum-derived antibodies until 12 to 14 weeks. Because many of the clinical syndromes associated with FIV infection can be due to opportunistic infections, further diagnostic procedures may determine treatable causes. For example, many FIV-seropositive cats with endogenous uveitis are coinfected by *T. gondii.*

Feline Infectious Peritonitis
Rare Indications ● Feline infectious peritonitis (FIP) is an appropriate differential diagnosis in

cats with fever, uveitis, keratitic precipitates, retinal hemorrhage, nonseptic abdominal or pleural exudates, anemia, hyperglobulinemia, and renal, hepatic, or neurologic abnormalities. However, currently available serologic tests cannot diagnose clinical FIP. Serologic testing is indicated for use as a screening procedure in breeding colonies that are coronavirus antibody negative.

Analysis, Artifacts, and Interpretation ● Circulating antibodies against coronaviruses are detected in feline serum by IFA and ELISA.

Antibody to coronavirus indicates prior exposure to a coronavirus in the FIP antigenic group. Enteric coronaviruses cause cross-reacting antibodies. A positive titer does not diagnose FIP or protect against disease. Feline vaccines containing bovine serum may occasionally cause false-positive results. Cats with FIP can have negative results because of rapidly progressive disease with a delayed rise in titer, disappearance of antibody in terminal stages of the disease, or immune complex formation. A positive coronavirus antibody titer does not predict whether a cat will ever develop FIP.

Distinguishing enteric coronavirus from FIP has been attempted using titer magnitude (Pedersen, 1987). IFA titers > 1:3200 have been associated with noneffusive FIP. Titers 1:100 to 1:3200 are commonly associated with the effusive form and occasionally with the noneffusive form but may also be due to enteric coronavi-

---

*Cite feline immunodeficiency virus antibody test kit, ID-EXX Corp., Portland, ME 04101.

†Cite Combo, IDEXX Corp., Portland, ME 04101.

rus. Titers of 1:256 or lower may be due to fulminating effusive FIP, enteric coronavirus, and recent vaccination for coronavirus. A kinetics-based ELISA test (KELA) is available (see Appendix I). A KELA titer > 1:250 in conjunction with appropriate clinical and laboratory signs is suspect for FIP. Repeat testing in 2 to 3 weeks to look for an increased titer is probably not clinically useful.

Definitive diagnosis requires histopathologic evaluation of tissues. Hyperproteinemia and polyclonal gammopathy (detected by electrophoresis, see Chapter 12) can occur, particularly in the noneffusive form. Monoclonal gammopathy rarely occurs. Classic nonseptic pyogranulomatous exudate with high protein and relatively low cell count (see Chapter 10) is a common basis for a presumptive diagnosis. Electrophoresis can also be performed on body fluids; a gamma globulin fraction ≥ 32% is highly suggestive of FIP (Shelly et al., 1988). If the albumin:globulin ratio of body fluid is > 0.81, FIP can probably be ruled out (Shelly et al., 1988). Kittens can be seropositive owing to colostrum-derived antibodies until 9 weeks of age. If kittens are infected by adult cats in the environment, antibodies can be detected again 8 to 14 weeks later. Virus can be secreted by antibody-positive healthy cats (Addie and Jarret, 1992). Titers may be determined if the diagnosis is doubtful, but interpretation is done in conjunction with clinical signs and laboratory data.

Canine Distemper

Rare Indications ● Dogs with appropriate signs of CNS disease can have antibodies against canine distemper virus measured concurrently in CSF and serum.

Analysis, Artifacts, and Interpretation ● CSF and serum IgG antibodies against canine distemper virus can be measured by serum virus neutralization, IFA, or ELISA. Serum IgM antibodies can be measured by ELISA (see Appendix I for availability of testing).

CSF antibodies to distemper virus are increased in some dogs subsequently diagnosed by histopathologic examination as having distemper encephalitis. False-positive results can occur in CSF samples contaminated with blood. Concurrent measurement of serum antibody concentrations can be helpful; if CSF concentrations are greater than serum concentrations, the antibody in CSF had to be produced locally and is consistent with CNS distemper. Detection of

serum IgG antibodies is of minimal diagnostic value because a positive titer could develop secondary to vaccination or previous exposure. A fourfold increase in serum IgG titer over a 3 to 4 week period is suggestive of recent infection. Detection of IgM antibodies in serum is consistent with recent infection but not clinical disease.

Definitive diagnosis requires demonstration of viral inclusions by cytologic analysis (Color Plates 1D and 1E), direct fluorescent antibody staining of cytology specimens, or histopathologic evaluation. In acute canine distemper, immunofluorescence of conjunctival scrapings can be helpful; fluorescence may be detected 5 to 21 days after infection (Greene and Appel, 1990). Antigen is present in buffy coat smears for only 2 to 9 days after infection; therefore, it is usually inapparent when clinical signs occur. The duration of persistence of CSF antibodies is unknown. CSF evaluation in dogs with canine distemper may reveal increased protein and leukocytes, with lymphocytes predominating. A presumptive diagnosis of distemper encephalitis can be made with increased CSF protein and leukocytes, with lymphocytes predominating and a positive CSF antibody titer in a sample not contaminated with peripheral blood.

Enteric Viruses

Determining serum antibodies to feline parvovirus and canine parvovirus or coronavirus is rarely performed clinically because of difficulty in interpreting positive results. However, detecting fecal shedding of canine parvovirus viral antigen by electron microscopy, virus isolation, fecal hemagglutination, fecal LA, or ELISA is more useful. An in-office ELISA for canine parvovirus in feces* seems to detect fecal shedding of parvovirus in acute cases accurately (see Chapter 9). Virus isolation or electron microscopy is required to identify canine coronavirus or feline parvovirus.

DIAGNOSIS OF DIROFILARASIS
(*Dirofilaria immitis*)

Cytology (Knott's Test or Filter Test)

Common Indications ● Cytologic evaluation for microfilaria is indicated in dogs with signs con-

---

*Cite canine parvovirus test kit, IDEXX Corp., Portland, ME 04101.

sistent with heartworm disease (right-sided heart disease, coughing, respiratory distress, eosinophilia, polyclonal hyperglobulinemia, or protein-losing nephropathy), in dogs about to begin prophylatic therapy (with diethylcarbamazine, ivermectin, or milbemycin), and rarely in cats with signs consistent with heartworm disease (respiratory disease, cardiomegaly, or unexplained vomiting). Advantages: very specific (microfilaria morphology differentiates *D. immitis* microfilaria from those of *Dipetalonema reconditum*), quick, and inexpensive; all concentration techniques (Knott's and filter tests) are much more sensitive than is examination of fresh blood smears and are reasonably sensitive in dogs that have not been treated with filaricidal drugs. Disadvantages: Up to 40% of dogs have spontaneous occult dirofilariasis (Zimmerman, 1992) and must be diagnosed by serologic testing and radiographic examination. The Knott's test and filter tests have poor sensitivity in cats.

Analysis, Artifacts, and Interpretation ● A positive test result diagnoses heartworm disease except in juveniles < 4 to 5 months of age, which could have received the microfilaria by transplacental transfer. Negative results in dogs that have not received microfilaricidal drugs is reasonable evidence of lack of infection; however, if microfilarial numbers are low, two or three tests are sometimes needed. Also, up to 40% of infected dogs are amicrofilaremic. Infected dogs receiving ivermectin or milbemycin as heartworm preventive are commonly amicrofilaremic. Clinical or laboratory signs of heartworm disease despite one or more negative microfilaria tests indicate serologic testing for circulating heartworm antigen and chest radiographs.

Heartworm Adult Antigen Titer

Common Indications ● Dogs with signs consistent with dirofilariasis (coughing, respiratory distress, exercise intolerance, ascites, eosinophilia, polyclonal hyperglobulinemia, or protein-losing nephropathy) but amicrofilaremic should be tested for adult antigens of *D. immitis*. Dogs on ivermectin or milbemycin preventive can have sterile female adult worms and be amicrofilaremic. The test can also be used to assess the efficacy of adulticide treatment. There is limited applicability in feline dirofilariasis. Advantages: greater sensitivity when compared with microfilaria detection techniques. Disad-

vantage: more expensive than microfilaria detection techniques.

Analysis, Artifacts, and Interpretation ● Circulating heartworm antigen is detected in serum by ELISA.* IFA and ELISA can detect circulating antibodies to microfilariae and adults, respectively, but have low sensitivity and specificity.

Intestinal parasites, *D. reconditum*, hemolysis, and concurrent use of diethylcarbamazine, ivermectin, or milbemycin do not alter results of antigen assays. The test may be positive as early as 5 to 6 months and is usually positive 6 to 7 months after infection. False-negative results usually occur in early stages of infection with nongravid females and may occur in single-sex infections or in animals with low worm burdens (fewer than five worms). Retesting in 2 to 3 months should be performed to detect dogs that test negative in the early stages of infection. After successful adulticide treatment, test results become negative in approximately 12 weeks.

In cats, serologic testing for circulating antigen is of limited value because the low worm burdens (i.e., one to five worms) may result in false-negative results. In experimental infections, cats that tested positive did so about 8 months after infection (Dzimianski et al., 1986). Therefore, a positive test result is specific for infection, but a negative result does not rule out dirofilariasis.

Definitive diagnosis requires detecting circulating microfilariae, characteristic radiographic signs (i.e., right-sided cardiac enlargement, increased diameter ± tortuosity of pulmonary arteries, and pulmonary interstitial infiltrate), or circulating heartworm antigen. Dogs that are amicrofilaremic but have clinical signs of disease should be evaluated serologically and with thoracic radiographs. In a previously infected and treated dog, it may be impossible to differentiate "new" from "old" radiographic lesions. In such cases, serologic testing is indicated. In cats, both Knott's test and serologic evaluation can have negative results, and results should be interpreted in concert with thoracic radiographs.

Bibliography

Addie DD, Jarrett O: A study of naturally occurring feline coronavirus infections in kittens. Vet Rec 1992;130:133–137.

*Cite Semi-quant canine heartworm test kit, IDEXX Corp., Portland, ME 04101.
Cite Snap canine heartworm kit, IDEXX Corp., Portland, ME 04101.
Assure/ CH, Synbiotics Corp., San Diego, CA 92127.
Dirochek, Synbiotics Corp., San Diego, CA 92127.
UNI-TEC CHW, canine heartworm antigen test kit, Synbiotics Corp., San Diego, CA 92127.

Anderson BE, Green CE, Jones DC, et al: *Ehrlichia ewingii* sp. nov., the etiologic agent of canine granulocytic ehrlichiosis. Int J Syst Bacteriol 1992;42:299–302.

Barlough JE, Stoddart CA: Cats and coronaviruses. JAVMA 1988;193:796–800.

Barr SC: American trypanosomiasis. *In* Greene CE (ed): Infectious Diseases of the Dog and Cat. Philadelphia, WB Saunders, 1990, pp 763–768.

Barr SC, Dennis VA, Klei TR: ELISA for detection of anti-*Trypanosoma cruzi* antibody in dogs (abstract). Proceedings, Annual Meeting American College of Veterinary Internal Medicine, New Orleans, LA, May 1991, p 893.

Barsanti JA: Cenitourinary tract infections. *In* Greene (ed): Philadelphia, WB Saunders, 1984, pp 157–183.

Barsanti JA: Histoplasmosis. *In* Greene CE (ed): Clinical Microbiology and Infectious Diseases of the Dog and Cat. Philadelphia, WB Saunders, 1984, pp 687–699.

Barsanti JA, Jeffrey KL: Coccidioidomycosis. *In* Greene CE (ed): Infectious Diseases of the Dog and Cat. Philadelphia, WB Saunders, 1990, pp 696–706.

Berg et al: Identification of the major coagulase-positive *Staphylococcus* sp of dogs as *Staphylococcus intermedius*. Am J Vet Res 1984;45:1307–1309.

Breitschwerdt EB: Laboratory diagnosis of tick-transmitted diseases in the dog. *In* Kirk RW, Bonagura JD (eds): Current Veterinary Therapy XI. Philadelphia, WB Saunders, 1992, pp 252–255.

Buhles WG, Huxsoll DL, Ristic M: Tropical pancytopenia: Clinical, hematologic and serologic response of dogs to *Ehrlichia canis* infection, tetracycline therapy, and challenge inoculation. J Infect Dis 1974;130:357–367.

Calvert CA, Dow SW: Cardiovascular infections. *In* Greene CE (ed): Infectious Diseases of the Dog and Cat. Philadelphia, WB Saunders, 1990, pp 97–113.

Calvert CA, Greene CE: Bacteria in dogs: Diagnosis, treatment, and prognosis. Comp Cont Ed Pract Vet 1986;8:179–187.

Carmichael LE, Greene CE: Canine brucellosis. *In* Greene CE (ed): Infectious Diseases of Dog and Cat. Philadelphia, WB Saunders, 1990, pp 573–584.

Cox HU, Hoskins JD, Newman SS, et al: Temporal study of staphylococcal species on healthy dogs. Am J Vet Res 1988;49:747–751.

Davidson MG, Breitschwerdt EB, Walker DH, et al: Identification of rickettsiae in cutaneous biopsy specimens from dogs with experimental Rocky Mountain spotted fever. J Vet Intern Med 1989;3:8–11.

Dow SW, Jones SL: Anaerobic infections. Comp Cont Ed Pract Vet 1987;9:827–839.

Dubey JP, Koestner A, Piper RC: Repeated transplacental transmission of *Neospora caninum* in dogs. J Am Vet Med Assoc 1990;197:857–860.

Dzimianski MT, McCall JW, McCall CA: Evaluation of heart worm immunodiagnostic test kits using well defined cat sera. Proceedings, Heartworm Symposium '86, Washington, DC, American Heartworm Society, 1986, pp 159–161.

Feder DM, Joseph RJ, Moroff SD, et al: *Borrelia burgdorferi* antibodies in canine cerebrospinal fluid (abstract). Proceedings, Annual Meeting, American College of Veterinary Internal Medicine, New Orleans, LA, May 1991, p 892.

Fox JG: Campylobacteriosis. *In* Greene CE (ed). Infectious Diseases of the Dog and Cat. Philadelphia, WB Saunders, 1990, pp 538–542.

French TW, Harvey JW: Serologic diagnosis of infectious cyclic thrombocytopenia in dogs using an indirect fluorescent antibody test. Am J Vet Res 1983;44:2407–2411.

Greene CE (ed): Clinical Microbiology and Infectious Diseases of the Dog and Cat. Philadelphia, WB Saunders, 1984.

Greene CE: Rocky Mountain spotted fever and ehrlichiosis. *In* Kirk RW (ed): Current Veterinary Therapy IX. Philadelphia, WB Saunders, 1986, pp 1080–1084.

Greene CE, Appel MJ: Canine distemper. *In* Greene CE (ed): Infectious Diseases of the Dog and Cat. Philadelphia, WB Saunders, 1990, pp 538–542.

Greene CE, Breitschwerdt EB: Rocky Mountain spotted fever and Q fever. *In* Greene CE (ed): Infectious Diseases of the Dog and Cat. Philadelphia, WB Saunders, 1990, pp 519–433.

Greene CE, Marks A, Lappin MR, et al: Comparison of latex agglutination, indirect immunofluorescent antibody, and enzyme immunoassay methods for serodiagnosis of Rocky Mountain spotted fever in dogs. Am J Vet Res 1990;54:20–28.

Greene CE, Schotts EB: Leptospirosis. *In* Greene CE (ed): Infectious Diseases of the Dog and Cat. Philadelphia, WB Saunders, 1990, pp 498–507.

Hardy WD, Zuckerman EE: Comparison of ELISA, IFA and immunoblot tests for detection of feline immunodeficiency virus infection. Proceedings, First International Conference of Feline Immunodeficiency Virus Researchers, Davis, CA, September 1991, p 56.

Hirsh DC, Ruehl WW: Clinical microbiology as a guide to the treatment of infectious bacterial diseases of the dog and cat. *In* Scott FW (ed): Contemporary Issues in Small Animal Practice. Vol 3. Infectious Diseases. New York, Churchill Livingstone, 1986, pp 1–28.

Jameson P, King LA, Lappin MR, et al: Canine lower respiratory *Mycoplasma* infections: Clinical signs, diagnostic findings, and clinical outcome in 65 cases. JAVMA, 1993, in press.

Jones RL: Laboratory diagnosis of bacterial infections. *In* Greene CE (ed): Infectious Diseases of the Dog and Cat. Philadelphia, WB Saunders, 1990, pp 453–460.

Lappin MR: Immunodiagnosis and management of clinical feline toxoplasmosis. Proceedings, Waltham Feline Medicine Symposium, Orlando, FL, January 20, 1993, pp 19–26.

Lappin MR, Greene CE, Winston S, et al: Clinical feline toxoplasmosis: Serologic diagnosis and therapeutic management of 15 cases. J Vet Intern Med 1989;3:139–143.

Lappin MR, Roberts SM, Davidson MG, et al: Enzyme-linked immunosorbent assays for the detection of *Toxoplasma gondii* specific antibodies and antigens in the aqueous humor of cats. JAVMA 1992;201:1010–1016.

Legendre AM: Blastomycosis. *In* Greene CE (ed): Infectious Diseases of the Dog and Cat. Philadelphia, WB Saunders, 1990, pp 669–678.

Lewis GE, Huxsoll DL, Ristic M, et al: Experimentally induced infection of dogs, cats, and nonhuman primates with *Ehrlichia equi*, etiologic agent of equine ehrlichiosis. JAVMA 1975;36:85–88.

Lindenmayer J, Weber M, Bryant J, et al: Comparison of indirect immunofluorescent-antibody assay, enzyme-linked immunosorbent assay, and Western blot immunoblot for the diagnosis of Lyme disease in dogs. J Clin Microbiol 1990;28:92–96.

Lindsay DS, Dubey JP: Immunohistochemical diagnosis of *Neospora caninum* in tissue sections. Am J Vet Res 1989;50:1981–1983.

Ling GV, Branam JE, Ruby AL, et al: Canine prostatic fluid: Techniques of collection, quantitative bacterial culture, and interpretation of results. JAVMA 1983;183:201–211.

Ling GV, Nyland TG, Kennedy PC, et al: Comparison of two sample collection methods for quantitative bacteriologic culture of canine prostatic fluid. JAVMA 1990;196:1479–1482.

Loar AS: FeLV: Current issues. Proceedings, 6th Annual Veterinary Medical Forum, American College of Veterinary Internal Medicine, Washington, D.C., May 26–29, 1988, pp 672–676.

Macy DW, Gasper PW: Plague. *In* Greene CE (ed): Infectious Diseases of the Dog and Cat. Philadelphia, WB Saunders, 1990, pp 621–627.

Martin CE: Ocular infections. *In* Greene CE (ed): Infectious Diseases of the Dog and Cat. Philadelphia, WB Saunders, 1990, pp 197–212.

McKiernan BC, Smith AR, Kissil M: Bacterial isolates from the lower trachea of clinically healthy dogs. JAAHA 1984;20:139–142.

Medleau L, Marks AM, Brown J, et al: Clinical evaluation of a cryptococcal antigen latex agglutination test for diagnosis of cryptococcosis in cats. JAVMA 1990;196:1470.

Pedersen NC: Coronavirus diseases (coronavirus enteritis, feline infectious peritonitis). *In* Holzworth J (ed): Diseases of the Cat. Philadelphia, WB Saunders, 1987, pp 193–214.

Perille AL, Matus RE: Canine ehrlichiosis in six dogs with persistently increased antibody titers. J Vet Intern Med 1991;5:195–198.

Rentko VT, Ross LA: Canine leptospirosis. *In* Kirk RW, Bonagura JD (eds): Current Veterinary Therapy XI. Philadelphia, WB Saunders, 1992, pp 260–263.

Rohrbach BW: Tularemia. JAVMA 1988;193:428–432.

Sharp NJH: Canine nasal aspergillosis/penicilliosis. *In* Greene CE (ed): Infectious Diseases of the Dog and Cat. Philadelphia, WB Saunders, 1990, pp 714–718.

Shelly SM, Scarlett-Kranz J, Blue JT: Protein electrophoresis on effusions from cats as a diagnostic test for feline infectious peritonitis. JAAHA 1988;24:495–500.

Troy GC, Forrester SD: Canine ehrlichiosis. *In* Greene CE (ed): Infectious Diseases of the Dog and Cat. Philadelphia, WB Saunders, 1990, pp 404–418.

Turner S, Kaufman L, Jalbert M: Diagnostic assessment of an enzyme-linked immunosorbent assay for human and canine blastomycosis. J Clin Microbiol 1986;23:294–297.

Wasmoen TL, Sebring RW, Blumer BM, et al: Examination of Koch's postulates for *Borrelia burgdorferi* as the causative agent of limb/joint dysfunction in dogs with borreliosis. JAVMA 1992;201:418.

Yamamoto JK, Sparger E, Ho EW, et al: Pathogenesis of experimentally induced feline immuodeficiency virus infection in cats. Am J Vet Res 1988;49:1246–1258.

Zenger E, Wolf AM: An update on feline retrovirus infections. *In* Kirk RW, Bonagura JD (eds): Current Veterinary Therapy XI. Philadelphia, WB Saunders, 1992, pp 272–277.

Zimmerman G: False negatives. Heartworm screening tests: Which one should you be using? Pet Vet April/March, 1992, pp 15–21.

Harold Tvedten

16 Cytology of Neoplastic and Inflammatory Masses

Diagnostic cytology is popular and useful. Major advantages of cytologic diagnosis include the following: Minimal equipment is needed, so cytology is possible in any practice; an essentially immediate cytologic conclusion is possible and obviates waiting one or more days for a histologic diagnosis; fine-needle aspirates are minimally invasive and minimally stressful for a patient; and cytology may save the expense of anesthesia and surgery. This chapter discusses cytologic evaluation of masses. The cytologic analysis of fluid, vaginal secretions, semen, respiratory tract material, and specific organs is described in the appropriate chapters.

Cytology can alter or eliminate the surgical approach. Obviously benign masses, such as lipomas and epidermal inclusion cysts, need not be removed immediately; if they are removed, a close resection (i.e., "shelling it out") is adequate, whereas wide excision is indicated for potentially malignant neoplasms. Any cytologic evidence of malignancy (e.g., possible carcinoma or sarcoma) dictates surgical removal for firm histologic diagnosis and a search for metastasis. Metastasis may obviate surgical removal. Neoplasms that are too vascular or invasive for surgery may require cytology for diagnosis instead of histopathology. If a specific tumor diagnosis is made certain, treatment combinations may be stated early. Diagnosis of lymphosarcoma usually initiates chemotherapy rather than surgery.

Cytology does have limitations. Histopathology is usually more diagnostic and definitive, since more information is available from a histologic section than from the smaller number of cells on a cytologic smear that lack tissue's architectural patterns. Cytology should be thought of as rendering a tentative diagnosis requiring histologic confirmation, especially for diagnosis of specific neoplasms. Cytologic diagnoses are more general (e.g., carcinoma) than are histologic diagnoses (e.g., thyroid adenocarcinoma). Of 147 skin tumors, only 105 (71%) cytologic diagnoses agreed with histologic diagnoses (Griffiths et al., 1984). Radical steps (e.g., euthanasia) should await confirmed diagnosis when possible.

There are exceptions in which cytology is as diagnostic as histology or more diagnostic (e.g., individual cell detail of leukemias is as diagnostic as tissue patterns). Cytology was correct in 60 of 64 round cell tumors and occasionally more diagnostic than histology (Duncan and Prasse, 1979). The cytologic and histologic diagnoses agreed on all of the following tumors: 37 mast cell tumors, 11 melanomas, 2 histiocytomas, and 1 cutaneous lymphosarcoma (Griffiths et al., 1984). Accurate cytologic diagnoses were also made for squamous cell carcinomas, lipomas, and metastasis to lymph nodes.

CYTOLOGIC TECHNIQUES

Slide Preparation

The major goal is to obtain a significant number of well-stained, intact cells that reflect the composition of the mass. Consider the site that is being sampled. An aspirate or impression smear should reflect the primary disease. Samples of a body surface are easier to obtain but are often misleading (Fig. 16–1). Samples of deeper tissue are more likely to be diagnostic. Epithelial cells at the edge of ulcers appear anaplastic, since they are actively proliferating to cover the ulcer (e.g., corneal ulcers can cytologically resemble squamous cell carcinoma). Ulcerated surfaces often have secondary inflammatory and septic changes. Soft centers of a mass may be necrotic or hemorrhagic, so a smaller firm mass or a more viable appearing area at the edge of a mass may be more diagnostic.

A fine-needle aspirate need obtain only one or more small drops of fluid to streak out like a blood smear. The smear must have a thin area where cells may settle flatly and expose a large surface area to view (Fig. 16–2). If the smear is thick, the cells are supported more upright on the slide and have a smaller diameter. Cells in thick areas are taller and thus stain darker. Proteinaceous and necrotic debris in the dried fluid surrounding cells interferes with staining. If the fluid is viscous, a squash preparation may be necessary to get a thin smear. A drop of fluid is placed between two slides, and as the drop spreads to its maximum diameter, the slides are slid apart while their surfaces are kept pressed together. This creates a smear on each slide.

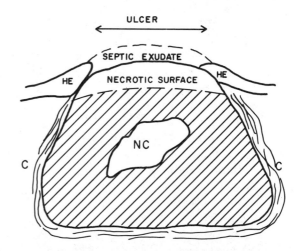

Figure 16–1 Sampling sites from a mass. Different cell populations are retrieved from different sites. Cells from the mass (hatched area) are representative and diagnostic. Samples from the surface may be only necrotic, septic exudate. Immature-appearing hyperplastic epithelial cells (HE) from the edge of an ulcer may mimic a carcinoma. Material from a necrotic center (NC) may resemble only debris. Cells from the boundary (C) may be fibroblasts from the capsule or a local inflammatory response. Mature fat or blood may be collected from adjacent normal tissue.

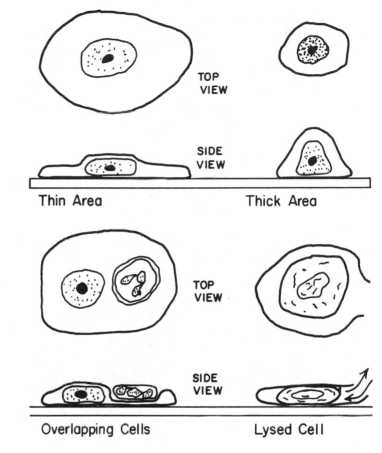

Figure 16–2 Cell morphology in three dimensions. The cell on the upper right is in the thick part of a smear so it fails to spread out over a large surface area. It appears smaller and darker from the top compared with the cell on the upper left, which has spread out in a thin area of a smear, allowing proper evaluation. The epithelial cell in the lower left has a neutrophil dimpled into its surface. The neutrophil appears to be in the cell when viewed from above. The partially lysed cell on the lower right has a swollen, enlarged nucleus and nucleolus, which may appear malignant instead of only damaged.

For impression smears, a freshly cut surface of a representative area of the specimen is gently touched to several areas of glass slides without any twisting or rubbing motion. Excess fluid is first removed by blotting the tissue with a paper towel. Check to see if cells exfoliated well before placing the tissue in formalin, which should always be stored in another area. Fibrous masses usually do not release cells easily and may need to be scraped with a scalpel to obtain enough cells for diagnosis. The moist material on the blade is streaked on slides.

Patient identification and the date must be noted on the slide so patients will get the right diagnosis. A description of the site is needed to interpret the results, especially if multiple sites are sampled. Mailing containers for slides should be too large (e.g., small box) to fit through the post office's automatic stamp canceling machine. The thin two-slide cardboard slide boxes that fit in an envelope often arrive with crushed glass slides even when marked "Hand Cancel."

Smears are air dried for Wright's-type stains and new methylene blue (NMB) staining. Alcohol fixation is required for Papanicolaou's

(Pap's) or Sano's stain. Air drying of cells slowly in a moist environment may cause cell distortion. Although rarely used, a hair dryer speeds drying. Hold the dryer far enough away from the smears to avoid "cooking" them. Prevent exposure to dust during storage. Flies eat unstained cells. Touch only the sides of the slides, or squamous cells from fingerprints can contaminate the smears and interfere with the interpretation.

Formalin exposure is a common problem causing excessive blue staining of smears stained with Wright's stain. Tissue used for impression smears should not have been placed in formalin before the slides were made. Formalin should not be stored near the stains or smears. Formalin should not be submitted in the same package with cytologic smears, where the fumes may act on unstained cells. Heparin anticoagulant also causes a blue discoloration of Wright's-stained cells.

The Stains

Most practices need only a modified Wright's-type stain and NMB. The Wright's stain has blue and orange dyes. The dyes stain acidic structures such as nucleic acids (DNA and RNA) in nuclei blue or purple and basic structures like proteins (e.g., hemoglobin in erythrocytes [RBCs]) orange. Obviously, pH changes in rinse water can affect staining characteristics. The "quick" stains are not true Wright's or Giemsa's (i.e., Romanovsky's) stains but have blue and orange dyes to give similar staining characteristics. Diff-Quik stain is popular because one can easily adjust the color of the cells. The blue and orange dyes are in separate jars, and by increasing or decreasing the number of times one dips the slide in a color, one can increase or decrease intensity of blue or orange. A Diff-Quik staining kit from Baxter Scientific Products (B4132-1) was priced at $80.85, and five premeasured vials of NMB cost $25 in 1992. The Diff-Quik stain illustrates distemper inclusion bodies well on blood smears. It may occasionally fail to stain granules in some mast cells, in contrast to routine Wright's stain (Rebar, 1978).

NMB is a monochrome stain with variably intense blue staining. It is used as a wet mount by placing a drop on the smear and applying a coverslip. To prevent retention of an air bubble over the most diagnostic part of the smear, use the coverslip gently to pull the drop of NMB over the cells to moisten them before slowly applying the coverslip. Staining is immediate. NMB stains nuclear material well and demonstrates distinct chromatin patterns. This nuclear detail is useful in determining malignant criteria. The transparent nature of NMB is a major advantage, since one can focus the microscope through different depths of tissue fragments to judge individual cell detail and architectural patterns in three dimensions. Tissue fragments are often the most diagnostic material on smears from neoplasms but stain too darkly to evaluate with Wright's stain. The fragments are like tiny biopsy sections that allow evaluation of how cells were oriented in the mass. These architectural patterns help identify the tissue type. One can evaluate adjacent cells for true variability that suggests malignancy, compared with the variability of isolated cells on a smear that may have come from different areas or cell types in the mass.

In summary, Wright's stain is best for inflammatory lesions, since the stained appearance of leukocytes (white blood cells [WBCs]) is similar to that in blood smears and bacteria are stained a characteristic, variable blue color. NMB is excellent for neoplasms, tissue cells in general, and fungi. The use of both Wright's and NMB stains for the same lesion is recommended, since different characteristics of the cells are illustrated by each stain. Cytoplasmic structures often show best on Wright's stain. Nuclear detail is best with NMB. Organisms not prominent on one stain usually are seen on the other. Use of only one stain may contribute to missing a diagnostic feature.

Other stains may be used. A combination of a drop of NMB and Sudan's or other oil stain selectively stains lipid and gives adequate cell detail. This stain combination is useful for fatty livers (Color Plate 3F), chylothorax (Color Plate 4B), aspiration pneumonia, or lipid granulomas. The NMB stains the nucleus and other cell structures blue, and the Sudan stains lipid red.

Gram's stain differentiates gram-negative from gram-positive bacteria, which may help in choosing antibiotics. Caution is suggested because staining is variable and must be done often to have confidence in it. It is not sensitive for screening cytologic smears for low numbers of gram-negative (i.e., red) bacteria in a red, proteinaceous background. Wright's stain is recommended to find bacteria and define their size and shape. Gram's stain is useful if bacteria are easily found. Acid-fast stain is rarely needed, since mycobacterial infections are uncommon.

Pap's stain or a modified Sano's trichrome stain is routinely used in human medicine. Specific malignant criteria have been established for cells stained with these stains (Allen et al., 1986). Pap's stain is a transparent stain that permits evaluation of tissue fragments and fine evaluation of nuclear characteristics like the NMB stain. The use of Pap's stain in the author's practice was discontinued because tumor diagnoses were made with the more rapid NMB and Wright's stains before the technician could finish the Pap's staining procedure, and the diagnoses were not changed by examining the Pap's smears.

Microscopes

A good quality, well-maintained microscope is needed for cytologic work. A binocular microscope is more comfortable for long periods of work. Four objectives are recommended. Use 4 × and 10 × for scanning a smear. Use the 50 × oil and 100 × oil for fine detail. Objectives of similar magnification may be substituted. The cost of a properly equipped, good quality microscope is about $1000 to $1800.

A 50 × oil planachromatic objective (40 × – 60× oil) pays for itself ($350–$400) by the time it saves. The magnification is sufficient for most detail, and more cells can be seen in a shorter time. Having more cells in the field of view allows better comparison of variations among cells and easier identification. The whole field of view is in focus with the more expensive plan-achromatic lenses, whereas with the achromatic lenses the perimeter is out of focus. With a wider field of view, less time is needed to find abnormal cells. A second oil objective (50 × and 100 ×) avoids the need to coverslip smears. Wright's-stained cells observed with a 40 × high dry objective appear fuzzy, since the cells are surrounded by air. Using mounting media with a coverslip or oil eliminates the air-cell interface and the poor cell detail. Adding a drop of oil is much faster than coverslipping all smears. Oily smears are, however, more messy to store and less permanent.

The microscope should be cleaned and lubricated by a trained repair person every 1 to 3 years, but daily cleaning is required. A cover prevents dust accumulation. Kimwipes are lint-free tissues that are satisfactory for cleaning microscope objectives not used for photomicroscopy. Kimwipes absorb oil better than does lens paper and thus clean more effectively. Oil should be removed from lenses at the end of a work period, since oil remaining on a lens can penetrate behind the lens to make the image permanently out of focus. Debris that dries on the surface may require xylene or lens cleaner to remove. The final polishing of the objective lens should be with lens paper. Avoid sharp vibrations such as dragging the microscope along the surface of a desk or setting it down hard. This can knock the prism out of alignment and cause a double image.

The condenser must be in the proper position for optimal detail. To position the condenser near the optimal setting (Köhler's illumination), first position the condenser close beneath the glass slide on the stage. While at high power, focus on the cells on a smear. Then slightly move the condenser to get the brightest light. If you are at optimal positioning, any dust on the condenser or light is in view. The aperture diaphragm in the condenser (i.e., the small lever extending from the condenser) is left all the way open (i.e., brightest light), or else the cells appear refractile.

Some people avoid the optimal position if the light is too bright for them, but it is better to use a neutral density filter, a less-bright bulb, or a more controllable light source than to suffer through poor cell detail to retain eye comfort. The "swing-in" condenser lens on Reichert (American Optical) microscopes should be swung out except at low power (2.5 × and 4 × objectives). When morphologic detail is not needed and the viewer wants only to easily find objects like parasite ova, urinary casts, or platelets in a hemocytometer, then the condenser is moved to the lowest position. This position gives structures more contrast.

There are several common problems with microscopy. When cells are in focus at medium power (10 × or 40 ×) but not with the oil objective, check to see if the slide is upside down. The cells are often on the underside of the slide. If the coverslip or mounting medium is too thick, one also cannot focus at high magnifications. If the fine focus will not turn any farther in the direction needed, it is often because the fine focus is turned too far in one direction. Adjust the coarse adjustment past the plane of focus needed and then turn the fine focus knob in the opposite direction to regain focusing ability. If the cells look refractile and have poor detail, the lighting is probably wrong. Adjust the condenser by opening the aperture diaphragm or raising the condenser up near the slide.

CYTOLOGIC CONCLUSIONS

The usual composition of a mass is a proliferation of tissue cells, an accumulation of inflammatory cells, or both. Miscellaneous masses include hematomas, cysts, or focal areas of necrosis. Characteristics of each type and its variants follow and are briefly summarized in Figure 16-3.

Slide Reading Approach

Veterinarians have had ample microscopy and pathology training, so most can read cytologic smears as long as they recognize their limitations and constantly train themselves. One form of continuing education is to perform cytology on excised masses and compare your descriptions and conclusions with histopathology reports. Cytologic evaluation is a visual task, so one should obtain one or more cytologic atlases for visual comparisons (Rebar, 1978; Perman et al., 1979). An organized approach to an aspirate or impression smear of an abnormal mass is necessary for consistent conclusions. A summary of steps follows, and details are in later sections. Normal structure may be sampled inadvertently. For example, a common error is to aspirate the submandibular salivary gland instead of the lymph node. These smears have mature acinar

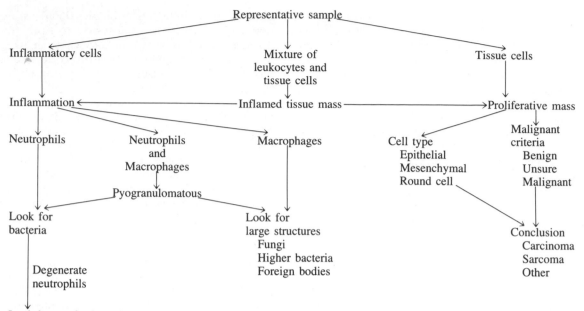

Figure 16–3 General cytologic approach. Most diagnostic samples are initially divided into an inflammatory or a proliferative pattern or both. Inflammatory samples are examined for likely causative organisms. Degenerative changes in neutrophils stimulate a longer search for bacteria. Proliferative patterns are evaluated for cell type and evidence of malignancy. Summary statements are then made. With an inflamed tissue mass, one pursues an inflammation approach or a proliferative mass approach based on the predominant cell type.

and ductal structures with foamy epithelial cells. The liver may be inadvertently sampled while obtaining "thoracic" aspirates.

Slide Reading Summary

1. First establish that a sufficient number of intact, properly stained cells are present.
2. Scan the smears at low power to determine variation in distribution and content.
3. Begin fine evaluation of cells in an area with intact cells of good staining quality.
4. Determine whether the cell population is primarily inflammatory. If so, attempt to identify the etiologic agent.
5. Determine whether a large enough population of noninflammatory (tissue) cells is present, indicating a proliferative tissue mass.
6. With proliferative tissue masses (e.g., neoplasia or hyperplasia), determine the cell type(s) present and the amount of evidence indicating malignancy.

The initial effort should be to screen the smears grossly for those most likely to be diagnostic. In tumor cytology, the slides with small fragments of tissue are most promising and should be stained with NMB or other transparent stain. The most cellular smears, which are most likely diagnostic, stain bluest since they have the most nuclei. Hemodiluted smears with few nucleated cells appear orange grossly with Wright's stain, which suggests a lower chance of a diagnostic smear.

Too often one goes immediately to the 100 × oil objective and stays at that power until fatigued. The scanning power must be used first and often to locate productive areas of the smear, which are then evaluated with an oil objective power. Promising areas are characterized by being thin and having intact, well-stained individualized cells. Cells poorly stained with Wright's stain have an altered blue color. The color and streaked-out appearance of necrotic, lysed cells indicates an area to avoid. Very diagnostic structures (e.g., bacterial and fungal colonies) may be rare and isolated, so take time to scan the smears and do not spend all the time at high magnification in a few areas. Similarly, tissue fragments that have the valuable architectural patterns of tiny "histopathologic sections" are irregularly distributed and found by scanning.

Finally, determine and record the cell population in terms of the percentage of various cell types. A hematology differential counter is useful to keep track of various cell types. Consistently describing the cell populations aids the mental process of forming conclusions. Writing a description keeps the mind active and avoids the problem of not knowing what to do next. Do not expect to identify all cells. Experts often use a category of "other" cells for unidentified cells and then morphologically describe the cells and suggest their origin. If the smears are moderately to markedly cellular and 99% of the cells are WBCs, including 90% neutrophils, then the conclusion is obviously that the mass is inflamed, perhaps an abscess. If only 1% are large mesenchymal cells, they would most likely be reactive cells (e.g., fibroblasts in an inflamed mass), not a sarcoma. It is common to have a few unidentified "active-appearing cells" in inflammatory masses. If they are few, they are ignored. On the contrary, if 50% of the cells are spindle-shaped mesenchymal cells, the conclusion would be that the mass is a connective tissue proliferation.

If the evidence indicates a neutrophilic inflammatory mass, one would look for the most likely etiologic agent (i.e., bacteria). Other inflammatory patterns suggest other causes. If the intermediate conclusion is that the mass is a connective tissue proliferation, one would determine and record the variety and magnitude of the malignant criteria. The amount of cytologic evidence of malignancy is then used to differentiate a sarcoma from a benign proliferation, such as a fibroma or granulation tissue.

Inflammatory Masses

Inflammation is diagnosed much more frequently with cytology than is neoplasia. Cytologic diagnosis simply requires an adequate number of inflammatory cells. The number of cells sufficient for diagnosis varies with the sample. A rare plasma cell and phagocytic macrophage aspirated from the eye indicate inflammation, whereas in pus there are thousands of neutrophils. In hemodiluted samples, one considers the number and type of WBCs usually found in blood. Blood has about a 500:1 RBC:WBC ratio, with mainly neutrophils and lymphocytes. More WBCs (e.g., 20:1 ratio) or WBCs not found in blood (e.g., plasma cells and phagocytic macrophages) must be present on hemodiluted samples to diagnose inflammation. Based on the predominant WBC type, different terms are used and different causes are suspected.

Neutrophilic Inflammation

Neutrophilic infiltrates (e.g., exudation, suppuration, abscess formation, and purulent inflammation) are so frequent that they are almost synonymous with inflammation. Neutrophils are the most motile WBCs and are the first to infiltrate an area. Some term neutrophilic inflammation acute inflammation even though neutrophils may be prominent in active, chronic lesions. Pus is composed mainly of neutrophils in a loose, fluid matrix of proteinaceous cell debris, so these cells are most easily obtained from an aspirate or impression smear of a mass. Other cells in an inflammatory mass may not exfoliate as easily, especially fibroblasts, if scarring is present. A neutrophil migrating between stratified squamous epithelial cells may indent into the surface of a squamous cell and appear as if it is in the squamous cell when it exfoliates (see Fig. 16–2).

Bacterial Sepsis • Neutrophils are associated with bacterial infections and some yeast infections (e.g., *Candida*), so neutrophilic inflammation indicates a search for bacteria. The best place to search is in the cytoplasm of neutrophils (Color Plate 4D). One reason is that the cytoplasm of neutrophils is usually clear and free of granular debris that may be confused with bacteria. This is not true of macrophages, which often contain phagocytized cell debris that can mimic bacteria. Bacteria are more prominent in the clear neutrophilic cytoplasm, and the phagocytic vacuole may help outline the organism.

Bacteria have uniform shapes and sizes, in contrast to granular debris on smears. The formation of uniform pairs, tetrads, and chains identifies the structures as bacteria. Wright's stain precipitate is coccoid in appearance and may mimic coccoid bacteria. Irregular size of the precipitate, a more purple color than the blue of bacteria, and a refractile appearance differentiate stain precipitate from bacteria (Fig. 16–4).

The description of bacterial sepsis should include number, location (e.g., in neutrophils), appearance, and whether a pure or mixed population is present. These observations permit certain conclusions. For example, a pure population of large cocci in pairs and tetrads within neutrophils from an abscessed lymph node suggests an infection (e.g., *Staphylococcus*), whereas a mixed population of variably sized large rods and cocci in neutrophils in abdominal fluid suggests sepsis from a ruptured gut. Branching, beaded filamentous organisms indicate a higher bacteria (e.g., *Actinomyces*) (Color Plate 4E).

Phagocytosis of bacteria indicates that the bacteria were probably significant. Bacteria free in the background are less convincing evidence

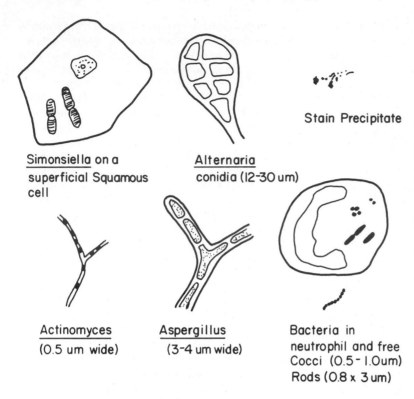

Stain Precipitate

Simonsiella on a superficial Squamous cell

Alternaria conidia (12-30 um)

Actinomyces (0.5 um wide)

Aspergillus (3-4 um wide)

Bacteria in neutrophil and free Cocci (0.5-1.0um) Rods (0.8 x 3 um)

Figure 16–4 Miscellaneous cytologic structures. The top row includes non-pathologic structures potentially confused with etiologic agents. *Simonsiella*, illustrated as two pairs of bacteria that resemble footprints, is normal flora of the oral cavity. *Alternaria* is composed of septate hyphae and is a common contaminant. Its conidia are club shaped with chambers. Stain precipitate is too irregular in shape and size to be the bacteria illustrated below it. *Actinomyces* is much narrower than fungal hyphae, such as *Aspergillus*.

of infection, since there could have been contaminant overgrowth in the stain or during handling of the sample. Bacteria on stratified squamous epithelial cells are usually normal flora from a body surface. A normal flora of the oral cavity of dogs is *Simonsiella*. Finding this huge bacterium localizes the sample to the mouth and pharynx (see Fig. 11–10 and Fig. 16–4).

Degenerative Neutrophils • How long should one search for bacteria in neutrophilic exudate? Bacteria may be in every field or in very low numbers. Antibiotic treatment may reduce the bacterial count below levels detected by cytology. A useful key is the appearance of the neutrophils. One should search for bacteria longer than usual if the neutrophils appear degenerate. Bacterial toxins cause rapid neutrophil death, with degenerative changes that suggest but do not prove sepsis. On the contrary, a predominance of nondegenerate neutrophils suggests a nonseptic environment and indicates a shorter (i.e., 10- to 15-minute) search for bacteria. However, some bacteria seem less toxic to neutrophils, and bacteria may even be found in nondegenerate neutrophils.

Morphologically degenerate neutrophils are characterized by swelling of the nucleus (karyolysis) and cytoplasm, reflecting rapid cell death. Karyolysis appears as a wider, more irregularly shaped, lighter staining nucleus that lacks the dark granular chromatin pattern and thin lobulated shape of viable nuclei (Color Plate 4E). The cytoplasm is foamy. Severely degenerate neutrophils may hardly resemble neutrophils as they swell and lyse into "globs" of nuclear debris. The degenerative changes due to bacteria must be differentiated from partial lysis due to storage of the sample, trauma to fragile cells during streaking of the smear, or nonbacterial toxic effects (e.g., urine). Inexperienced cytologists tend to overidentify degenerative neutrophil changes by examining partially lysed cells. Pus always has a variable number of damaged neutrophils, but one must evaluate only intact, undamaged cells. If the neutrophils with intact cell boundaries appear nondegenerate, then lysed neutrophils on the slide are probably artifactually broken rather than degenerate from bacterial toxins.

Nondegenerate neutrophils resemble normal cells in a blood smear with clear cytoplasm and a dark, thin, lobulated nucleus. A lack of bacterial toxins permits cells to live longer. Old neutrophils become hypersegmented and are good evidence of a nontoxic environment. Nondegenerate neutrophils dying slowly of old age also have pyknotic or karyorrhectic nuclei, which appear as dense, dark purple-staining round masses in cells or free in the background.

Incidentally, karyorrhectic nuclear material mimics yeast and must be recognized as such.

Necrosis • Viscous necrotic material is abundant in pus. Streaks of nuclear debris are commonly misidentified as mucus or fungal hyphae unless the streaks are traced back to a partially lysed nucleus. Necrosis is suggested by numerous lysed cells but is proved by cellular debris phagocytized by macrophages. Cholesterol crystals reflect breakdown of certain lipids and appear like panes of glass (i.e., clear rectangular crystals). The crystals are unstained and only outlined by other material taking the stain. Blood pigments and crystals occur with necrosis of RBCs.

Granulomatous and Pyogranulomatous Inflammation

When the inflammatory population is mainly macrophages (granulomatous) or a mixture of neutrophils and macrophages (pyogranulomatous), one must consider an etiologic agent bigger than bacteria. If an agent is not found, only a morphologic conclusion of subacute to chronic inflammation is reached. Neutrophils exfoliate more easily than do macrophages and therefore are more numerous in exudate or impression smears than in tissue sections. Similarly, cytologic reports describe more neutrophils than do histopathologic reports of granulomas. Fungi, higher bacteria, foreign bodies, and cell debris are predominantly phagocytized by macrophages.

Scanning of the smears is critical to find large, abnormal structures like burdock awns (golden brown, linear, barbed plant material) in samples from a lingual foreign body granuloma. Gross inspection may locate fungal colonies as a spot in one area of a smear, or they may be initially noted as off-white, yellow, or green flecks in a fresh sample. Macrophages are inspected for phagocytized material. In organized hematomas, they contain hemosiderin and RBCs. Macrophages from necrotic lesions contain nuclear fragments and cellular debris. In traumatized lipomas, they contain oil droplets or rarely yellow fat crystals. The combination of a drop of a fat stain (e.g., Sudan's) and a drop of NMB demonstrates lipid in macrophages. Yeast and hyphae usually stain blue on NMB and Wright's stain, but if they stain poorly, their shape is usually outlined by background material. To confirm the presence of an unstained organism, try another stain. Mycobacteria do not stain and appear as clear slits (i.e., rod-shaped ghosts) in macrophages. Smears may be sent to a referral laboratory for acid-fast staining.

Chronic Inflammation

Chronic inflammatory lesions that lack the abundance of macrophages in the preceding granulomatous category have a mixture of inflammatory cells including plasma cells, lymphocytes, macrophages, neutrophils, and occasional fibroblasts. This pattern is expected in canine lick "granulomas," in the later stages of healing of an inflammatory lesion (e.g., an old abscess), or in a chronic low-grade inflammatory disease (e.g., proliferative synovitis). Smears from very fibrous lesions are often acellular and might be mistaken for a poor aspirate. Repeat sampling yields similarly acellular samples. Since fibroblasts exfoliate poorly, use plasma cells as a cytologic indicator of chronicity (Perman et al., 1979).

Eosinophilic Inflammation

Inflammation is usually classified by the most numerous type of WBC. Since eosinophils are normally rare, eosinophils on smears need only exceed 20% to 30% of a significantly large population of WBCs to diagnose eosinophilic inflammation. Eosinophilic granuloma complex in cats and Siberian husky dogs is diagnosed when the cytologic smears from a typical lesion in the expected area indicate eosinophilic inflammation with a variable component of macrophages, plasma cells, and mast cells. In cats, the eosinophilic plaque and linear granuloma likely have eosinophilic infiltrates, whereas the eosinophilic ulcer may not (Scott, 1975). Parasites (e.g., *Paragonimus kellicotti*) (see Fig. 11–12) and allergic reactions should be considered as differential diagnoses based on the area and history, but neoplastic (e.g., canine mast cell tumor, see Color Plates 3A and 3B) and various infectious/inflammatory diseases may also have eosinophilic infiltrates (see Eosinophilia in Chapter 4).

Lymphocytic Inflammation

A small mass or elevation of a surface may consist of well-differentiated lymphocytes and a variable number of plasma cells. These occur in the nasopharyngeal area, vagina, and intestine, where one might not expect a lymph node or focal lymphoid tissue. This lymphoid hyperplasia may be focal (e.g., focal lymphoid hyper-

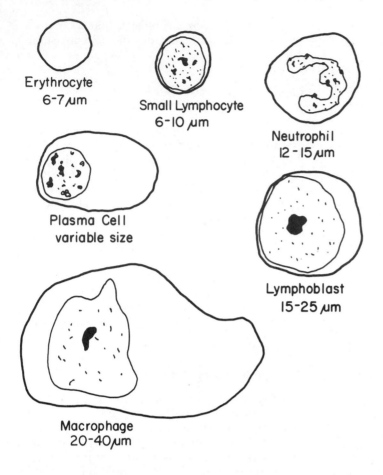

Erythrocyte
6-7 μm

Small Lymphocyte
6-10 μm

Neutrophil
12 - 15 μm

Plasma Cell
variable size

Lymphoblast
15-25 μm

Macrophage
20-40 μm

Figure 16–5 Cell sizes. Certain cells on smears may be used as micrometers to judge the size of infectious agents and maturity of unknown cells. These cells are drawn to scale.

plasia in vagina) or diffuse (e.g., lymphocytic rhinitis). Possible causes of this immune stimulation include viral or mycoplasma infections, but many agents are possible.

Selected Etiologic Agents

Descriptions of several organisms follow to aid in cytologic diagnosis of these agents. A microbiology text with an atlas is useful (Beneke and Rogers, 1970). Granulomatous or pyogranulomatous inflammation suggests larger organisms, but the type of inflammation is not a major differentiating feature of the various agents. Definitive diagnosis is by culture of the organism. Some laboratories have fluorescein-labeled antiglobulins specific for various fungi. Many organisms have distinct geographic distributions (e.g., salmon disease in Washington, Oregon, and northern California). Anatomic location of the infection (e.g., cryptococcosis in feline nasal cavity) also aids in diagnosis.

The dimensions are often given in micrometers (μm). One can buy a micrometer to fit the microscope's eyepiece. The micrometer's units

may be calibrated for each objective by using the grid of a hemocytometer. A simpler way is to use RBCs and WBCs for size estimation. Recall that depending on the thickness of the smear, cells vary in diameter (see Fig. 16–2), so these values are only approximate. Canine RBCs are about 7 μm, and feline are about 6 μm. The approximate diameters of WBCs on blood smears are as follows: neutrophils, 14 μm; eosinophils, 16 μm; small lymphocytes, 6 to 10 μm; large lymphocytes, 12 to 15 μm; blast-transformed lymphocytes, 15 to 25 μm; monocytes, 14 to 20 μm; and macrophages, 20 to 40 μm (Fig. 16–5).

Fungal Characteristics • Most of the organisms described in this section are fungi. The first nine are yeast or spherical structures (Fig. 16–6). Yeast are characterized by the formation of buds on uniformly sized round to oval structures. Spherules like *Coccidiodes*, *Rhinosporidium*, and *Prototheca* form endospores. The organisms are differentiated by size, appearance of buds or endospores, shape, capsule, and location in the body. Other structures may mimic yeast, such as oil droplets, especially when two droplets touch

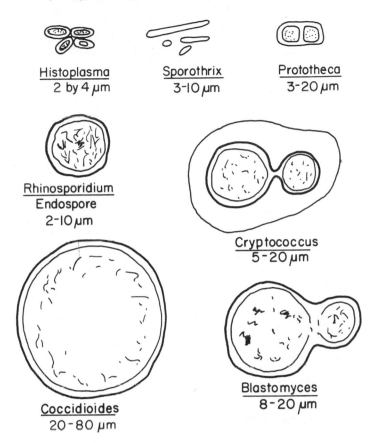

Figure 16-6 Comparative morphology of selected yeast and spherical organisms. These are drawn to scale; size is useful for differentiation.

to resemble budding. Unlike yeast, oil droplets are of various sizes and are refractile.

Fungal hyphae have two parallel cell walls and form branches. Hyphae are 3 to 20 μm thick, may have distinct septa, and may form spores or fruiting bodies (sporophore). Streaks of nuclear debris and lint may mimic hyphae. *Alternaria* is a common contaminant in the air, dust, and smears. It has golden septate hyphae that are fairly characteristic by themselves, but the diagnostic club-shaped conidia reminiscent of *Microsporum* are often present. Disregard an occasional fungal hypha on smears, especially if *Alternaria* is present. Pathogenic fungi are likely to be phagocytized or intermixed with inflammatory cells. Contaminant fungi are found anywhere on a slide, including areas away from tissue imprints or fluid smears. If a colony of fungi is found, check the stain for fungal contamination by applying the stain to a blank slide.

Histoplasmosis • *Histoplasma capsulatum* in cats is most consistently found in bone marrow aspirates (Clinkenbeard et al., 1987). Blood smear analysis is not a sensitive diagnostic test, but yeast may be found in phagocytes in any body fluid. Buffy coat smears concentrate WBCs for

examination. *Histoplasma* may be diagnosed in dogs and cats by cytology or histopathology of enlarged lymph nodes, liver, or other organs (e.g., colonic scrapings). The small (2–5 μm) yeasts are in macrophages and occasionally in neutrophils (see Fig. 16–6). It may be difficult to note budding when the yeast fills a phagocyte (Color Plate 2E).

Sporotrichosis • *Sporothrix schenckii* is abundant in samples of draining, ulcerated lesions of cats but is difficult to demonstrate in canine lesions. In cats, the yeast is very pleomorphic with round, oval, and cigar-shaped 3- to 10-μm forms (see Fig. 16–6) in macrophages, in neutrophils, and free in the background (Dunstan et al., 1986) (Color Plate 2F). Note: People acquire this infection from animals more easily than they do other mycoses.

Cryptococcosis • *Cryptococcus neoformans* may be found in various tissues. A nasal mass in cats is a classic presentation. This yeast is best identified by the variably thick gelatinous capsule that often doubles the size of the cell (see Fig. 11–5 and Fig. 16–6). Budding is from a narrow base, in contrast to *Blastomyces*, which has broad-based buds. Cells vary from 5 to 20 μm in diameter. *Rhinosporidium seeberi* occurs in the nose of dogs and produces endospores (2–10 μm) that may be confused with cryptococcosis. *Cryptococcus* yeast is demonstrated on NMB-stained smears, so messy india ink preparations are unnecessary. Inflammation may be absent, and the lesion just a glistening mass of yeast.

Rhinosporidiosis • *R. seeberi* infects the nasal cavity of dogs with the formation of recurrent nonneoplastic polyps. The huge trophic stages (60–120 μm) and sporangia (100–300 μm) are diagnostic on histologic sections. The smaller 2- to 10-μm endospores from ruptured sporangia are seen on cytologic preparations (see Fig. 16–6). The spherical endospores lack budding and the characteristic capsule associated with *Cryptococcus*.

Coccidioidomycosis • *Coccidioides immitis* is recovered from pulmonary or disseminated lesions in dogs. It is characterized by large size and internal endospores. Spherical sporangia are 20 to 80 μm in diameter (see Fig. 16–6). Endospores (2–5 μm in diameter) are usually in the bigger spherules. *Coccidioides* organisms tend to be surrounded by neutrophils on smears (Perman et al., 1979). The arthrospores formed in fungal cultures are highly infectious, so warn the microbiologist.

Blastomycosis • *Blastomyces dermatitidis* is an 8- to 20-μm-diameter thick-walled budding yeast infecting the lungs or other tissues in dogs and occasionally cats. With Wright's stain, the yeast cells are dark blue and are often collapsed and wrinkled from the alcohol dehydration step but appear more typical with NMB stain. They are best found by scanning the slides. Since the yeasts are large, they are often pushed to the end of the smears (see Fig. 11–13 and Fig. 16–6).

Candidiasis • *Candida albicans* is a normal flora. Rarely it infects a surface (i.e., thrush or moniliasis) or may be disseminated. It is a typical thin-walled budding yeast about 2 to 6 μm in diameter. It is differentiated from other yeasts by the formation of pseudohyphae (3–4 μm thick), which look like short septate hyphae. Pseudohyphae found in parakeratotic skin scabs resulted in the diagnosis of moniliasis that would have been missed in a diabetic dog that had hyperadrenocorticism and poor resistance to infection.

Pityrosporum • *Pityrosporum* (*Malassezia*) is a small budding yeast resembling *Candida* (Color Plate 4F). It is abundantly found in ear swabs of dogs with chronic otitis that has been nonresponsive to antibiotic therapy. Being able to diagnose chronic yeast otitis alone justifies cytology in private practice.

Protothecosis • *Prototheca* is rarely disseminated in dogs. Signs are related to lesions in the skin, eye, and intestine. The 3 to 20 μm in diameter (usually just smaller than a neutrophil) round to oval algae have a clear cell wall and may have two or more endospores (see Fig. 16–6). Cytologic and histologic diagnosis is confirmed by culture and immunofluorescent tests on tissues.

Aspergillosis • *Aspergillus* sp. is the most common fungus associated with canine nasal infections. It is critical to scan many smears to find the fungal colony, since a majority of the smear is exudate with secondary bacterial sepsis. Finding a septic exudate may suggest a bacterial cause and terminate the slide evaluation before the primary problem is found. Grossly finding a green (*Aspergillus fumigatus*) or brown (*Aspergillus niger*) mass (i.e., the fungal colony) to use for cytology improves the probability of diagnosis. On scanning, the fungal colony resembles a clump of debris; but on high power, it is a mass of septate, branching hyphae of comparably uniform thickness (3–4 μm) (Color Plate 2D). This is good evidence of aspergillosis. The center of an *Aspergillus* colony may not stain, thus requiring examination of its perimeter. The large (300 μm) branching conidiophore with 2.5- to 3-μm spherical conidia is diagnostic if found. A cytologic smear may occasionally have only the small, green spherical spores. See the discussion above on hyphae under Fungal Characteristics to differentiate nonpathogenic forms like *Alternaria*.

Mycetoma • Cutaneous fungal granulomas have a confusing array of identities (eumycotic mycetomas, maduromycosis, and chromoblastomycosis) and are caused by a wide variety of fungi (*Drechslera*, *Allescheria*, *Madurella*, *Cladosporium*, *Fonsecaea*, and others). Cytologic diagnosis is limited to identification of a granulomatous or pyogranulomatous lesion with one or more fungal forms (i.e., hyphae or spherules). The shape, size, and color noted on an unstained slide should be recorded. Fungal culture is required for specific etiologic diagnosis.

Mucormycosis • *Mucor* and similar fungi may be found in canine gastric ulcers or other tissues.

The hyphae are nonseptate, branching, and wider (15–20 μm) than those of *Aspergillus* sp. Confirm by culture.

Alternaria • *Alternaria* is a ubiquitous contaminant found in various microscopic preparations. One must recognize the large, golden brown septate hyphae and characteristic club-shaped conidia with longitudinal and transverse septa to avoid confusion with truly pathogenic fungi (see Fig. 16–4). Rarely, *Alternaria* may be considered pathogenic if it invades deeper tissues.

Dermatophytes • Cytology for dermatophytes is covered in Chapter 15.

Higher Bacteria • *Actinomyces, Nocardia,* and *Dermatophilus* are higher bacteria with a branching structure suggestive of fungi. Their thin width of 0.5 to 1.0 μm distinguishes them from thicker fungal hyphae, which have two distinct cell walls separated by obvious space (Fig. 16–4). Due to the much higher frequency of *Actinomyces viscosus* than of *Nocardia* sp., no cytologic attempt is made to differentiate them in our practice. *Actinomyces* is characterized by long, branching filaments with a beaded appearance on Wright's stain (i.e., variable staining intensity along the filaments). Scanning smears hastens the detection of darkly stained bacterial colonies, which appear as "sulfur granules." *Actinomyces* may be coated with an eosinophilic material and form "clubs" radiating out from the colony. Other organisms with the eosinophilic clubbing around colonies are *Staphylococcus* (botryomycosis), *Actinobacillus, Coccidioides,* and *Aspergillus.* The colonies in the exudate appear as white to yellow granules and should be collected for the smear. Mixed bacterial infections may accompany *Actinomyces* and *Nocardia.*

Dermatophilus congolensis causes cutaneous infections in dogs less frequently than in other species. It is identified by soaking skin scabs in saline and then rubbing the underside of the scabs on glass slides. On Wright's stain, characteristic railroadlike patterns of parallel and longitudinal rows of zoospores (0.5–1.0 μm) forming variably thick branching structures on squamous cells are found.

Mycobacteriosis • *Mycobacterium lepraemurium, Mycobacterium fortuitum, Mycobacterium bovis,* and some other mycobacteria cause subcutaneous or cutaneous masses in cats and less frequently in dogs (Gross and Connelly, 1983). Feline leprosy (*M. lepraemurium*) lesions occur anywhere on a cat; atypical mycobacteriosis tends to cause fistulous tracts on the ventral abdomen. The organisms are demonstrated by impression smears of the granulomas or smears of the draining tracts stained with acid-fast stains. Mycobacteria do not stain with Wright's stain and appear as clear slits or "ghosts" in macrophages. Mail the smears to a cytologist or microbiologist for staining.

Notify the histopathologist, because documentation of mycobacteria requires special processing. The organisms tend to localize in clear lipid droplets in the center of granulomas and are lost during alcohol and xylene steps in routine slide preparation. Frozen sections retain the organisms and their staining ability. Culture is required to differentiate feline leprosy from atypical mycobacteriosis. Advise the microbiologist to use media for atypical mycobacteria. Cytology, histopathology, and culture may need to be repeated.

Salmon Disease • *Neorickettsia helminthoeca* may be identified in macrophages from lymph nodes of infected dogs. A moderate to large number of coccoid to rod-shaped bodies (0.3-μm diameter) are spread through the cytoplasm of macrophages. Macchiavello's stain is excellent for rickettsiae, but Wright's-type stains may be used. Trematode eggs are in a dog's feces a week after the infested fish have been eaten.

Ehrlichiosis • An *Ehrlichia canis* morula (raspberry-like cluster of tiny bodies) in circulating WBCs, cytologic smears of lung, or synovial fluid is diagnostic but is found too rarely to be relied on. It is most likely seen in the acute stage of the disease (see *E. canis* discussion in Chapters 5 and 15).

Toxoplasmosis • *Toxoplasma gondii* is found too rarely in macrophages and neural, ocular, or muscle tissue to serve as a useful diagnostic test. The actively dividing forms (tachyzoites) are crescent shaped (2–4 μm by 4–7 μm) with a nucleus at one end. The shape may not be discerned when several are packed in a cell but becomes apparent when freed from a ruptured cell. Smaller bradyzoites are in stable tissue cysts that remain infective for a long time. Similar protozoa to consider are *Sarcocystis* and *Leishmania.* Active *Toxoplasma* infection is best diagnosed by serology (see Chapter 15). Small (10–12 μm) coccidial oocysts of *Toxoplasma* are briefly (i.e., 2 weeks) shed in feces by cats after ingestion of infected meat. This suggests the enteric infection but is too transient for consistent diagnosis. Other coccidial oocysts are usually larger (20–40 μm).

Proliferative Masses (Neoplasia)

Initial Decisions

The major initial conclusions are (1) that the smears represent the mass and (2) that the lesion is a noninflammatory proliferation (e.g., benign neoplasm, malignant neoplasm, focal hyperplasia, or normal tissue). These conclusions must be made before considerations of the tissue type or the cytologic malignancy of the mass. The presence of a moderate to large number of cells of one type should be representative of the mass. For mammary neoplasm cytology, more than 100 cells per slide were considered adequate for evaluation (Allen et al., 1986). When a small number of tissue cells are present, one is less confident that they represent the mass, especially if they are a minor component compared with blood or exudate.

The observed cells indicate a proliferative tissue mass if they are noninflammatory tissue cells of one type (i.e., a monomorphic population). This conclusion is often made difficult by concurrent inflammation and necrosis in many neoplasms. The higher the percentage of inflammatory cells in the population, the lower one's confidence that the mass is not primarily inflammatory. A majority of many tissue cells of one cell type indicates a proliferative mass.

Cell Typing

The shape of the cells, their association with other cells, especially in tissue fragments, and cytoplasmic features are used to indicate the tissue of origin. Do not expect to routinely identify the exact cell type by cytology; rather, determine whether it is an epithelial, a mesenchymal (i.e., connective tissue), or a round cell tumor. Additional information such as location (e.g., mammary tumor) usually suggests a specific diagnosis. Some very malignant neoplasms, for example, may lack differentiating features to identify the cell type, but the cytologic conclusion of "malignant neoplasm—type undetermined" is sufficient. A mass may be composed of multiple tissue types (e.g., an epithelial mass often has some connective tissue stroma). Melanoma is a neoplasm that may have an epithelial or a connective tissue appearance.

Epithelial cells are best indicated by distinct cell-cell junctions (Fig. 16–7). Cell shapes are illustrated better with NMB than with Wright's stain. Epithelial cells form surfaces with tight cell junctions that persist to a variable degree on smears. Be cautious of interpreting adjacent, crowded cells on a thick part of the smear as having epithelial junctions where the cells simply flatten along edges of contact. Look for distinct linear junctions complete with formation of corners. Nonepithelial adjacent cells often

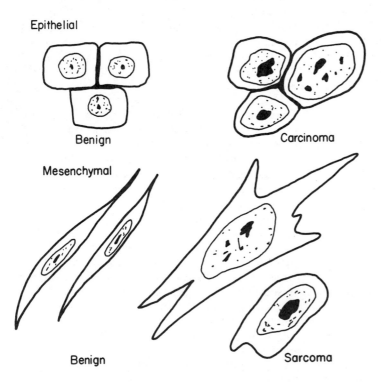

Figure 16–7 Benign and malignant examples of epithelial and mesenchymal cells. Note the tight intercellular junctions of epithelial cells and the elongated spindle or stellate shapes of mesenchymal cells. Malignant nuclei are larger, are more variable, and have more irregular nucleoli and chromatin.

form holes (windows) at corners. The multiple adjacent desmosomes (cell-binding sites) may appear like teeth of a comb as the cells pull apart. Epithelial cells may form layers, so an epithelial cell may be identified in a pocket formed by an adjacent epithelial cell, as one hand fits in the "palm" of another. Tissue fragments in NMB-stained smears may have acinar structure with lumina (glandular origin) or papillary structures (fingerlike epithelial projections with a central core of connective tissue stroma). Well-differentiated epithelial cells may retain squamous, polyhedral, cuboidal, or columnar shapes and cilia. Secretory material such as mucus, granules, or vacuoles suggests epithelium.

Some other tissues such as mesothelium form surfaces and may mimic epithelial tissue. This fact plus the anaplastic appearance of reactive mesothelial cells causes many misdiagnoses of carcinoma in pleural and peritoneal fluids. Mesothelial cells can form epithelial-type papillae, which are mesothelial cell–lined, fingerlike projections formed during irritation of a surface (e.g., villous proliferation in *Actinomyces* pleuritis). Synovial cells, endothelial cells, and melanocytes may also mimic epithelial cells.

Cells are classified as mesenchymal (e.g., fibrous, osseous, muscle, or neural connective tissue) mainly by an elongated shape forming tail-like or conical extensions (see Fig. 16–7). Two tails are found on spindle-shaped cells (Color Plate 3D). Three or more tails are on stellate cells. Nuclei tend to be more oval. Mesenchymal cells are usually individualized or discrete cells that lack sharply defined cell borders. Occasionally, if a tissue fragment is present, mesenchymal cells may be trapped in the matrix that they form (e.g., pink osteoid). Cytoplasmic structures suggest the specific cell type. Melanocytes usually have a fine brown to black pigment. Hemosiderin may be mistaken for melanin but is usually larger and may be mixed with the green or yellow pigment that is more easily recognized as hemosiderin or accompanies erythrophagocytosis. Osseous cells sometimes have prominent pink cytoplasmic granules. Columnar epithelial cells may mimic spindle cells, since the point where the cell pulled away from its attachment to the basement membrane often pulls out to a thin tail. The other end of the columnar cell has a flat surface with cilia to indicate its true type.

The round cell category includes four specific tumors and some tumors without differentiation. These individualized cells do not form distinct cell-cell attachments or the spindle to stellate shapes. Four tumors in this category are

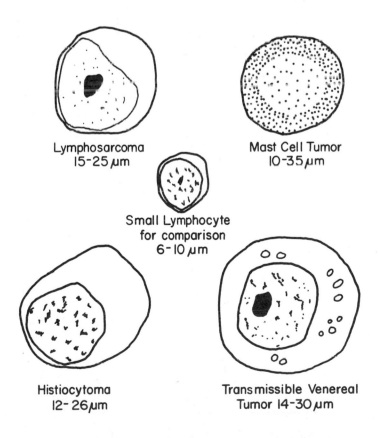

Figure 16–8 Round cell tumors. Cell characteristics of the four round cell tumors are illustrated with a small lymphocyte for size comparison.

Lymphosarcoma
15-25 μm

Mast Cell Tumor
10-35 μm

Small Lymphocyte
for comparison
6-10 μm

Histiocytoma
12-26 μm

Transmissible Venereal
Tumor 14-30 μm

lymphosarcoma and other hematopoietic cell neoplasms, mast cell tumor, transmissible venereal tumor, and canine histiocytoma. Characteristics of these are illustrated in Figure 16–8 and described later. Do not limit the differential to these, since anaplastic melanomas and carcinomas may cytologically have discrete round cells with few or no differentiating features.

Malignant Criteria

After deciding that the cytologic population represents a proliferative mass, one evaluates malignant criteria. One should routinely record the malignant criteria of the smear and quantitate the amount (small, moderate, or great) to improve one's consistency. A written checklist (Table 16–1) helps avoid missing points and permits an easier step-by-step approach to a conclusion than does a mental checklist. When a checklist is finished, the relative abundance of

Table 16–1 CYTOLOGIC CHECKLIST FOR LIKELY NEOPLASMS

	Indication of Amount or Severity		
	Small	Moderate	Great
Smear's characteristics			
Total cellularity			
Amount of tissue cells			
Amount of inflammation			
Type of inflammation			
Cell type			
Cell description			
Epithelial evidence			
Mesenchymal evidence			
Round cell evidence			
Malignant criteria			
Nuclear			
Large size			
Variable size			
Variable shape			
High N:C ratio			
Chromatin			
Irregular shape			
Variable size			
Irregular parachromatin clearing			
Nucleolar			
Large size			
Variable number			
Irregular shape			
Mitotic figures			
Atypical forms			
Large number			
Final impression			

evidence is more apparent. Based on the strength of the sum of evidence, a conclusion is made with an indication of one's confidence (e.g., carcinoma, probable carcinoma, possible carcinoma, or no cytologic evidence of malignancy).

How are malignant criteria converted into a conclusion? Grading systems attempt to convert subjective observations into quantitative measures. A scoring system for malignancy of canine mammary neoplasm has been critically evaluated (Allen et al., 1986). It allows objective consideration of how conclusions are made. More critical reviews of veterinary cytology, which is often more art than science, are needed. One point was added for each of 10 cytologic criteria shown to correlate significantly with histopathologic conclusions of malignancy. A score of 0 to 3 was benign, 4 to 7 was inconclusive, and 8 to 10 was malignant. It is apparent that several malignant criteria are required, and many samples have inconclusive amounts of evidence. Therefore, do not try to make a diagnosis from every sample. This system had few false malignant diagnoses (i.e., high specificity), but the sensitivity in identifying malignancy was only 17% to 25%. When the cutoff for a test is set high for best specificity (i.e., few false-malignant diagnoses), the sensitivity is usually lower (i.e., more false-benign diagnoses). High specificity is preferred to sensitivity, especially if euthanasia may be determined by the diagnosis.

One should not expect simply to count malignant criteria until a "magic" number is reached. Even with rigid definitions of each malignant criterion, the mammary neoplasm scoring system had a wide inconclusive range. The number of malignant criteria noted in each case varies because cytologists vary. A nucleus that appears large to one observer may seem normal to another. People vary in thoroughness. Use of a numbering system is weakened if equal weight is given when a few cells barely have the change as when most cells have great alterations. No single feature or group of features always proves malignancy, and the conclusion is a subjective impression.

Malignancy is best indicated by nuclear variability (Color Plate 3C). Variation in nuclear size (anisokaryosis) and very large nuclear size are obvious even on poor quality smears. The greater the nuclear size and anisokaryosis, the stronger the evidence of malignancy. Anaplastic cells tend to have large nuclei and minimal cytoplasm, resulting in a high nuclear: cytoplasmic (N:C) ratio. Nuclear shape variation, if bizarre, such as with pseudopods and marked convolutions, is strong evidence. Multinucleation in cells not normally multinucleated occurs in malignant and reactive cells. Molding of a nucleus around the nucleus of an adjacent cell is evidence that the cells grew next to each other rather than a criterion of malignancy.

Variation in intranuclear structures is best evaluated with a nuclear stain like NMB, Sano's trichrome, or Pap's. Variable chromatin pattern is strong evidence of malignancy. Malignant chromatin patterns are characterized by variability in the size, shape, and distribution of chromatin. Irregular parachromatin clearing appears as an area of clear space separating the chromatin granules unevenly. The variability gives a coarse, irregular chromatin pattern. Well-differentiated cells have uniform chromatin with even distribution. Some malignant nuclei have variably thick nuclear margins from irregular margination of chromatin along the nuclear membrane, which can be noted with Pap's stain. Active nuclei have fine chromatin and increased clear space between chromatin (i.e., parachromatin area). This makes the nucleus appear lighter than a smaller, well-differentiated nucleus with condensed chromatin. Active nuclei occur in malignant and nonmalignant cells.

Malignant cells often have prominent nucleolar variation, such as excessive variation in the number of nucleoli (varying from one to five or more), large nucleolar size (may become as large as an RBC), variation in nucleolar shape (jagged, sharply pointed, or irregular nucleoli), and variation in size of nucleoli even within the same nucleus. Malignant nuclei lack uniformity among themselves. Benign cells have consistent numbers (e.g., one, two, or three) of small to moderate-sized round nucleoli. A few mitotic figures are often given excessive weight as malignant criteria (i.e., they are commonly found in nonneoplastic macrophages in exudates). Mitotic figures indicate malignancy if they are numerous or abnormal. Abnormal mitotic shapes include excessive numbers of chromosomes (e.g., tripolar metaphase plate instead of the normal two rows of chromosomes) and lag chromatin (i.e., a chromosome separated from the other chromosomes in the mitotic figure).

Cytoplasmic changes are weak indicators of malignancy. A basophilic cytoplasm indicates active protein synthesis and abundant RNA. A large nucleolus also indicates active RNA synthesis and thus protein synthesis. Protein synthesis is often high in malignant cells but also in active nonneoplastic cells (e.g., hyperplasia or reactive change). Malignancy of a mast cell tumor is partially indicated by variability in the number, size, and distribution of cytoplasmic granules. Abundance of cytoplasm and differentiated features (e.g., retaining a columnar shape or cilia) are benign features.

Degenerative changes mimic malignant changes. Nuclei and nucleoli swell with cell damage (see Fig. 16–2), and the large nuclear size, light nuclear color, and nucleolar prominence make the damaged cell appear malignant. Do not evaluate cells with broken cytoplasmic boundaries or with partial leakage of nuclear material out of the nucleus! Even apparently intact cells may be swollen and degenerating. The best indication of cell death is chromatin that has lost its granular, stippled appearance on Wright's stain and appears streaked or smudged. The degeneration is less obvious on NMB-stained cells, so it is easier to mistake the degeneration for malignancy.

Cells degenerate quickly in certain fluids like unbuffered saline and urine. Cells from bronchial brushings, for example, have much better cell detail than do cells collected with a saline flush. Cells degenerate within minutes in saline, which is acidic (pH 6) and lacks inorganic ions and glucose for cellular metabolism. Hanks' balanced salt solution (HBSS) preserves cell morphology and is the best fluid to retrieve cells when cell detail is critical (e.g., neoplastic diagnosis). The cost of HBSS prevents its routine use. Mediocre cell detail is adequate for evaluation of exudates and sepsis, so HBSS is not needed. To prevent excessive cell degeneration, make smears as quickly as possible, avoid prolonged cell storage in fluids, use the fluid most hospitable to cells (e.g., lactated Ringer's solution is probably better than saline but not as good as HBSS), and stain the smears quickly unless unstained smears are to be sent to a cytologist.

Selected Cytologic Diagnoses

Mammary Neoplasms

Cytologic evaluation of mammary masses is used to plan surgical removal. Lack of cytologic evidence of malignancy permits local resection for histologic diagnosis and possible cure. Cytologic evidence of malignancy or the gross presentation of the neoplasm may indicate more radical surgery.

Ten cytologic criteria were significantly correlated to histopathologic conclusion of malignancy (Allen et al., 1986). Cytologic evaluation was modified by Sano's trichrome stain of smears fixed in 95% ethanol while still wet. The malignant criteria were variable nuclear size, giant nuclei (more than two times normal), distortion of nuclear or cytoplasmic membranes, high N:C ratio (>1:2), irregular chromatin shapes, variable chromatin size, parachromatin clearing (i.e., a discrete pale area in a dense chromatin pattern), variable nucleolar number (more than three), abnormal nucleolar shape, and macronucleoli (more than two times normal). Abnormal nucleolar shape was defined as "not round or oval." Nuclear membrane distortion was indentation of the nuclear shape by a cytoplasmic organelle like a vacuole in contrast to nuclear molding, which was the molding of a nucleus about another cell's nucleus without cell crowding.

Abnormal mitotic figures (e.g., asymmetric or trisomy) always denoted malignancy but were rare. Similarly, cytoplasmic projections indicated malignancy but were infrequent. Neither nuclear molding, irregularly thick nuclear margins, cellularity of the smear, poor intercellular cohesion, nor multinucleation allowed differentiation between benign and malignant neoplasms. Fine-needle aspirates of mammary tumors were more cellular and had better tissue architecture than impression smears, scrapings, or nipple secretions. Spindle cells on smears did not differentiate simple from complex or mixed tumors. In another survey, only eight of 19 histologically confirmed mammary carcinomas were identified as such by fine-needle cytology (Griffiths et al., 1984). This again demonstrates that cytology should be used for tentative diagnoses, with histopathology as the definitive procedure.

Perianal Gland Tumor

Cells of perianal gland tumor (hepatoid tumor) resemble hepatocytes with a square or polyhedral shape and abundant cytoplasm (Color Plate 3E). The cytoplasm has characteristic granularity with Wright's stain. Round nuclei have one or two prominent nucleoli. Clusters of cells may retain the typical long columnar pattern seen in tissues. The site of the mass aids in identification. Rare metastasis may occur (i.e., lung), but the cells remain distinctive. Malignancy is determined not by cytologic criteria but by histologic evidence of vascular invasion.

Transitional Cell Carcinoma

Transitional cell carcinoma is diagnosed by finding significant numbers of well-preserved, malignant-appearing epithelial cells in urine. Cells in urine rapidly degenerate and swell, causing nuclear and nucleolar enlargement mimicking neoplasia. Other carcinomas may shed malignant cells into urine, but transitional cell carcinoma is the most common one.

Lipoma

Diagnosis is rapid and simple. Smears grossly have clear droplets of lipid that do not dry. These could be stained with Sudan's or another fat stain and counterstained with NMB, but this is not necessary. The stained smears usually lack cells except for a variable number of adipocytes singly or in tissue fragments. Adipocytes are large cells with a small dark nucleus on one edge. The thin cell membrane appears wrinkled, since alcohol in Wright's stain removes the lipid. Mature fat has the same appearance as a lipoma. Lipomas may be traumatized, hemorrhagic, fibrotic, or inflamed. These changes are indicated by macrophages, other inflammatory cells, blood, and fibroblasts.

Mast Cell Neoplasms

Mast cell neoplasms are confidently diagnosed by finding a moderate to large population of mast cells with a variable number of eosinophils in a mass. The round, distinctly granular cells with round nuclei are easily identified on Wright's stain (see Fig. 16–8) (Color Plate 3A). A Diff-Quik stain may fail to stain mast cell granules in some mast cell tumors (Rebar, 1978). Malignancy is indicated by the degree of mast cell differentiation. Histologic grading of canine cutaneous mast cell tumors has been associated with differences in survival. Classification was from grade 1 (well-differentiated, round monomorphic cells with no mitotic activity and round nuclei with condensed chromatin) to grade 2 (intermediate) to grade 3 (pleomorphic cells with irregularly shaped cells, vesiculated nuclei with one or more prominent nucleoli, binucleation, frequent mitotic figures, and cytoplasmic granules that were indistinct, fine, or not obvious) (Color Plate 3B).

Feline cutaneous mast cell tumors without splenic involvement are usually benign, and survival in a small survey of 14 cats did not correlate with a grading system similar to the canine system (Buerger and Scott, 1987). A histiocytic-like cutaneous mast cell tumor in young Siamese cats may have granules that are difficult to find (see also Mastocytemia in Chapter 4).

Cytologically, cutaneous mast cell tumors are

subclassified by degree of differentiation. Some of the nuclear criteria of malignancy may be hard to identify on Wright's-stained cytologic smears, since the nuclei may be obscured by granules and often stain poorly owing to the heparin content of the mast cell. NMB is better for nuclear detail. Cytoplasmic characteristics of malignancy in dogs include variation in the size, density, and prominence of the granules. Malignant cells have fewer and finer granules. Granules may polarize to one end of malignant cells. Anaplastic cells are larger (12–35 μm instead of the normal 10–20 μm), with mitotic figures and binucleation (Duncan and Prasse, 1979).

Histiocytoma

A histiocytoma can be a troublesome cytologic diagnosis because the cells are not distinctive. Cells may exfoliate poorly, and secondary inflammation may be present. The cells are 12 to 26 μm, round to oval with distinct cell boundaries. They occasionally have indented nuclei without apparent nucleoli (Duncan and Prasse, 1979). Chromatin is fine, and mitotic activity is present. Cytoplasm on Wright's stain is pale blue. The N:C ratio varies and is usually 1:1. This benign tumor may be considered malignant by human pathologists unfamiliar with it. Lymphosarcomas may have a histiocytic appearance and be confused with a histiocytoma, so caution is advised if the presentation is not typical for histiocytoma (i.e., a small dome-shaped mass in a young dog).

Transmissible Venereal Tumor

Transmissible venereal tumor cells have morphologic features similar to lymphoblasts. Cytoplasm has the pale hyaline blue of lymphoid cells but has distinct vacuoles. Transmissible venereal tumor is a round cell tumor with discrete cells but can also have epithelial-type sheets of cells. The round cells are 14 to 30 μm in diameter. Round to oval nuclei have a prominent nucleolus and linear, cordlike chromatin (Duncan and Prasse, 1979). Mitotic activity is common. Location of the mass on the body, plus being from an endemic area, supports the diagnosis.

Epidermal Inclusion Cyst

Epidermal inclusion cysts are common skin lumps in dogs. The contents of the cyst mainly consist of mature stratified squamous epithelial cells, so the diagnosis is made by finding large numbers of squames (very mature, nonnucleated squamous cells) and keratinized debris on aspirate smears. Recall that squames are common contaminants on slides, mainly from fingerprints. Other debris, including cholesterol crystals, may be present. Traumatized cysts may be inflamed or hemorrhagic.

Hematoma/Seroma

Hematomas are fluctuant masses containing fluid with a variable amount of blood in variable states of degeneration. Recently formed hematomas have aspiration smears resembling a blood smear. Platelets, if present, suggest active bleeding because platelets are rapidly lost from fluid. With time the RBCs are ingested and converted to various blood pigments by infiltrating macrophages (Color Plate 4C). The granular or crystalline pigments have various colors (blue, green, black, gold, and yellow). The proteinaceous fluid from a seroma has few RBCs.

Hepatic Cytology

Hepatocytes have abundant granular cytoplasm and a round nucleus with a prominent nucleolus. Hepatocytes are readily identified by normal binucleation (i.e., diploid). Common alterations include vacuolar degeneration (e.g., fatty liver and glucocorticoid hepatopathy), inflammation (e.g., chronic active hepatitis), cholestasis, and neoplasia. Aspiration cytology can identify these processes, although histopathology better identifies and quantitates the disorders. When hepatocyte vacuoles are seen, fatty change is identified by applying one to two drops of Sudan's stain and counterstaining with one to two drops of NMB (Color Plate 3F). Canine glucocorticoid hepatopathy vacuoles are not fat positive. Cholestasis is indicated by swollen, green bile canaliculi between hepatocytes and by the blue-green granular pigment within hepatocytes. Inflammation may be difficult to prove cytologically because inflammatory infiltrates are minimal. If only a few lymphocytes or neutrophils are on a bloody smear, it is hard to tell whether the WBCs are from peripheral blood or a mild inflammatory infiltrate. Since plasma cells and vacuolated macrophages are not found in peripheral blood and are not caused by hemodilution of tissue cells, they are more consistent indicators of inflammation than are neutrophils and lymphocytes. Extramedullary hematopoiesis is indicated by nucleated RBCs and megakaryocytes. Neoplasia is diagnosed by previously described criteria.

Lymph Node Cytology/Lymphosarcoma

Aspiration cytology is the initial test to evaluate enlarged lymph nodes. Cytology may provide evidence of metastasis and other disorders even in the absence of lymph node enlargement. Since lymphoid cells are fragile and large lymph nodes are often necrotic, many smears may not be diagnostic if inadequate numbers of intact cells are present. Scan the smears for variation in distribution. Then a differential cell count is performed in a thin area with good cell morphologic detail, and other areas are examined to ensure that the differential count is representative. Based on the population's composition, one makes one or more of the conclusions in Table 16–2.

The lymphoid cells in a normal lymph node are about 10% lymphoblasts and 75% to 90% small to medium-sized, well-differentiated lymphocytes. Plasma cells are infrequent (0–3%) except in some commonly reactive nodes (e.g., gut and submandibular). Criteria used to differentiate lymphoblasts from well-differentiated, small to medium lymphocytes vary. Lymphoblasts are as large as neutrophils or larger and have a light, fine nuclear chromatin pattern and a nucleolus. In contrast, the small lymphocyte is just larger than an RBC and the nucleus has coarser and darker chromatin (see Fig. 16–5). Medium-sized lymphocytes are grouped with small lymphocytes as well-differentiated cells if they have a mature, coarse chromatin pattern. Prolymphocytes are immature lymphoid cells with large nuclear size and immature chromatin patterns and are included with the lymphoblasts despite their apparent lack of nucleoli.

Lymph node cytology is commonly diagnostic

Table 16–2 CYTOLOGIC LYMPH NODE CONCLUSIONS

Conclusion	Cytologic Features
Normal	Normal cell population, no lymph node enlargement
Hyperplastic	Normal cell population, enlarged lymph node
Reactive	Similar to hyperplastic but suggests slight increases in plasma cells, lymphoblasts, leukocytes, or macrophages with hemosiderin or debris
Lymphadenitis	Large population of one or more nonlymphoid leukocytes, organisms may be present
Metastatic neoplasia	Population of nonlymphoid cells with cytologic evidence of malignancy, excessive numbers, or atypical location
Lymphoid neoplasia	Usually a majority of lymphoblasts and/or prolymphocytes

for lymphosarcoma (see Chapter 4). The percentage of lymphoblasts or other obviously immature forms is the major diagnostic criterion in lymphosarcoma, in which there is usually a majority of lymphoblasts or other immature cells. The higher the percentage of lymphoblasts, the greater one's confidence in a diagnosis of lymphosarcoma. Atypical morphology, other than immaturity, is not a consistent or sensitive indicator of lymphosarcoma. When present, features like bizarre nuclear and cytoplasmic shapes, numerous mitotic figures, or irregular chromatin patterns add to the confidence one has in a diagnosis of malignancy.

The frequent necrosis in lymph nodes affected with lymphosarcoma can cause aspiration and impression smears to be too thick, since cells in a loose necrotic matrix readily exfoliate. The background of excessive cell debris on aspirate and impression smears interferes with staining. One often finds only a small percentage of intact and well-stained cells around the thin perimeter of the smear. Lysed cells (i.e., "naked" nuclei) and partially lysed normal cells have swelling of the nucleus and nucleolus. This creates a large, light-stained nucleus with a prominent nucleolus resembling a lymphoblast. Failure to ignore these damaged cells leads to an erroneously high percentage of lymphoblasts and an incorrect conclusion of lymphosarcoma. Skip the damaged cells. Repeated aspiration may be required to obtain a diagnostic sample.

Chronic lymphocytic leukemia (CLL) is not diagnosed by immaturity of the population, since the neoplastic lymphoid cells are well differentiated and "mature" in appearance. CLL is uncommon but should be considered as a cause of lymphadenopathy if a cytologically monotonous lymphoid population is present. CLL would be best diagnosed by histopathology of the affected lymph nodes, spleen, bone marrow or by complete blood count.

Highly reactive lymph nodes may have an increased percentage (e.g., 10–25%) of lymphoblasts and some very large lymphoblasts to suggest lymphosarcoma. The heterogeneity of the population is a useful indication of a reactive/hyperplastic node compared with the monotonous population in lymphosarcoma. An admixture of small to medium lymphocytes with the lymphoblasts and an increased number of plasma cells supports the more conservative diagnosis of a reactive lymph node.

Reactive and hyperplastic lymph nodes are essentially the same: a benign, expected response to some irritant in its drainage field. A hyperplastic lymph node has a normal lymphoid population but is increased in size owing to an immunologic stimulus (e.g., *Demodex* in the skin). If the stimulus is associated with hemorrhage or inflammation so that the node has hemosiderin-ladened macrophages, a few neutrophils and eosinophils, or an excessive number of lymphoblasts, the diagnosis tends to be reactive lymph node.

If the majority of the cells from the lymph node are nonlymphoid WBCs, then lymphadenitis is diagnosed. The predominant WBC determines the type of inflammation (neutrophilic, granulomatous, pyogranulomatous, or eosinophilic). The likely causes were discussed earlier under Inflammatory Masses.

Metastatic neoplasia is diagnosed if adequate numbers of malignant-appearing nonlymphoid cells are present. A few large anaplastic cells can occur in nonneoplastic reactive nodes, and unless the cells are very distinctive (e.g., forming definite epithelial patterns), a confident diagnosis requires many cells (e.g., perhaps 50–100). Occasional mast cells are normal in lymph nodes and can undergo hyperplasia so that many mast cells are required to diagnose metastasis. Macrophages with hemosiderin mimic melanocytes, so be careful diagnosing metastatic melanoma. Inflamed lymph nodes may be fibrotic, so accept a few fibroblasts without diagnosing sarcoma. A few cells prove metastasis if they are foreign to the lymph node, such as perianal gland cells and melanocytes.

Bibliography

Allen SW, Prasse KW, Mahaffey EA: Cytologic differentiation of benign from malignant canine mammary tumors. Vet Pathol 1986; 23:649–655.

Beneke ES, Rogers AL: Medical Mycology Manual. 3rd ed. Minneapolis, Burgess Publishing Co, 1970.

Buerger RG, Scott DW: Cutaneous mast cell neoplasia in cats: 14 cases (1975–1985). JAVMA 1987;190:1440–1444.

Clinkenbeard KD, Cowell RL, Tyler RD: Disseminated histoplasmosis in cats: 12 cases (1981–1986). JAVMA 1987;190:144–148.

Duncan JR, Prasse KW: Cytology of canine cutaneous round cell tumors. Vet Pathol 1979;16:673–679.

Dunstan RW, Reimann KA, Langham RF: Feline sporotrichosis. JAVMA 1986; 189:880–883.

Griffiths GL, Lumsden JH, Valli VEO: Fine needle aspiration cytology and histologic correlation in canine tumors. Vet Clin Pathol 1984;13:13–17.

Gross TL, Connelly MR: Non-tuberculous mycobacterial skin infections in two dogs. Vet Pathol 1983;20:117–119.

Perman V, Alsaker RD, Riss RC: Cytology of the Dog and Cat. South Bend, American Animal Hospital Association, 1979.

Rebar AH: Handbook of Veterinary Cytology. St Louis, Ralston Purina, 1978.

Scott DW: Observations on the eosinophilic granuloma complex in cats. JAAHA 1975;11:261–270.

Appendix I
Listing of Referral Laboratories

Harold Tvedten

This appendix contains a noncomprehensive list of laboratories used by Michigan State University's Veterinary Clinical Center's clinical pathology laboratory and some of the other authors. These are referral laboratories that are often used by a veterinary college's laboratory. Most common clinical pathology tests are omitted because they are performed by most veterinary laboratories. Specific clinical pathology tests are discussed in appropriate chapters. The information available from this listing often includes the name of the laboratory, laboratory director, service role, service range, address, phone number, fees, and how to submit certain types of samples. Parts of this information are often absent if not readily available in the author's files.

The reader should contact any laboratory for current, correct information concerning submission, techniques, fees, and reference values for each laboratory before submitting samples. Note that all laboratories perform many more tests than are listed here. Under a specific test listing, only one or a few laboratories are arbitrarily included, although many laboratories offer that test.

DISCLAIMER

The list was included to provide some basic, practical information. There was no intent to advertise or certify these laboratories at the expense of unlisted laboratories or to create a comprehensive list of referral laboratories in North America or describe how to submit samples for all useful tests. This listing does not assure the reader that the laboratories will be able to process their samples or that the information included may still be current and appropriate. Fees are frequently changed. Submission procedures recommended by the particular laboratory for various tests may vary with those recommended in the rest of the book, and a laboratory may change its recommendations. This is especially true of endocrine tests.

ORGANIZATION OF THE LIST

The addresses and full description of laboratories are only listed once. Laboratories with multiple listings are described in the first section. Only a partial address of these laboratories is then given in the later alphabetical list of individual tests, so readers must refer back to the alphabetical listing of these laboratories for addresses and phone numbers. The second section on individual tests is grouped into subsections on endocrine, immunologic, serologic, toxicologic, and other tests. Laboratories only listed with one individual test have their address and other descriptions included with that test.

The following is a list of American Association of Veterinary Laboratory Diagnosticians, Inc. (AAVLD) accredited laboratories (there may be additions or deletions to this list):

County of Los Angeles
Department of Health Service Division
Comparative Medical and Veterinary Public Health Service
Downey, CA

Colorado Veterinary Diagnostic Laboratory System
Fort Collins, CO: Grand Junction, CO; Rocky Road, CO

Department of Pathobiology, Avian Species
University of Connecticut
Storrs, CT

Florida Veterinary Medicine Diagnostic Laboratory System
Florida Department of Agriculture
Kissimmee, FL

Division of Comparative Pathology
University of Miami
Miami, FL

Diagnostic Assistance Laboratory
College of Veterinary Medicine
University of Georgia
Athens, GA

Diagnostic and Investigational Laboratories
Tifton, GA

Laboratories of Veterinary Diagnostic Medicine
College of Veterinary Medicine
University of Illinois
Urbana, IL

Illinois Department of Agriculture Laboratory System
Centralia, IL; Galesburg, IL; Springfield, IL

The Division of Diagnostic Laboratories
School of Veterinary Medicine
Tufts University
Jamaica Plains, MA

Indiana Animal Disease Diagnostic Laboratory and Southern Indiana Purdue Agricultural Center
Purdue University
West Lafayette, IN

Iowa Veterinary Diagnostic Laboratory
College of Veterinary Medicine
Iowa State University
Ames, IA

Kansas Veterinary Diagnostic Laboratory
Department of Veterinary Diagnosis
College of Veterinary Medicine

Kansas State University
Manhattan, KS

Murray State University
Veterinary Diagnostic and Research Center
Hopkinsville, KY

Louisiana Veterinary Medical Diagnostic Laboratory
School of Veterinary Medicine
Louisiana State University
Baton Rouge, LA

Animal Health Diagnostic Laboratory
College of Veterinary Medicine
Michigan State University
P.O. Box 30076
East Lansing, MI

Minnesota Veterinary Diagnostic Laboratory
University of Minnesota
St. Paul, MN

Mississippi Veterinary Diagnostic Laboratory
Mississippi Department of Agriculture
P.O. Box 4389
Jackson, MS

Veterinary Medical Diagnostic Laboratory
College of Veterinary Medicine
University of Missouri
Columbia, MO

State of Montana Animal Health Division
Diagnostic Laboratory
Bozeman, MT

Nebraska Veterinary Diagnostic Laboratory System
Department of Veterinary Science
University of Nebraska
Lincoln, NE; North Platte, NE

North Carolina Veterinary Medical Diagnostic Laboratory
System
North Carolina Department of Agriculture
Raleigh, NC

North Dakota State Veterinary Diagnostic Laboratory
Department of Veterinary Science
North Dakota State University
Fargo, ND

Oklahoma Animal Disease Diagnostic Laboratory
College of Veterinary Medicine
Oklahoma State University
Stillwater, OK

Pennsylvania Department of Agriculture
Bureau of Animal Industry Laboratory
Summerdale, PA

Animal Disease Research and Diagnostic Laboratory
South Dakota State University
Brookings, SD

Texas Veterinary Medical Diagnostic Laboratory
Texas A&M University System
P.O. Box 3200
Amarillo, TX

Texas Veterinary Diagnostic Laboratory

Texas A&M University System
College of Veterinary Medicine
College Station, TX

Washington Animal Disease Diagnostic Laboratory
College of Veterinary Medicine
Washington State University
Pullman, WA

Central Animal Health Laboratory
Wisconsin Department of Agriculture
Mineral Point Road
Madison, WI

Wyoming State Veterinary Laboratory
Department of Veterinary Science
Laramie, WY

Another listing of animal disease laboratories arranged by state and city is available from the source below. Information provided includes the name of the laboratory, director, address, phone, affiliation, who may submit specimens, major species accepted for examination, and the services offered. This source may be used to locate referral laboratory testing nearest to the reader. Send correspondence to

National Veterinary Services Laboratories
Biometrics and Data Systems
P.O. Box 844
Ames, IA 50010

LABORATORY DESCRIPTIONS

Note that the full addresses listed here are not repeated under the descriptions of individual tests later.

APL Veterinary Laboratories
4230 S. Burnham Ave.
Suite 250
Las Vegas, NV 89119
Phone (702) 733-7866
(800) 433-2750

Director of Clinical Pathology ● Dr. J.K. Klaassen

Service Role ● Commercial.

Service Range ● Clinical and anatomic pathology, endocrinology, serology, toxicology, and microbiology.

Animal Health Diagnostic Laboratory (AHDL)
Michigan State University
P.O. Box 30076
Lansing, MI 48909-7576
Phone (517) 353-1683

Director ● Dr. W.M. Reed

Service Role • State-supported diagnostic laboratory serving mainly Michigan veterinarians and animal owners.

Service Range • Pathology, clinical pathology, endocrinology, field investigation, immunology, microbiology, nutrition, parasitology, and toxicology.

Clinical Immunology Laboratory
University of Pennsylvania
Room 4102
School of Veterinary Medicine
3850 Spruce Street
Philadelphia, PA 19104
Phone (215) 898-6882

Director • Dr. Robert Schwartman

Service Role • University.

Service Range • Immunology (rheumatoid factor, Coombs', immunoglobulins, immunofluorescent biopsy), endocrinology, FIP and FeLV titer, *Aspergillus* antigen, and ELISA for atopic disease.

Comparative Hematology Laboratory
Wadsworth Center for Labs and Research
New York State Department of Health
Box 509, Empire State Plaza
Albany, NY 12201-5090
Phone (518) 869-4507
Fax (518) 869-4533

Director • Dr. James Catelfamo (518-869-4501)

Consultant • Dr. Marjory Brooks (518-869-4537)

Consultant • Dr. Jean Dodds (310-828-4804)

Service Range (Hemostasis) • Individual factor analysis, coagulation screening tests, coagulation inhibitor assays, von Willebrand's factor, platelet aggregation.

Diagnostic Laboratory
College of Veterinary Medicine and Biomedical Sciences
Colorado State University
Fort Collins, CO 80523
Phone (303) 491-1281

Service Range • Wide range of tests.

Diagnostic Laboratory
New York State College of Veterinary Medicine
Cornell University
P.O. Box 786
Ithaca, NY 14850
Phone (607) 253-3900

Director • Donald H. Lein

Hansen Veterinary Immunology
450 Porter Road
Suite C
Dixon, CA 95620
Phone (916) 678-9680

Director • Dr. H. Hansen

Service Role • Commercial.

Service Range • Immunologic testing such as ANA, immunofluorescence of tissue, titers for canine distemper, FIP, FIV, heartworm, feline leukemia, and FOCMA.

Immunology Laboratory
College of Veterinary Medicine
University of Florida
Box J-126, Health Center Building 215
J.H.M.H.C.
Gainesville, FL 32610
Phone (904) 392-4751

Infectious Disease Laboratory
University of Georgia
Department of Small Animal Medicine
College of Veterinary Medicine
Athens, GA 30602-7390
Phone (706) 542-6484
(706) 542-7474
Fax (706) 542-6460

Director • Dr. Craig Greene

Service Role • Veterinary school affiliated laboratory.

Service Range • Serologic texting for tick-borne diseases (*Ehrlichia canis*, RMSF, Lyme disease), canine and feline toxoplasmosis, FIV, and *Cryptococcus*.

Louisiana Veterinary Medical Diagnostic Laboratory
P.O. Box 25070
Baton Rouge, LA 70894

Phone (504) 346-3193
Fax (504) 346-3390

Professional Animal Laboratory, Inc.
17672A Cowan Ave., Suite 200
Irvine, CA 92714
Phone (800) 745-4725 in USA
        (800) 542-1151 in California
        Fax (714) 752-4935

President ● Dr. Lon J. Rich

Consultant ● Dr. Jean Dodds

Service Role ● Commercial.

Service Range ● Clinical and anatomic pathology, serology, endocrinology, etc.

Protatek Reference Laboratory
574 East Alamo Street, Suite 90
Chandler, AZ 85225
Phone (602) 545-8499

Southwest Veterinary Diagnostics, Inc.
13633 North Cave Creek Road
Phoenix, AZ 85022
Phone (602) 971-4110

Pathologist ● Dr. Robert Bartsch

Service Role ● Commercial.

Service Range ● Clinical pathology, serology, histopathology, endocrinology.

Texas Veterinary Medical Diagnostic Laboratory
Texas A&M University System
College of Veterinary Medicine
P.O. Drawer 3040
College Station, TX 77841-3040
Phone (409) 845-3414
Fax (409) 845-1794

Director ● Dr. A.K. Eugster

Service Role ● State diagnostic laboratory system.

Service Range ● Clinical and anatomic pathology, bacteriology, virology, toxicology, etc.

Tick Borne Diseases Laboratory
College of Veterinary Medicine
North Carolina State University
Raleigh, NC 27606
Phone (919) 829-4357

Veterinary Medical Research and Development
P.O. Box 502
Pullman, WA 99163
Phone (509) 334-5815
        (800) 222-8673
        Fax (509) 332-5356

Vice President ● Robert E. Wildes

Service Role ● Commercial.

Service Range ● Primarily immunoglobulin quantitation (bovine, equine, and canine), also CBC, Coombs', and histopathology.

VetPath, Inc.
2062 North Center
Saginaw, MI 48603
Phone (800) 292-0363 (for sample pickup)

Service Role ● Commercial.

Service Range ● Very wide range of clinical pathology tests.

Comments ● VetPath is part of MedPath, Inc., and a toll-free number (800-631-1390) gives client service and a local laboratory.

ENDOCRINE TESTS

Laboratory
Endocrine Diagnostic Section
Animal Health Diagnostic Laboratory
Michigan State University
Phone (517) 353-0621

Director ● Dr. R. F. Nachreiner

Service Role ● Endocrinology, therapeutic drug monitoring.

General Preparation of Samples ● Thyroid hormones are stable and need no refrigeration. Other hormones should be sent on ice packs. Do not send whole or clotted blood. Let blood clot at room temperature and quickly centrifuge for serum collection. If the sample is stored longer than an hour, place on ice. Plasma collected in an EDTA tube should be centrifuged within 15 minutes, and the plasma refrigerated immediately.

Serum Thyroid Profile • Sample—1.5 ml of *serum* for T_3, T_4, free T_3, and free T_4. One milliliter of serum for only the T_3 and T_4 and 0.5 ml of serum for reverse T_3.

Thyroid Hormone Therapy Check • T_3 at 3 hours after Cytobin, or T_4 4 to 8 hours after Soloxine. Indicate the therapy, dose, animal's weight, and sample time. Wait 1 month after discontinuing therapy before reevaluating thyroid function.

Charge • Thyroid profile $14; T_3 + T_4 $12; reverse T_3 $8.

TSH Stimulation • Sample—Include a presample of 1½ ml for a thyroid profile and a 1-ml sample for T_3 and T_4 8 hours after IM injection of Dermathycin (TSH) at a dose of 5 IU for dogs < 50 pounds and 10 IU for bigger dogs.

Charge • $22.

Cortisol • Sample—0.5 ml of plasma per sample on ice. For combined dexamethasone suppression-ACTH response test, collect a pretest sample, inject 0.1 mg of dexamethasone/kg IV, and obtain a 2- or 4-hour postdexamethasone sample, then inject 2.2U ACTH gel (HP Acthar)/kg IM and collect 1-hour and 2-hour post-ACTH samples. For low-dose dexamethasone suppression, collect a pretest sample, inject 0.01 mg of dexamethasone/kg IM, and obtain 6- and 8-hour post-dexamethasone samples.

Charge • Combined dexamethasone suppression/ACTH response $28; low-dose dexamethasone suppression $23; urinary cortisol $7.

Insulin • Sample—1 ml of serum per sample. For insulinoma, collect samples before and 1 and 5 minutes after 0.03 mg of glucagon/kg IV, or collect samples before and 15, 30, 45, and 60 minutes after 1 g of glucose/kg IV given over 30 seconds to a dog fasted for 24 hours.

Charge • Pre $10; post $7.

Aldosterone • Sample—0.5 ml of plasma/sample before and 2 hours after 2.2U ACTH gel/kg IM.

Charge • $17.

Gastrin • Sample—0.5 ml of serum/sample on ice. Include a resting sample after a 24-hour fast, then 15, 30, 45, and 60 minutes after feeding ½ can P/D and ½ can beef broth or a whole can if the dog is > 40 pounds.

Charge • $10 pre; $7 post.

Parathormone • Sample—Remove at least 0.5 ml of serum within 2 hours after collecting the blood. Ship on ice by express delivery.

Charge • $25.

Testosterone • Sample—1.0 ml of serum/sample on ice. For GnRH (Cystorelin) response, obtain pretest sample, inject 0.1 µg GnRH/pound IV, and obtain 1- and 2-hour postsamples.

Charge • $10.

Catecholamine, Somatomedin, and Others • Sample—Contact the laboratory.

Estradiol (Estrogen)

Laboratory • Diagnostic Laboratory
Cornell University

Sample • 1 ml of serum.

Charge • $15.

Laboratory • Rothgerber Endocrinology Laboratory
Veterinary Teaching Hospital
Colorado State University
Fort Collins, CO 80523

Service Role • University.

Service Range • Wide variety of hormones including estradiol.

Sample • Contact laboratory for information.

Charge • Contact laboratory.

Endogenous ACTH

Laboratory • Professional Animal Laboratory, Inc.

Sample • 1.0 ml of frozen plasma in siliconized or plastic tube.

Charge • $35.

Laboratory • Animal Health Diagnostic Laboratory
Michigan State University
Endocrinology Section

Sample • Call laboratory.

Charge • Call laboratory.

IMMUNOLOGIC TESTS

ANA

Laboratory • Immunology Laboratory
College of Veterinary Medicine
University of Florida
(will phone results in 7 to 10 days, if requested)

Sample • 0.5 ml of frozen serum.

Charge • $20.

Laboratory • Professional Animal Laboratory, Inc.

Sample • 1.0 ml of serum or synovial fluid.

Charge • $16.

Laboratory • Attn: Referral Services
Clinical Pathology Laboratory
A215 Veterinary Teaching Hospital
Michigan State University
215 Veterinary Medical Center
East Lansing, MI 48824-1314

Director • Dr. J. Stickle

Sample • 1 ml of serum (dog, cat, horse).

Charge • $15.

Antithyroid Antibody

Laboratory • Immunology Laboratory
University of Florida
College of Veterinary Medicine

Sample • 0.5 ml of serum with a cold pack.

Charge • $15.

Blood Typing or Pedigree Testing

Laboratory • Immunohematology and Serology Laboratory
Department of Medicine
B228 Life Sciences Building
Michigan State University
East Lansing, MI 48824-1317
Phone (517) 355-4616
Fax (517) 353-5436

Director • Dr. Robert Bull
Canine RBC typing for identifying blood donors.

Sample • 5 ml of whole blood in acid-citrate-dextrose or EDTA. Ship cool, not frozen, by 24-hour courier. Results available 24 to 48 hours afer receiving sample.

Charge • $35 per animal for complete typing.
Feline RBC typing for identifying blood donors.

Sample • 3–5 ml of EDTA blood. Ship cool, not frozen, by 24-hour courier. Results available in 24 to 48 hours after receiving sample.

Charge • $35 per animal for complete typing.
Molecular genetic pedigree substantiation (dog).

Sample • Must call for arrangements. Results in 30 days.

Charge • $50.

Immunoglobulin Quantitation

Laboratory • Veterinary Medical Teaching Hospital
College of Veterinary Medicine
University of Florida

Sample • 0.2 ml (minimum) per antibody type to be tested.

Charge • $15 per class of immunoglobulin tested (IgA, IgM, IgG).

Laboratory ● Clinical Immunology Laboratory
Veterinary Animal Disease Diagnostic Laboratory
1243 Veterinary Pathobiology Building
Purdue University
West Lafayette, IN 47907
Phone (317) 494-9676

Director ● Dr. Paul Snyder

Sample ● 1 ml of serum.

Charge ● $9 per immunoglobulin.

Immunofluorescence of Tissue

Laboratory ● Veterinary Medical Teaching Hospital
Immunology Laboratory
College of Veterinary Medicine
University of Florida

Sample ● Biopsy in Michel's medium.

Charge ● $24.

Laboratory ● Clinical Immunology Laboratory
University of Pennsylvania

Sample ● Tissue in Michel's fixative.

Charge ● $20.

Rheumatoid Factor

Laboratory ● Immunology
College of Veterinary Medicine
University of Florida

Sample ● 2 ml of serum.

Charge ● $15 for dogs; $23 for cats.

Laboratory ● Clinical Immunology Laboratory
School of Veterinary Medicine
University of Pennsylvania

Sample ● Serum from 10-ml clot tube.

Charge ● $10.

Myasthenia Gravis

Acetylcholine Receptor Antibody

Laboratory ● Comparative Neuromuscular Laboratory
Basic Science Building
Room B200
University of California, San Diego
LaJolla, CA 92093-0614
Phone (619) 534-1537

Director ● Dr. Diane Shelton

Sample ● 1 ml of serum with cold pack.

Charge ● $25.

SEROLOGIC TESTS

Borreliosis—Lyme Disease

Laboratory ● Infectious Diseases Laboratory
University of Georgia

Sample ● 0.5 ml of serum for ELISA.

Charge ● $18 for IgM and IgG titers.

Laboratory ● Diagnostic Laboratory
Colorado State University

Sample ● 0.5 ml of serum for ELISA.

Charge ● $17.

Laboratory ● Animal Health Diagnostic Laboratory
Michigan State University

Sample ● 1 ml of serum or clot tube.

Charge ● $18 for IgM and IgG.

Laboratory ● Tick Borne Diseases Laboratory
North Carolina State University

Sample ● 1 ml of serum.

Charge ● $13.

Laboratory ● Southwest Veterinary Diagnostics, Inc.

Sample ● 1 ml of serum for IFA.

Charge ● $17.

Laboratory ● Protatek Reference Laboratory

Sample ● 1 ml of serum for IFA.

Charge ● $24.

Babesiosis

Laboratory ● Tick Borne Diseases Laboratory
North Carolina State University

Sample ● 1 ml of serum.

Charge: ● $10 to 13 for initial sample and convalescent.

Laboratory ● Texas Veterinary Medical Diagnostic Laboratory

Sample ● 0.5 ml of serum.

Charge ● $20.

Laboratory ● Protatek Reference Laboratory

Sample ● 1 ml of serum for IFA.

Charge ● $24.

Canine Brucellosis

Laboratory ● Diagnostic Laboratory
Cornell University

Sample ● 2 to 3 ml of serum.

Charge ● $6.

Laboratory ● Diagnostic Laboratory
Colorado State University

Sample ● 0.5 ml of serum.

Charge ● $17.

Canine Distemper Titer

Laboratory ● Diagnostic Laboratory
Cornell University

Sample ● Minimum of 0.1 ml of frozen cerebrospinal fluid (in dry ice).

Charge ● $12.50.

Laboratory ● Diagnostic Laboratory
Colorado State University

Sample ● 0.5 ml of serum for serum neutralization.

Charge ● $17.

Laboratory ● Animal Health Diagnostic Laboratory
Michigan State University
Virology Section—Dr. Maes

Sample ● 2 ml of serum.

Charge ● $6.

Canine Parvovirus Titer

Laboratory ● Diagnostic Laboratory
Cornell University

Sample ● 1 ml of serum for serum neutralization.

Charge ● $12.

Laboratory ● Animal Health Diagnostic Laboratory
Michigan State University
Virology Section—Dr. Maes

Sample ● 1 ml of serum, prefer paired samples. The section accepts samples for various feline and canine viruses.

Charge ● $6.

Laboratory ● Diagnostic Laboratory
Colorado State University

Sample ● 0.5 ml of serum for serum neutralization.

Charge • $17.

Ehrlichia Canis Titer

Laboratory • Veterinary Diagnostic Medicine
P.O. Box U
Urbana, IL 61801
Phone (217) 333-1620 (phone/fax
results in 1–2 days if requested)

Director • Dr. Ibulaimu Kakoma

Sample • 1 ml of serum (cold packed—not frozen).

Charge • $24.

Laboratory • Tick Borne Diseases Laboratory
North Carolina State University

Sample • 1 ml of serum.

Charge • $15.

Laboratory • Infectious Diseases Laboratory
University of Georgia

Sample • 0.5 ml of serum.

Charge • $18.

Note • A tick-borne disease panel for RMSF,
Lyme disease, and *E. canis* requires 2 ml of
serum and costs $45.

Laboratory • Protatek Reference Laboratory

Sample • 1 ml of serum.

Charge • $24.

Laboratory • Southwest Veterinary Diagnostic,
Inc.

Sample • 1 ml of serum.

Charge • $17.

Laboratory • Texas Veterinary Medical Diagnostic Laboratory

Sample • 1 ml of serum.

Charge • $14 for screen; $30 for titer.

Ehrlichia Platys Titer

Laboratory • Louisiana Veterinary Medical Diagnostic Laboratory

Sample • 3-ml clot tube.

Charge • $15.

Laboratory • Protatek Reference Laboratory

Sample • 1 ml of serum.

Charge • $24.

Ehrlichia Risticii and Ehrlichia Equi Titers

Laboratory • Protatek Reference Laboratory

Sample • 1 ml of serum.

Charge • $24.

Feline Infectious Peritonitis
(Note: see Chapter 15 about this test)

Laboratory • Infectious Disease Laboratory
University of Georgia

Sample • 1 ml of serum for indirect fluorescent
antibody.

Charge • $11.

Laboratory • Diagnostic Laboratory
Cornell University

Sample • 1 ml of serum for kinetics-based ELISA.

Charge • $14.

Laboratory • Texas Veterinary Medical Diagnostic Laboratory

Sample • 0.5 ml of serum.

Charge • $10 (out-of-state fee).

Feline Leukemia Virus

Laboratory ● Hansen Veterinary Immunology

Sample ● Three air-dried, unfixed blood smears for fluorescent antibody.

Charge ● $10.

Sample ● 1.0 ml of serum for ELISA.

Charge ● $10.

Laboratory ● National Veterinary Laboratory, Inc.
P.O. Box 2329
Franklin Lakes, NJ 07417
Phone (201) 891-2992

Director ● Dr. William Hardy

Sample ● Three air-dried, unfixed blood smears for fluorescent antibody.

Charge ● $10 ($10 each for first two tests, then $5 each if from multiple-cat households).

Laboratory ● Feline Retrovirus Research Laboratory
Colorado State University
Department of Pathology
Fort Collins, CO 80523

Director ● Dr. Edward Hoover

Sample ● Three air-dried, unfixed blood smears for fluorescent antibody.

Charge ● $15.

Sample ● 1 ml of serum for ELISA.

Charge ● $10.

Sample ● 1 ml of serum for Western blot.

Charge ● $20.

Sample ● Contact laboratory for virus isolation.

Charge ● $30.

Feline Oncornavirus Cell Membrane Antigen (FOCMA D53)

Laboratory ● Hansen Veterinary Immunology

Sample ● 1.0 ml of serum.

Charge ● $10.

Feline Immunodeficiency Virus

Laboratory ● Hansen Veterinary Immunology

Sample ● 1 ml of serum.

Charge ● $15.

Note ● Western blot requires 1 ml of serum and costs $20.

Laboratory ● Feline Retrovirus Research Laboratory
Colorado State University

Sample ● 1 ml of serum for ELISA.

Charge ● $10.

Sample ● 1 ml of serum for Western blot.

Charge ● $20.

Sample ● Call laboratory for virus isolation.

Charge ● $30.

Laboratory ● National Veterinary Laboratory, Inc.

Sample ● 1 ml of serum for ELISA.

Charge ● $10.

Sample ● 1 ml of serum for Western blot.

Charge ● $20.

Fungal Titer (Coccidioidomycosis, Cryptococcosis, and Blastomycosis)

Comment ● The State Health Department Laboratories have access to other laboratories to evaluate animal samples if human exposure is involved.

Laboratory ● Southwest Veterinary Diagnostic Laboratory (for coccidioidomycosis)

Sample ● 3 to 4 ml of serum.

Charge ● $13.

Laboratory ● Medical Microbiology Laboratory (for coccidiomycosis)
University of California at Davis
P.O. Box 1440
Davis, CA 95617
Phone (916) 752-1757

Director ● Dr. Demosthenes Pappagianis

Sample ● 2 to 3 ml of serum.

Charge ● $22 for immunodiffusion and $27 for quantitative immunodiffusion.

Laboratory ● Texas Veterinary Medical Diagnostic Laboratory

Blastomycosis AGID ● 0.5 ml of serum, $8.

Coccidioidomycosis AGID ● 0.5 ml of serum, $8.

Cryptococcus Antigen ● 1.0 ml of serum—screen $15, titer $28 (out-of-state fees).

Aspergillosis AGID ● 1.0 ml of serum, $8.

Laboratory ● Infectious Disease Laboratory (for Cryptococcus)
University of Georgia

Sample ● 1 ml of serum, CSF, or aqueous humor.

Charge ● $11.

Laboratory ● Diagnostic Laboratory
Cornell University

Sample ● 1 ml of serum.

Charge ● $15.

Heartworms (IFA/ELISA for Occult Dirofilariasis)

Laboratory ● Animal Health Diagnostic Laboratory
Michigan State University

Sample ● 1 or 2 ml *nonhemolyzed* serum.

Charge ● $10.

Laboratory ● Diagnostic Laboratory
Colorado State University

Sample ● 0.5 ml of serum.

Charge ● $17.

Leptospirosis Titer

Laboratory ● Animal Health Diagnostic Laboratory
Michigan State University

Sample ● 10 ml of serum (acute and convalescent titers).

Charge ● $4.

Rocky Mountain Spotted Fever Titer

Laboratory ● Infectious Disease Laboratory
University of Georgia

Sample ● 0.5 ml of nonhemolyzed canine serum on a frozen pack.

Charge ● $18 for screen, $24 for exact titer (IgM and IgG).

Laboratory ● Tick Borne Disease Laboratory

Sample ● 1 ml of serum.

Charge ● $15.

Toxoplasmosis Titer

Laboratory ● Animal Health Diagnostic Laboratory
Michigan State University

Sample ● Minimum of 2 ml of chilled or frozen serum.

Charge ● $10.

Laboratory ● Infectious Disease Laboratory
University of Georgia

Sample ● 1 ml of serum for both IgG and IgM.

Charge ● $18.

Laboratory ● Diagnostic Laboratory
Colorado State University

Sample ● 1 ml of serum for both IgG and IgM, 0.3 ml of aqueous humor or CSF in EDTA.

Charge ● $17 for serum, $25 for aqueous humor or CSF.

Sample ● 1 ml of serum, 0.3 ml of aqueous humor or CSF in EDTA for *Toxoplasma* antigen.

Charge ● $17.

Neosporosis Titer

Laboratory ● Dr David Lindsay
Room 122
Green Hall
College of Veterinary Medicine
Auburn University
Auburn, AL 36849-5519

Sample ● 0.25 ml serum.

Charge ● $20.

Tularemia Titer

Laboratory ● New Mexico Department of Agriculture
Veterinary Diagnostic Services
700 Camino de Salud, NE
Albuquerque, NM 87106
Phone (505) 841-2576

Sample ● 1 ml for tube agglutination.

Charge ● Call laboratory.

Laboratory ● Must contact local public health laboratories.

Trypanosomiasis

Laboratory ● Texas Veterinary Medical Diagnostic Laboratory

Sample ● 1 ml of serum.

Charge ● $10.

THERAPEUTIC DRUG MONITORING

Laboratory ● Endocrine Diagnostic Section
Animal Health Diagnostic Laboratory
Michigan State University

Sample ● Dilantin or phenobarbital: 0.5 ml of serum/sample collected 2 to 3 hours after pill and just before next pill at 8 hours.

Digoxin ● 0.5 ml of serum/sample collected 8 hours after pill and just before next pill at 24 hours.

Charge ● $10 pre; $7 post.

Laboratory ● Clinical Pharmacology Laboratory
College of Veterinary Medicine
Texas A&M University
College Station, TX 77843
Phone (409) 845-9184

Director ● Dr. Dawn Boothe

Sample ● Contact laboratory for amount of serum and time relative to drug administration. Currently has assays for gentamicin, amikacin, phenobarbital, phenytoin, potassium bromide, benzodiazepines, and digoxin.

Charge ● Contact laboratory.

TOXICOLOGIC TESTS

Laboratory ● Animal Health Diagnostic Laboratory
Michigan State University
Toxicology Laboratory

Director ● Dr. W. E. Braselton

Anions (Water) (Chloride, Nitrite, Nitrate, Sulfate)

Sample ● 100 ml of water in bottles provided by an Extension agent or public health official.

Charge ● $8.

Anthelmintics (Avermectin, Benzimidazoles, Levamisole)

Sample ● 50 g of liver; 50 of g muscle; 5 ml of serum.

Charge ● $25.

Anticoagulants (Brodifacoum, Bromadiolone, Chlorphacinone, Coumafuryl, Dicumarol, Diphacinone, Pindone, Warfarin)

Sample ● 50 g of liver, stomach contents, bait; 5 ml of whole blood or serum.

Charge ● $18.

Cholinesterase (Blood)

Sample ● 1 ml of whole blood (EDTA or heparin), chilled, not frozen.

Charge ● $12.

Cholinesterase (Brain)

Sample ● ½ brain (frozen).

Charge ● $12.

Cyanide

Sample ● 100 g of forage; 20 g of muscle; 5 ml of blood.

Handling ● Samples must be quick frozen and received frozen.

Charge ● $10.

Drugs, Pesticides, Industrial Chemicals (Gas Chromatography/ Mass Spectrometry Screen)

Sample ● 10 ml of whole blood; 50 g of brain; 100 g each of rumen or stomach contents, liver,

and kidney; 10 g of body fat; 400 g of suspected material.

Charge ● $25.

Ethylene Glycol

Sample ● 1 ml of serum; 50 g of liver; 5 ml of urine.

Charge ● $25.

Insecticides (Chlorinated Hydrocarbons)

Sample ● 50 g of brain; 100 g each of stomach or rumen contents, liver, and kidney; 10 g of body fat.

Charge ● $25.

Lead (Blood)

Sample ● 2 ml of whole blood.

Minerals (Tissue and Water)

Sample ● Minerals in tissue or water for Al, Sb, As, Ba, B, Ca, Cd, Cr, Co, Cu, Fe, Hg, K, Mg, Na, P, Pb, Se, Tl, and Zn. Submit 100 g each of stomach contents, liver, kidney, and suspect material; 2 to 10 ml bile, 1 L of water in special bottles provided by an Extension agent or public health official.

Charge ● Tissue minerals $18; serum or bile minerals $12.

Sample ● Minerals in urine for Ar, Hg, and thallium: submit 10 ml of urine.

Charge ● $12.

Minerals (Serum) (B, Ba, Ca, Cu, Fe, Mg, P [Total]), Na, Zn

Sample ● 2 ml of serum.

Charge ● $12.

Minerals (Urine) (As, Tl, Hg)

Sample ● 10 ml of urine.

Charge ● $12.

Mycotoxins (Aflatoxin, Zearalenone, T2, Diacetoxyscirpenol [DAS], Vomitoxin, Ochratoxin)

Sample ● 500 g of feed, kept dry or frozen.

Charge ● $23 (qualitative screen); $23 (quantification of identified mycotoxin).

Polybrominated Biphenyls

Sample ● 50 g of brain.

Charge ● $20.

Strychnine

Sample ● 50 g of liver, stomach contents, bait.

Charge ● $13.

OTHER TESTS

Alkaline Phosphatase Isoenzymes

Laboratory ● Laboratories of Veterinary Diagnostic Medicine
University of Illinois at Urbana-Champaign
P.O. Box U, 2001 South Lincoln Ave.
Urbana, IL 61801

Director ● Dr. W. Hoffman

Sample ● 1 ml or more of serum. The alkaline phosphatase activity should be three to four times normal before submitting this test.

Charge ● $22.

Calculus Analysis

Laboratory ● Minnesota Urolith Center
Department of Small Animal Clinical Sciences
College of Veterinary Medicine
University of Minnesota
St. Paul, MN 55108
Phone (612) 625-4221

Director ● Carl Osborne

Sample ● Calculi(us) shipped dry in unbreakable container. Contact center for preservation of urethral plugs.

Charge ● Complete questionnaire on case.

Laboratory ● Urinary Stone Analysis Laboratory
Department of Medicine
School of Veterinary Medicine
University of California at Davis
Davis, CA 95616

Supervisor ● Annette Ruby

Sample ● Calculi(us) shipped dry in sealed plastic bag within a mailing tube.

Charge ● Crystallography $35; bacterial culture and sensitivity $22.50.

Coombs' Test

Laboratory ● Professional Animal Laboratory, Inc.

Sample ● 2 to 3 ml of EDTA blood.

Charge ● $15.

Fecal Fat (24-Hour)

Laboratory ● Human hospital laboratories may perform test.

Sample ● Weighed 24-hour sample in preweighed container.

Hemostatic Testing

Laboratory ● Comparative Hematology Laboratory
New York State Department of Health
Albany, NY

Sample • Contact laboratory for complete instructions before submission. Two milliliters of citrated plasma for coagulation and vWF:Ag assays. One milliliter of citrate or EDTA plasma for vWF:Ag assay only. Plasma with hemolysis or clots is unacceptable. Special shipping with dry ice or frozen cold packs is necessary.

Charge • None.

Consultation •
   Dr. Marjory Brooks (518) 869-4537, clinical management of hemostatic disorders
   Dr. James Catalfamo (518) 869-4501, platelet function and hemostasis
   Dr. Jean Dodds (310) 828-4804 (fax 310-828-8251), all areas of hemostasis

Pyruvic Kinase

Laboratory • VetPath, Inc.

Sample • 7 ml of EDTA whole blood (specify test #J-15).

Charge • $26.

Pyruvate Transketolase

Laboratory • VetPath, Inc.

Sample • 4 ml *frozen* heparinized blood (specify test #899).

Charge • $27.50

Trypsin-Like Immunoreactivity

Laboratory • Comparative Toxicology Laboratories
   Veterinary Clinical Science Bldg.
   Kansas State University
   Manhattan, KS 66506
   Phone (913) 532-5679

Sample • 1 ml of serum from dog fasted 12 hours. Also offer cobalamin (B$_{12}$) and folate testing.

Charge • $20.

Laboratory • GI Laboratory
   1248 Lynn Hall
   Department of Veterinary Clinical Sciences

Purdue University
West Lafayette, IN 47907
Phone (317) 494-0331
Fax (317) 494-8640

Director • Dr. David Williams

Sample • 0.5 ml of serum from dog fasted 12 to 18 hours.

Charge • $20 to $30.

Comment • Serum cobalamin (B$_{12}$) and folate concentrations available on 1.0 ml of nonhemolyzed serum from fasted dog for $20. Feline fecal proteolytic activity and TLI available.

Vitamin E, Selenium, and Vitamin A

Laboratory • Clinical Nutrition Section
   Animal Health Diagnostic Laboratory
   Michigan State University

Director • Dr. H. Stowe

Sample • 0.5 ml of serum per vitamin, 1 ml serum for selenium.

Charge • $6 per vitamin in serum; $8 in liver; $8 per selenium in serum; $10 in liver.

von Willebrand's Factor

Laboratory • Comparative Hematology Laboratory
   New York State Department of Health
   P.O. Box 509
   Albany, NY 12201-0509

Sample • 1 ml of citrated plasma; special mailing requirements—20-gauge needle or larger, 3.8% citrate, no hemolysis permitted but lipemia and icterus are acceptable.

Charge • no charge.

Laboratory • Professional Animal Laboratory, Inc.

Sample • 1 ml of citrated plasma as above.

Charge • $17.

Appendix II
Reference Values
Harold Tvedten

These reference values are used by the Veterinary Clinical Center at Michigan State University. Literature values are referenced. *One preferably should use reference values specific for the laboratory or instrumentation used for deriving data for one's patients.* See appropriate chapters for details about tests, including full names for those abbreviated here. Canine values were derived from 120 apparently normal dogs and 40 apparently normal cats and using a Technicon H-1 analyzer.

HEMATOLOGY REFERENCE VALUES TECHNICON H-1 HEMATOLOGY ANALYZER

	Test	Units	Canine	Feline
C O M P L E T E B L O O D C O U N T	WBC	× 10³/µl	6.02–16.02	4.87–20.10
	RBC	× 10⁶/µl	6.15–8.70	6.12–11.86
	Hemoglobin	g/dl	14.1–20.0	9.0–15.6
	Hematocrit	%	43.3–59.3	29.3–49.8
	MCV	fl	63.0–77.1	41.9–54.8
	MCH	pg	21.1–24.8	12.5–17.6
	MCHC	g/dl	29.9–35.6	28.1–32.0
	Platelets	× 10³/µl	164–510	26–470*
	MPV†	fl	3.9–6.1	4.1–8.3
	RDW†	%	11.9–14.9	14.2–17.6
	HDW†	g/dl	1.49–2.17	1.71–2.41

*See other platelet range of 230–680 × 10³/µl listed later, which is a more accurate range. This reference range extends down into the thrombocytopenic range, which illustrates the problems of automated platelet counts on routinely collected feline blood samples.
†Using the multispecies software 2.0.

ABSOLUTE DIFFERENTIAL LEUKOCYTE COUNTS

	Test	Units	Canine	Feline
D I F F E R E N T I A L	Neutrophils	× 10³/µl	3.23–10.85	2.5–12.5
	Lymphocytes	× 10³/µl	0.53–3.44	1.5–7.0
	Monocytes	× 10³/µl	0.0–0.43	0.0–0.85
	Eosinophils	× 10³/µl	0.0–1.82	0.0–1.50
	Basophils	× 10³/µl	0.01–0.54	0
	LUC*	× 10³/µl	0.26–2.09	N/A

Canine reference ranges are based on automated leukocyte differential counts of a Technicon H-1 analyzer on blood from 120 apparently normal dogs.
Note: Do not use automated differential leukocyte count reference ranges for interpreting manual differential leukocyte counts.
*LUC, large unstained cell in automated leukocyte differential (Technicon H-1).
(Feline manual total leukocyte differential cell counts are from Jain NC: Schalm's Veterinary Hematology. 4th ed. Philadelphia, Lea and Febiger, 1986.)

COAGULATION REFERENCE VALUES

	Test	Units	Canine	Feline
C O A G U L A T I O N	Platelets†	× 10³/µl	166–575	230–680
	PT	seconds	5.1–7.9	8.4–10.8
	APTT	seconds	8.6–12.9	13.7–30.2
	Fibrinogen	mg/dl	100–245	110–370
	FDP	µg/ml	<10	<10

*Coagulation tests are performed on the Fibrometer System.
†Actual range/manual count.
(Feline values are from Killingsworth C: Screening coagulation tests in the cat. Vet Clin Pathol 1985;14:19–23.)

CHEMISTRY REFERENCE VALUES

Test	Units	Canine	Feline
Arterial blood gas			
pH		7.36–7.44	7.36–7.44
P_{CO_2}	mm Hg	36–44	28–32
P_{O_2}	mm Hg	90–100	90–100
T_{CO_2}	mEq/L	25–27	21–23
HCO_3	mEq/L	24–26	20–22
Venous blood gas			
pH		7.34–7.46	7.33–7.41
P_{CO_2}	mm Hg	32–49	34–38
P_{O_2}	mm Hg	24–48	35–45
T_{CO_2}	mEq/L	21–31	27–31
HCO_3	mEq/L	20–29	22–24
A:G ratio (calculated)		0.89–2.68	0.80–1.68
Albumin	g/dl	3.2–4.7	3.0–4.6
ALP (alkaline phosphatase)	IU/L	0–90	4–81
ALT (SGPT)	IU/L	10–94	23–109
Ammonia (resting)	ug/dl	25–92	30–100
Amylase	IU/L	371–1,503	531–1,660
AST (SGOT)	IU/L	10–62	14–41
Bile acid (fasting)	umol/L	0.0–15.3	0.0–7.6
Bile acid (2 hour)	umol/L	0.0–20.3	0.0–10.9
Bilirubin—total and direct	mg/dl	0.1–0.6	0.1–0.7
BSP		0–5%	0–5%
BUN	mg/dl	7–32	18–41
Calcium	mg/dl	9.0–11.9	8.4–11.5
Cholesterol	mg/dl	116–317	64–229
CPK	IU/L	51–529	91–326
Creatinine	mg/dl	0.5–1.4	0.7–2.2
Electrolyte profile			
Sodium (Na)	mEq/L	146–156	153–162
Potassium (K)	mEq/L	3.9–5.5	3.6–5.8
Chloride (Cl)	mEq/L	113–123	119–132
T_{CO_2}	mEq/L	16.9–26.9	12.5–24.5
Anion gap	mEq/L	9–22	10–27
Gamma GT	IU/L	1–6	1–3
Globulin	g/dl	1.5–3.5	2.1–4.0
Glucose	mg/dl	53–117	57–131
LDH	IU/L	42–130	63–193
Lipase	U/L	90–527	
Lipase	Sigma-Tietz units	0.1–1.3	0.1–0.4
Magnesium	mg/dl	1.36–2.09	1.38–2.36
Osmolality—serum			
Calculated	mOsm/Kg	302–325	219–371
Determined	mOsm/Kg	293–321	290–320
Osmolality—urine	mOsm	200–2,000	200–2,000
Phosphorus	mg/dl	1.9–7.9	2.9–8.3
SDH	IU/L	5.4–33.3	0.4–10
Total protein	g/dl	5.3–7.6	5.5–7.7
Triglyceride	mg/dl	10–500	10–500
Uric acid	mg/dl	0–1	0–1
Serum iron (Abbott)	μg/dl	61–255	34–122
Iron profile*			
Total iron	μg/dl	84–233*	68–215
UIBC	μg/dl	142–393	105–205
TIBC	μg/dl	284–572	†
Saturation	%	20–59	†

*Harvey JW, French TW, and Meyer DJ: Chronic Iron Deficiency Anemia in Dogs. JAAHA 18:946–960.
†Values not directly determined.

SELECTED FACTORS TO CONVERT COMMONLY USED UNITS TO THE INTERNATIONAL SYSTEM OF UNITS

Substance	Common Unit	×	Conversion Factor	=	International Unit
Albumin (proteins)	g/dl		10		g/l
Ammonia	μg/dl		0.554		μmol/L
Bicarbonate	mEq/L		1		mmol/L
Bile acids	μg/ml		2.45		μmol/L
Bilirubin	mg/dl		17.1		μmol/L
Calcium	mg/dl		0.25		mmol/L
Total CO_2	mEq/L		1		mmol/L
P_{CO_2}	mmHg		0.133		KPa*
Cholesterol	mg/dl		0.026		mmol/L
Chloride	mEq/L		1		mmol/L
Creatinine	mg/dl		88.4		μmol/L
Folate	ng/ml		2.27		nmol/L
Glucose	mg/dl		0.055		mmol/L
Insulin	μIU/ml		0.0417		μg/l.
Iron	μg/dl		0.179		μmol/L
Magnesium	mg/dl		0.411		mmol/L
P_{O_2}	mmHg		0.133		kPa*
Phosphate	mg/dl		0.323		mmol/L
Potassium	mEq/L		1		mmol/L
Sodium	mEq/L		1		mmol/L
Urea nitrogen	mg/dl		0.357		mmol/L
Xylose	mg/dl		0.067		mmol/L
Enzymes	IU/L		0.017		μkat/L†
Amylase	Somogyi units/dl		1.85		IU/l
ALT (SGPT)	Karmen units/ml		0.48		IU/L
Lipase	Cherry-Crandall units/ml		278		IU/L
Blood cells	Cells/μl		1,000,000		cells/L‡

*kPa, kilopascal.

†1 kat, 1 katal (i.e., 1 mol/sec), is for reporting enzyme activity, but most laboratories report serum enzyme activity in international units of IU/L or U/L (i.e., 1 μmol/min).

‡Reported as 10^9 cells/L.

(Modified from Kaneko JJ: Clinical Biochemistry of Domestic Animals. 3rd ed. New York, Academic Press, 1980, pp 785–791; Lehmann HP and Henry JB: SI units. In Henry JB (ed): Clinical Diagnosis and Management by Laboratory Methods. 17th ed. Philadelphia, W.B. Saunders, 1984, pp 1428–1450.

Index

Note: Page numbers in *italics* refer to illustrations; those followed by a *t* refer to tables.

ISBN 0-7216-5202-6

90038